URGENT CARE MEDICINE

URGENT CARE MEDICINE

EDITORS

Tanise I. Edwards, MD, FAAEM

Medical Consultant
Urgent Care and Emergency Medicine
Medical Consultant
Optum Division
UnitedHealth Group
McLean, Virginia

Thom A. Mayer, MD, FACEP, FAAP

Professor of Emergency Medicine and Pediatrics
Georgetown University School of Medicine
George Washington University School of Medicine
Washington, D.C.
Chair, Department of Emergency Medicine
Inova Fairfax Hospital
Falls Church, Virginia

McGraw-Hill
MEDICAL PUBLISHING DIVISION

New York   Chicago   San Francisco   Lisbon   London   Madrid   Mexico City
Milan   New Delhi   San Juan   Seoul   Singapore   Sydney   Toronto

McGraw-Hill

A Division of The **McGraw·Hill** *Companies*

URGENT CARE MEDICINE

1234567890   AGMAGM   098765432

ISBN 0-07-022068-9

This book was set by V&M Graphics Incorporated.
The editors were Andrea L. Seils and Muza Navrozov.
The production supervisor was Lisa Mendez.
The index was prepared by Alexandra Nickerson.
The designer was Marsha Cohen/Parallelogram.
Quebecor World Martinsburg was printer and binder.

This book is printed on acid-free paper.

Library of Congress Cataloging-in-Publication Data

Edwards, Tanise I.
   Urgent care medicine / authors, Tanise I. Edwards, Thom A. Mayer.
      p. ; cm.
   Includes bibliographical references and index.
   ISBN 0-07-022068-9
   1. Emergency medicine. 2. Ambulatory medical care. I. Mayer, Thom A. II. Title.
   [DNLM: 1. Emergency Medical Services—organization & administration. 2.
   Ambulatory Care Facilities—organizations & administration. 3. Emergency
   Treatment—methods. WX 215 E26u 2002]
   RC86.7.E39 2002
   616.02′5—dc21
                                                                                    2001031616

"Unless the Lord builds the house, its builders labor in vain."

Psalm 13:6

This book is dedicated with all my love to my parents, Mattie and Zeno Edwards; my sister, Colette; Mark, my husband; and my children, Briana and Brendan, whose hugs, kisses, and smiles bring a never-ending joy to my world.

Tanise I. Edwards

CONTENTS

CONTRIBUTORS*

Bill Bosley, PA-C [7]
Physician Assistant
Emergency Physicians of Northern Virginia
Inova Fairfax Hospital
Falls Church, Virginia

Robert J. Cates, MD, MS [5]
Vice Chair
Department of Emergency Medicine
Inova Fairfax Hospital
Falls Church, Virginia

Anne Boland Docimo, MD, MBA [2]
Chief Medical Officer
UPMC Health Plan
Pittsburgh, Pennsylvania

Stephen J. Dresnick, MD [1]
Clinical Professor of Emergency Medicine
University of North Carolina at Chapel Hill
Chapel Hill, North Carolina
President
Symbiont Partners
Coral Gables, Florida

Glenn G. Druckenbrod, MD FACEP [17]
Medical Director
Department of Emergency Medicine
Inova Fairfax Hospital
Falls Church, Virginia

Tanise I. Edwards, MD, FAAEM [3, 6, 10, 11, 13, 19, A1, A2]
Medical Consultant
Urgent Care and Emergency Medicine
Medical Consultant
Optum Division
UnitedHealth Group
McLean, Virginia

Z. Colette Edwards, MD, MBA [14]
Vice President and Senior Medical Director
CIGNA Healthcare of Ohio
Cleveland, Ohio

J. Mark Evans, MD, FAAOS [15]
Hand and Orthopedic Surgeon
Department of Orthopedic Surgery
Fairfax Hospital
Commonwealth Orthopedics and Rehabilitation
Fairfax, Virginia
Leesburg, Virginia

Louis Kofi Essandoh, MD, FACC [9]
Assistant Professor of Medicine
Johns Hopkins University School of Medicine
Baltimore, Maryland
Director
Cardiac Consultants
Annapolis, Maryland

Daphne G. Golding, MD, FAAP [16]
Private Practice
Chestnut Hill Medical Center
Philadelphia, Pennsylvania

Susan Gregory, MD [10]
Clinical Assistant Professor of Medicine
Pennsylvania Hospital
Philadelphia, Pennsylvania

Dan Hanfling, MD, FACEP [4]
Inova Fairfax Hospital
Operational Medical Director
Fairfax County Fire and Rescue Department
and Inova Medical AirCare Helicopter
Medevac
Falls Church, Virginia

---

*The numbers in brackets following the contributor name refer to chapter(s) authored or coauthored by the contributor.

John Howell, MD, FACEP [20, 21]
Clinical Professor of Emergency Medicine
Georgetown University School of Medicine
Washington, D.C.
Director
Academic Affairs
Department of Emergency Medicine
Inova Fairfax Hospital
Falls Church, Virgina

Safy John, MD [10]
Assistant Professor of Clinical Medicine
New York Medical College
Valhalla, New York

Gary D. Johnson, MD [18]
Clinical Associate Professor
Department of Neurosciences
Brown University School of Medicine
Neurologist Miriam Hospital
Providence, Rhode Island

Deborah A. Loney, MD [8]
Private Practice
Sterling, Virginia

Thom A. Mayer, MD, FACEP, FAAP [1, 4,
    5, 7, 12, 20, 22, 23]
Professor of Emergency Medicine
    and Pediatrics
Georgetown University School of Medicine
George Washington University School
    of Medicine
Washington, D.C.
Chair
Department of Emergency Medicine
Inova Fairfax Hospital
Falls Church, Virginia

Michael Mortiere, PA-C [23]
Physician Assistant
Alexandria Hospital
Assistant Clinical Professr
Department of Health Care Sciences
Georgetown University Hospital
Washington, D.C.

Lynn M. Schnapp, MD [10]
Associate Professor
Department of Medicine
Division of Pulmonary
    and Critical Care Medicine
University of Washington School of Medicine
Harborview Medical Center
Seattle, Washington

Jesse Wardlow, MD [8]
Clinical Assistant Professor
Department of Otolaryngology
Loyola University Medical Center
Maywood, Illinois

The practice of urgent care medicine is unique in that it encompasses aspects from both the fields of emergency medicine and traditional office-based ambulatory medicine. The urgent care physician must be knowledgeable and capable of handling a variety of conditions—medical, surgical, and trauma—that can present in the urgent care setting. As in the practice of emergency medicine, the physician working in this setting must be fully capable of stabilizing patients with all disease processes and presentations. The practitioner must also be capable of handling the unpredictability of the practice, including fluctuating patient volumes and lack of control over patient flow and patient characteristics; he or she must also have the skills that will be needed at any given time to treat a patient. Additionally, patients seen in the urgent care setting may be completely unknown to the physician, thus requiring the urgent care physician to possess the ability to rapidly establish a rapport while simultaneously assessing the patient's needs. On the other hand, unlike the case in emergency medicine, there is no available in-house specialty "backup," no facilities for complex diagnostic testing, and no critical care unit (CCU) or surgical suite for patients requiring admission or advanced care. When further evaluation or more complex or ongoing treatment is needed, patients in the urgent care setting must be transported from the urgent care facility to the appropriate setting. Also in contrast to the practice of emergency medicine and more similar to that of ambulatory medicine, most patients seeking care in the urgent care setting have more routine medical complaints. Patients may present requesting a routine physical exam, an update of immunizations, or evaluation for a simple sinus infection or rash. Consequently, at any given time, the acuity level in urgent care medicine can vary from the high-severity acute myocardial infarction to the 2-week-old sprained ankle.

The demands of urgent care medicine, therefore, require a certain balance between the practices of emergency and ambulatory medicine. This book was designed to supplement the knowledge of those physicians who are practicing in the urgent care setting but who may not have had training specific to the requirements of this field. For instance, emergency medicine–trained physicians are fully capable of treating and triaging patients with acute problems, but have little background in the requirements of a Department of Transportation Physical Examination. On the other hand, the internal medicine–trained physician may be fully capable of providing the more routine care that represents the bread and butter of urgent care medicine while having little experience in the evaluation and treatment of acute surgical disease, the reduction of an acute ankle dislocation, or illnesses that are unique to the pediatric population.

The purpose of this book, therefore, is to serve as a quick and practical clinical reference to the practice of urgent care medicine. It attempts to cover the wide spectrum of disease commonly seen in the urgent care setting. Each section covers disease presentations by history and physical examination, appropriate urgent care management, and criteria for hospital transfer or outpatient management. Also included under the various diagnoses are specific "Errors to Avoid," designed to help avoid many of the pitfalls that can pose problems in clinical practice. The "Key Points of Documentation" have been incorporated to serve as a reminder of specific documentation that should be recorded on the chart of every patient who presents with that particular complaint.

Appendix 1 is a list of differential diagnoses by organ system or presenting symptoms; it is intended to help formulate a differential for patients presenting with one of the listed complaints. It allows the physician to review the listed differential diagnoses based on patient history and physical examination. Use of this appendix should act as a reminder of the various diagnoses that should be ruled out in order to avoid missing potentially life-threatening conditions or conditions requiring acute intervention. If a conclusive diagnosis cannot be determined or the acute diagnoses listed cannot be reasonably eliminated, further evaluation of the patient is needed.

Appendix 2, "Radiographic Signs and Symptoms," serves as an overview in outline form of radiology in the urgent care setting. It is divided into two parts; the first presents standard and additional radiographic views that may aid in patient evaluation; the second discusses radiographic findings by disease, injury, or the individual parts of the body and provides information that can be used to evaluate specific radiographic films.

As previously discussed, the practice of urgent care medicine is demanding and exacting. Nonetheless, this field affords many opportunities to experience the gratification of providing easily accessible and unencumbered patient care. The urgent care physician fills a vital role in the practice of medicine, particularly given the great mobility of today's society. The urgent care physician—who is required to evaluate such a wide spectrum of presenting complaints and such diverse patient populations—must always maintain a high degree of vigilance, although it is impossible for any one physician to meet the demands of every aspect of medical practice. In summary, in order to provide safe and optimal care in the field of urgent care medicine, it is important, in approaching each patient, for the urgent care physician to *"recognize what one knows, recognize what one doesn't know, and care enough about the patients to seek consultation whenever needed."*

Tanise I. Edwards

I

MANAGEMENT

DEFINITION OF FAST-TRACK AND URGENT CARE MEDICINE

Stephen J. Dresnick / Thom A. Mayer

THE HISTORY OF URGENT CARE CENTERS

Emergency medicine initially evolved in response to a publicly defined need for expert episodic evaluation and treatment of acute illnesses and injuries. Similarly, urgent care medicine has evolved from a publicly defined need for treatment of less severe illnesses and injuries, with the added incentives of clean, pleasant surroundings as well as avoidance of the frequent delays and unpredictable service experienced in many hospital emergency departments.

Many patients who present to emergency departments do so because they are unable to get appointments in a timely fashion with their personal physicians. As the population has become more and more mobile, fewer than 20 percent of people even have what they could call a personal physician. Studies also indicate that 70 to 80 percent of patients seen in hospital emergency departments could be seen in an alternative and less costly setting. Although the marginal cost of seeing nonacute patients in an emergency department has been studied, it is obvious that a different level of skill is required to treat a patient with otitis as compared with one who has been a victim of multiple trauma. It is also evident that hospital space is more expensive per square foot—both to construct and to operate—because of the need to comply with regulatory and licensing requirements.

Nonetheless, over the past 30 years, the volume of patients seen in hospital emergency departments has continued to rise, at a time when the actual number of acute care hospitals with emergency departments has declined. This increase in volume has occurred at the same time that hospital capital spending has largely been unavailable to keep up with the volume. As a result, alternatives to the traditional emergency department have emerged. As early as the 1980s, facilities that called themselves "free-standing emergency centers" began to appear. Unfortunately, this occurred just when emergency medicine was attempting to gain primary board status, having been approved only as a "conjoint-modified" board several years earlier. Medical organizations such as the American

Medical Association expressed concerns that patients with heart attacks might inadvertently present to these facilities after hours and might suffer increased morbidity or even mortality as a result. Some centers began using the term *minor emergencies* to describe what they did, but this did little to appease the medical establishment. Rather than fight the battle, the fledgling trade organization that had been formed to promote the concept of urgent care soon encouraged its members to change their name, and the organization followed suit, changing its name to the National Association of Urgent Care Centers. This seems to have been the first use of the term *urgent care.*

By 1986, there were almost 2000 urgent care centers in the United States, and predictions at the time suggested that there would be 10,000 within the next 10 years. Needless to say, hospitals became concerned that these centers, particularly when they were located near a hospital facility, would siphon off the paying patients who had minor emergencies. This became of particular concern when Congress enacted the "antidumping" law now known as the Emergency Medical Treatment and Active Labor Act (EMTALA). This law, even in its earliest form, required hospitals to evaluate patients regardless of their ability to pay in order to screen for "medical emergencies." Hospitals became increasingly concerned that these two factors would leave them with few patients to see other than those with true emergencies, such as multiple trauma and gunshot wounds, as well as the medically indigent, who would use the emergency department as a free clinic.

Hospitals began to realize that many patients would actually prefer to go to a hospital for medical care, but only if they could be treated quickly and efficiently. Thus in the mid-1980s, many hospitals, as a defensive strategy, began to develop "fast tracks." These were designed to attract and retain workers' compensation patients and those with minor illnesses who were able to pay and preferred to be treated promptly within the hospital. After all, the 1980s became known as the "now" generation, as this clearly was the decade that saw the emergence of fast food, convenience stores, self-pump gas stations, and other forms of fast, convenient services.

Ideally, "fast tracks" or urgent care facilities should be able to see large volumes of patients who need minimal diagnostic testing and few therapeutic procedures. Therefore, while urgent care centers and hospital fast tracks may differ in location, the similarity between the two is based on the types of patients seen, the dedication of specific resources for such patients, and the clearly defined focus on that market segment. By choosing to avoid the typical emergency department (in urgent care, this is self-triage by the patient who opts to be seen in that setting), these patients can be seen and treated in less than an hour, as they will not have to wait for their turn for lab and x-ray services. Similarly, satisfaction among patients who can be seen in a hospital-based fast track is high. This can be a tremendous advantage to a facility that is trying to enhance its reputation in the community. Therefore, patients and families of patients with true emergencies expect to spend several hours in an emergency department and rarely get upset waiting for lab, x-ray, or consultations. But those with minor complaints generally expect to be seen promptly.

Of note, while the types of patients seen in both the urgent care setting and the emergency department fast track are similar, these facilities differ in payment mechanisms; hospital emergency departments have traditionally billed in a different fashion and with different "common procedural terminology" codes than those used by urgent care centers.

THE FUTURE OF URGENT CARE MEDICINE

Having emerged from the need for timely, professional, accurate, and customer-focused service for minor illness and injuries, what is the future of urgent care medicine in our changing health care system? There are many reasons to believe that urgent care centers will not only survive but flourish in the changing health care environment. First, to the extent that urgent care centers compete with other market segments in health care, such competition is most likely to be with primary care practices primarily and to a lesser extent with hospital-based fast-track services. While payment mechanisms in health care are constantly changing, the predominant mechanism for compensating primary care physicians at the present time is through some form of capitation or a modified capitation model. Although there are a number of mechanisms intended to keep patients "in plan" with their managed care organizations, there are still a substantial number of patients who are willing to spend a limited part of their discretionary income for the convenience of immediate urgent care. There is also substantial evidence to indicate that current managed care and capitation structures lead patients to feel that they are obliged to wait too long for appointments with their primary care physicians. In such an environment, it is likely that urgent care centers will continue to have a place—if they are appropriately operated and marketed—to deal with patients who want a more immediate response to their urgent care needs.

In addition, many urgent care centers have established contractual or noncontractual relationships with managed care organizations to handle the "overflow" of patients presenting to the managed care plan. Demand management (telephone triage) systems can be put in place to help assure that patients who are part of a defined plan can be sent to specific urgent care centers with which the managed care organization has a contractual relationship. Such relationships are helpful not only from a physical standpoint but also in assuring that patient information, continuity, and quality improvement activities are coordinated with the plan.

It is also important for all urgent care centers to develop referral relationships to hospitals, primary care practices, and emergency departments in their areas. Strategic affiliations are key to the success of urgent care centers, particularly as the payment mechanisms for urgent care change (see below.). The management and professional staff of the urgent care center should establish both informal and formal relationships with area primary care practices and emergency departments—which will help to assure the success of the urgent care facility.

Other factors that augur well for well-situated, well-designed, and well-operated urgent care centers include growth of the economy and the patient population base. While the rapid recent expansion will almost certainly see some future reciprocal downturn, there is every reason to believe that the economy will continue to support the payment of discretionary income (if necessary) for the convenience of the prompt, accurate, and courteous treatment of minor illnesses and injuries.

There are, however, two potential threats to urgent care centers, both of which loom large. The first is the tendency for some organizations to resist change. As health care undergoes technological and operational advances, it is essential that urgent care centers and their staffs be capable of dealing rapidly and efficiently with change and master the important skills of change management. All organizations within health care must have the capacity to combine administrative, managerial, ownership, and operational interests in a strategically guided effort to change appropriately. For example, the emergence of telephone triage demand management systems has presented both an opportunity and a threat to urgent care centers. Such telephone triage systems are a threat in that, if appropriately and effectively utilized, they can proactively triage patients to health care settings other than urgent care. In the past, such patients might have used an urgent care center because of its location and proximity, the patient's prior experience, and so on. With the advent of telephone triage to manage demand, patients may be guided elsewhere. These systems, however, can also represent an opportunity for those urgent care centers that recognize the phenomenon, actively pursue strategic alliances with other organizations, and retain the capacity to manage the volume patients seen because of such referrals.

The second major threat to urgent care centers arises from the August 2000 implementation of Ambulatory Payment Classifications (APCs). This new system signals a rapid and radical departure from past reimbursement structures for hospital services. The implementation of APCs is expected to have a somewhat positive effect on reimbursement for emergency departments, but it will likely also have a important impact on hospital-owned urgent care centers. While APCs are projected to increase total payments to hospitals for Medicare outpatient services by 4.6 percent (with nonteaching hospitals expected to realize an estimated 5.0 percent increase and major teaching hospitals an increase of 2.6 percent), it is also anticipated that hospital or hospital system participation in freestanding ambulatory or urgent care centers will be sharply curtailed because of declining levels of reimbursement for these facilities under the APC system. Management and staff of ambulatory care centers need to be prepared for this change, as it is quite likely that hospitals will simply sell or spin off their urgent care centers to physician or investor groups. Thus, urgent care physicians need to be prepared to change from being "intrapreneurs" to entrepreneurs who take an active part in owning and managing the urgent care center. While this certainly involves some change, it is also potentially a great opportunity to help develop and expand the urgent care practice.

2

THE URGENT CARE CENTER

Anne Boland Docimo

THE MISSION

Urgent care centers have developed in response to demands in the medical marketplace. Patients, as consumers, seek convenience and affordability when selecting a provider for minor illnesses and injuries. Unable to accurately judge the technical aspects of medical care, patients substitute service as the chief indicator of satisfaction.[1] Managed care organizations (MCOs) seek low-cost alternatives to traditional emergency departments to meet members' urgent care needs. Employers want low cost as well as convenient care for drug screens, preemployment physicals, and on-the-job injuries.

An urgent care center (UCC), whether freestanding or as part of a hospital-based emergency department, should respond to all of these needs. In fact, the mission of any urgent care center is to provide convenient and affordable quality care for minor episodic health care needs.

(For purposes of clarity, this chapter will focus on freestanding centers unless otherwise noted. In general, the same concepts apply to hospital-based departments.)

> **Long waiting time** is the most frequent complaint logged by emergency department patients.

FACILITY: LOCATION, LOCATION, LOCATION

Patients value convenience and efficiency when they are seeking care for minor illnesses and injuries. The center, therefore, should be well located and easily accessed, with adequate, well-lit parking. Attractive, clean facilities are pleasing to patients and staff. The architectural design can have a positive effect on the patient mix, services provided, and the financial operations of the facility.[3]

Urgent care facilities should be designed with each customer's needs clearly in mind—patients, referring physicians, and payers. Related services should be provided in contiguous areas to simplify patient flow. Referring physicians prefer sending patients to nearby locations that are easily accessible. If specialists such as orthopedists and plastic surgeons will be performing procedures in the center, they may request specific equipment and instruments. Payers will value centers that are convenient for their members, with organized billing and medical records departments.

Most urgent care centers are freestanding buildings. Some are located in medical office buildings and may be affiliated with other providers in the building. Approximately 80 percent are located in the suburbs, near residential areas.[4] In choosing a site for a new center, demographic and insurance data should be analyzed carefully to ensure that a sufficient number of eligible residents would be able to use the center's services. Areas with new construction and a growing population are preferred. People residing in the area less than 3 years and households with children are more likely to use urgent care centers.[5] Neighboring physician practices, competing centers, and the managed care market must also be evaluated. If the managed care penetration is high, availability of contracts must be determined.

Urgent care facilities vary in size (roughly 4000 to 10,000 sq ft), depending on the services offered. In addition to traditional office space and examination rooms, most have procedure rooms, laboratories, and x-ray capabilities. Additionally, some centers offer acute physical therapy on-site. Last, adequate storage space for supplies, medications, and paperwork is essential to keep the center well organized and neat.

Supplies will vary by location and by acuity of patients seen. In addition to the supplies found in a traditional office-based practice, an urgent care center must be equipped to treat lacerations and minor fractures and to perform minor surgical procedures. Oxygen, suction, pulse oximeter, peak flow meters, and nebulizers are needed. Intravenous equipment, fluids, and frequently used medications (IM, IV, and PO) should be available. Equipment to test vision and hearing is necessary for preemployment physicals. All urgent care facilities should have life-support capabilities including a "crash cart" in case of an emergency, though this is not the mission of the center. Any unstable or emergent patient should be transferred via 911 to an emergency department.

A freestanding facility is similar to a physician's office in that no certification is needed; each practitioner must simply have a license to practice medicine. Additional regulations, however, are being considered in some states.

PATIENT PROFILE

In a study by Kinney and Gerson of patients presenting to an urgent care center, the average age was 33.2 years and 71 percent had a primary care physician. One-third sought care for an injury. The remainder had an illness.[6] Snell and others found that patients choosing urgent care centers over emergency departments tended to have higher incomes. When surveyed about where they would seek care in a given circumstance, patients correctly chose the emergency department for a serious illness or injury.[7]

Most patients presenting to urgent care centers have "self-triaged" and present with symptoms of minor illnesses and injuries. The National Ambulatory Medical Survey identified the most common problems seen in the urgent care setting, which, in descending order of frequency, follows: cough, throat symptoms, back symptoms, stomach pain, headache, chest pain, skin rashes, and musculoskeletal aches from trauma or overuse.[8] Common diagnoses include viral syndromes, pharyngitis, sinusitis, otitis media, bronchitis, and gastroenteritis. Sprains, strains, overuse syndromes, and lacerations are common trauma diagnoses. Additionally, all centers will have a mix of higher-acuity patients, such as acute asthma exacerbations, pneumonia, headaches, and abdominal pain. Despite the evidence that most patients who visit urgent care centers do not have emergent conditions, it is important that the providers not become complacent. It is not uncommon for a patient to present with seemingly minor symptoms but to require extensive evaluation or hospital admission.

Urgent care centers affiliated with multispecialty group practices or practicing under capitation contracts may treat higher-acuity patients more frequently. The UCC affiliated with a health maintenance organization (HMO) will be considered the alternative to the emergency department by the MCO. Telephone triage nurses or demand management firms may direct patients to the center instead of to an emergency department. If a center is located adjacent to a group practice, it may have more extensive ancillary services available, such as computed tomography (CT) scanners and ultrasound. The providers in these settings must feel comfortable with the higher-acuity patient mix.

Other centers market extensively to employers for workers' compensation injuries, preemployment physicals, drug screens, etc. These centers may have higher volumes and a lower average acuity level.

Hours of operation

Most centers are open 365 days a year, 12 h per day, according to a nationwide survey of urgent care centers. In the northeastern and southeastern regions, centers were open an average of 9 h per day on weekends and holidays.[9,10] Exact hours of operation will vary by location, contractual requirements, and patient mix. Centers located in business districts, performing preemployment physicals and treating on-the-job injuries, may have restricted hours.

In general, urgent care centers are open into the evening and on weekends and holidays to serve patients after traditional physician office practices have closed. An analysis of patient arrival times to determine peak times should be used to adjust the hours of operation and staffing as needed.

Some centers take patients by appointment in addition to accepting walk-in patients. Appointments may be concentrated during hours of the day that may have been identified as "slow periods." However, mixing walk-in patients and those with appointments may be difficult from a patient satisfaction perspective. Patients prefer the convenience of walk-in care and may be surprised to find that others have appointments. Patients with appointments will not appreciate waiting while unscheduled patients are seen. To avoid excessive wait times, ample open time must be left in the schedule to accommodate the expected walk-in volume. In order to be successful, the urgent care center should not schedule appointments during the busiest hours of the day.

Staffing

It is essential to stress the urgent care mission when staff are being recruited, hired, and trained. Physicians, nurses, technicians, and office personnel must understand the importance of high-quality, friendly, and efficient service in the urgent care setting.

Ambulatory patients choose their providers and will recommend services to their friends and neighbors. Patients appreciate friendly service and will provide immediate feedback to the staff. With this in mind, everyone's job description should include "whatever else your job entails" to provide a positive, caring experience for the patients. Staff will also enjoy working as a team in a cooperative, service-oriented environment.

Providers

Physicians who enjoy providing episodic care for illnesses and injuries are ideal for the urgent care setting. The North American Association for Ambulatory Urgent Care (NAFAC), a trade association, had a nationwide survey conducted on a variety of issues. This survey found that 100 percent of ambulatory urgent care centers were staffed by licensed physicians at all times. The clinical training of urgent care medical directors was in family or general practice (51 percent) and emergency medicine (32 percent).[10] In the northeastern region of the country, the clinical training for medical directors was somewhat different: family practice (43 percent), emergency medicine (30 percent) and internal medicine (19 percent).[9,10]

The most important criterion for practicing in the urgent care setting is that the physician be skilled in the evaluation and management of patients with acute medical needs in a setting with limited resources. The physicians must be capable of providing an initial reading of x-rays and be skilled in interpreting laboratory data as well as ECGs. Providers must also demonstrate competence in performing such common procedures as administering local anesthesia, laceration repair, and splinting.

Providers in this setting will usually be seeing patients previously unknown to them and will therefore probably have no access to the patients' medical records. Limited ancillary services are available. To provide efficient and cost-effective service, laboratory and x-ray studies should be ordered only if the results will affect the patient's immediate diagnosis and treatment.[11] Therefore, in this setting, providers must often rely on the accuracy of the history and physical to make decisions.

Providers must also guard against becoming complacent in the urgent care setting. Most patients will have minor injuries and self-limited illnesses.[12] However, some patients with minor complaints may have serious underlying illnesses. For example, mild "indigestion" may be a patient's only symptom of underlying coronary artery disease. It is essential for providers to remain alert and rule out serious illness in every patient.

On the other hand, the urgent care setting is designed and staffed to provide episodic care—not long-term care of chronic illnesses. Attempts to fully evaluate and treat chronic conditions in the urgent care setting are frustrating for both the patient and the provider. Lengthy workups will undermine the efficiency of the center. Patients in need of continuing care should be referred to a primary care provider (PCP). Patients with emergent health care needs beyond the scope of the urgent care setting should be transferred to the hospital emergency department.

Some urgent care facilities are affiliated with or located near primary care practices. In these settings, the urgent care center serves as the front door to the primary care practice. Many patients seeking urgent care services do not have an identified PCP. If ongoing health issues are identified, patients are referred to a continuing care provider. Simultaneously, during peak times of the day, the PCPs may refer patients to be seen in the UCC for acute, unscheduled health care needs. Both patients and providers will appreciate the service. This arrangement also has staffing advantages, as the PCPs may work occasional shifts in the UCC or may work there while "building up" their practices.

Physician staffing should be appropriate for the center's patient volume. When a center first opens, single-physician coverage should be adequate. Provider productivity will depend on patient acuity mix. If patients present for drug screens, vaccinations, and allergy injections, more patients can be seen per provider hour. With adequate support staff and low patient acuity, the provider may be able to treat four to five patients per hour. Patients undergoing procedures such as laceration repair or abscess drainage will require more time and the provider will be able to see fewer such patients per hour. Although tracking of relative value units (RVUs) may be a more accurate means of measuring patient acuity and provider productivity, these parameters are not easily monitored in most settings. The center's overall patient acuity can be estimated by using the evaluation and management (E&M) billing codes. Patient volumes, turnaround time, and overall acuity should all be considered in determining necessary provider coverage.

Physician compensation is dependent on the relationship between the physicians and the center. Over half of urgent care centers are owned and operated by a single physician or a physician group.[10] Compensation arrangements include percentage of revenues generated, fixed salary, and hourly rates. Any arrangement can be modified to include incentives and profit sharing as motivating tools. Physicians with a sense of ownership will work to market the center within the community and among fellow physicians.

Physician Extenders

Physician assistants and nurse practitioners work well in the urgent care setting and should be considered when patient volumes rise and double coverage is needed. Physician extenders (PEs) are lower-cost providers, and studies have shown that they are well received by patients in the acute care setting.[13,14] In a survey of emergency departments using PEs, 27.7 percent required the PE to discuss the case with a physician before ordering any medication and 39.6 percent of the facilities required the physician to see the patient before discharge.[15] In a few remote and rural areas, PEs may be the sole providers available. Patients seen by a PE may be subject to lower reimbursement schedules unless a licensed physician directly supervises the care and signs the patient record.

Support Staff

The importance of providing excellent service to patients cannot be stressed enough. It should be considered in the recruitment, training, and evaluation of all clinical and support staff. Patients seeking care in this setting are seeking service and convenience. All staff must work together to meet each patient's service expectations.

Clinical Support Staff

The type of clinical support staff in a center may vary depending on patient acuity, community needs, and local standards of care. A registered nurse (RN) or licensed practical nurse (LPN) can provide nursing support, but state licensing boards may limit the LPN's scope of practice and require a RN for certain procedures. An x-ray technician will be needed to take and process films. Depending on the complexity of the lab, a nurse, x-ray technician, or medical assistant can be trained to perform stat lab tests.

The provider and clinical support staff should function as a team to expedite each patient's care.

The technical staff in lab and x-ray should be cross-trained as medical assistants to take vital signs, stock and clean rooms, set up suture trays, etc. The techs should be able to assist throughout the center and not be limited to performing specialized functions. As such, they become valuable members of the patient care team. Also, as staff salaries will represent over 50 percent of the center's operating budget, each individual should be as productive as possible.

In performing all functions, the focus is patient care. The support staff is an important part of the care team, enabling the provider to be more efficient. The provider will be able to see more patients with the support of a strong staff. Incentive plans and bonuses can be designed for the support staff. Both bonuses and incentive plans can be based on patient volumes, patient satisfaction survey results, repeat patient visits, patient referrals, etc.

Administrative Support Staff

The front-office staff must be courteous and competent. Accurate registration and insurance information is essential for reimbursement. The center's administrator must make sure that the front office staff receives adequate training, supervision, and support. At peak hours, additional front-office coverage will be needed to answer phones, register patients, and collect copayments.

The business officer/administrator may have a medical or business background. Knowledge of the business of medicine—managed care, coding, billing, and payer requirements—is essential. The medical director will have to work closely with the office administrator in supervising the staff and ensuring that clinical standards are upheld. If the center is part of a network or hospital system, many of the administrative and business functions can be performed off site in a central office. In that case, the administrative overhead can be shared by several centers.

PATIENT FLOW

Patients presenting to urgent care centers are seeking efficient service. As soon as possible after registration, a clinical staff member should greet the patient and escort him or her to the treatment area. If a room is not available, the chart should be placed in a rack in the clinical area. This will serve as a constant visual reminder that there are patients waiting for treatment. With electronic records, a tracking system will serve the same purpose.

Upon arrival in the urgent care area, the nurse should briefly assess the patient, noting the chief complaint, pertinent past medical history, medications, and brief history of present illness. Any relevant clinical findings may be noted, e.g., "lungs clear" or "swollen wrist, neurovascularly intact."

The nurse should also initiate the patient workup using written standing orders. This will greatly decrease the patient's length of stay. Most urgent care patients present with straightforward complaints. Protocols for ordering lab tests and x-rays may be developed for common clinical situations. (For example, a patient with burning on urination should have a urinalysis.) Also, patients should be appropriately prepared to be seen by the provider—e.g., back pain patients should be undressed with pants and shoes off. If the nurse is unsure about whether to order a study, the provider should be consulted. Staff should remember that the sooner the workup begins, the shorter the length of stay.

Paperwork should be minimized. Clinical notes, orders, and results should all be recorded on the same medical record. No separate nursing assessment forms, order sheets, or progress notes should be needed in the urgent care setting.

A key concept in patient flow is that all activity should be directed toward serving the patient's needs while maximizing good use of the provider's time. The "rate-limiting steps" must be identified and streamlined. Lab tests and x-rays should be ordered as soon as possible to shorten the overall stay. Every patient comes to be seen by the provider, so systems should be designed to facilitate provider productivity. If the provider is asking patients to put on a gown, taking vital signs, obtaining specimens, and transporting patients to x-ray, she or he cannot be very productive. The fewer times the provider must interact with each patient, the more efficient the provider will be. In addition, patients will appreciate time spent with a provider who is able to focus on their medical needs rather than multiple ancillary tasks.

LABORATORY

The availability of stat results from an on-site laboratory increases the physicians' ability to evaluate and treat a wide range of patients in an urgent care setting. In the NAFAC survey, 80 percent of ambulatory urgent care centers had general laboratory capability on site.[10] Laboratory testing, however, can be a significant bottleneck to patient through-put. Most urgent care patients can be completely evaluated without any lab studies. In an effort to deliver efficient and cost-effective care, only studies affecting patient disposition should be ordered in the urgent care setting.

At times, however, referring physicians may request that additional routine studies be performed. Some contracts may require special studies, such as drug screens in pre-employment physicals. Every effort should be made to streamline the process. While patients generally do not need to wait in the center for routine results, a strict follow-up process must be in place to ensure that the results are reported to the patient as well as his or her physician or employer.

Laboratory Regulations

In 1988 Congress passed the Clinical Laboratory Improvement Amendments (CLIA), establishing standards for quality and reliability of patient test results. The regulations define three categories of tests: waived, of moderate complexity (including the subcategory of provider-performed microscopy), and of high complexity. CLIA set specifications for quality control, patient test management, personnel, and proficiency testing.

Eight simple tests are waived from specific CLIA requirements:

- Dipstick or tablet urinalysis
- Fecal occult blood
- Ovulation test using visual color comparison
- Urine pregnancy test using visual color comparison
- Erythrocyte sedimentation rate

- Hemoglobin by copper sulfate method or single-analyte method
- Spun microhematocrit
- Blood glucose using a device approved by the U.S. Food and Drug Administration (FDA) for home use

If only the tests listed above are performed, a certificate of waiver must be obtained. Although specific CLIA regulations do not apply to the performance of these tests, the manufacturer's instructions must be followed.[16]

Tests not listed as waived are either moderate- or high-complexity tests. Examples of moderate-complexity tests include the following:

- Microscopic analysis of urinary sediment
- Direct-antigen tests for group A streptococci
- Gram stains, hematology
- Chemistry conducted on fully automated instrument

A laboratory of moderate complexity is sufficient for an urgent care setting, but labs performing high-complexity tests will have to comply with tougher standards in regard to quality control and personnel training.

CLIA regulations require that a moderate-complexity lab have a lab director, clinical consultant, technical consultant, and testing personnel. The laboratory director of a moderate-complexity lab must be a doctor of medicine, osteopathy, or podiatry with at least 1 year of experience supervising a lab or training equivalent to 20 continuing medical education (CME) hours in laboratory medicine. The laboratory director can also serve as the clinical consultant who aids in reporting and interpreting test results as needed.[16]

The technical consultant is responsible for technical and scientific oversight of the laboratory and must have an undergraduate degree in sciences and 1 or 2 years of specific laboratory training or experience. The technical consultant will establish specific laboratory procedures, develop a quality control program, enroll in an approved proficiency-testing program, and train and evaluate staff. Testing personnel for moderate-complexity labs must have a minimum of a high school diploma and documented training appropriate to the level of testing performed in the clinical laboratory.

CLIA regulations include detailed specifications for preparing a procedural manual, the necessary quality control measures, and proficiency testing. During the first 2 years after registering with the Health Care Financing Administration (HCFA) as a moderate-complexity lab, an inspection will occur. The Commission on Office Laboratory Accreditation (COLA) is a federally recognized private accrediting agency with similar regulations. Labs accredited by COLA fulfill federal requirements.[9,16]

Some states have separate CLIA-approved licensing programs. In those states, the lab may obtain a state license and comply with state regulations. In general, state and CLIA requirements are similar. Before establishing a physician's office laboratory, the medical director should review the applicable state and federal regulations.

Laboratory Reimbursement

In contracting for urgent care services, it is essential that stat labs not be carved out. If the contract requires the provider to send simple lab studies to an outside reference lab, the value of the services provided in the urgent care center is greatly diminished. Lab turnaround time would be unacceptable, and in some cases, patients would have to be referred to the hospital for a complete evaluation. Urgent care centers must therefore provide efficient and complete service to be successful. The contract for urgent care services should include a list of stat lab tests to be performed in the on-site laboratory. If contracting is done by capitation or case rate, the cost of stat lab tests may be included.

Laboratories in Emergency Department Fast-Track Centers

For fast-track centers within emergency departments, some point-of-service testing results in quicker lab turnaround times and shorter length of stay for patients. Rapid strep tests, urinalysis, and urine pregnancy tests represented 78 percent of the laboratory studies used in one fast-track setting.[17] Emergency department or lab personnel can perform point-of-service testing. The hospital lab director can assist with the necessary training, quality control, and proficiency testing.

RADIOLOGY SERVICES

Radiology services are essential in the urgent care setting. Minor trauma, sprains, and possible fractures represent a significant portion of presenting complaints. A registered and licensed radiology technologist and a fully functional x-ray room are needed to provide this service. Since most patients presenting for care will not require films, the technologist should be cross-trained to perform other clinical and clerical duties.

The physician on duty reads all films at the urgent care center. Initial treatment decisions will be based on this initial reading. All films, however, should be overread by a radiologist. Patients should be informed of the initial results, told that a specialist will review the films, and assured that any change in the reading will be communicated to them promptly.

A careful system must be in place to check for any discrepancies between the urgent care provider's reading and that of the radiologist. This is important not only for acute findings but also for incidental findings—e.g., a possible lung mass noted on a shoulder film. Patients should be contacted as soon as possible regarding any discrepancy, and the necessary treatment changes or follow-up arrangements should be made for the patient. All communication with the patient must be clearly documented in the medical record.

In contracting for urgent care services, it is important that x-ray services not be carved out of the contract. As with the lab, x-rays should be available on site during all hours of operation. If the patient must go to another facility for films, the care is neither convenient nor efficient.

The urgent care center charges for x-ray service and then contracts with the radiology group to provide the overreads. Usually the radiology contract is on a per-film basis. A time frame within which all overreads should be completed—ideally 24 h—should be specified in the contract. The growing field of telemedicine may prove valuable in this setting, particularly in rural areas. This option should be explored when purchasing radiographic equipment and contracting for services.

PHARMACY

Many centers dispense prepackaged pharmaceuticals. A limited formulary of frequently prescribed medications should be developed. The list of commonly prescribed medications found in Table 2-1 could be used as a starting point in preparing a formulary. Physicians practicing in the center should contribute to the formulary preparation and

TABLE 2-1

COMMONLY PRESCRIBED MEDICATIONS

Antibiotics
Amoxicillin
Amoxicillin/clavulinic acid (Augmentin)
Cephalexin
Dicloxacillin
Doxycycline
Erythromycin
Trimethoprim/sulfamethoxazole (Bactrim)
Macrodantin
Metronidazole
Penicillin

Ophthalmic antibiotics
Erythromycin ophthalmic ointment
Gentamicin ophthalmic solution
Sodium Sulamyd ophthalmic solution
Tobramycin ophthalmic solution/ointment

Otologic mediations
Cortisporin otic solution
Triethanolamine otic solution (Cerumenex)

Analgesics
Acetaminophen
Acetaminophen with codeine
Acetaminophen with oxycodone
Aspirin
Butalbital, aspirin, and caffeine (Fiorinal)
Butalbital, acetaminophen, and caffeine
   (Fioricet)
Codeine
Ibuprofen
Indomethacin
Naproxen

Anti-fungals
Clotrimazole cream
Clotrimazole and betamethasone cream
   (Lotrisone)
Clotrimazole vaginal suppositories
Miconazole vaginal cream, suppositories
Mycostatin topical cream (Nystatin)

Asthma
Albuterol inhalers (Proventil, Ventolin)
Albuterol solution
Triamcinolone inhaler

Other
Bisacodyl suppositories (Dulcolax)
Diazepam
Diphenhydramine
Diphenoxylate atropine (Lomotil)
Guaifenesin (Robitussin, Humabid)
Guaifenesin with codeine (Robitussin AC)
Hydroxyzine
Magnesium hydroxide (Milk of Magnesia)
Magnesium hydroxide, aluminum
   hydroxide (Maalox)
Meclizine (Antivert)
Naphazoline and pheniramine (Naphcon-A)
Phenazopyridine (Pyridium)
Prednisone
Prochlorperazine (Compazine)
Promethazine (Phenergan)
Pseudoephedrine and tripolidine (Actifed)
Psuedoephedrine (Sudafed)

Other topical medications
Bacitracin
Hydrocortisone cream
Triamcinolone cream

revise it as necessary. Both prescription and nonprescription medications can be available. Prepackaged medications can be purchased from pharmacies and dispensed by the physician on duty. Some states may require each physician to obtain a separate license to dispense medications. Medications must be stored in a locked cabinet. A careful inventory-control procedure, such as end-of-shift counts, is essential for narcotics and controlled substances.

Patients appreciate the convenience of on-site pharmacy services. Since many insurance programs cover prescription costs, patients may prefer to purchase their medications from pharmacies that participate in third-party payment contracts. However, many commonly prescribed medications are inexpensive, and patients may prefer to fill these prescriptions on site even if they have some insurance coverage. Patients should pay for their medications before leaving the center.

Some centers offer "starter packs" or samples from the pharmaceutical companies with a 1- to 2-day supply of medication. This lower-cost alternative is a valuable service to patients. The patients avoid late-night trips to the pharmacy and are able to start treatment immediately.

In dispensing any medications, the provider must comply with state regulations. Medications must be labeled with the patient's name and the date as well as instructions that the patient can understand. The prescribing physician's name and dispensing location are also required. State regulations will vary and must be considered before initiating a dispensing service.

SPECIALTY BACKUP AND REFERRALS

Some patients presenting to the urgent care center will require a specialist's care—immediately or in follow-up. If a center is affiliated with a hospital system or network, there may be a designated physician on call for each service. Most urgent care centers, however, operate like private physicians' offices. The provider is free to contact any available specialist in the patient's network. The specialty groups that provide the best service usually receive the most referrals. Orthopedics, plastic surgery, ear-nose-throat, and internal medicine are contacted most frequently for immediate consultation or to arrange follow-up for a patient.

In some instances the specialist will be able to come to the center and provide definitive care. If the plastic surgeon is willing to see a patient on site for laceration repair, that is a valuable service to the patient. The center's support staff should assist with any procedures. The patient will receive a bill from the urgent care center's provider for the initial evaluation and any ancillary studies. The specialist will bill directly for the consultation or procedure. Under these arrangements, the patient avoids a trip to the emergency department and a possibly long wait for service. The specialist will appreciate the opportunity to provide the service in a streamlined fashion and will be happy to receive calls from the center. Both the patient and the specialist are potential sources for future referrals to the center.

Most patients referred to a specialist can be seen in follow-up at a later date. Scheduling of appointments for patients before discharge is not easily accomplished—especially if the patient is being seen after traditional office hours. If there are certain services receiving a high volume of referrals from the center, such as family medicine or orthopedics, a system can be developed to streamline those appointments. For example, willing orthopedic groups could be "on call" for the center and provide a schedule template with designated openings for center patients requiring follow-up. At discharge, a patient requiring follow-up would be given one of the available appointments. The completed template would then be sent by fax to the participating specialist.

Patients requiring wound checks, suture removal, and so on may be seen in follow-up at the center as long as there are no restrictions in the contract. It is important that the proper referral procedure for each MCO is followed so that those patients are not held responsible for a specialist's charges. Some MCOs insist that all follow-up be provided in the PCP's office, and that all specialty care be arranged by the PCP. The provider should have access to referral requirements for each MCO. To streamline the referral process, a directory should be kept at the nurses' station with physicians and their insurance participation organized by specialty. A provider manual from each contracting payer should be kept in the center as a reference. If the referral guidelines are unknown or not clear, it is best to have MCO patients check referrals with their PCP first. Eventually, the providers and support staff will be familiar with the policies of the most frequent payers. In a center with computerized medical record or practice management systems, MCO-specific referral information should be available on "HELP" screens in the system.

Patients who present to the urgent care center who are unstable or who are found to have more serious medical needs will require transfer to the hospital via the Emergency Medical System (EMS). The urgent care provider should speak with the emergency physician on duty regarding the patient. Copies of any medical records, ECGs, lab results, and x-rays should be sent with the patient. (See Chapter 4, "Interfacility Transport of Patients.") The PCP can be informed before or after the transfer. A call should be placed to the patient or family members the next day to check on the patient's outcome.

CONTRACTING/REIMBURSEMENT

It is important to the financial success of a center that people living in the area have access to the services through their existing insurance coverage. Urgent care services should be marketed to as many payers as possible: insurers, employers, and the general public. Insurance contracts may be written as fee for service, case rate, or capitated reimbursement. In fee-for-service contracts, the center is paid its charges (or a percentage of charges) covering the professional fee and any ancillary studies. In case-rate contracts, a single negotiated amount is paid to the center for each patient visit. Variations on case-rate contracts exist. Tiered case rates based on patient acuity can be negotiated. The case rate includes professional fees and some or all ancillary services. Capitated rates involve a set monthly payment for all services provided to the contracting organization's membership. The payment is usually a set amount per member per month (PMPM). This rate is paid regardless of how many members seek care. In general, this method would only be used in a large center or a center associated with a primary care or multispecialty group.

Freestanding urgent care facilities are similar to physicians' offices and generally do not require state licensing or certification. The bills are for professional services and ancillary studies. No facility fee is charged. Hospital-based urgent care centers charge facility fees. They may use the same facility code as the emergency department or the code for the outpatient facility. This depends on the physical location of the center and the type of services provided. Centers within or next to the emergency department often bill using emergency facility codes.

If certain services are carved out of a contract, the payer will not reimburse the center for them. For example, if lab and x-ray studies were carved out of the contract, the center would not be paid for those services. Patients would have to be directed to a participating lab or radiology practice to have the tests performed. Carving ancillary services out of an urgent care center contract limits the provider's ability to treat the patient and significantly reduces the level of service the center is able to provide to patients. Stat labs and x-rays should be included in any contract to provide urgent care services.

An urgent care center may contract directly with employers for preemployment physicals, drug screening, and work-related injuries. Some employers have specific needs regarding preemployment physicals. These should be stated in the contract and be readily available to the treating provider. Department of Transportation (DOT) physicals are quite specific but vary from state to state. The patient may bring the paperwork, but extra forms should be available on site. Drug screening has chain-of-custody and patient verification requirements. The reference lab that performs the test will provide the necessary materials and instructions for collecting and submitting specimens.

Most on-the-job injuries can be treated safely and efficiently in the urgent care setting. Employers want patients to be seen quickly and to see them return to work as soon as possible. Written instructions regarding treatment, follow-up, and return-to-work information should be given to the patient and employer. At some centers, work-related visits comprise a significant share of the overall business. Some have physical therapy available on site. These centers market their cost-efficient and convenient services to area employers.

EMTALA

Privately owned freestanding urgent care centers are considered physician offices, not hospital emergency departments. As such, they are not subject to the Emergency Medical Treatment and Active Labor Act (EMTALA). This law was crafted to prevent hospitals from refusing to treat or transferring patients based on their ability to pay. EMTALA applies to all hospitals participating in the Medicare program.[18]

The law requires that the hospital provide a medical screening examination to all patients requesting emergency care to determine whether an emergency medical condition exists. The hospital is obligated to provide treatment to stabilize the patient in the case of an emergency. If no emergency medical condition is detected, the hospital is under no obligation to provide routine or nonemergent medical care.

The EMTALA regulations do apply to urgent care centers located on a hospital campus and to off-campus sites that are hospital-owned and operate under the hospital's Medicare provider number. Patients presenting to a hospital-owned facility or any location on the hospital campus requesting emergency care are entitled to a medical screening examination and stabilizing treatment if necessary.

Hospitals may direct patients requesting emergency care to urgent care facilities on campus for medical screening examinations as long as all persons with the same medical condition are directed to that site regardless of their ability to pay. It is appropriate to redirect patients with minor illnesses and injuries from the emergency department to a hospital-based urgent care clinic as long as all similar patients are treated in the same fashion.

Before any urgent care center goes into operation, an attorney familiar with EMTALA regulations should be consulted.

MEDICAL RECORDS

The medical record should present an accurate, complete accounting of the patient's visit. Providers are quite familiar with the standard contents of the "SOAP" note: subjective, objective, assessment, and plan. These components are essential, but a well-designed record—whether paper or electronic—should also serve to document physicians' orders, procedures, telephone consultations, discharge instructions, etc. In addition, the HCFA documentation requirements should be considered in selecting or designing a patient record-keeping system.

The provider is responsible for reviewing all data on the record. Chief complaint, vital signs, allergies, medications, and additional data such as visual acuity and pulse oximetry should be clearly documented on the same record used by the provider. Information should be available when and where it is needed. The record should promote complete documentation by being straightforward and easy to use. Orders should be timed and space provided to record results of studies; also, records of telephone consultations should be provided. Discharge time and condition should be documented.

HCFA mandates that providers carefully document their care before billing Medicare for professional services. Two sets of documentation guidelines have been released; either set may be used to support the evaluation and management codes used in professional billing. Medicare requires this level of documentation, and other payers may follow suit. A full explanation of these requirements is beyond the scope of this text. Detailed sources are available from HCFA and professional organizations. Since most patients seen in the urgent care setting have minor illnesses and injuries, the documentation guidelines are not too burdensome. Neither a lengthy review of systems nor a complete physical exam is necessary in most cases. Some commercially available records are designed to assist the provider in meeting HCFA documentation guidelines.

Discharge instructions are critical in an urgent care practice. In most cases, the provider is meeting the patient for the first time and discharging the patient home with treatment. There is no continuing physician-patient relationship. Discharge instructions should clearly state what to do if a condition fails to improve or becomes worse. The provider should carefully document any instructions given to the patient at the center, including follow-up plans with the PCP or specialist.

Preprinted instruction sheets are available from professional associations, drug companies, and textbooks for most common diagnoses and symptoms. If a diagnosis-specific instruction sheet is given to the patient, that should be recorded on the medical record—e.g., "Abdominal pain sheet given." Calls to patients after discharge should also be documented in the medical record.

In markets with a high penetration of managed care payers, follow-up and consultation are not always straightforward. The provider should be sure that any referrals are made to participating providers in the patient's insurance plan. The patient may be held responsible for any charges from a nonparticipating provider.

Sophisticated computerized medical record systems are now available for outpatient practices. Many would satisfy the requirements of an urgent care practice. These systems simplify documentation, order entry, results reporting, prescriptions, discharge instructions, referral networks, and follow-up calls to patients after discharge. Computerized patient records afford advantages to all aspects of clinical documentation. Patient records are immediately available, including lab results, x-ray results, and consultant's notes. Clinical guidelines can be incorporated into many of the electronic systems. Records can be automatically sent by fax to referring providers.

Computerized practice management systems are excellent tools for patient registration, billing, and all the business functions of the center. Reports can be generated to assist with many aspects of the practice, including scheduling appropriately for patient volumes, monitoring productivity, marketing, and contracting.

PATIENT FOLLOW-UP AFTER DISCHARGE

Some patients will have lab results and final x-ray readings pending at the time of discharge. The treating physician may not be at the center when the results are reported. A reliable system must be in place enabling all lab and x-ray results to be reviewed and acted upon promptly. The physician on duty should review, document, and date all results the day they are reported. Patients should be contacted as soon as possible and instructed about any necessary change in treatment. All calls to and from patients must be documented in the medical record. If the center is unable to reach a patient by phone, the attempted calls should be documented in the record, and a registered letter sent to the patient's address.

Most patients seen in the urgent care setting have acute signs and symptoms that will resolve with the treatment and follow-up arranged by the provider. Some patients— such as those with a febrile illness, asthma, etc.—may benefit from a call the next day to check on their status or to review the discharge instructions. A simple system can be set up to facilitate this process. The provider places a completed "call-back form" in a nursing report binder. The nurse on duty the next day places the call as instructed on the form and places the completed form in the patient's medical record. Since staff will vary from day to day, this binder can also be used to communicate about patients who will be returning for wound checks, dressing changes, and so on.

In a computerized system the tickler "To Do" list would be generated automatically each day. Follow-up calls would be easily documented in the patient's record.

PATIENT SATISFACTION

Freestanding centers attract patients by providing excellent service and convenient care. Patients are best at judging the level of service and the caring attitudes of the staff. Most patients are not qualified to judge the technical components of their care, so they judge the quality of care based on their total experience in the center. These judgments will determine whether or not the patient returns and refers other patients to the center.

Measuring patient satisfaction has become an industry in itself. However, a simple comment card can be an inexpensive source of immediate feedback. It is important to recognize that patients are not uniform in their expectations. The data will be very subjective and may be ambiguous. However, feedback may identify areas needing improvement. Comments and complaints offer an opportunity to improve these processes.

Patients appreciate good service and routinely compliment the staff when their expectations are met or exceeded. Positive comments from patients and public recognition for providing excellent service is a powerful motivator. Financial incentives such as bonuses based on patient satisfaction measures should be considered. A qualified staff motivated to provide excellent service will help to make a center successful.

REFERENCES

1. Banker N: Convenient care in the hospital emergency department. *J Hosp Mktg* 1:113, 1987.
2. *The Clockwork ED.* Washington, DC: Advisory Board; 1998.
3. Dunn A: History of ambulatory care facilities from a roving hospital administrator's point of view. *J Ambul Care Mgt* 22:8, 1999.
4. Berliner H, Burlage R: The walk-in chains: the proprietarization of ambulatory care. *Int J Health Services* 17:585, 1987.
5. Gregory D et al: Emergency service: a strategy for hospital-sponsored ambulatory care satellites. *Hosp Health Services Admin* 111, 1984.
6. Kinney TJ, Gerson L: Utilization of a freestanding emergency center by patients with and without private physicians. *Ann Emerg Med* 12:762, 1983.
7. Snell F et al: Factors in choosing an urgent care center versus an emergency department. *J Emerg Nurs* 13:355, 1987.
8. Schappert S: National Ambulatory Medical Care Survey: 1991 summary. *Vital Health Stat* 116:1, 1994.
9. Wenmark W: *Hot Opportunities for Emergency Medicine Urgent Care.* Minneapolis, MN: North American Association for Ambulatory Urgent Care; 1998.
10. Hays R: *Preliminary Findings from the Factor IV Statistical Report.* Jupiter, FL: Haysmar, Inc; 1993.
11. Schriger D: Toward a philosophy of testing: the utilization of diagnostic tests in the emergency department, in Cantrill S, Karas S (eds): *Cost-Effective Diagnostic Testing in Emergency Medicine.* Dallas: American College of Emergency Physicians; 1994:11.
12. Wong J: Efficiency and effectiveness in the urgent care clinic. *Postgrad Med* 99:161, 1996.
13. Sturmann K et al: Physician assistants in emergency medicine. *Ann Emerg Med* 19:304, 1989.
14. Rhee K, Dermeyer A: Patient satisfaction with a nurse practitioner in a university emergency service. *Ann Emerg Med* 26:130, 1995.
15. Ellis G, Brandt T: Use of physician extenders and fast tracks in United States emergency departments. *Am J Emerg Med* 15:229, 1997.
16. Health Care Financing Administration: *CLIA Updates.*
17. Meislin H et al: Fast track: urgent care within a teaching hospital emergency department. Can it work? *Ann Emerg Med* 17:45, 1988.
18. *Emergency Medical Treatment and Active Labor Act (EMTALA) Enforcement Guidelines.* Washington DC: Health Care Financing Administration; 1998.

DOCUMENTATION

Tanise I. Edwards

Documentation in the urgent care setting, as in all aspects of medicine, must be complete, accurate, and consistent. This type of documentation is best achieved when the urgent care center's chart has designated fields to be completed as well as specialized forms available when additional charting is required (i.e., consent-for-transfer forms or "against medical advice" documents). Chart documentation must appropriately represent the patient's stay while in the urgent care facility as well as accurately describe the patient's chief complaint, illness, or injury. Additionally, documentation should support the patient's discharge diagnosis as well as his or her clinical condition. All consultations, procedures, and treatments rendered in the urgent care center as well as the response to care must be included in the chart documentation.

Standard charts should be used for almost all patients who present for treatment in the urgent care center, including first-time visits for patients requesting allergy injections and blood pressure checks. Under certain circumstances, the standard chart may not have to be completed. This may be the case when a patient presents with a form for a sports, employment, or department of transportation (DOT) physical that will encompass the same documentation that would be completed in the standard chart.

URGENT CARE CHARTS

A well-designed chart (see Fig. 3-1) will include fields for the patient's name and chart/medical record numbers on *each* page. There should be areas to be completed for vital signs (blood pressure, pulse, respiratory rate, and temperature), allergies, medications, and past medical history. There should also be an area to document the last menstrual period as well as the date of the last tetanus shot. Additionally, there should be ample space for nursing assessment, physician assessment, any treatments or orders (including lab tests and x-rays), and results. The primary chart should also include space in which to document time of discharge, the patient's condition at discharge, any discharge instructions that were given, and the physician's signature. Space for reassessment and any specialty consultations can be included either on the main chart or, in some cases, on an addendum chart. All recorded data should be accompanied by a time notation.

Date_____

Patient:_____ Social Security #: _____ - __ - _____ Age:_____ Sex: _____

Reason for Visit:_____

Allergies:_____

Medications:_____

PMH:_____

_____

Nursing History: _____

_____

_____

Time			
Temp			
B. P.			
Pulse			
Resp.			

LNMP:_____   Last Tetanus:_____   Weight:_____

Physician History and Examination:

_____
_____
_____
_____
_____
_____
_____
_____
_____
_____
_____
_____
_____
_____
_____
_____

LABS   □ CBC   □ Rapid Strep   □ Throat Culture
        □ UA   □ Urine Culture   □ HCG
        □ Chem 7   □ ECG   □ Peak Flow
        □ Other

X-RAYS: _____
_____

MEDICATION/ORDERS		
Time Ordered	Medication/Treatment	Time Given

Reassessment/Lab Results:

Discharge Instructions:
_____
_____
_____

Physician Signature:_____   Time of Discharge: _____

Discharge Condition		
□ Improved	□ Unchanged	□ Worsened
□ Transferred to:		
□ 24 Hour Check		

FIGURE 3-1   Sample urgent care chart.

Not only does such documentation allow for accurate recording of the patient's stay but it also serves as a prompt for reevaluation and a means of recording delays in patient management that should be addressed.

Each time a patient presents for treatment or evaluation, a current list of medications and allergies should be recorded as well as an updated past medical history. It is important for patients to be questioned regarding this information at *each* visit; the examiner should avoid the habit of simply transcribing information from previous visits. Medications, allergies, and the medical history can all change, sometimes over the course of days. Similarly, patients should have their blood pressure, pulse, respiratory rate, and temperature checked at each visit. If a center decides not to check a specific vital sign under certain circumstances (for instance, some centers do not check the temperature of patients who present with a minor, acute injury), this should be uniformly understood among the staff. Staff should be encouraged, however, to use clinical judgment as indicated by the given situation. Except as accepted procedure, no field on a chart should be left blank. If no information is needed in the field, "N/A" can be entered. If all fields are required to be completed, errors of omission can be reduced or avoided.

In addition to the standard charting, certain conditions require documentation of additional information. For instance, all patients with visual/eye complaints require a documented visual acuity examination both before and after treatment; wounds require assessment of tetanus status; extremity injuries require documentation of neurovascular status; women of childbearing years should have a last menstrual period (LMP) noted; potential surgical patients require information on when they last ate.

When the physician is reviewing the patient chart—either prior to or during evaluation—it is important that he or she review all nursing data. At times, key information, which may be vital to patient assessment, may be provided during the nursing assessment yet not shared during the physician evaluation. Additionally, if the nursing assessment records information that is not in keeping with the physician's evaluation, this must be addressed directly through documentation. For example, if during the evaluation of a 6-month-old, the nurse notes that the child is irritable or lethargic, this is an indication of a sick child who may require a spinal tap and admission. If, however, upon physician evaluation the child is found to be playful, happy, alert, and interactive, it should be documented as such, including the fact that no irritability or lethargy was noted.

The history and physical examination in the urgent care setting should be complete but problem-oriented and documented as such. For instance, a patient who presents for removal of an isolated splinter foreign body does not require a complete review of systems or general physical examination. Problem-focused examination and history is key to providing the patient flow needed to render time-conscious care. When patients present with vague or ambiguous complaints or have multiple underlying medical problems, a more detailed, comprehensive examination and history may be in order. Consultation with the primary care physician may also prove beneficial.

If, during nursing assessment, an electrocardiogram (ECG) is performed or oxygen saturation is measured, this must be documented along with physician notification of the results. Whenever any medications or treatments are ordered, the time when the order was placed and the time when the order was completed should be documented. It must also be noted whether the patient was able to tolerate the treatment and the patient's response to the treatment, if any. Documented pre- and post- measurements, particularly when nebulizer treatments are administered, are a must. If pain medication is ordered, it is important to use a consistent pain scale to document response to treatment. The scale most frequently used rates pain on a scale of 1 to 10, with 1 being virtually no pain and 10 representing excruciating or unbearable pain. This type of documentation helps everyone to understand both the patient's subjective level of pain and his or her response to treatment.

When procedures are to be performed, it is important to document any discussions with the patient prior to beginning the procedure and to note that appropriate consent was obtained. This will include discussing both the risks and benefits of the procedure and the risks associated with not performing the procedure. All aspects of the procedure should be documented, including type of anesthesia used, if applicable (i.e., lidocaine versus bupivacaine; with or without epinephrine), size of needle used to administer anesthesia, location of injection, etc. It should be noted that the area was prepped and that the procedure was performed under sterile conditions if so performed. It should also be noted whether the procedure was well tolerated or if there were any difficulties, complications, or unexpected findings. Pre- and postprocedure evaluation is key and must be documented, including neurovascular status and x-ray results when indicated (i.e., reduced dislocations, foreign-body removal, etc.).

When patients refuse care, it is important to document that the risks have been discussed with them and that they are aware of said risks. To this end, it is important to also document that the patient is competent to make an informed decision. Under these circumstances, it is imperative to have a witness included in the discussion. The witness is also to sign the refusal-of-care form attesting that the patient was informed and aware but refused treatment. When the witness can be a family member of the patient, this is ideal.

When there has been a consultation with either a patient's primary physician or a specialist, a detailed account of the conversation should be documented in the patient's chart. It is important to note that the patient's case was discussed with the consulting doctor exactly as written in the patient's record, including all available results. Any recommendations from the consulting clinician for additional testing, direction of care, or follow-up instructions should be carefully documented. It is absolutely imperative, however, to note that the urgent care physician is the treating physician and is ultimately responsible for the patient and the consequences of the care provided. Therefore, while telephone consultations may be helpful, if there is any concern regarding the patient's condition or diagnosis or about the recommended treatment plan, further evaluation or additional consultation should be sought.

Discharge instructions are another important component of documentation in the urgent care setting. Many facilities use commercially designed instruction sheets for many diagnoses. When these forms are used, the chart should document that the instruction form was given and reviewed with the patient prior to discharge. Also, when standard forms are used, it is important to review them for medications that may be contraindicated for the particular patient being seen. If any contraindications are present, the patient must be instructed not to use the medication (and it must be documented that this was done).

In other facilities, the treating physicians may provide discharge instructions of their own preference. Whatever system is used, however, it is important that what has been discussed with the patient be documented. When non-English-speaking patients are being cared for, it is also important to document that instructions were either given to them in their own language or reviewed with them via a translator. It does no good to provide instructions that patients cannot understand.

In addition to providing clinical information regarding the patient's urgent care visit, accurate charting also serves as a means of verification for ICD-9 coding and billing information. The level of care rendered, the time when the care was provided, treatments administered (including patient reassessment), as well as the complexity level of the patient's diagnosis all provide information for insurance billing. Simple, problem-focused complaints, such as that of a child with an uncomplicated sore throat, will not require the same level of assessment as the case of an elderly diabetic who is complaining of chest pain. Certain criteria must be met to satisfy the requirements for accurate billing. For instance, it is important in the documentation of a laceration to include the type of laceration, length, depth, and involvement of adjacent structures, as well as anesthesia used for repair, the number of stitches placed, and any special care (such as irrigation, debridement, packing, foreign-body removal, etc.) that was rendered. Failure to provide adequate documentation may lead to underpayment or rejection of the claim.

4

INTERFACILITY TRANSPORT OF PATIENTS FROM THE URGENT CARE SETTING

Dan Hanfling / Thom A. Mayer

INTRODUCTION

Patients who present for evaluation and treatment at an urgent care facility may sometimes exceed the capabilities that are available on site. Certain patients may require transfer to an emergency department for additional diagnostic evaluation that is not possible in the urgent care setting. Others will need admission to the hospital for definitive care of a diagnosed illness or injury. With the advent of observation units in hospitals, some patients may require transfer in order to undergo clinical observation and diagnostic testing for periods of up to 23 h. These situations demand a previously developed and thoughtfully considered transfer policy in order to expedite the ongoing care of such patients.

An established transfer protocol will contribute to improved care of the sickest patients likely to be seen in an urgent care facility. This must include a triage system that allows the health care providers to recognize early which patients are likely to need transport to the local emergency department or hospital. It must also incorporate communication with the accepting physician, who will ultimately have medical and legal responsibilities for the care of the transferred patient. A transfer protocol must also detail what additional care ought to be provided while awaiting arrival of the transferring emergency medical services (EMS) unit; this should be specific with regard to the transfer of care to the EMS practitioners. Such medical oversight can comprise both direct, or "on-line," medical control and indirect, or "off-line," medical control.

This chapter presents the elements required to establish a transfer protocol, reviews the types of patients requiring transfer for definitive diagnosis or treatment, describes the legal setting in which transfer of a patient occurs, and highlights the differences between the types of EMS transport available.

OPTIONS FOR PREHOSPITAL TRANSPORT

Patients who are in need of further evaluation in the emergency department or of admission to the hospital will require transfer from the urgent care facility, which ought to be accomplished under previously established transfer protocols. This entails understanding of the resources available for transport and the mechanism by which they are accessed. Such transfers are often performed under previously established referral patterns to the local hospitals, including those facilities that may provide specialty care in the setting of trauma, cardiac disease, pediatrics, obstetrics, psychiatry, and the like.

Development of a transfer protocol is governed under the established guidelines of the American College of Emergency Physicians (ACEP). Optimal planning for the transfer of a patient begins with an understanding of the medical requirements for that individual patient. It must also take into account the capabilities of the personnel and EMS system or agency to be used for the transfer. In a policy statement addressing these matters, the ACEP noted that the transferring physician is responsible under federal law for assuring that qualified personnel using appropriate equipment transfer the patient.[1]

There are various levels of prehospital services that may be used for an interfacility transport (Table 4-1). These include private vehicle, prehospital ground or air medical EMS service, or dedicated specialty transport service. Patients who require no medical care en route, such as those who may be transferred for elective diagnostic procedures or treatment, may wish to travel by private vehicle with or without accompanying family or friends. The vast majority of patients, however, will require some degree of prehospital medical support.

TABLE 4-1

LEVELS OF PATIENT TRANSPORT

LEVEL	STAFFING	TYPES OF PATIENTS
Private vehicle (POV)	None	Minor illnesses or injuries requiring subspecialty evaluation (i.e., orthopedics, ophthalmology, ENT, plastic surgery)
Basic life support (BLS)	EMT-B	Stable patients not requiring intravenous drip or medications (i.e., extremity fractures, lacerations)
Advanced life support (ALS)	EMT-CT, EMT-I, EMT-P (depending on state regulations)	Acutely ill or injured patients (i.e., chest pain, asthma, congestive heart failure, abdominal pain)
Specialty care teams (aeromedical or ground)	EMT-P, RN, MD	Severely ill or injured patients, particularly those with special needs (i.e., neonatal or pediatrics, burns, trauma, acute myocardial infarction)

Key: EMT-B, Emergency Medical Technician—Basic; EMT-CT, Emergency Medical Technician—Cardiac Technician; EMT-I, Emergency Medical Technician—Intermediate; EMT-P, Emergency Medical Technician—Paramedic; MD, medical doctor; POV, privately owned vehicle; RN, registered nurse.

Basic life support (BLS) ambulances are staffed by personnel trained as basic emergency medical technicians (EMT-B). They are capable of performing cardiopulmonary resuscitation (CPR) and providing other first aid treatments but may not administer oxygen or administer medications and have no training in performing invasive procedures. Such services may be sufficient for the transport of stable patients in whom the likelihood of a life-threatening emergency does not exist. Advanced life support (ALS) ambulances are manned by emergency medical technicians trained to the intermediate (EMT-I), cardiac care (EMT-CT), or paramedic (EMT-P) levels. These staff possess the training and authorization to administer drug therapy and perform invasive procedures, including the initiation of intravenous access, interpretation of 12-lead electrocardiograms (ECGs), and the use of endotracheal intubation for definitive airway management. These transferring units may belong to either a local municipal agency or a private service transport entity.

These transporting units and their personnel operate by established medical protocol, often under the direct and indirect medical oversight of an agency operational medical director. One consequence of their being called upon to provide a level of care outside the scope of their training or as allowed by medical protocol is that such transporting units may render suboptimal medical care. Furthermore, overuse of field units for interfacility transfers makes them unavailable for prehospital response.[2] As a result of such limited critical care capability in the traditional prehospital EMS model, the use of specialty care transport systems arose. The advent of interhospital transport teams was initially concentrated upon the use of air medical transport of trauma patients. This has evolved to include cardiac, pediatric, and neonatal patients, among others. Care for these patients may also be facilitated by dedicated critical care ground transport services, which employ the use of mobile intensive care units (ICUs).

In some areas of the country, all ambulance and medical unit transports from urgent care centers are processed as 911 emergency calls. This is in contrast with regions in which the availability of private ambulance companies has led to all but the most time-sensitive of their transports being handled by such private companies. Furthermore, in areas with heavy penetration of managed care organizations (MCOs), transports may need to be preapproved or arranged with specific ambulance companies with which the MCO has contractual arrangements. However, in no case should timely patient care be compromised for financial or administrative reasons.

TYPES OF PATIENTS REQUIRING TRANSFER

Although urgent care centers, by definition, are not designed to care for patients with severe illnesses and injuries, such patients nevertheless arrive at urgent care centers for evaluation. By virtue of such a center's limited resources, certain types of patients who present for initial evaluation to an urgent care facility will require transfer to a local hospital emergency department, regional trauma center, burn center, or children's hospital for definitive diagnosis, treatment, and care. It is important to have a sense early in the initial evaluation of an urgent care patient who will require transfer to another health care setting. Because certain medical conditions are considered time-dependent emergencies and because the transfer is also a time-dependent event, early recognition of such patients is crucial.

Trauma

Patients who present with traumatic injuries may require a level of care beyond that delivered in the urgent care setting. Patients with evidence of closed head injury, possible cervical spine injury, thoracoabdominal trauma, or severe orthopedic injury—especially in the context of a mechanism of injury supporting the possibility of morbidity—should be transferred to a trauma center for additional evaluation and care. The American College of Surgeons has clearly identified patients who may require a higher level of care and has set forth guidelines to promote the transfer of such patients (Table 4-2). Such patients include those with closed head injury with documented or suspected loss of consciousness or presentation with altered mental status in the setting of a traumatic mechanism of injury. Chest injuries, including altered ventilatory status due to pneumothorax or pulmonary contusion, will require definitive surgical care, as will the evaluation of a widened mediastinum on chest x-ray. Abdominal pain suggestive of solid organ injury will require definitive evaluation. Significant orthopedic injuries, especially those involving disruption of the pelvic ring or long bone fractures, will require transfer to the regional trauma center. Of course, any evidence of spinal cord injury will also necessitate the provision of a higher level of care. Finally, serious burn injuries will require specialized care at a regional burn center. This includes those injuries occurring in patients at the extremes of age, full-thickness burns involving 5 percent of body surface area, partial-thickness burns involving from 10 to 20 percent of body surface area, burns involving particular body parts, and other criteria as set forth by the American Burn Association (Table 4-3).[3]

TABLE 4-2

INTERFACILITY TRAUMA TRIAGE CRITERIA

Central nervous system/head injury	Penetrating injury or depressed skull fracture Loss of consciousness > 5 min Glasgow Coma Scale (GCS) score < 14 or deterioration in GCS score
Central nervous system/spinal cord injury	Focal neurologic deficits
Chest trauma	Widened mediastinum Major chest wall injury Suspected cardiac injury
Abdominal trauma	Abdominal pain with or without hemodynamic instability
Orthopedic trauma	Long bone fractures Pelvic ring disruption
Evidence of high-energy impact	Motor vehicle crash or pedestrian injury with velocity > 25 mph Passenger compartment intrusion Ejection of patient or rollover Death of occupant in same car
Comorbid factors	Age < 5 years or > 55 years

Source: Adapted from ACS,[3] with permission.

TABLE 4-3

CRITERIA FOR BURN CENTER REFERRAL

TYPE OF BURN	ANATOMIC INVOLVEMENT
Partial-thickness burn	Greater than 10% of total body surface area (BSA) in patients < 10 years or > 50 years of age Greater than 20% total BSA in other age groups Involvement of face, eyes, ears, hands, feet, genitalia, or perineum or of skin overlying major joints
Full-thickness burn	Greater than 10% total BSA in patients < 10 years or > 50 years of age Greater than 20% total BSA in other age groups Involvement of face, eyes, ears, hands, feet, genitalia, or perineum or of skin overlying major joints Greater than 5% BSA in any age group
Electrical burns (including lightning injury)	Strong likelihood of deep tissue destruction
Chemical burns	Strong likelihood of deep tissue destruction
Inhalation injury	Suspected or confirmed airway involvement

Source: Adapted from ACS,[4] with permission.

Cardiac

Chest pain is a common complaint in the urgent care setting. Differentiation between chest pain of cardiac versus noncardiac origin often requires evaluation, observation, and definitive diagnosis, which can only be provided in the hospital setting. These patients can often be initially stabilized in the urgent care setting, including the use of intravenous nitrates and heparin therapy if available. If these medications are not available, the patient should receive appropriate stabilizing therapy including oxygen, relief of chest pain with sublingual or topical nitrates, and aspirin. Occasionally, patients with chest pain in the urgent care setting will actually have demonstrable ECG evidence of acute myocardial infarction. If indicated, these patients may require thrombolytic therapy in addition to the aforementioned treatment regimen. When criteria for thrombolytic therapy are present (Table 4-4), this information should be clearly communicated to the EMTs and to the emergency physician at the receiving hospital. In addition, a copy of the ECG should be sent with the patient or faxed to the emergency department. Regardless of whether the patient with chest pain is being considered for admission to rule out a myocardial infarction, experiencing unstable angina, or having the real thing, rapid transport to the local hospital for eventual admission to the intensive care or coronary care unit will be required.

Medical

A significant number of medical conditions will also require transport to the local emergency department or hospital for definitive evaluation and treatment. These include but are not limited to conditions calling for the immediate attention and care of specialty

TABLE 4-4

USE OF THROMBOLYTICS IN ACUTE MYOCARDIAL INFARCTION

INDICATIONS	CONTRAINDICATIONS	RELATIVE CONTRAINDICATIONS
Chest pain suggestive of ischemia	Active internal bleeding	Age > 75 (increased incidence of hemorrhagic stroke)
ST-segment elevation > 1 mm in two or more contiguous leads	Suspected aortic dissection	History of cerebrovascular accident
	Recent history of hemorrhagic stroke	Delayed presentation (> 12 h)
New onset of LBBB in setting of ischemic symptoms	Recent trauma or surgery (2 weeks)	Uncontrolled hypertension (SBP > 180 mmHg or DBP > 110 mmHg)
	Known intracranial neoplasm	Active peptic ulcer disease
Presentation within 12 h of onset of symptoms	Pregnant or menstruating female	
	Previous allergic reaction to lytic agent	

Key: LBBB, left bundle branch block; SBP, systolic blood pressure; DBP, diastolic blood pressure.
Source: Adapted from AHA,[10] with permission.

physicians. Patients diagnosed with gastrointestinal bleeding, for example, may need ICU admission. So, too, will patients presenting to the urgent care center after taking an intentional overdose of medications that require specific antidote therapy and supportive care. In addition to those medical patients who require admission to the hospital, a number of patients may require additional diagnostic studies that are available only in the emergency department setting.

Obstetric and Gynecologic

Few patients in active labor would be expected to present in an urgent care setting. However, it is clear that by federal law any patient in active labor who is unstable may not be transferred in such a state. Such patients may be transported prior to delivery, but only as long as such a transfer would have a clear benefit.[5] More commonly evaluated, though, is the patient in the beginning stages of a pregnancy, where the onset of vaginal bleeding with or without abdominal pain may represent a surgical emergency. A pregnant patient with a possible ectopic pregnancy will require diagnosis by ultrasound, which is usually not available in the urgent care facility.

Pediatric

Depending upon the degree of training of the urgent care health care provider staff, their level of comfort in treating pediatric patients, and the presenting symptoms and complaints, certain pediatric patients will require transfer to the local emergency department or regional children's hospital for further evaluation and care. Among patients who are initially stabilized in the urgent care setting, those requiring continued intravenous therapy or other inpatient treatment or diagnosis will also require transfer.

Psychiatric

Patients who present to the urgent care setting with behavioral or psychiatric problems will often need admission to the hospital for such conditions. Following the medical clearance and stabilization of these patients, transfer to an accepting facility can be initiated. Most of these patients should not require additional treatment during transport, which should facilitate the disposition of these patients. One exception would be the need for physical restraints. Such cases might require the presence or accompaniment of law enforcement personnel.

MECHANISM FOR INTERFACILITY TRANSFER

The decision to transfer a patient out of the urgent care facility and to the hospital is ultimately a matter of experience and medical judgment. Once this decision is made, the transfer should proceed without delay so as to expedite the ultimate care of the patient being transferred. Any additional diagnostic studies that may delay transport should be deferred for completion at the receiving institution.

Responsibilities for the transfer of patients between medical facilities are well delineated. The referring physician is responsible for the initiation of the transfer process to the receiving institution and for the selection of an appropriate mode of transportation and level of care required for optimal management of the patient en route. This includes the discussion of the case with an accepting physician, who will ultimately be responsible for the ongoing medical care of the transferred patient. Together, both physicians can outline any additional steps required to stabilize a patient prior to transport. If needed, the receiving physician can also assist in arranging for the transportation from urgent care to the hospital.

All interfacility transfers will require the completion of mandatory documentation, which includes a description of the patient's diagnosis, summary of treatment course and interventions, the names of the transferring and accepting physicians, and the risks and benefits associated with the patient's transfer. In addition to conveying the necessary information regarding the transfer, this documentation serves as legal protection for the transferring institution. Finally, included with the patient should be a copy of all pertinent laboratory or radiographic data for evaluation and review at the receiving institution.

CHECKLIST FOR PATIENT TRANSPORT

The following steps should be taken by the urgent care management to assure smooth transfer of care to patients. Because of the number of physicians and EMS contacts, it is usually preferable to have the medical director of the urgent care center handle or initiate these steps.

- Prospectively contact the emergency department chairperson or emergency department medical director in order to discuss transfer arrangements and to establish a professional relationship
- Prospectively meet with the emergency department nursing director
- Identify and meet with the EMS medical director and the appropriate administrative personnel from the local EMS agencies

- Clarify local medical control policies and procedures
- When transports are necessary, specify the following steps in the transfer policy:

Call the local EMS agency on either the nonemergency or 911 line, as appropriate. For private ambulance or specialty team transports, contact them directly.

Clearly state the nature of the clinical problem, the level of transport required (ALS, BLS, etc.), and the treatment anticipated en route.

Contact the emergency physician at the receiving hospital to discuss the patient's care.

PATIENT TRANSFER AND THE LAW

Interfacility transport and the movement of patients from one health care setting to another are governed by a strict set of legal parameters. In response to the inappropriate transfer of uninsured patients from one hospital to another, Congress passed the Emergency Medical Treatment and Active Labor Act (EMTALA) in 1986. This became a part of the Consolidated Omnibus Budget Reconciliation Act (COBRA) enacted into legislation the year before. These laws clearly govern the transfer of patients from the urgent care setting to the local hospital.

EMTALA mandates that any patient who presents to a facility that receives Medicare funds and describes itself as providing emergency care must provide a medical screening examination to all patients who so desire. The required medical screening examination is provided in order to determine the presence or absence of an emergency medical condition. Nursing triage alone is not considered a sufficient level of medical screening. If the required screening examination reveals an emergency medical condition, the urgent care providers are responsible for stabilizing the patient within their means and may not transfer the patient unless it is clear that the benefits of transfer outweigh the risks.[5]

If an unstable patient is transferred, federal law makes it clear that an appropriate level of care must be provided to the patient while en route from one facility to another. This is clearly the responsibility of the transferring physician. Occasionally, the transferring physician from the urgent care facility or another designated health care provider may elect to accompany an unstable patient to the hospital.[6] This can be done to assist the transporting EMS crew while also providing a higher level of care than would be available from the prehospital providers alone.

CONCLUSION

Expeditious and safe transport of patients from an urgent care facility to the hospital is ultimately dependent upon the transferring physician. Each transport situation, however, will vary given the type of patient, distance to be traveled, and skills of the prehospital providers. Knowledge of the availability and types of EMS transport available to the urgent care facility will be paramount to ensuring a successful transport. Contact numbers for the EMS and specialty transport services should be readily available. The skills and capabilities of providers in these systems should be understood. Logistic issues such as location of the medical facility and directions to it—as well as parking or landing zones to be used by ground or air transport units and availability of certain types of equipment—should all be worked out beforehand. This may best be facilitated by pre-arranged visits by representatives of the EMS agencies to the urgent care facility.[7,8]

Transport of patients from the urgent care setting to the hospital becomes the choice of the transferring urgent care physician. This choice can be summarized by the following three questions: *How quickly must the patient be transferred? What level of care must be provided to assure a safe medical transport? And does the transport violate any legal requirements?*[9]

REFERENCES

1. American College of Emergency Physicians: Medical direction of interfacility patient transfers. *Ann Emerg Med* 31:154, 1998.
2. Meador S, Low R: Interfacility transports, in Kuehl AE (ed): *Prehospital Systems and Medical Oversight.* Baltimore: Mosby; 1994:414–419.
3. American College of Surgeons, Committee on Trauma: Stabilization and transport, in Alexander RH, Proctor HJ (eds): *Advanced Trauma Life Support.* Chicago: American College of Surgeons; 1993:295–301.
4. American College of Surgeons, Committee on Trauma: Injuries due to burns and cold, in Alexander RH, Proctor HJ (eds): *Advanced Trauma Life Support.* Chicago: American College of Surgeons; 1993:255.
5. Maggiore A: Avoid COBRA's fangs. EMTALA: Legislating appropriate critical care transports. *JEMS* 24(8):66–74, 1999.
6. Wuerz R, Meador S: Adverse events during interfacility transfers by ground advanced life support services. *Prehosp Disaster Med* 9(1):50–53, 1994.
7. Woodward G, King B: "Interfacility" transport from the home or office. *Pediatr Emerg Care* 13(2):164–168, 1997.
8. Davis C, Rodewald L: Use of EMS for seriously ill children in the office: a survey of primary care physicians. *Prehosp Emerg Care* 3:102–106, 1999.
9. Clemmer T, Thomas F: Transport of the critically ill." *Crit Care Med* 28(1):265–266, 2000.
10. American Heart Association: Guidelines 2000 for Cardiopulmonary Resuscitation and Emergency Cardiovascular Care, Part 7, Section 1, Acute Coronary Syndromes (Acute Myocardial Infarction). *Circulation* 102(8):172–203, 2000.

CUSTOMER SERVICE IN URGENT CARE MEDICINE

Thom A. Mayer / Robert J. Cates

Urgent care centers (UCCs) are by nature and definition health care organizations in a highly competitive environment. The patients who use UCCs do so primarily based on quality of care and convenience but also on the service provided. It is essential for successful urgent care centers to understand the importance of a commitment to customer service as a part of the fundamental mission of the center. This is not to say that quality of care and convenience of the operation are not important, but simply that those aspects of health care in general and UCCs in particular are assumed by the patient—who wants a facility that combines quality of care, convenience, and excellent customer service.[1]

This chapter presents the approach to customer service that has been utilized at the Inova Fairfax Hospital Emergency Department and its affiliated emergency care centers. The fundamental program was designed in 1994 and was developed as the "Emergency Department Survival Skills" program. After this course had been taught to all emergency and emergency care center staff, there was a dramatic improvement in customer service ratings. Patient complaints dropped from 2.4 to 0.4 per 1000 visits. Patient compliments rose from 0.6 visits to over 5.7 per 1000 emergency department (ED) visits.[2] Patient satisfaction scores saw a similar increase in all areas that were key quality indicators (Table 5-1). However, although all of these indicators improved dramatically, two in particular improved so dramatically as to seem to defy statistical reality. The areas that showed this great improvement involved (1) the skill of the physician and (2) the skill of the nurse. In short, the patients' perception of the quality of their care—based on customer service training, orientation, and commitment—was greatly improved. Equally important, employee satisfaction scores rose substantially during the same time period, verifying that customer satisfaction improves employee satisfaction.

TABLE 5-1

PATIENT SATISFACTION SURVEY FOR INOVA FAIRFAX HOSPITAL EMERGENCY
DEPARTMENT AND EMERGENCY CARE CENTERS—IMPROVED TRENDS

1. Staff's efforts to keep family informed
2. Overall respect shown to patient
3. Overall quality of medical care
4. How quickly seen by triage nurse
5. Explanation provided by triage nurse
6. Triage nurse's sensitivity to patient pain
7. Doctor's ability to explain condition, diagnosis, and treatment options
8. Skill of the emergency doctor
9. Wait time to be seen by a doctor
10. Skill of emergency department nurses
11. Caring and courtesy of emergency department nurses
12. Nursing staff's ability to keep patient informed
13. Medical needs were met

WHY DEVELOP CUSTOMER SERVICE PROGRAMS?

Aside from the importance from a competitive standpoint of developing a customer
service focus for UCCs, there is a long list of reasons that customer service should be
initiated in emergency department and urgent care settings (Table 5-2). These include
improved clinical care, reduced stress, improved morale, better relationships with referral agencies, improved financial profiles, better risk management, quality improvement,
etc. However, none of these is the most important reason to get customer service right
in the health care setting, which is that *it makes the job easier!*

Through customer service programs presented at over 200 health care facilities
nationwide, organizations which have been successful in implementing customer service
programs have one thing in common: they all agree that the primary reason for their success is that customer service skills and initiatives make the job easier for the clinicians
providing care on a day-to-day basis. Thus, as psychologists have indicated for years,

TABLE 5-2

EFFECTS OF PATIENT CARE/CUSTOMER SERVICE PHILOSOPHY

1.	Makes clinician's job easier	3.	Reduces stress
2.	Improves clinical care	4.	Improves morale
	• Patient compliance	5.	Improves reputation
	• Patient/family understanding	6.	Improves long-term resources
	• Origins of medicine/nursing	7.	Improves risk management
		8.	Improves interdepartmental relations

intrinsic motivation is a much stronger force than extrinsic motivation—it is better for the staff to hold themselves accountable for customer service than for management to try to "beat it into their heads."

ARE THEY PATIENTS OR ARE THEY CUSTOMERS?

In designing and implementing the survival skills course, customer service training programs in various businesses and industries across the nation were researched. Almost without exception, the types of courses that were available, even in health care settings, fit into one of two types of programs. The first of these had a central message: "Smile, be nice, even when it hurts!" This type of course faced substantial resistance from health care providers because it implies that the solution is simply to be nicer, work harder, "get your act in gear," and that it is simply a matter of smiling more to make things better. Experienced staff realize that this is not the case, and that such a simplistic approach is intrinsically demeaning. Finally, such programs simply do not work, even in the health care environment.

The second type of course that is often taught has a slightly different but related message: "Stop calling them patients—start calling them customers!" While somewhat less offensive to health care workers, such courses again miss the point by assuming that a simple change in vocabulary will result in improved outcomes for our patients, their families, and the staff who care for them on a day-to-day basis. Rather than rely on such simplistic solutions, the survival skills course includes an exercise designed to help health care professionals realize that they have their own inherent and intuitive definitions of customers and patients, even if those definitions have not been clearly articulated. As Fig. 5-1 illustrates, imagine a gauge with a needle pointing toward either *Patient* or *Customer*, depending solely on the reaction of the health care workers to various scenarios to which they are exposed. After hearing each clinical scenario, the respondents are simply asked whether they would classify the other person as a patient or as a customer.

Scenario 1: A 55-year-old woman presents with severe substernal chest pain with radiation to the jaw and the left arm. An electrocardiogram (ECG) is rapidly obtained and is noted to show substantial ST-segment elevation, indicating an acute anterior myocardial infarction. Is this a patient or a customer?

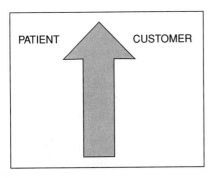

FIGURE 5-1   The patient–customer gauge. In this thought exercise, health care providers are presented with three distinct clinical scenarios (see text) and asked to indicate whether the needle on the gauge points toward *patient* or *customer*.

Scenario 2: A 3-year-old child is brought to the urgent care center by his parents, having been seen by the pediatrician on the morning of the same day. The pediatrician diagnosed left otitis media and started the patient on antibiotics and fever control measures. The parents state that they "can't get the fever down," although the boy's temperature is 37.5°C. Is this a patient or a customer?

Scenario 3: Scenario 3 is the same as scenario 2 with one exception—this child is *your child*. Is this more of a patient or more of a customer?

Among the over 20,000 health care professionals who have responded to this exercise, who have diverse backgrounds and live in broad geographic locations, the results are strikingly consistent. The woman in scenario 1 is universally recognized as a patient, while the child in scenario 2 is identified as a customer (with the parents invariably being identified as the primary customers). Scenario 3 invariably causes health care professionals to question whether they would classify their own child as a patient or a customer, despite the low degree of severity of the illness, because of the personal nature of the case.

Further, when health care professionals are questioned as to why they rate the woman in the first scenario as a patient, they invariably answer that she is more acutely ill, needs immediate technical intervention, has less choice, and has a time-dependent problem. The child in scenario 2 is rated more of a customer because he is less severely ill, has more choice, and requires more service skills (Table 5-3). Simply stated, patients have more time- and technical-dependent problems and customers have more service- and "art of medicine"–dependent problems. It is extremely important to note that both emergency department and UCC professionals, almost without exception, have also noted that they have a high degree of clarity in knowing how to take care of patients, who primarily require technical expertise to care for their illnesses or injuries. This is in contrast to the lack of clarity with regard to how to approach the customer, largely because physicians and nurses have had very little training in formal customer service skills and techniques. This clarity in caring for patients and confusion in caring for customers presents a paradox in that research strongly suggests that the service needs of patients are surprisingly uniform, cutting across cultural, economic, and geographic boundaries as well as the various levels of illness severity and acuity. Cleary and Edgman-Levitan have delineated specific dimensions that patients seek, which include individualizing care, coordinating care, improving communication, enhancing physical comforts, providing support to patients, giving patients choices, and ensuring smooth transitions in care.[3] What remains to be done is to clearly delineate how these dimensions can be applied at the bedside in various settings, including urgent care.

However, based on experience in the survival skills course, it is clear that health care professionals in all settings, even without extensive experience or specific customer service training, can and do make such patient/customer diagnoses in the daily course of delivering health care in their respective settings. All of us, as clinicians, assess patients routinely and make an internal, entirely nonscientific (but no less accurate) judgment of whether they are primarily patients or primarily customers usually according to a simple diagnostic rule: "The more horizontal they are, the more they are patients. The more vertical they are, the more they are customers."

While the point is simple, direct, and obvious, it has nonetheless not been stated widely enough to be put into practical use at the bedside: "Just as all patients have a clinical diagnosis requiring technical expertise, they also have a customer service diagnosis requiring excellent service skills."

Treating one while ignoring or neglecting the other predictably results in either poor clinical outcomes or less than desired patient satisfaction. This is not a new and revolutionary concept but simply an understated and neglected one. In addition, as the patient's clinical status improves because of appropriate use of technical skills, and as patients move from the horizontal to the vertical position, aspects of customer service excellence assume increased importance.

To return to the scenarios in the exercise for a moment, is the woman with the myocardial infarction only a patient? Are the boy and his parents only customers? To answer these questions, another exercise is needed. Imagine performing a "patient–customer autopsy" on any given person at any given time. If we could dissect what percentage is patient and what percentage is customer, what would the results tell us? Although most physicians tend to think of a woman with a myocardial infarction as a 100 percent patient, more careful scrutiny and thought would indicate that there are parts of her, however small, that are also customer. In addition, such "100 percent patients" also have family members and friends who have customer service needs to be addressed as well. Similarly, the child with the fever and his parents are never quite 100 percent customers either. The degree to which they are considered patients or customers is an indirect reflection of how horizontal versus vertical we diagnose them to be. This relationship is reflected in Fig. 5-2, which indicates that if a person is about 20 percent customer, they are probably about 80 percent patient. Conversely, those who are quite ill and are deemed by health care professionals to be 80 percent patient are still about

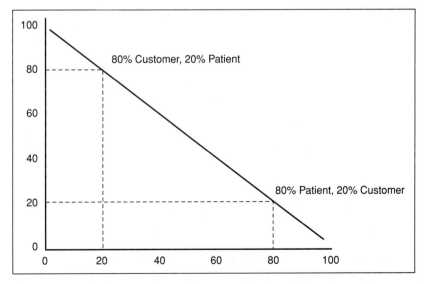

FIGURE 5-2 Assessing the percentage of patient versus customer. In assessing clinical versus customer service diagnosis, participants are asked to answer the questions "What percent patient is this? What percent customer is this?" Answers from physicians consistently demonstrate a nonscientific but linear relationship of customer versus patient diagnoses.

TABLE 5-3

HEALTH CARE PROFESSIONALS' DISTINCTIONS BETWEEN THEIR DEFINITION
OF PATIENTS VERSUS CUSTOMERS

PATIENT	CUSTOMER
Acutely ill or injured	Less severely ill
Dependent on physician	Independent
Power/control with clinician	Power/control with customer
Less choice	More choice
Technical expertise required	Service skills required
Greater satisfaction for clinician	Less satisfaction for clinician
High clarity of treatment	Less clarity of treatment
Time-dependent	Service-dependent

SOURCE: Mayer and Cates,[1] with permission.

20 percent customer. *The bottom line is that they are all* people, *who have both clinical and customer service needs to be met if we are to fulfill our role as health care providers.*

Therefore, the answer to the question "are they patients or are they customers?" is that they are always both, to varying degrees, depending upon factors that are intuitively known by health care professionals and that center around issues of patient illness, level of choice, and dependency (Table 5-3). Just as patients have clinical diagnoses, they also have customer service diagnoses comprising a set of hopes and expectations regarding their clinical care. And, as the third scenario demonstrates, it is never surprising that if the person is a member of our own family, we tend to have a different assessment of how vertical versus horizontal the person is and therefore how much of a customer he or she represents and how much of a patient.

CUSTOMER SERVICE CORE COMPETENCIES

Experience in "Survival Skills" customer service training has led to the conclusion that there are three core competencies that must be met in providing health care and in combining technical excellence and customer service excellence:

1. Making the customer service diagnosis and offering the right treatment.
2. Negotiating agreement and resolution of expectations
3. Building moments of truth into the clinical encounter

The First Survival Skill: Making the Customer Service Diagnosis and Offering the Right Treatment

As indicated in the patient–customer thought exercise presented above, just as every patient has a clinical diagnosis requiring our technical expertise, every patient also has a customer service diagnosis to which we should apply appropriate skills and techniques.

Urgent care and emergency department physicians and nurses are among the best and most accurate diagnosticians in health care, routinely seeing up to 50 to 60 patients per shift and accurately assessing and treating their medical needs. These diagnostic skills can also be put to use in making the customer service diagnosis as well. Let us look at some examples, which are summarized in Fig. 5-3. In scenario 2 above, a 3-year-old child is brought in with a clinical diagnosis of fever—but what is the family's biggest fear or concern? In other words: *What is their customer service diagnosis?* For parents with febrile young children, their concern is not the fever per se but rather the fear that the child has meningitis or will develop seizures or brain damage. Thus, while our clinical diagnosis may be occult bacteremia, acute otitis media, pharyngitis, or some other clinical entity, the customer service diagnosis and treatment are to assure the parents that the child does not have a serious life- or limb-threatening illness and is not likely to develop one. Thus, treating only the clinical diagnosis and ignoring the customer service diagnosis may be "good science," but has it provided good medical care? If a patient presents to the UCC with chest pain, what is his or her biggest concern? Health care providers around the country have stated without equivocation that the patient fears that the chest pain is due to a heart attack.[4] Thus, we, as clinicians, not only need to rule out a myocardial infarction from a clinical standpoint, we also need to speak in direct and clear language to our patients, whether or not we feel they have had a heart attack or whether they need to be referred for further studies to determine this diagnosis. As a rule, patients with abdominal pain are primarily concerned about possible appendicitis. We can certainly diagnose and treat that illness, but we also need to speak specifically to the reasons that they have abdominal pain. As in emergency departments, abdominal pain is one of the top reasons for seeking care in a UCC, so we should be very proficient not only in diagnosing the clinical problem accurately but also in addressing customer service concerns regarding the abdominal pain. Finally, if a young child is brought in with a facial laceration, we certainly know how to treat that from a clinical standpoint, but we also need to know how to reassure the parents that there will be a minimal scar and that we will do everything we can to minimize that scar even further by the treatment that we provide. Thus, we need to treat the customer service diagnosis as well as the clinical diagnosis.

Additional ways in which we can help to make the customer service diagnosis and offer the right treatment include anticipating experiences from the customer's viewpoint rather than from the viewpoint of the health care provider. Data from The Advisory

Clinical Diagnosis	Customer Service Diagnosis
Pediatric Fever	Meningitis/Seizures
Chest Pain	Heart Attack
Abdominal Pain	Appendicitis/Cancer
Facial Laceration	Scarring, Guilt, Pain

FIGURE 5-3 **Making the customer service diagnosis versus the clinical diagnosis. In addition to having a clinical diagnosis, illustrated on the left, patients/customers also have a customer service diagnosis, which must also be addressed during the course of their care (on the right).**

Board and other sources indicate that the number one time interval the patients assess in determining quality in health care is "How long does it take to see the doctor?"[5] When we realize this, it becomes important to get the patient back to a room as rapidly as is feasible and to design our processes to help eliminate any non-value-added or extraneous steps. For example, emergency departments and UCCs across the country have often changed the process to in-room registration, which helps move the patients through the process more quickly and lets them see a physician faster. Similarly, if the physician is busy seeing other patients, advanced standing orders for certain clinical problems such as extremity trauma can be helpful in assuring that x-ray and/or laboratory studies are ordered, many times before the patient even sees the physician. All of these are ways in which we can anticipate, from the customer's viewpoint, how best to move patients through the system to provide a pleasing result.[6]

Experienced UCC physicians and nurses also learn to anticipate the customer's perspective by grouping diagnostic information into common themes. As indicated previously, the majority of patients presenting with abdominal pain have at least some concern as to whether this may represent appendicitis. (Patients over the age of 50 years often have a different concern—whether they have cancer.) Patients with ankle injuries want to know whether a bone is broken. By using our clinical experience and combining it with making the customer service diagnosis as well, we can redesign our interaction with patients to address not only their clinical problems but also the customer service or "art of medicine" aspect as well. The more we can translate those needs into the way our system operates on a daily basis, the better off we are, and the more satisfied our patients/customers will be.

In addition, there are a number of verbal skills we can utilize that can also be helpful in caring for such patients. These are summarized in Table 5-4. Therefore, the first "survival skill core competency" is to make not only the clinical diagnosis but also the customer service diagnosis, assuring that the patient receives the right treatment for both the clinical and customer aspects of care.

TABLE 5-4	
	VERBAL SKILLS—COMMUNICATE REASONABLE EXPECTATIONS

1. Introduce yourself in a professional fashion.
2. Explain what will happen.
3. Address family members—bring them into the encounter.
4. Establish a high level of professionalism and courtesy.
   - Sit down whenever possible.
   - Listen *actively*.
   - High level of manners (courtesy).
5. Provide information as it becomes available—frequent updates.
6. Check the patient's progress (multiple brief encounters).
7. Never underestimate the value of pillows, blankets, water, OJ.
8. "Are there any other problems I can help you with?"

The Second Survival Skill: Negotiating Agreement and Resolution of Expectations

When we make the diagnosis that a woman with severe chest pain has a myocardial infarction, we determine that she is nearly "100 percent patient." Do the woman and her family agree with us? Quite frankly, the more horizontal the patients are, the more likely they are to agree with us that they are patients and the more dependent they will be on us for their care. What about the child with the "fever"? We diagnosed this as a nearly 100 percent customer scenario. Do the parents agree with us? Of course they do not. In all likelihood they would not have come to the UCC or emergency department with a child that they did not think constituted a potentially serious emergency. In this case, our customer service diagnosis does not agree with theirs. Stated another way, *they have a different set of expectations for their encounter than we do as health care providers*. In these circumstances we need to negotiate our expectations back toward resolution of those expectations. How do we do that? Table 5-5 lists the skills necessary for negotiation of agreement and resolution of expectations. We start by being sure that we have a clear sense of what our expectations are for that specific clinical encounter—a step too seldom taken by health care providers. We follow this by discovering the patients' expectations, which can be done in the simplest possible way—by asking them what their expectations are. Nothing can replace a straightforward, simply worded question to patients regarding their expectations concerning their clinical condition. Once we have a clearer sense of how our expectations vary from the patients' expectations, we can assess those differences and begin to employ appropriate negotiation skills and strategies.

A number of books present negotiation courses that can be helpful. These are listed in the Selected Readings at the end of this chapter. All of these books provide excellent strategies for negotiation. The simplest and most straightforward is in *Getting to Yes*. It is only through negotiating effectively with our patients that we can ever hope to resolve the differences in our expectations. Further, health care providers will always be well served by having a finely honed and ongoing process of obtaining and utilizing negotiation skills. A good portion of our lives is spent in negotiation, whether at home, at work, or in our day-to-day interactions with our friends and family. When we refer a patient from the urgent care center to the emergency department or to a physician's practice, that is a form of negotiation, including obtaining a timely consult and appointment. We negotiate with our patients with regard to their acceptance of our diagnosis and treatment, including the specific treatment plan that we will utilize, appropriate follow-up care, and any questions they may have regarding further expectations for their illness or injury.

TABLE 5-5

NEGOTIATING AGREEMENTS AND RESOLVING EXPECTATIONS

Discovering expectations: ours	Teaching the customer how to be right
Discovering expectations: theirs	Negotiation skills and strategies
Assessing the differences	Dialogue and inquiry skills

The Third Survival Skill: Building Moments of Truth into the Clinical Encounter

Jan Carlzon, who at the time was president of Scandinavian Airlines System (SAS), introduced the concept of the "moments of truth." When he assumed the presidency of SAS, he was faced with revitalizing a major airline in the midst of a massive organizational crisis. His first management strategy was a stroke of customer service genius. He addressed the employees of SAS, speaking to them many hundreds to thousands at a time in hangars across Europe. With the aid of large video screens to project his image, he noted that the airline had previously defined itself primarily according to its business functions. For example, the airline flew a certain number of aircraft along specified routes with load capacity and revenue capacity geared toward maximizing use and profitability as well as market share. Carlzon challenged the airline and its employees to redefine themselves as follows: "SAS is 'created' 50 million times a year, 15 seconds at a time. These 50 million 'moments of truth' are the moments that ultimately determine whether SAS will succeed or fail as a company. They are the moments when we must prove to our customers that SAS is their best alternative."[7]

This constituted a radical shift from defining the company from a strictly business and process standpoint to focusing on the concept that the individuals making up the organization literally redefined their organization daily through these moments of truth. While the concept has become more widely accepted in many customer service industries, it originated with Carlzon and his challenge to the employees of SAS. This concept is easily applied to the health care environment, in that each team member redefines the facility on a daily basis by the moments of truth that occur between him or her and our customers, including patients, family, the medical staff to whom we refer, and the entire health care community in which we exist.

The brilliance of Carlzon's strategy goes further. Not only do the employees redefine the company on a daily basis, but they are free to tap into their own creativity by using empowerment strategies. He challenged his employees to ask a simple question about each of the activities that they undertake during the course of the day: "Does what I'm doing support the overall strategy of serving the customer?"

How do we build moments of truth into the clinical encounter? There are several ways it can be done (Table 5–6). The first is ensuring that we are managing the clinical encounters and the perceptions thereof. Patients need to have explanations for delays and for the process through which we put them. One of the core strategies for developing moments of truth in the clinical encounter is ensuring that information is exchanged accurately and frequently and that expectations are created and met at every stage of the health care process. Even upon checking into the urgent care center, the patients should be offered a time estimate of when they might be expected to be moved into a room, seen by the physician, and have treatment completed. From companies such as Walt Disney, we can learn the importance of "expectation creation" and assuring that we create expectations that we expect to be able to exceed. For example, if we estimate that the patient will be put into a room within 10 min and in fact we expect to be able to do so within 5 min, we have created an expectation that we not only hope but expect to exceed, which will please both patient and family.

TABLE 5-6

BUILDING MOMENTS OF TRUTH INTO THE CLINICAL ENCOUNTER

Managing clinical encounters and perceptions

Service transitions

Service fail-safes

Service recovery

Creating customer loyalty

Building customer service into the "bricks & mortar"

The ongoing search for customer service excellence

An additional way of building moments of truth into the clinical encounter is to understand the concept of service transition. Research in health care and in other environments has indicated that a primary source of patient satisfaction and dissatisfaction is service transitions, wherein service is handed off either from one individual to another or from one service to another. In the urgent care center environment, there are numerous service transitions, from check in at the counter, to initial evaluation by the nurse, to evaluation by the physician, to potential evaluation through lab or x-ray, which is then handed back to the nurse and physician for further service transitions. Viewed in this way, it is important to be sure that these transitions are managed prospectively so that the handoffs from one service area to the other can be handled as effectively as possible.

PUTTING IT TO WORK IN THE URGENT CARE CENTER

Effectively creating customer service in the UCC requires several key steps. First, there has to be a clear commitment toward customer service in addition to clinical care in the competitive UCC environment. In most cases, the urgent care center should have a clear model or mission statement that decisively states why it exists. Figure 5-4 shows the mission statement of the INOVA Fairfax emergency departments and UCCs which focuses not only on clinical care but on customer service as well. This statement clearly delineates the specific goal to be the best not in the state, not in the region, but in the entire nation. That is a high goal, but if it is not clearly stated and stated in an effective fashion, none of the staff will understand precisely how important it is. That mission statement appears in every treatment room in which patients are seen. That is the level of commitment that is necessary to build a customer service environment.

In addition, there has to be a complete dedication to processes that help serve the customer, with an understanding of the importance of constantly questioning how we might be able to provide better service to our patients. The best way to obtain this information is simply to ask them directly and clearly, either in the form of surveys, or in simple verbal conversations or follow-up telephone calls with our patients. How can we do this better? That is what we want to know and that is what we are committed to.

Finally, it is necessary to assure that this becomes a part of the entire fabric of the operation, from hiring staff through orientation, and in follow-up meetings with the

Fairfax Hospital
Emergency Department

Our goal is to offer our patients *the best* patient care and customer service of any Emergency Department in the country.

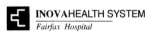 INOVAHEALTH SYSTEM
Fairfax Hospital

FIGURE 5-4   The goal of the urgent care center should be clearly stated and prominently displayed for patients and staff members alike.

staff. Are customer compliments and complaints and customer surveys discussed at every staff meeting or are they simply something that management sees alone? In a truly empowered customer service environment, all compliments and complaints as well as all survey information should be fed back to the staff with their input as well. The staff should be involved in hiring new staff to assure that those people who will be working at the facility are dedicated to its clinical and customer service initiatives.

The staff should also be practicing in an empowered environment, which recognizes that the strength of the organization is through the moments of truth, created by the staff on a daily basis, and not by the owners or managers of the facility alone. Once that type of environment has been created, it begins to build on itself, so that patients, family members, and the urgent care center team begin to work together to define even better ways in which quality of clinical care and excellence in customer service can be combined.

References

1. Mayer T, Cates RJ: Service excellence in healthcare. *JAMA* 282:1281–1283, 1999.
2. Mayer T, Cates RJ, Mastorovich MJ, Royalty D: Emergency department patient satisfaction: customer service training improves patient satisfaction and ratings of physician and nurse skill. *J Health Mgt* 43:427–440, 1998.
3. Cleary PD, Edgman-Levitan S: Healthcare quality: incorporating the patient's perspective. *JAMA* 278:1608–1612, 1997.
4. Mayer TA, Cates RJ, Royalty D: Customer service in triage. *Topics Emerg Med* 19:28–39, 1997.
5. Thompson DA, Yarnold PR, Williams DR, Adams SL: Effects of actual waiting time, perceived waiting time, information delivery, and expressive quality on patient satisfaction in the emergency department. *Ann Emerg Med* 28:657–665, 1996.

6. Walsh DP, Seff LR, Mayer TA: Customer relations in the emergency department, in Salluzzo R, Mayer TA, Strauss R, Kidd P (eds): *Emergency Department Management: Principles and Applications.* St. Louis: Mosby; 1997.

7. Carlzon J: *Moments of Truth: New Strategies for Today's Customer-Driven Economy.* New York: HarperCollins; 1987.

SELECTED READINGS

Fischer R, Ury W, Patton B: *Getting to Yes: Negotiating Agreement Without Giving In.* New York: Penguin Books; 1991.

Shell GR: *Bargaining for Advantage: Negotiation Strategies for Reasonable People.* New York: Viking; 1999.

Marcus LJ: *Renegotiating Healthcare: Resolving Conflict to Build Collaboration.* San Francisco: Jossey-Bass; 1995.

II

CLINICAL PRACTICE

PHYSICAL EXAMINATION

Tanise I. Edwards

PHYSICALS IN THE URGENT CARE SETTING

Many patients present to urgent care centers requesting evaluation for a general physical examination. Patients seeking the services of the urgent care center for a physical are usually meeting the requirements for school entrance, employment, international travel, or sports participation. Patients who do not have a relationship with a primary care physician will often turn to the urgent care physician to meet this need. Additionally, patients who do have a primary physician but who are unable to secure an appointment in a timely fashion may also seek out the services provided in the urgent care setting. Each type of physical has its own specific requirements that must be met in order for the patient to meet the criteria set forth by the company, state, school, etc. In performing a physical, the physician must be aware of these criteria and any special conditions that may exist; a full understanding of the activities in which the patient will be involved is key. This chapter includes an overview of sports, school and camp, Department of Transportation, and preemployment physicals; these are the most commonly seen requests in the urgent care setting. Patients requesting physical examination for foreign travel may have additional requirements. At times these may be beyond the scope of an urgent care facility. In such circumstances, a division of travel medicine in the Department of Public Health may be able to meet these needs as well as to provide any special immunizations. When wilderness or arduous conditions are involved, evaluation must include assessing the patient's ability to meet the conditions of such environments.

- *When patients are requesting a general medical or annual physical, it may be prudent for the patient to be referred to a primary care physician.* A primary care physician will then be capable of treating any ongoing or chronic medical conditions as well as helping to establish a primary care relationship with the patient.

DEPARTMENT OF TRANSPORTATION PHYSICALS

There are over 6 million drivers who operate commercial vehicles involved in interstate commerce,[1] and Department of Transportation (DOT) physicals are designed to evaluate the fitness of these drivers to perform their duties safely. DOT physicals are performed under the regulations and general guidelines set by the Federal Motor Carriers Safety Regulations, which require medical certification for interstate commercial drivers. Unlike most situations in which patients seek medical care and evaluation, the primary obligation of the physician performing the DOT examination is to protect the safety and well-being of the public.[2] While performing a DOT physical, the physician is specifically evaluating the driver for any conditions that may impair his or her ability to safely perform the duties of interstate commercial driving. These duties may include not only the ability to stand up to conditions associated with long-distance driving but also the ability to load and unload cargo upon reaching the desired destination. Strict criteria are outlined and must be met in order for the driver to be certified (Table 6-1). In performing

TABLE 6-1

**FEDERAL MOTOR CARRIER SAFETY REGULATIONS
U.S. DEPARTMENT OF TRANSPORTATION**

**Physical Qualifications for Drivers
Subpart E—Physical Qualifications and Examinations
§392.41 Physical qualifications for drivers.[3]**

(a) A person shall not drive a commercial motor vehicle unless he/she is physically qualified to do so and, except as provided in 391.67, has on his/her person the original, or a photographic copy, of a medical examiner's certificate that he/she is physically qualified to drive a commercial motor vehicle.

(b) A person is physically qualified to drive a commercial motor vehicle if that person–

(b)(1) Has no loss of a foot, a leg, a hand, or an arm, or has been granted a waiver pursuant to 391.49;

(b)(2) Has no impairment of:

(b)(2)(i) A hand or finger which interferes with prehension or power grasping; or

(b)(2)(ii) An arm, foot, or leg which interferes with the ability to perform normal tasks associated with operating a commercial motor vehicle; or any other significant limb defect or limitation which interferes with the ability to perform normal tasks associated with operating a commercial motor vehicle; or has been granted a waiver pursuant to 391.49.

(b)(3) Has no established medical history or clinical diagnosis of diabetes mellitus currently requiring insulin for control;

(b)(4) Has no current clinical diagnosis of myocardial infarction, angina pectoris, coronary insufficiency, thrombosis, or any other cardiovascular disease of a variety known to be accompanied by syncope, dyspnea, collapse, or congestive cardiac failure;

(b)(5) Has no established medical history or clinical diagnosis of a respiratory dysfunction likely to interfere with his/her ability to control and drive a commercial motor vehicle safely;

(b)(6) Has no current clinical diagnosis of high blood pressure likely to interfere with his/her ability to operate a commercial motor vehicle safely;

(b)(7) Has no established medical history or clinical diagnosis of rheumatic, arthritic, orthopedic, muscular, neuromuscular, or vascular disease which interferes with his/her ability to control and operate a commercial motor vehicle safely;

(continues on next page)

TABLE 6-1

FEDERAL MOTOR CARRIER SAFETY REGULATIONS
U.S. DEPARTMENT OF TRANSPORATION

((b)(8) Has no established medical history or clinical diagnosis of epilepsy or any other condition which is likely to cause loss of consciousness or any loss of ability to control a commercial motor vehicle;

b)(9) Has no mental, nervous, organic, or functional disease or psychiatric disorder likely to interfere with his/her ability to drive a commercial motor vehicle safely;

(b)(10) Has distant visual acuity of at least 20/40 (Snellen) in each eye without corrective lenses or visual acuity separately corrected to 20/40 (Snellen) or better with corrective lenses, distant binocular acuity of at least 20/40 (Snellen) in both eyes with or without corrective lenses, field of vision of at least 70° in the horizontal meridian in each eye, and the ability to recognize the colors of traffic signals and devices showing standard red, green, and amber;

(b)(11) First perceives a forced whispered voice in the better ear at not less than 5 feet with or without the use of a hearing aid or, if tested by use of an audiometric device, does not have an average hearing loss in the better ear greater than 40 decibels at 500 Hz, 1,000 Hz, and 2,000 Hz with or without a hearing aid when the audiometric device is calibrated to American National Standard (formally ASA Standard) Z24.5 1951;

(b)(12)(i) Does not use a controlled substance identified in 21 CFR 1308.11 Schedule I, an amphetamine, a narcotic, or any other habit-forming drug;

(b)(12)(ii) Exception. A driver may use such a substance or drug, if the substance or drug is prescribed by a licensed medical practitioner who:

(b)(12)(ii)(A) Is familiar with the driver's medical history and assigned duties; and

(b)(12)(ii)(B) Has advised the driver that the prescribed substance or drug will not adversely affect the driver's ability to safely operate a commercial vehicle; and

(b)(13) Has no current clinical diagnosis of alcoholism.

the DOT examination, the physician should keep in mind that the purpose of the examination is to assess potential medical problems that could "affect the driver's ability to operate a motor vehicle safely,"[2] not to diagnose or treat specific conditions. When medical diagnoses are discovered that require treatment or further assessment, the driver should be given the option of a full evaluation or a referral for further evaluation if appropriate. When a full evaluation is performed, this should be written up separately from the DOT physical. In fact, if the DOT examination is paid for by the employer, any evaluation beyond that required by the DOT examination should be performed as a separate evaluation and a new chart generated with the appropriate billing data.

The DOT examination form is divided into three sections: the health history, the physical examination, and the medical examiner's certificate (Fig. 6-1). Before evaluation begins, it is important that the driver's photo identification be checked to make sure that the person to be examined corresponds with the person listed on the examination and that the examinee holds a valid commercial driver's license (CDL). The driver should also sign a form attesting to the fact that all information provided is accurate.

(text continues on page 61)

Medical Examination Report
FOR COMMERCIAL DRIVER FITNESS DETERMINATION

649-F (6045)

1. DRIVER'S INFORMATION
Driver completes this section.

Driver's Name (Last, First, Middle)						New Certification ☐ Recertification ☐ Follow Up ☐	Date of Exam
Address	Social Security No.		Birthdate M / D / Y	Age	Sex ☐ M ☐ F		
	City, State, Zip Code	Work Tel: ( ) Home Tel: ( )	Driver License No.			License Class ☐ A ☐ C ☐ B ☐ D ☐ Other	State of Issue

2. HEALTH HISTORY
Driver completes this section, but medical examiner is encouraged to discuss with driver.

Yes No
- ☐☐ Any illness or injury in last 5 years?
- ☐☐ Head/Brain injuries, disorders or illnesses
- ☐☐ Seizures, epilepsy
- ☐☐ medication
- ☐☐ Eye disorders or impaired vision (except corrective lenses)
- ☐☐ Ear disorders, loss of hearing or balance
- ☐☐ Heart disease or heart attack; other cardiovascular condition
- ☐☐ medication
- ☐☐ Heart surgery (valve replacement/bypass, angioplasty, pacemaker)
- ☐☐ High blood pressure ☐ medication
- ☐☐ Muscular disease
- ☐☐ Shortness of breath

Yes No
- ☐☐ Lung disease, emphysema, asthma, chronic bronchitis
- ☐☐ Kidney disease, dialysis
- ☐☐ Liver disease
- ☐☐ Digestive problems
- ☐☐ Diabetes or elevated blood sugar controlled by:
  - ☐ diet
  - ☐ pills
  - ☐ insulin
- ☐☐ Nervous or psychiatric disorders, e.g., severe depression
- ☐☐ Loss of, or altered consciousness

Yes No
- ☐☐ Fainting, dizziness
- ☐☐ Sleep disorders, pauses in breathing while asleep, daytime sleepiness, loud snoring
- ☐☐ Stroke or paralysis
- ☐☐ Missing or impaired hand, arm, foot, leg, finger, toe
- ☐☐ Spinal injury or disease
- ☐☐ Chronic low back pain
- ☐☐ Regular, frequent alcohol use
- ☐☐ Narcotic or habit forming drug use

For any YES answer, indicate onset date, diagnosis, treating physician's name and address, and any current limitation. List all medications (including over-the-counter medications) used regularly or recently.

_____

_____

_____

I certify that the above information is complete and true. I understand that inaccurate, false or missing information may invalidate the examination and my Medical Examiner's Certificate.

_____   _____
Driver's Signature   Date

Medical Examiner's Comments on Health History (The medical examiner must review and discuss with the driver any "yes" answers and potential hazards of medications, including over-the-counter medications, while driving.)

_____

_____

_____

_____

FIGURE 6-1   Sample Department of Transportation physical examination form. (© 1994 & published by J.J. Keller & Associates, Inc., Neenah, WI. Used with permission.)

TESTING (Medical Examiner completes Section 3 through 7)

3. VISION

Standard: At least 20/40 acuity (Snellen) in each eye with or without correction. At least 70° peripheral in horizontal meridian measured in each eye. The use of corrective lenses should be noted on the Medical Examiner's Certificate.

INSTRUCTIONS: *When other than the Snellen chart is used, give test results in Snellen-comparable values. In recording distance vision, use 20 feet as normal. Report visual acuity as a ratio with 20 as numerator and the smallest type read at 20 feet as denominator. If the applicant wears corrective lenses, these should be worn while visual acuity is being tested. If the driver habitually wears contact lenses, or intends to do so while driving, sufficient evidence of good tolerance and adaptation to their use must be obvious. Monocular drivers are not qualified.*

Numerical readings must be provided.

ACUITY	UNCORRECTED	CORRECTED	HORIZONTAL FIELD OF VISION
Right Eye	20/	20/	Right Eye °
Left Eye	20/	20/	Left Eye °
Both Eyes	20/	20/	

Complete next line only if vision testing is done by an ophthalmologist or optometrist

Applicant can recognize and distinguish among traffic control signals and devices showing standard red, green and amber colors? ☐ Yes ☐ No

Applicant meets visual acuity requirement only when wearing:
☐ Corrective Lenses

Monocular Vision: ☐ Yes ☐ No

Date of Examination _____ Name of Ophthalmologist or Optometrist (print) _____ Tel. No. _____ License No./State of Issue _____ Signature _____

4. HEARING

Standard: a) Must first perceive forced whispered voice ≥ 5 ft., with or without hearing aid, or b) average hearing loss in better ear ≤ 40 dB

☐ Check if hearing aid used for tests. ☐ Check if hearing aid required to meet standard.

INSTRUCTIONS: *To convert audiometric test results from ISO to ANSI, -14 dB from ISO for 500 Hz, -10 dB for 1,000 Hz, -8.5 dB for 2,000 Hz. To average, add the readings for 3 frequencies tested and divide by 3.*

Numerical readings must be recorded.

		Right Ear			Left Ear		
a) Record distance from individual at which forced whispered voice can first be heard.	Right Ear Feet	Left Ear Feet					
b) If audiometer is used, record hearing loss in decibels. (acc. to ANSI Z24.5-1951)		500 Hz	1000 Hz	2000 Hz	500 Hz	1000 Hz	2000 Hz
		Average:			Average:		

5. BLOOD PRESSURE / PULSE RATE

Numerical readings must be recorded.

Blood Pressure	Systolic	Diastolic
Driver qualified if ≤ 160/90 on initial exam.		

Pulse Rate	☐ Regular
	☐ Irregular

GUIDELINES FOR BLOOD PRESSURE EVALUATION

On initial exam	Within 3 months	Certify
If 161-180 and/or 91-104, qualify 3 mos. only.	If ≤ 160 and/or 90, qualify for 1 yr. Document Rx & control the 3rd month. _____,	Annually if acceptable BP is maintained
If > 180 and/or 104, not qualified until reduced to < 181/105. Then qualify for 3 mos. only.	If ≤ 160 and/or 90, qualify for 6 mos. Document Rx & control the 3rd month. _____,	Biannually

Medical examiner should take at least 2 readings to confirm blood pressure.

6. LABORATORY AND OTHER TEST FINDINGS

Numerical readings must be recorded.

Urinalysis is required. Protein, blood or sugar in the urine may be an indication for further testing to rule out any underlying medical problem.
Other Testing *(Describe 'and record)*

URINE SPECIMEN	SP. GR.	PROTEIN	BLOOD	SUGAR

FIGURE 6-1 (*continued*)

7. PHYSICAL EXAMINATION

Height: _____ (in.)   Weight: _____ (lbs.)

The presence of a certain condition may not necessarily disqualify a driver, particularly if the condition is controlled adequately, is not likely to worsen or is readily amenable to treatment. Even if a condition does not disqualify a driver, the medical examiner may consider deferring the driver temporarily. Also, the driver should be advised to take the necessary steps to correct the condition as soon as possible particularly if the condition, if neglected, could result in more serious illness that might affect driving.

Check YES if there are any abnormalities. Check NO if the body system is normal. Discuss any YES answers in detail in the space below, and indicate whether it would affect the driver's ability to operate a commercial motor vehicle safely. Enter applicable item number before each comment. If organic disease is present, note that it has been compensated for.

See Instructions to the Medical Examiner for guidance.

BODY SYSTEM	CHECK FOR:	YES*	NO
1. General Appearance	Marked overweight, tremor, signs of alcoholism, problem drinking, or drug abuse.		
2. Eyes	Pupillary equality, reaction to light, accommodation, ocular motility, ocular muscle imbalance, extraocular movement, nystagmus, exophthalmos, strabismus uncorrected by corrective lenses, retinopathy, cataracts, aphakia, glaucoma, macular degeneration.		
3. Ears	Middle ear disease, occlusion of external canal, perforated eardrums.		
4. Mouth and Throat	Irremediable deformities likely to interfere with breathing or swallowing.		
5. Heart	Murmurs, extra sounds, enlarged heart, pacemaker.		
6. Lungs and chest, not including breast examination.	Abnormal chest wall expansion, abnormal respiratory rate, abnormal breath sounds including wheezes or alveolar rales, impaired respiratory function, dyspnea, cyanosis. Abnormal findings on physical exam may require further testing such as pulmonary tests and/or xray of chest.		

BODY SYSTEM	CHECK FOR:	YES*	NO
7. Abdomen and Viscera	Enlarged liver, enlarged spleen, masses, bruits, hernia, significant abdominal wall muscle weakness.		
8. Vascular System	Abnormal pulse and amplitude, carotid or arterial bruits, varicose veins.		
9. Genito-urinary System	Hernias.		
10. Extremities - Limb impaired. Driver may be subject to SPE certificate if otherwise qualified.	Loss or impairment of leg, foot, toe, arm, hand, finger. Perceptible limp, deformities, atrophy, weakness, paralysis, clubbing, edema, hypotonia. Insufficient grasp and prehension in upper limb to maintain steering wheel grip. Insufficient mobility and strength in lower limb to operate pedals properly.		
11. Spine, other musculoskeletal	Previous surgery, deformities, limitation of motion, tenderness.		
12. Neurological	Impaired equilibrium, coordination or speech pattern; paresthesia, asymmetric deep tendon reflexes, sensory or positional abnormalities, abnormal patellar and Babinski's reflexes, ataxia.		

*COMMENTS: _____

_____

_____

Note certification status here. See Instructions to the Medical Examiner for guidance.

☐ Meets standards in 49 CFR 391.41; qualifies for 2 year certificate

☐ Does not meet standards

☐ Meets standards, but periodic evaluation required

Due to _____ driver qualified only for:

☐ 3 months   ☐ 1 year
☐ 6 months   ☐ Other

☐ Temporarily disqualified due to (condition or medication): _____

Return to medical examiner's office for follow up on _____

☐ Wearing corrective lenses

☐ Wearing hearing aid

☐ Accompanied by a _____ waiver/exemption

☐ Skill Performance Evaluation (SPE) Certificate

☐ Driving within an exempt intracity zone

☐ Qualified by operation of 49 CFR 391.64

Medical Examiner's Signature _____

Medical Examiner's Name (print) _____

Address _____

Telephone Number _____

If meets standards, complete a Medical Examiner's Certificate according to 49 CFR 391.43(h). (Driver must carry certificate when operating a commercial vehicle.)

FIGURE 6-1 *(continued)*

Health History and Initial Screening

The health history section should be completed prior to examination of the patient. It has been found, however, that up to 10 to 15 percent of drivers do not give an accurate health history.[2] The health history section, therefore, must be reviewed with the driver prior to completing the evaluation. A review of the health history will help to clarify the conditions listed as well as any positive responses. Often statements that are initially reported as negative by the driver will be positive upon review. At times, the manner in which questions are asked may shed better light on a driver's health history and uncover conditions not originally listed. Additionally, the driver should be questioned regarding any medications that are taken (either over the counter or prescribed). A medication history may often provide valuable information on the driver's health; the use of all medications should be documented on the patient's chart.

On the initial examination, which can be performed by support staff prior to the physician's evaluation, the history should be reviewed (as outlined above). Vital signs (including height, weight, blood pressure, and a pre- and postexercise pulse), a visual check (including both acuity and color vision), and a hearing assessment should all be performed. Vision testing must include testing of visual acuity, distant binocular acuity, visual fields, and color testing for standard red, green, and amber. Hearing can be checked either by a forced whisper test or with an audiometer. If a forced whisper is used, the driver should be capable of perceiving a forced whisper in the better ear at "not less than 5 feet with or without the use of a hearing aid."[3] Audiometer evaluation, when available, may be more accurate, especially in those circumstances when an abnormal or ambiguous result is noted on forced whisper. Urine can also be collected at this time, as well as urine for drug screening if required. This initial evaluation can often reveal limiting conditions that obviate the need for further evaluation by the physician in the urgent care setting either due to conditions that would prompt an automatic failure of certification or secondary to conditions that will need further primary care evaluation before certification. Protocols should be set up by the urgent care center to handle cases in which failure is evident at this junction of the examination. Many patients may choose to abort further evaluation if failure is evident, especially if further evaluation would otherwise be needed. Others may decide to have the evaluation completed, particularly if they will pursue a waiver for the disqualifying condition.

 Physical Examination

The first step in the physical examination should be review of the health history and all data collected on the initial screening. This approach will allow additional focus on any information of concern that may require a more in-depth evaluation. During the physical examination, it is important to keep in mind that the evaluation is specifically targeted toward any aspects, physical, mental, or organic, that can influence safe operation of a commercial vehicle.[3]

General Appearance and Development

Evaluation should note any evidence of gross abnormalities, including body habitus and posture, and any stigmata of general medical conditions such as alcoholism, intravenous drug use, anorexia, anemia, thyrotoxicosis, etc. Any localized or generalized adenopathy should also be noted.

Vision

In addition to visual acuity and color vision, the examination should include evaluation for evidence of visual field deficits, monocular vision, diplopia, ptosis, use of a prosthesis, end-organ damage, and other abnormalities that may interfere with a driver's vision. Conjunctiva should be checked for evidence of anemia. If corrective lens are needed (including use of contact lenses), certification must include checking the statement, "Qualified only when wearing corrective lenses."

Hearing

In addition to hearing, the ears should be checked for evidence of middle- or inner-ear disease and peripheral vertigo. If a hearing aid is needed to meet DOT requirements, certification must include checking the statement, "Qualified only when wearing a hearing aid."

Throat

Evaluation should note any evidence of abnormalities that may produce difficulty with swallowing or breathing.

Thorax

Examination should include evaluation for evidence of murmurs, dysrhythmias, cardiovascular disease, particularly congestive heart failure (CHF), cardiomyopathy or hypertrophic cardiomyopathy, which could predispose to syncope, dyspnea, dysrhythmias, infarction, or cardiac failure. Lungs should be evaluated for evidence of pulmonary disease, including chronic obstructive pulmonary disease (COPD), chronic asthma, tuberculosis (TB), or pulmonary fibrosis, which could interfere with the physical demands of commercial driving.

Abdominal/Gastrointestinal

Examination should include evaluation for evidence of tenderness, scars, injury, hernia, and masses, which, if present, may warrant further evaluation prior to certification.

Genitourinary

Examination should include evaluation for evidence of inguinal hernias and a urinalysis.

Neurologic

Examination should include evaluation of reflexes, motor strength, gait, and any tremors that may be present. Pupils should be checked for pupillary reflexes, both to light and accommodation. A Romberg's test must also be done, with positive or negative results documented.

Extremities

Any amputations, deformities, impairments, weakness, or atrophy should be noted. Examination should include evaluation of the ability to grasp objects and to perform the plantarflexion and dorsiflexion required to operate the pedals of a vehicle. Range of motion should be checked, particularly in the shoulder, elbows, and wrists.

Spine
Examination should evaluate range of motion as well as evidence of disk herniation, sciatica, or previous spinal surgery. Neck evaluation for range of motion should also be included during this part of the examination.

Certification

Certification can be for a standard 2-year period if all criteria are successfully met. Certain diagnoses, however, prompt automatic failure of certification (see Table 6-1), while other conditions may require special waivers or specialty clearance in order for the driver to pass medical certification. In the urgent care setting, most conditions that require further evaluation or a waiver in order to meet qualification for certification should be referred to the patient's primary care physician. Depending on the reasons for further evaluation, drivers may be qualified for a period of time that is less than 2 years. This may allow temporary qualification while awaiting further evaluation by a primary physician. An example of such a situation would be a driver requiring follow-up for borderline blood pressure elevation; in this case, a 3-month certification could be given while starting medication and assessing response.

Waivers

Waivers allow certification of drivers when criteria for certification routinely would not be met. Waivers require application to the Federal Highway Association by the driver and are best left to the driver's primary care physician or specialist.

Further information on DOT physicals can be obtained from The U.S. Department of Transportation Federal Highway Administration or via The Federal Motor Carrier Safety Administration Web site at http://www.fmcsa.dot.gov/rulesregs/fmcsr/medical.htm. Any physician who performs DOT physicals must be fully versed in the requirements for certification. When a driver is disqualified, appropriate documentation of specific objective medical evidence should be included in the patient's record. Accurate documentation is key should there be legal questions regarding either certification or the criteria used for failure to certify. A full copy of the DOT form should also be kept on record at the urgent care center along with any additional patient information. Under all circumstances, however, medical records must be kept confidential unless the appropriate release has been signed.

PREPLACEMENT EMPLOYMENT EVALUATIONS

In addition to DOT physicals, adult patients often seek physical examination in the urgent care setting for reasons of employment. In some cases, businesses may contract with the urgent care center to provide preplacement evaluation for their employees; in the majority of cases, however, individuals present independently for evaluation as a condition of their employment. It is important for both the examiner and the patient to realize that the preplacement evaluation differs from the recommended preventive health physical or a patient's "annual" physical. The express purpose of this examination is to evaluate the suitability of a potential employee for the specific duties of the position for which the exam is performed. (Thus, the type of evaluation that is an integral part of an annual physical may be conspicuously absent from these examinations.) Preplacement examinations, in addition to assessing physical suitability, can also supply a baseline for various conditions that may require future monitoring secondary to exposures or hazards of a given occupation; it may also identify preexisting medical conditions that may have an accelerated course or be made worse by duties of the workplace. This identification can then allow for recommendations for accommodations that alleviate aggravating factors. In order to properly assess the suitability for employment, the examining physician must be fully knowledgeable on the particular duties and requirements of the position for which the applicant will be responsible, and the examination performed must take into account all of the requirements of the job.

In conducting a preplacement evaluation, much like a DOT physical, the physician-patient relationship is not automatic. This is particularly true when the employer retains the physician for the evaluation. In addition to an understanding of whether a physician-patient relationship is present, it is also important for physicians performing preplacement evaluations to be acutely aware of the parameters set forth by the Americans with Disabilities Act (ADA). Decisions regarding fitness for the position must be made based on the applicant's ability to perform the essential duties of the position without personal risk or risk to others; evaluation must also take into account whether "reasonable accommodations" can be made if needed. It should be noted that the ADA does not allow for inquiry into a person's medical history, impairments, or previous injuries *prior* to the job offer; in order to avoid such a situation, particularly if the place of employment has retained the physician, it is best for the urgent care center to perform these evaluations *only* after a job offer has been made to the applicant but preceding the commencement of employment.

Prior to evaluation, the applicant should sign a release that allows the physician to discuss any relevant findings of the evaluation with the future employer; this is particularly important when an applicant independently seeks an evaluation. However, in discussing the evaluation with the employer, medical conditions that are not relevant to employment should not be included. As medical confidentiality is still required, there must be a specific person to whom the results of evaluation can be forwarded or with whom they can be discussed. When the place of employment retains the physician, the name of this contact person should be made known, along with a detailed description of the duties of the position being offered. When an individual requests the evaluation, he or she must provide not only a written description of the responsibilities of the position (of which a copy should be kept in the patient's chart), but also the name of the specific individual to whom the results of the evaluation are to be sent.

Physical Examination

The type of physical examination conducted will reflect the requirements for the position sought; thus not all preplacement evaluations will be the same. If manual labor is required, for instance, a detailed musculoskeletal examination with special attention to the back may be required. Similarly, evidence of cardiac disease may be important, depending on the contractual obligations of the position. Some preplacement evaluations may require an electrocardiographic (ECG) evaluation, chest x-ray evaluation (particularly as a baseline), tuberculosis testing, or pulmonary function testing. Other physical examinations may require evaluation of an applicant's mental status. What is required for a satisfactory evaluation, therefore, must be known prior to beginning the examination. Under certain circumstances, preplacement physicals, such as Federal Aeronautics Administration (FAA) physicals or physicals for positions that require the use of a respirator, have specific certification requirements that are beyond the capability of an urgent care center; these evaluations are best left to occupational health physicians.

Regardless of the specific criteria that must be met during the evaluation, it is very important to be aware that *all* physicals performed for the same position within a company must entail the *same* evaluation and meet the *same* requirements for all applicants.

School physics

As with other physicals that may be requested, parents often seek school physicals in the urgent care setting because of its convenience, lack of a physician relationship, or time constraints that limit the parents' ability to schedule a physical with their primary physician. These physicals are generally required prior to a child's first attendance in the school system. Some schools require that an annual physical be on record prior to admission each school year. The purpose of the school physical is twofold. First, it is a means by which medical conditions that may pose problems for the child in the school setting can be identified, thereby allowing the parents to seek appropriate help or accommodations (i.e., vision impairment, deafness, etc.). Second, the school physical provides verification that immunization requirements have been met and that certain communicable diseases, such as tuberculosis, which may put a school population at risk, are not present. As such, there must be adequate documentation or verification of the child's immunization history prior to the completion and signing off of this section of the examination form.

Most public school districts as well as most private schools have specific physical examination forms. These forms generally require the following of the examining physician: verification of the immunization history or exemption reasons (medical or religious), height, weight, head circumference (if applicable by age of child), vision testing, hearing testing, and blood pressure level. Date of tuberculin testing, with the results, may be requested, as well as hemoglobin or hematocrit and results of a urinalysis for sugar and protein. In addition to the standard general pediatric examination, an assessment of the child's behavioral state and estimated development level may often be requested. Parents or guardians are generally asked to provide information regarding the child's past medical history, ongoing or chronic medical conditions, allergies (medication, food, insects, etc.), as well as any medications or medical devices (i.e., prostheses, glasses, etc.) that the child uses. It is important to review the information provided as well as to obtain a complete review of systems (including developmental and behavioral history) prior to conducting the physical examination. A complete physical should then be performed, looking particularly for any undiagnosed conditions or areas of concern that would affect the school environment or the child's ability to learn. All abnormalities should be discussed with the guardian and appropriate referral made.

SUMMER CAMP PHYSICALS

Summer camp physicals often combine the requirements set forth in the school physical and the preparticipation sports physical. Depending on the nature of the camp, more specific requirements may have to be met. The specific activities in which the child will be involved should be discussed and documented in the chart prior to giving medical clearance.

SPORTS PHYSICALS

Students commonly present to the urgent care setting requesting preparticipation physicals as required by their school or sports team. As previously mentioned, many athletes present either because of convenience, unavailability of their primary care physician (PCP), or lack of an established relationship with a PCP. For many players, this evaluation may be the only preventive health care that they receive. Unfortunately, the preparticipation physical examination is not the same as a comprehensive physical examination and is not meant to be a replacement for either regular health maintenance or the preventive education that accompanies a "traditional" physical. The intent of the sports physical is to evaluate the athlete for safe participation in the selected activity. The examination is designed to screen for life-threatening conditions (there are up to 1 in 200,000 sudden cardiac deaths each year among high school athletes),[4] for conditions that may put an athlete at risk for injury, and for conditions that may require modification or limitation of participation. The preparticipation examination should also evaluate an athlete's level of fitness, need for rehabilitation of previous injury, and any requirement for special protective sports gear, such as protective eyewear. Unfortunately, any disqualification or even limitation on an athlete's participation may often put the examiner at direct odds with the athlete, the coach, and the parents. The focus of the examination, however, must always remain on safe participation.

Causes of Sudden Death in the Younger Athlete

- Hypertrophic cardiomyopathy (found in up to one-third of cases of sudden death)
- Unsuspected congenital cardiovascular disease (congenital artery anomalies such as anomalous origin of the left main coronary artery)
- Myocarditis
- Aortic stenosis
- Dilated cardiomyopathy
- Long-QT syndrome
- Arrhythmogenic right ventricular dysplasia
- Cardiac arrest secondary to blunt trauma to the chest from high-velocity projectiles such as baseballs or soccer balls

The Older Athlete

In contrast with younger athletes, the older athlete must be more closely evaluated for ischemic and atherosclerotic disease, including risk factors for coronary artery disease

(CAD). Other causes of sudden death in the older athlete include cerebral aneurysms and bronchial asthma, both of which should be screened for during the examination.

Health History

Athletes typically present with the form that requires completion for participation. Many forms are of limited value in that they request little information that can reasonably clear a player for participation. There is marked variability between forms and many forms are wholly inadequate for clearance for participation. It is therefore incumbent upon the examining physician to evaluate and document an examination based on appropriate medical criteria. A comprehensive history is the initial component of the examination, and a detailed history may reveal important information that could potentially limit safe participation for an athlete. Therefore, in addition to obtaining a general health history, questions should be asked that are specifically geared to evaluating risk factors for participation. Each athlete should be questioned regarding any history of the following:

- Chest pain
- Heart murmurs
- Syncope or near syncope
- Palpitations
- Dyspnea
- Hypertension
- Medication use
- Alcohol use/illicit drug use/cigarette or cigar use
- Allergies
- Limitation of activity or exertion by shortness of breath or fatigue that is extreme, unexpected, or inexplicable
- Asthma, either intrinsic or exercise-induced
- Last normal menstrual period (in the female athlete)
- Hospitalizations and surgeries (including retinal surgery)
- Previous limited sports participation
- Ongoing illness
- Illnesses of more than 1 week's duration (such as infectious mononucleosis)
- Use of appliances (glasses, braces, hearing aids, contact lens)
- Previous head trauma
- Coagulopathy
- Frequent or recurrent musculoskeletal injuries
- Previous fractures (including stress fractures), sprains, joint laxity, dislocations (including dates)
- Last tetanus shot

The family history should also be checked, noting any history of death at an early age due to cardiac pathology, hypertrophic or dilated cardiomyopathy, long-QT syndrome, Marfan's disease, or significant arrhythmias.

If the athlete's form does not include a detailed section on health history, the urgent care center should have a checklist form that the examining physician can use to help eliminate any potential for missed information. On most preparticipation forms, the health history section requests that the parent complete the section prior to examination. It is imperative that the form be completed by a parent and not a minor student in order to avoid obtaining a limited or inaccurate history. It is also imperative that the examining physician review the history with a parent. Many statements that are initially checked off as negative on the form will often come to light as suggesting a significant problem during direct questioning. To this end, questions should be asked in such a manner as to be understood by the athlete and the parent (i.e., do not ask the athlete if he or she has ever experienced dyspnea; rather, ask about any episodes of shortness of breath). When athletes present to an urgent care center unaccompanied by a parent, the physician may have to review the health history with the parent via phone.

 ## Physical Examination

The physical evaluation on a sports examination should focus on those areas that may be indicative of undiagnosed cardiac disease or predisposing conditions that may call for limited participation.

Vital Signs

Vital signs should be checked and documented, including a resting pulse, an immediate post-exercise pulse, and a 1-min post-exercise pulse. The nurse can have the athlete jog in place for 2 min to determine the exercise pulse rates. Hearing, visual acuity, height, and weight should also be checked as part of the baseline vital signs.

General Appearance

The participant's overall appearance should be noted, including evidence of the stigmata of Marfan's syndrome, anorexia, obesity, or congenital abnormalities.

- Anorexia may be found in athletes of either sex and in any sport, but it has been noted particularly in wrestling, gymnastics, diving, and cross-country running.[5]

Specific Organ Systems

Each organ system should then be evaluated for abnormalities, with special attention to the cardiovascular and musculoskeletal examination.

Eyes: Proper symmetry of the pupils is checked (this is very important if anisocoria is noted, for future reference if a head injury should occur); the examiner also checks for full range of extraocular motion, intact visual fields, and intact peripheral vision. Any need for corrective lenses or protective eyewear is noted.

Ears: Any tympanic membrane abnormalities or ruptures and any evidence of otitis externa or cauliflower ear are noted.

Nares: Septal deviation or deformity is noted (septal erosions may be a sign of cocaine abuse, which, among other concerns, could predispose to arrhythmias).

Oral Pharynx: Use of appliances or braces is noted, also the presence of any missing, avulsed, or fractured teeth.

Cardiac: The presence or absence of any murmur is noted and documented; if a murmur is present, the examiner should note the effect of position changes (supine, sitting, leaning forward, squatting) and the Valsalva maneuver on the murmur; the quality and symmetry of distal pulses in both the upper and lower extremities is checked; resting heart rate is checked for bradycardia or tachycardia; and the presence of any arrhythmias (including sinus arrhythmia or bradycardia) is documented.

Pulmonary: The applicant is checked for asymmetry, excursion, and the presence of abnormal lung findings on auscultation, particularly the presence of bronchospasm.

Abdomen: Any scars, bruits, organomegaly, or masses are noted as well as any tenderness to palpation.

- Hernias may require strict limitations of activity or suspension of activity until repair.

Genitalia: Male athletes are examined for bilaterally descended testes, masses, and hernias; female athletes generally do not require a pelvic examination unless specifically stated or directed by concerns elicited on history or physical examination. Ideally, a urinalysis should be obtained for evaluation of hidden renal disease noted by significant proteinuria or hematuria.

Adenopathy: Any evidence of localized or general adenopathy is noted.

Skin: The examiner evaluates for bruising (particularly evidence of easy bruising indicative of a coagulopathy), lesions, and impetigo.

Back and Neck: Range of motion and flexibility are evaluated as well as tenderness to palpation or tenderness on range of motion. Any scoliosis or abnormal curvature should also be noted.

Musculoskeletal: All extremities should be checked for symmetry, deformities, muscular atrophy, and strength; all joints should be checked for full range of motion; reflexes should be checked as well as gait, balance, and Romberg testing.

Medical Clearance

Clearance for sports participation may include clearance for full participation, limited participation, limited participation pending further evaluation, or failed medical clearance. Any significant cardiac symptoms on history or any cardiac abnormalities—including arrhythmias, new murmurs, or changes in previously diagnosed murmurs—must be further evaluated, generally with a referral to a PCP or a cardiologist. Other, noncardiac conditions or abnormalities may also require further evaluation by the athlete's PCP or the appropriate specialist. For instance, a history of recent mononucleosis may preclude participation in contact sports (see Table 6-2, "Contact and Limited Contact Sports"), as

TABLE 6-2

CONTACT AND LIMITED CONTACT SPORTS[a]

Baseball	Handball	Skiing
Basketball	Hockey	Soccer
Boxing	Horseback riding	Softball
Canoeing	Lacrosse	Squash
Cheerleading	Martial arts	Surfing
Diving	Racquetball	Volleyball
Football	Rugby	Wrestling
Gymnastics	Skating	

[a]This list has been modified from the Committee on Sports Medicine and Fitness, American Academy of Pediatrics: Medical conditions affecting sports participation. *Pediatrics* 4:757, 1994. It is not meant to be inclusive of all contact or limited contact sports.

would a history of recent or multiple episodes of head trauma. Patients with symptoms of exercise-induced asthma or hypertension without previous evaluation may also benefit from limited participation until further evaluation is undertaken. Similarly, many orthopedic injuries may require rehabilitation before clearance for full participation. For some athletes, full clearance for participation may be based on the provision that certain conditions are met, such as "full clearance only with the use of corrective lenses," or "full clearance with use of inhaler prior to participation." Under no circumstances, however, should an athlete ever be cleared for participation if there is any doubt or concern regarding the athlete's ability to participate in the given activity safely.

REFERENCES

1. Pommerenke F: DOT examinations: practical aspects and regulatory review. *Am Fam Physician* 58(2): August, 1998, pp. 415–426.
2. Hartenbaum NP: The DOT Medical Examination: a guide to commercial driver's medical certification. Beverly, MA: OEM Health Information, 1997.
3. Federal Motor Carrier Safety Regulations, 49 CFR, Part 391.41–49; Subpart E—Physical Qualifications and Examination. U.S. Department of Transportation, 1997.
4. Maron BJ: Cardiovascular risks to young persons on the athletic field. *Ann Intern Medicine* 129:379–386, 1998.
5. Rice SG: Preparticipation physical examinations: giving an athlete the go-ahead to play. *Consultant* 34(8): August, 1994, pp. 1129(9).

BIBLIOGRAPHY

Committee on Sports Medicine and Fitness, American Academy of Pediatrics: Medical conditions affecting sports participation. *Pediatrics* 4:757–758, 1994.

Federal Motor Carrier Safety Regulations, 49 CFR, Part 391.41–49; Subpart E—Physical Qualifications and Examination. U.S. Department of Transportation, 1997.

Glover DW, Maron BJ: Profile of preparticipation cardiovascular screening for high school athletes. *JAMA* 10:1829–1830, 1998.

Hartenbaum NP: The DOT Medical Examination: a guide to commercial driver's medical certification. Beverly, MA: OEM Health Information, 1997.

Maron BJ et al: Cardiovascular preparticipation screening of competitive athletes. *Circulation* 94(4):850–856, 1996.

Maron BJ: Cardiovascular risks to young persons on the athletic field. *Ann Intern Med* 129: 379–386, 1998.

McCunney RJ: *A Practical Approach to Occupational and Environmental Medicine.* Boston: Little, Brown; 1988.

Pommerenke F et al: DOT examinations: practical aspects and regulatory review. *Am Fam Physician* 58(2): August, 1998, pp. 415–426.

Rice SG: Preparticipation physical examinations: giving an athlete the go-ahead to play. *Consultant* 34(8): August, 1994, pp. 1129(9).

Rom WN: *Environmental and Occupational Medicine,* 3rd ed. Philadelphia: Lippincott-Raven; 1998.

Rosenstock L: *Clinical Occupational Medicine.* Philadelphia: Saunders; 1986.

7

NONTRAUMATIC AND TRAUMATIC EYE DISORDERS

Thom A. Mayer / Bill Bosley

INTRODUCTION

Ocular complaints are a frequent cause of visits to the urgent care center (UCC) and all physicians staffing such centers should be proficient in the evaluation and management of patients with both traumatic and nontraumatic ophthalmologic problems. The majority of eye disorders presenting to UCCs are due to mild, largely self-limited diseases such as conjunctivitis, corneal abrasions, hordeola, and inflamed chalazia. Nonetheless, complaints involving the eye are extremely frightening to patients, often cause a great deal of pain, and in fact comprise a group of patients who may present with ophthalmologic problems requiring urgent therapy, intervention, and referral. For all of these reasons, it is extremely important that UCC physicians not only be comfortable with the examination of the eye but also have a ready reference available to assist them in evaluating and managing such patients. This chapter is written expressly for that purpose.

Because people are extremely sensitive about their eyes and the potential loss or limitation of sight, UCC physicians must be prepared to carefully evaluate and manage such patients as well as be prepared to spend significant time explaining the diagnosis and treatment to the patient. In addition, all UCCs should have clear lines of referral to ophthalmologists and area emergency departments (EDs) to make sure that patients can be appropriately referred and seen in follow-up in a timely fashion. The management of the UCC should make sure that there is adequate equipment for evaluation and treatment of the eye and that referral sources with ophthalmologists are prospectively determined and carefully cultivated.

Clinical Assessment and Initial Stabilization

Patients with ophthalmologic complaints fall into three broad categories:

1. Pain, discomfort, or foreign-body sensation
2. Visual disturbances
3. Abnormal appearance of the eye or its surrounding structures

Simply stated, these patients' complaints can be summarized as follows:

- Feels funny—pain or discomfort
- Sees funny—change or loss of vision
- Looks funny—abnormal appearance

With any of the three types of symptoms, a careful history should determine whether the symptoms are acute, subacute, or chronic; whether there is an association with nonocular complaints or chronic medical problems; and whether the complaint is resolving, static, or progressive. Additional history should include current and past medications, surgical treatment, past ophthalmologic disorders, and systemic diseases (including diabetes, hyperthyroidism, collagen vascular disease, and HIV infection). A history of possible exposure to toxins such as salicylates, quinine, and methanol should also be obtained.

Feels Funny

Many patients complain of eye pain; in such cases the quality of the pain should be delineated and carefully documented in the chart. Itching or burning of the eye often indicates conjunctival disease, while foreign-body sensation suggests involvement of the cornea or conjunctiva. A chief complaint of pain usually indicates a problem in the anterior segment of the eye, particularly when burning pain or itching is described. Sharp, unremitting pain results from a corneal or conjunctival foreign body or from a corneal epithelial defect such as an abrasion or ulcer. Photophobia is common in corneal disease, iritis, uveitis, temporal arteritis, or scleritis. Pain associated with decreased vision, nausea, and vomiting often signals acute angle-closure glaucoma.

Sees Funny

Acute vision loss or visual disturbances ("sees funny") should be characterized as monocular or binocular, transient or persistent, and should be correlated with any additional findings on the physical examination. Figure 7-1 describes an algorithm for evaluation of patients with vision loss. *Transient monocular* vision loss may be due to amaurosis fugax or ophthalmic migraine. *Persistent monocular* vision loss is more common and may be due to central retinal artery occlusion, central retinal vein occlusion, vitreous hemorrhage, vitreous detachment, retinal tears or detachments, optic neuritis, or, more rarely, ischemic neuropathy or HIV retinopathy. *Transient binocular* vision loss may be caused by papilledema, migraines, or transient ischemic attacks. *Persistent binocular* vision loss may be caused by cortical blindness, functional blindness, toxic optic neuropathy, or chiasmal disease.

Visual disturbances not involving complete vision loss can also be characterized carefully by history. Sudden, persistent unilateral changes can be caused by angle-closure glaucoma, iritis, vitreous hemorrhage, temporal retinal artery or vein occlusion, optic neuritis, or retinal detachment. Gradual, persistent, unilateral changes can be caused by corneal opacities, glaucoma, cataracts, retinal detachment, macular degeneration, or intraocular inflammation. Visual disturbances lasting from a few seconds to

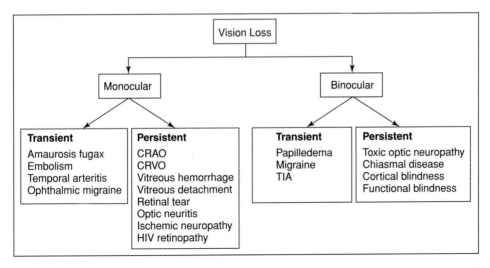

FIGURE 7-1   Algorithm for evaluation of vision loss. CRAO = central retinal artery occlusion; CRVO = central retinal vein occlusion; HIV = human immunodeficiency virus; TIA = transient ischemic attack.

minutes suggest emboli from a cardiac valve or a carotid artery plaque. All such complaints warrant immediate ophthalmologic consultation. Temporary visual changes followed by a headache may represent the aura of a migraine. Ophthalmologic migraine is a temporary visual change in the absence of valvular, carotid, or cerebral vascular disease, with no subsequent headache. Sudden loss of vision in both eyes is uncommon and suggests cortical or functional blindness.

Floaters are a form of visual disturbance that can be seen by the patient only when the eyes are open. Specks of various shapes and sizes, "spiderwebs," or "bug"-shaped lesions are commonly described by patients. Floaters are usually observed when the patient looks at a back-lit area such as the sky, a blank wall, or reading matter. They may represent harmless aging changes but can also herald vitreous hemorrhage associated with retinal tears or diabetic retinopathy. Such patients must be referred to an ophthalmologist within 24 to 48 h.

Photopsias are visual perceptions (specks, rings, lightning flashes, etc.) that occur in the absence of light stimuli and can be seen only with the eyes closed. When these are associated with a sudden shower of floaters, a retinal tear is the most likely cause. Photopsias also occur when the vitreous strikes the retina in a posterior vitreous detachment (PVD). This is more common with patients who are nearsighted or have had a cataract extraction. There is no specific treatment for PVD, but the initial presentation warrants referral to the ophthalmologist for a dilated eye examination.

Looks Funny

The most common abnormal appearance to the eye is redness. A red eye may be caused by anything from a simple subconjunctival hemorrhage to iritis, acute angle-closure glaucoma, corneal ulcer, foreign bodies, or abrasions. Injection of the eye accompanied by an associated purulent discharge implies bacterial or chlamydial disease. Swelling and erythema of the soft tissues without history of trauma or chemical splash suggests cellulitis or allergic phenomena, particularly when accompanied by chemosis, or swelling of the conjunctiva. Other abnormal appearances of the eye include pupillary irregularities or abnormal extraocular muscle problems.

ANATOMY, PHYSICAL EXAMINATION, AND PATIENT MANAGEMENT

This section details pertinent anatomy of the eye, appropriate physical examination, and appropriate treatment. The visual system, the eyebrows and eyelids, and the accessory structures of the eye include the globe, the optic nerve and its pathways to the occipital cortex, parasympathetic reflex pathways for pupillary constriction (miosis), sympathetic pathways for pupillary dilatation (mydriasis), midbrain and pontine nuclei, and pathways for control of conjugate eye movement. In addition, the bony orbit encases the globe as well as the structures passing through it, which include the six extraocular muscles, periorbital fat, blood vessels, lympathics, nerves, and the lacrimal gland (Fig. 7-2).

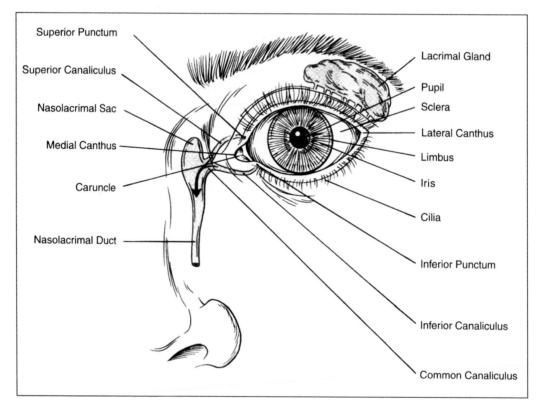

FIGURE 7-2   Anatomic diagram of the eye and adnexa. (From Tintinalli JE et al: *Emergency Medicine: A Comprehensive Study Guide,* 5th ed. New York: McGraw-Hill; 2000. With permission.)

General Principles of the Eye Examination

When a medical patient presents with a complaint, the first clinical information obtained is a set of vital signs. Likewise, the first objective data obtained from the eye patient is the visual acuity (VA). For medicolegal purposes, VA should be obtained and documented on the chart before any eye drops are instilled. This may not always be possible because of severe patient discomfort due to pain or photophobia. If an anesthetic agent is required to check VA, the reason should be documented. The only reason *not* to check VA is a chemical burn, which requires prompt irrigation with normal saline. By convention the right eye (OD) is documented above the left eye (OS), noting whether or not glasses were worn.

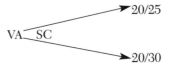

This notation indicates that the VA in the right eye was 20/25 and that in the left, 20/30. SC denotes "without corrective lenses." CC means "with corrective lenses."

VA is a test of macular function. A pinhole occluder is utilized so that only one eye at a time is tested. If the patient wears contact lenses or glasses, VA should be tested both with (CC) and without (SC) corrective lenses. (Patients with contact-lens problems rarely have a backup pair of glasses.) Individuals who wear corrective lenses but present without them should be screened using the pinhole occluder. VA should first be checked by looking through the large hole and then dropping down the pinhole disk and having the patient select one small opening through which to view the eye chart. This is a crude way of compensating for refractive error, in the same manner that squinting helps myopes to see better in the distance.

The smallest object that can be clearly seen and distinguished at a distance of 20 ft determines VA. The classic Snellen chart is designed so that the letters subtend a 5-min angle to the eye at 20 ft. This is converted to lay terms by expressing VA as a fraction. The numerator denotes the patient's distance from the chart letters, and the denominator denotes the distance from the chart at which a normal person can see the chart letters. VA of 20/40–2 means that the patient incorrectly identified two letters on the 20/40 line and from 20 ft is able to read only what a normal person would be able to read at 40 ft. If the patient is unable to read the large "E" at the top of the eye chart (20/400), the next step is to determine whether he or she can count fingers (CF) or see hand motion (HM) and at what distance. If the patient is unable to do either of these, then one may shine a light at his or her eye to determine whether light perception (LP) or no light perception (NLP) is present.

If a discrepancy of more than two lines is found between eyes, the patient is asked whether any difference in VA existed before the injury or problem developed. A history of amblyopia, commonly called "lazy eye," would change the plan and urgency for treatment. A decreased VA in the affected eye without a history of amblyopia points to a serious visual problem (central retinal artery occlusion, branch retinal vein occlusion, vitreous hemorrhage, optic neuritis) or obstruction along the visual axis (corneal foreign body, abrasion, iritis, cataract). After the measurement of VA, the rest of the eye is examined in a consistent, systematic way. The following sections give instructions and a recommended sequence in which this should be done.

External

The external exam begins with an overall inspection of the patient's face and eyes. The eyelids should cover the uppermost area of the iris. Is the white of the sclera interposed between the upper lid and the iris, giving the appearance of the eyes bulging out (proptosis)? If so, thyroid disease must be considered. Are the lids swollen and/or erythematous? That might suggest conjunctivitis, cellulitis, or an allergic reaction. Is the patient blinking normally with both eyes? If one eyelid does not seem to close completely or as often as the other eye, then Bell's palsy is a possibility. Is one eyelid droopy (ptosis)? This may be due to mechanical factors, Horner's syndrome, or myasthenia gravis. Is there a circumscribed, erythematous swelling? Within the lid proper, this might be a chalazion or, on the lid margin, a hordeolum. If conjunctivitis is suspected, the area anterior to the tragus should be palpated for tender preauricular lymph nodes associated with viral conjunctivitis. Look at the nature of the discharge—watery versus purulent (i.e., viral versus bacterial). If vesicular lesions are present on only one side of the face, they may be due to herpes zoster. When vesicular lesions involve the tip of the nose, there is or soon will be corneal involvement. Even if corneal dendrites are not visible on initial presentation, such patients should be referred to the ophthalmologist. Are there dry crusts at the bases of the eyelashes, flaking off erythematous lids? This may mean blepharitis. For traumatic injuries, their location must be documented, and one must always be aware of the accessory structures that lie deep to the skin—i.e., lacrimal gland, inferior canaliculus, lacrimal sac, or tarsal plate—where such injury may have negative long-term consequences functionally or cosmetically.

Pupils

The pupils should be round and equal in size. An irregular shape may be the result of previous eye surgery, trauma, or adhesions (synechiae) from prior inflammatory processes. Anisocoria, or different-sized pupils, may be physiologic or the result of using eyedrops. Physiologic anisocoria (usually <1 mm) is found in many patients, and the relative pupillary size will remain consistent throughout the examination. Anisocoria is most easily detected in blue-eyed individuals.

To check pupillary light reflexes, the patient is first directed to look at an object more than 15 ft away. It is preferable to document the diameter of the pupils in a dimly lighted room before shining light into the eye and then seeing to what diameter the pupil constricts after the eye is illuminated (direct response). Thereafter the other eye is quickly checked to see whether its pupil is also constricted (consensual response). This is documented in millimeters (mm), such that "OU 5 —> 3" means both pupils started at 5 mm and both constricted to 3 mm. Any variance should be noted—e.g., OD 5 —> 3, OS 5 —> 4 would designate that the left eye only constricted to 4 mm.

The most important abnormal pupillary response to rule out is the afferent pupillary defect (APD), also called the Marcus Gunn pupil. This is checked by rapidly swinging a flashlight from the right eye to the left and vice versa. The left eye should constrict in consensual response to light directed at the right eye; when the direct light swings to the left eye, the left pupil should stay constricted. Dilation of the left pupil signifies a positive APD. There can be some vacillation of pupillary diameter, but a true APD manifests itself by sustained pupil dilation. A positive APD indicates a serious problem somewhere along the optic nerve or retina, and VA in the affected eye should be significantly decreased or absent.

Extraocular Movements

With the patient looking straight ahead, the straightness of the eyes is assessed. Deviation of one eye temporally is exotropia and deviation nasally is esotropia. If asymmetry is observed, the patient is asked whether this is old or new. Extraocular movements (EOMs) are then checked. One method is to for the examiner to circumscribe the letter "H" in front of the patient with his or her index finger, having the patient move only the eyes, not the head, to follow the finger. It is important to watch for lack of conjugate movement. If any restriction of eye movement is detected, the patient must be asked whether this is associated with any double vision. In traumatic injury, limitation of upward gaze in the injured eye (entrapment) indicates an orbital floor fracture. One must observe carefully to detect this, because entrapment may be subtle and, with soft tissue swelling, difficult to perceive. Any lagging or inability to cross the midline suggests third nerve palsy. This requires further neurologic assessment, since internuclear ophthalmoplegia from multiple sclerosis (MS) or cerebral vascular aneurysm is in the differential.

The patient's eyes should be taken to extreme positions of gaze, in all directions, to check for nystagmus. These involuntary rhythmic eye movements may be either congenital or acquired. There are many varieties of nystagmus, but the jerk nystagmus is probably the type one thinks about in discussing this topic. It begins with a slow phase, where the eye slowly drifts in one direction; this is followed by the fast phase, where the eye quickly returns to its original position. The cycle then repeats itself. The examiner documents the direction of gaze (straight up, straight down, right or left) and states in which direction the slow and fast phases were present. Acquired nystagmus has a broad etiology, ranging from visual loss (secondary to trauma or a dense cataract), toxic or metabolic factors (secondary to alcohol, phencyclidine, lithium, salicylates, anticonvulsants, thiamine deficiency, or Wernicke's encephalopathy), neurologic problems (secondary to trauma, stroke, tumor, or MS), and nonphysiologic causes (intentional eye movements that the patient cannot sustain for more then 30 s without fatigue). Nonsustained nystagmus evoked on extreme horizontal gaze can be seen in normal individuals. However, sustained gaze-evoked nystagmus may be indicative of brainstem disease and requires prompt evaluation. Nystagmus due to vestibular disease (labyrinthitis, Ménière's disease) is usually accompanied by other symptoms—e.g., past pointing, tendency to fall, vertigo—and is frequently associated with autonomic nervous system involvement (e.g., nausea, vomiting, diaphoresis, hypotension, and tachycardia).

Visual Fields

The confrontation method of testing visual fields (VF) in the primary care office or the ED is only a rough screening method to identify defects. To check the nasal VF of the patient's left eye, the examiner sits about 3 ft away facing the patient. The patient is directed to fixate on the examiner's right eye while he or she fixates on the patient's left eye. This allows the examiner to know whether the patient is looking directly at the examiner's fingers. Both examiner and patient then occlude the other eye with the palm of the hand. The examiner then presents different numbers of fingers in all four quadrants at a position halfway between them. To check the patient's left temporal VF, the examiner must cover his or her left eye with the left palm, then present the fingers of the right hand. For ease of visualization, the examiner usually presents either one, two, or five fingers. This procedure is repeated for the patient's right eye. Any defect is documented with a visual field chart diagram.

Fundus

The direct ophthalmoscope is a hand-held instrument with a rheostat-controlled light source, a set of filters with different spot sizes and other illuminated openings, a viewing aperture, and a disk of rotating corrective lenses. A lighted window shows the lens power as either a "minus" red number to neutralize the nearsighted (myopic) eye or a "plus" white number to neutralize the farsighted (hyperopic) eye.

The direct ophthalmoscope is used to inspect the posterior pole of the eye or fundus. These two terms are frequently used interchangeably; however, the term *posterior pole* refers only to the optic nerve and macula, whereas the fundus includes the optic nerve, the retina and its blood vessels, the choroid, and the sclera. The direct ophthalmoscope gives an erect image, has a small field of view (5 degrees), and has a large magnification (14×); it is monocular. For comparison, the indirect ophthalmoscope used by the ophthalmologist gives an inverted and reversed image, has a large field of view (depending on the power of the hand-held lens, 45 to 50 degrees), and has small magnification (hand-held lens–dependent 3 or 2×); it is stereoscopic.

To examine the fundus, the room is first darkened. To view the patient's right fundus, the ophthalmoscope is held in the examiner's right hand with the index finger on the rotating dial and right eye used. Everything is then switched to the left for the patient's left eye. Both examiner and patient should be in a comfortable position, preferably with the patient seated and fixated on a distant, straight-ahead object, such as an "X" on a wall at the patient's eye level. To begin with, the dial lens is set at "O." The examiner then approaches the patient temporal to the visual axis, finds the red reflex, and then moves closer to the patient, directing his or her gaze slightly nasally to find the optic nerve. When this is found, the dial is rotated until the nerve head comes into sharp focus. A cataract, depending on its density, can make it difficult to obtain sharp focusing and sometimes will not even permit visualization of the fundus. Absence of the red reflex indicates the presence of a dense cataract. If a blood vessel is found, it should be followed back to the optic nerve, where a systematic examination can begin. The horizontal cup:disk ratio is documented; ratios greater than 0.5 or a difference between the eyes of more than 0.2 is suspect and should be referred to the ophthalmologist. The examiner looks for swelling of the optic nerve (papilledema) and venous pulsations. (Venous pulsations look like a balloon starting to be filled that is then deflated.) If venous pulsations are present, there is no increase in intracranial pressure (ICP); however, their absence does not imply increased ICP in an alert individual. A rim of black pigment around the nerve is a normal finding. The vascular arcades are inspected from the optic nerve out to the periphery. Any abnormalities, hemorrhages, exudates, or arteriovenous nicking is noted. Finally, the patient is told to look directly into the light; this will bring the macula and fovea into view. Although the fovea is a depression, it has the appearance of a yellowish projection up toward the viewer.

Slit Lamp

The slit lamp is a microscope that gives a magnified, erect, stereoscopic view of the anterior segment of the eye. Magnification ranges from about 10 to 500×.

A simple slit lamp has a frame to hold the patient's head, magnifying lenses, controls for light intensity and width and height of the slit beam, and a cobalt blue filter to be used for staining the cornea with fluorescein. A joystick located on the base controls up and down excursions and fine focusing. These basic controls are the only ones the nonophthalmologist need master. The other controls, lenses, and attachments are not used in the primary care setting.

The table height should be comfortable for both patient and examiner. The patient is positioned with the chin in the cup and the forehead against the headband. The height of the chin rest is adjusted so that the pupils are level with the eye-level marker. The oculars are set to the examiner's refractive error and the interpupillary distance is adjusted for the examiner's eyes. The lights in the room are then dimmed and the examination begins.

If only one eye is involved, the unaffected eye is examined first. Starting with low magnification and a wide beam, the lids, lid margins, and lashes are assessed. The presenting complaint directs what should be looked for and what is likely to be found.

The conjunctiva is examined while maintaining the same slit lamp settings used for the lids. The tarsal conjunctiva is examined first by everting the lids. Lower lid eversion is accomplished by pulling down on the skin below the lid margin. For upper lid eversion, while the patient is looking down, the examiner grasps some eyelashes with the thumb and forefinger, pulling the lid away from the globe. The tail end of a cotton-tipped applicator is then placed against the upper lid crease and the lid is lifted up and over the stick. Then, after the stick has been slid out, the examiner continues to hold the lid everted with the thumb that was used to grasp the eyelashes. The slightly concave shape of the everted lid as it faces the examiner is due to the tarsal plate. Foreign bodies, mucus, pus, papillae, and injection of the conjunctival blood vessels are sought. The patient is asked to look inferiorly in order to check the superior fornix and superiorly to check the inferior fornix. Next, the bulbar conjunctiva is examined by looking at the pattern of injection—whether it is diffuse (typical of the red eye seen with conjunctivitis, abrasion, foreign body, ulcer, herpes zoster ophthalmicus) or sectorial (wedge-shaped and localized).

To examine the cornea, the light source should be a narrow, tall beam. With mid-level magnification, the surface is scanned, looking for clarity, epithelial defects, foreign body, or infiltrate (focal white area in the stroma, looks like ground glass). Even if a corneal foreign body is found, this author always does upper and lower lid eversion to make sure that no other foreign bodies are trapped within the tarsal conjunctiva or the fornices.

The anterior chamber (AC) should be inspected for depth, flare, and cells before staining with fluorescein. Depth will be difficult for the nonophthalmologist to assess. Once one has examined a goodly number of normal eyes, the task of determining an abnormal AC seems like less of a challenge. If a clinical history for acute glaucoma is present, one may appreciate a billowing forward of the iris, giving the patient a shallow AC and a narrow angle. Flare has the appearance of a beam of light passing through fog and is visible when protein is in the AC. The light source should be turned up to its highest intensity with the slit at its shortest height and widest aperture, making the light source a round beam of light. When one looks for cells in the AC at this light setting, they have the appearance of specks of dust passing through a ray of sunlight. Cells are ranked on a scale of 1 to 4, the latter figure indicating the largest number of cells. With blood in the AC from trauma (hyphema), one can document the percent depth of layering of the cells at the base of the AC, i.e., 25 percent if the lower fourth of the AC contains red blood cells. In the healthy eye with normal depth and no flare or cells, this is documented as "AC–D&Q" for "deep and quiet."

Periorbital Soft Tissue and Retrobulbar Space

Periorbital soft tissue should be examined visually and by palpation prior to a more detailed examination of the eye. The most common findings in the periorbital space are infection and swelling due to acute allergic reactions (usually due to contact reactions). Edema, erythema, and tenderness of the periorbital soft tissue is found in both *periorbital* or *preseptal cellulitis*. This is in contrast to *orbital cellulitis*, where the deeper retrobulbar and postseptal soft tissues are involved. Periorbital cellulitis usually involves swelling, erythema, and tenderness but does not involve changes in extraocular motion or pupillary findings. This is in contrast to retrobulbar processes, in which there is pain with eye movement as well as proptosis, ophthalmoplegia, and afferent pupillary changes. Retrobulbar hematoma or cellulitis is most commonly due to complications from ophthalmologic surgery but may also be associated with hemophilia, leukemia, and hypertension.

One of the most important distinctions in urgent care and emergency medicine is distinguishing periorbital or preseptal cellulitis from orbital or postseptal cellulitis, since the latter carries a poor prognosis if not diagnosed and managed appropriately at the earliest possible time. *Orbital or postseptal cellulitis* is a true ophthalmologic emergency and usually occurs by direct extension of bacteria from either the ethmoid or maxillary sinuses following either acute or chronic sinusitis. Orbital cellulitis often progresses rapidly and patients have orbital pain, swelling, erythema, and conjunctival infection; they are both febrile and toxic. There is often pain with eye movements and patients also have symptoms of ptosis, ophthalmoplegia, and pupillary changes. These patients require prompt initial treatment and immediate referral to the ED for a computed tomography (CT) scan to confirm the diagnosis and delineate the extent of involvement. The most common organisms in this disease are *Streptococcus pneumoniae*, *Haemophilus influenzae*, and *Staphylococcus aureus*. If possible, the patient should be given broad-spectrum antibiotics prior to referral from the UCC—for example, ticarcillin-clavulanate 3.1 g IV or cefuroxime 5 to 3.0 g IV. *S. aureus* is the most common pathogen, although many of these infections are polymicrobial. In diabetics and immunocompromised patients, mucormycosis is also a possibility. The primary reasons for aggressive treatment and urgent referral for such patients include the risks of bacteremia and spread of the infection posteriorly to the cavernous sinus.

Periorbital or preseptal cellulitis is a more superficial infection that does not traverse the orbital septum. Because it is a limited infection of the periorbital soft tissues and does not extend to the retrobulbar space, visual acuity, pupillary reaction, and ocular motility are preserved. Headache is rare in such patients, and they are generally neither febrile nor toxic. While orbital cellulitis occurs from extension from infected sinuses in most cases, periorbital cellulitis usually results from either mild trauma to the area or extension of the soft tissue infection from the skin. The most common etiologic agent is *S. aureus*, although mixed infections are also common. While periorbital cellulitis is usually limited to the superficial areas, the possibility of extension to the orbital or postseptal space warrants aggressive treatment with oral antibiotics. Children should be treated with either amoxicillin-clavulanate (Augmentin) 20 to 40 mg/kg per day in divided doses or cefuroxime 50 mg/kg IM or IV followed by oral antibiotics. Patients should also use warm compresses and should receive a definite and prearranged referral to an ophthalmologist for follow-up care within 48 h to assure that the disease does not extend further. If such referral cannot be obtained, the patient should have a referral either back to the UCC or to an ED for a reexamination within the 48-h period. In addition, the patient should be clearly instructed to return immediately to the UCC, the ED, or the ophthalmologist if symptoms suggesting orbital cellulitis develop.

In children under 5 years of age, preseptal cellulitis may be associated with bacteremia and can in some cases be a prelude to sepsis and meningitis. In these children, more aggressive treatment, including a sepsis workup and blood cultures as well as intravenous antibiotics, should be considered. In most cases, it is best to discuss such cases with the pediatrician and the ophthalmologist to make sure that the child is aggressively diagnosed and treated.

Eyelids and Lacrimal Apparatus

The eyelids contain muscles for opening the eye, glands that contribute a viscous material to decrease the rate of tear film evaporation, and the tarsal plates, a cartilaginous skeleton that supports the eyelids. The eyelids offer protection to the front of the eye during the blink reflex and also serve to spread tear film across the surface of the cornea, keeping it moist. The lid margins (Fig. 7-3) on the surface of the eyelid contact each other when the eyes are closed, creating an effective seal across the eye and containing meibomian glands and the eyelashes. The tarsal plates attach to a layer of fascia, the

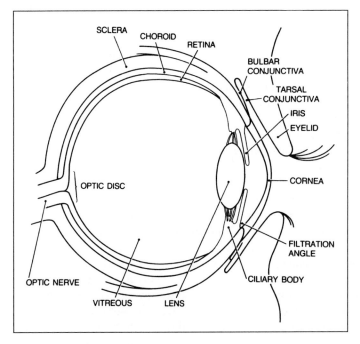

FIGURE 7-3 Horizontal cross-sectional diagram of the eye. (From Tintinalli JE et al: *Emergency Medicine: A Comprehensive Study Guide*, 5th ed. New York: McGraw-Hill; 2000. With permission.)

orbital septum, which is continuous with the periosteum at the edges of the orbit. This forms an important barrier between the outside and the inside contents of the orbit and delineates preseptal from orbital cellulitis.

The lacrimal gland is located in the upper temporal quadrant of the orbit (Fig. 7-2). The drainage system for tears, the lacrimal apparatus, is located nasally. Only the openings in the nasal aspect of the upper and lower lid margins (the puncta) are visible with the slit lamp. The rest of the system lies below the skin and within the nasal cavity. The superior and inferior puncta drain through the canaliculi into the lacrimal sac, located just nasal to the medial canthus. Tears then drain to the nasolacrimal duct, which empties through an opening just below the inferior meatus of the nose (which explains why the nose "runs" when one cries).

A wide range of signs and symptoms are attributable to the eyelids and lacrimal tissues. Ptosis is drooping or sagging of the upper eyelid, which may be bilateral or unilateral. It can be caused by decreased sympathetic tone (such as Horner's syndrome), muscle problems (such as myasthenia gravis or muscular dystrophy), changes associated with aging, and third nerve palsies, comprising a wide array of problems including botulinum toxin exposure, tumors, and aneurysms. Ptosis per se requires no specific treatment other than patient reassurance and, occasionally, patching of the eye for cosmetic reasons. However, the underlying cause of the ptosis must be determined with patient referral to the appropriate specialty. In new-onset ptosis, that workup should include a CT scan to exclude tumors and aneurysms. *Blepharitis* is inflammation of the lid margins, which is usually bilateral and most commonly chronic in nature. The lid margins are erythematous, slightly swollen, and often scaly. The most common causes are seborrhea and focal staphylococcal infection. *Lid edema* is a more generic term that technically includes blepharitis, but it is more of a nonspecific finding caused by a number of inflammatory and allergic processes. All patients with blepharitis, whether with staphylococcal infection or seborrheic dermatitis, should have warm, moist compresses placed on the eyes several times a day to help soften the scaling and crusting as well as to decrease inflammation. The scaling skin should be removed from the eyelids twice a day using gentle scrubs with baby shampoo; either the fingertips or cotton-tipped applicators are utilized, with care taken to avoid scratching the cornea. In cases of seborrheic blepharitis, antiseborrheic dandruff shampoos such as T-gel should be used on the scalp. Clinical findings (small ulcerations along the lid margins and purulence), history, and cultures may distinguish staphylococcal infection from seborrheic blepharitis. However, unless this distinction can be clearly made, an ophthalmic ointment effective against *S. aureus* should be placed on the lid margin twice a day for 10 to 14 days. Erythromycin or gentamicin ointments are effective in these cases, although fluoroquinolone eyedrops may be utilized in resistant cases. Patients with blepharitis should be referred for follow-up with either their primary care physician or the ophthalmologist.

One of the most common ophthalmologic presentations to UCCs and EDs is the stye, more technically known as a *hordeolum*, which is an infection of a meibomian gland (internal hordeolum) or superficial gland (external hordeolum). The presentation is quite distinctive in that the lid is focally inflamed and usually quite tender, with a focal soft eruption in the subcutaneous tissue. Both internal and external hordeola should be treated with warm, moist compresses and eye ointments effective against *S. aureus*, applied twice daily to the lid margins for 5 to 7 days. The majority of such cases will resolve within this time frame, although persistent or expanding lesions may need referral to the ophthalmologist.

A *chalazion* is a chronic granulomatous inflammation most commonly due to a persistent and inadequately treated internal hordeolum. A chalazion may look superficially like a hordeolum, but it is usually firmer and nontender, although it may become large enough to be cosmetically irritating or even interfere with vision. Most chalazions will require referral to an ophthalmologist for either topical or intralesional steroid therapy or, in rarer cases, incision, drainage, or cosmetic removal.

The lid margins may become everted (*ectropion*) or inverted (*entropion*); both of these conditions more commonly affect the lower lid than the upper lid, and they are most commonly seen with a loss of supporting tissue associated with aging. The most common presentation of patients with ectropion is either the cosmetic change ("looks funny") or problems with excessive tearing ("feels funny") due to displacement or obstruction of the punctum. In the latter cases, there may be inadequate tears retained within the eye to lubricate the cornea. Further, in some cases the eye will not be able to close adequately to protect the cornea, which can result in corneal abrasions, chronic corneal inflammation, and even, in some cases, corneal ulceration. Most patients with ectropion require the use of artificial tears to help lubricate the eye, but antibiotics are usually not necessary unless secondary infection has occurred. If corneal abrasions, infection, or ulceration have occurred, they should be treated appropriately with antibiotics. The most common presentation of entropion results from displacement of the eyelashes inward, which not only disrupts tear film mechanisms but can also irritate the cornea mechanically. When corneal irritation has occurred, the lid margins should be everted as much as possible and an eye patch, topical antibiotics, and cycloplegics applied prior to referral to an ophthalmologist within 24 to 36 h. The definitive treatment for both ectropion and entropion is surgical, so patients should be referred to the ophthalmologist for consultation. However, in many elderly patients, ectropion in particular is treated symptomatically, with surgical repair reserved for more severe or cosmetically concerning cases.

Blepharospasm is repeated, usually involuntary blinking or twitching of the eyelid. These symptoms are usually due to what is known as *essential blepharospasm*, which is bilateral and can present as either intermittent or persistent blepharospasm. Essential blepharospasm disappears during sleep and is a benign and self-limited process, but in rare cases it may require treatment. Blepharospasm can also be associated with involvement of additional facial muscles on the affected side. This condition can be due to serious intracranial disorders and requires referral for exclusion of these causes.

Infection of the nasolacrimal sac is known as *dacryocystitis* and presents with erythema, edema, and pain localized below the medial canthus. In acute infectious dacryocystitis, pressure near the punctum may express purulent material. In some cases, acute dacryocystitis can progress into orbital cellulitis and is therefore treated aggressively. All cases of dacryocystitis should be treated with warm compresses and oral antibiotics effective against *S. aureus, H. influenzae,* and beta-hemolytic streptococci. Options include amoxicillin-clavulanate or a third-generation cephalosporin. *Any* concerns regarding orbital cellulitis should be treated aggressively and referred immediately for evaluation and therapy.

Dacryoadenitis refers to infection and inflammation of the lacrimal gland, which is usually viral in nature and produces redness, tenderness, and swelling above the lateral canthus, which can be associated with both chemosis and injection of the conjunctiva. While dacryoadenitis is usually due to viral agents, bacterial infection may occur, so oral antimicrobials are usually prescribed to all patients.

Excessive tearing is known as *epiphora* and may be caused by chronic irritation or nasolacrimal duct obstruction due to tumors, infection, or mucosal inflammation. Nasolacrimal duct patency can be assessed by placing fluorescein in the affected eye, after which the dye should appear in either the nasal passages or the pharynx.

Keratoconjunctivitis sicca, or dry-eye syndrome, is usually caused by mechanical disruption of the tear film mechanism, resulting in irritation of the cornea and paradoxical epiphora. It is often associated with involvement of the lacrimal gland and sarcoid, Sjögren's syndrome, or medications with anticholinergic properties. Artificial tears should be prescribed for these patients and they should be referred to their primary care physician or the ophthalmologist.

Conjunctiva, Episclera, and Sclera

The palpebral conjunctiva covers the inner surface of the eyelid, while the bulbar conjunctiva covers the anterior surface of the globe, reflecting backwards on itself at both the inferior and superior fornices. The conjunctiva is invested with copious blood vessels, which are not apparent in the healthy eye. However, when the eye is inflamed, these vessels become engorged and visible, giving the eye a typical "bloodshot" appearance. In addition, the conjunctiva is attached at the junction of the cornea and the sclera but is otherwise loose and somewhat mobile; it reacts to edema and inflammation in a sometimes dramatic fashion. In acute allergic reactions, for example, a significant *chemosis* may occur, resulting in a fairly startling appearance of the eye, which is usually due to simple allergic inflammation. An important diagnostic maneuver involves the use of topical vasoconstrictors. These should produce a dramatic constriction of conjunctival vessels as opposed to episcleral vessels, which will not react to such vasoconstrictors.

Conjunctivitis is one of the most common presentations to UCCs and EDs and is due to bacterial, viral, chlamydial, or allergic causes, which can usually be roughly distinguished on clinical grounds (Table 7-1). *Bacterial conjunctivitis* classically presents as "pinkeye," with inflammation of the bulbar and palpebral conjunctiva and a sometimes copious mucopurulent discharge. Patients will often give the history of their eyes "being stuck together" when they awaken in the morning. Bilateral symptoms are common, particularly since the disease can be spread by contact by rubbing one eye and then the other. In many cases there may be a history of exposure to someone who has had similar symptoms. There may be swelling of the preauricular lymph nodes, but this is less common from bacterial than viral causes. All patients with conjunctivitis should have a careful physical examination, including fluorescein staining of the cornea to avoid missing a corneal abrasion, dendrite, or ulcer. Topical ophthalmic antibiotics should be utilized for 5 to 7 days, utilizing a broad-spectrum agent capable of covering the mixed flora that cause such infection. Trimethoprim and polymixin-B drops or ointment (Polytrim), macrolides (erythromycin), aminoglycosides (gentamicin or tobramycin), or fluoroquinolones such as ciprofloxacin (Ciloxan) or ofloxacin (Ocuflox) may be utilized. There is a small but discrete incidence of patients with allergies to sulfa and neomycin preparations, although those antibiotics are also utilized (Table 7-2). In patients who wear contact lenses, the contact lens should be removed until the eyes have cleared, but a more broad-spectrum antibiotic with coverage for *Pseudomonas* [Ciloxan, Ocuflox, Tobrex (tobramycin)] should be utilized. Gentamicin in the form of drops or ointment has also been utilized in the past, but the high incidence of inflammatory reactions to it have led to a decrease in its use.

In some cases, bacterial conjunctivitis can be distinguished from viral conjunctivitis, while in others it is difficult to make this distinction. The discharge in patients with

TABLE 7-1

DIFFERENTIAL DIAGNOSIS OF CONJUNCTIVITIS BY ETIOLOGY

	ONSET	ITCHING	PAIN	SWOLLEN LIDS	DISCHARGE (AMOUNT, QUALITY)	CONJUNCTIVAL INJECTION	HISTORY OF EXPOSURE
Bacterial	Acute	Common	Minimal	Common	Copious, purulent	Moderate to severe	Common
Viral	Acute, subacute	Rare	Minimal	Variable	Moderate, seropurulent	Moderate to severe	Common
Allergic	Acute	Very	None	Common	Moderate, clear	Moderate	None to patients, common to allergens
Chlamydial	Chronic	Rare	Minimal	Rare	Minimal, seropurulent	Moderate	Sexually transmitted disease

TABLE 7-2

OPHTHALMIC TOPICAL DRUG THERAPY

1. **Anesthetics**
   Proparacaine, 0.5% (preferred agent)
   Tetracaine, 0.5%

2. **Antibiotics**
   Bacitracin ointment, 500 U/g
   Ciprofloxacin (Ciloxan), 0.3%
   Erythromycin ointment, 0.5%
   Gentamicin ointment or solution, 0.3% (not preferred)
   Tobramycin (Tobrex) ointment or solution, 0.3%
   Neomycin/Polymyxin/Bacitracin ointment or drops (avoid using due to allergic reactions)
   Ofloxacin (Ocuflux), 0.3%
   Sulfacetamide ointment or solution, 10% (burning sensation on installation, topical sensitizer)

3. **Antipruritic and antiallergy medications**
   Mast cell stabilizer—cromolyn sodium, 4% (Opticrom)
   Nonsteroidal inflammatory—ketorolac (Toradol), 0.5% (burns on installation)
   Decongestant drops—naphazoline (Naphcon-A), 0.1%

4. **Cycloplegic-mydriatic agents**
   Cyclopentolate, 0.5%, 1.0%, 2.0% solutions
   Homatropine, 2.0%, 5.0% solutions
   Tropicamide, 0.5%, 1.0% solution

5. **Mydriatic agents**
   Phenylephrine, 2.5%

6. **Miotics**
   Pilocarpine, 0.5%–10%

viral conjunctivitis is often more seropurulent than mucopurulent and it may be somewhat less copious. In addition, preauricular nodes are more commonly swollen in viral cases. However, viral and bacterial cultures with or without Gram stains are the most definitive way to make a diagnosis, which takes several days to process. Because of this, most cases of viral conjunctivitis are also treated with ophthalmic antibiotics, since an absolute distinction between the two can be difficult to make. In both cases the cornea should be stained to avoid missing abrasions, ulcers, and dendrites, and similar antibiotic therapy should be utilized. In addition, in both viral and bacterial conjunctivitis, Naphcon-A (pheniramine maleate and naphazoline) may be prescribed at a dose of one drop three or four times a day as needed for itching or congestion of the conjunctiva. In both bacterial and viral conjunctivitis, the patient should have a complete ophthalmologic examination repeated 7 to 10 days after the initial therapy has begun to assure that complete healing has occurred and that no corneal ulcers are present.

The debate continues to rage whether ophthalmic drops or ointment is the preferred treatment for bacterial conjunctivitis. Some studies have indicated that ophthalmic antibiotic drops have a very short half-life within the eye because of dilution by the tearing mechanisms and that ointments provide both better penetration and longer duration of the antibiotic within the conjunctiva itself. However, there seems to be no difference in time to resolution of symptoms or occurrence of complications between the two, so it is generally felt that it is safe to prescribe either drops or ointment. Some ophthalmologists actually prescribe both, utilizing drops during the day and ointment at night.

The incidence of *allergic conjunctivitis* seems to be rising, perhaps because of broader exposure to allergens in general. The most dramatic presentation of allergic conjunctivitis is frank chemosis, in which there may be dramatic and, to the patient, alarming swelling of the conjunctiva. Allergic conjunctivitis often presents with a clear discharge, and patients usually have redness, tearing, and itching. Patients should be treated with cool compresses, artificial tears as needed, and decongestant/antihistamine drops such as Naphcon-A or Patanol (olopatadine). In cases with dramatic symptoms, nonsteroidal agents (ketorolac 0.5%) or mast cell stabilizers such as cromolyn sodium 4% may be utilized. In some patients with allergic conjunctivitis, secondary bacterial infection may also occur, which should be treated with appropriate ophthalmic drops or ointment.

Two other causes of conjunctivitis require consideration, as each necessitates specific treatment. *Chlamydial conjunctivitis* classically results in a mild to moderate inflammation that may often be mistaken for viral conjunctivitis. The discharge is seropurulent in nature and is mild to minimal, but the condition has a more chronic course. Over time, if allowed to persist, a chronic follicular reaction develops, with continuation of the seropurulent discharge. Outpatients with documented chlamydial conjunctivitis (up to 60 percent of men and 90 percent of women) have coexistent sexually transmitted diseases (STDs). Appropriate ophthalmologic and genitourinary cultures should be taken and systemic therapy for a proven STD should be offered. Topical erythromycin ointment has been shown to decrease the duration of ophthalmic symptoms but should be used only in combination with systemic therapy.

Neonatal conjunctivitis or *ophthalmia neonatorum* refers to conjunctivitis occurring within the first 28 days of life. Such cases are usually due either to *Neisseria gonorrhoeae* or *Chlamydia*, both of which are acquired during the process of vaginal childbirth. Neonates presenting with symptoms of conjunctivitis should have careful Gram staining of the eyes as well as a detailed examination to rule out systemic infection. Neonates with conjunctivitis usually have a fairly intense inflammatory reaction, and secondary corneal ulceration or even perforation must be carefully considered. Any patient with neonatal conjunctivitis seen in the UCC should be referred to the pediatrician or to the ED for further workup and possible admission.

A *pterygium* is a fibrovascular tissue growth extending over the cornea, usually occurring nasally, although it may also present in the temporal area. These growths often occur in patients exposed to environmental irritants or ultraviolet light, and are therefore more common in patients who work outside. Unless they are acutely irritated or inflamed or there is secondary bacterial infection, they require no immediate treatment and can be referred electively to the ophthalmologist, who may perform elective removal if clinically indicated. It is very common to have patients present to the UCC who have had a rupture of a conjunctival blood vessel, resulting in *a subconjunctival hemorrhage*, which sometimes presents as a dramatic redness of the eye with accumulation of blood on the bulbar surface. Symptoms often occur after a sudden Valsalva maneuver, typically after sneezing or coughing or a prolonged breath-holding spell. While the presentation is often dramatic, treatment is usually symptomatic unless the condition occurs in a patient with a known bleeding disorder. A *pinguecula* is similar to a pterygium but is a chronically thickened and yellowish waste area of the conjunctiva on either the nasal or temporal aspect of the limbus. These lesions are associated with aging and consist of atrophied and degenerated elastic tissue; they do not require acute treatment.

The sclera is in many respects the most visible aspect of the eye, consisting of a durable, white elastic collagen shell encasing the globe. The sclera is essentially avascular, with the blood supply being provided by the episclera and the choroid. It is encased by the episclera, comprising both parietal and visceral layers, each with distinct blood supplies.

The most important problem with scleral versus episcleral disease in UCCs and EDs has to do with distinguishing episcleritis from scleritis. *Episcleritis* refers to inflammation of superficial episcleral blood vessels, accounting for the classically described finding of a "salmon hue." Patients present most commonly either because of the change in color of the eye or because of a mild to moderate headache or aching pain in the eye ("feels funny"), which is often accompanied by photophobia and excessive tearing. The inflammation and injection of the episcleral vessels may be limited to one quadrant of the eye, resulting in a fairly striking clinical presentation. Causes of episcleritis include external irritants, viral disease, and idiopathic causes, although up to 40 percent of patients with episcleritis have an underlying collagen vascular disease or systemic inflammatory condition. Episcleritis is usually self-limited but may require oral pain medications for the headache and photophobia. It can persist for weeks or months or recur after treatment. Episcleritis is often distinguished from scleritis not only by its clinical presentation (see below) but also by the use of topical vasoconstrictors, which readily constrict the superficial vessels of episcleritis while the deep vessels involved in scleritis are resistant to such agents.

Scleritis is a more serious condition involving the deep scleral vessels, which produce a bluish rather than salmon-colored hue. The pain of scleritis is typically much more severe and is often described by the patient as "boring" in nature; it is usually accompanied by more dramatic photophobia and tearing. The majority of patients have some underlying systemic disease or collagen vascular disorder. All patients with scleritis should have appropriate treatment of their pain and referral to an ophthalmologist, since more extensive workup is necessary in these cases to clarify the cause. Most patients with scleritis also receive treatment with topical steroids and systemic anti-inflammatory medication as well.

Cornea

The cornea is a five-layered structure consisting of a thin outermost epithelium, Bowman's membrane, the stroma (the thickest layer), Descemet's membrane, and an endothelial layer. The total thickness of the cornea varies from 0.5 mm centrally to approximately 1.0 mm at the periphery. The horizontal diameter measures about 11 to 12 mm, which is slightly larger than its vertical diameter of approximately 10.5 mm. Knowing these dimensions helps in estimating pupil size. The epithelium of the cornea is highly invested with sensory nerves, which are branches of the ophthalmic division of the trigeminal nerve. This rich investment with sensory nerves accounts for the dramatic symptoms present when a corneal abrasion occurs. The healthy cornea is avascular, but the limbus has a rich network of branches from the anterior ciliary artery. These blood vessels, when inflamed, are hyperemic and present the classic "ciliary flush" seen with iritis. The limbus also contains the drainage system for removal of aqueous humor from the anterior chamber. The cornea is tightly adherent to the sclera at the limbus. Examination of the cornea can easily be performed with a hand-held ophthalmoscope or a slit lamp; fluorescein examination should be utilized at any time if corneal disease is suspected. The most common corneal problem presenting to UCCs is corneal abrasions, which are dealt with under the heading "Traumatic Injury," further on in this chapter. The most common nontraumatic problem involving the cornea is infection and inflammation of the cornea, referred to as keratitis. More commonly, the infection and inflammation involve not just the cornea but also the conjunctiva, producing *keratoconjunctivitis*. Patients with keratitis or keratoconjunctivitis present with injection and pain or headache. One of the most common causes of keratoconjunctivitis is ultraviolet exposure, either from flash exposure to the eye or prolonged exposure to the sun without appropriate ultraviolet-blocking sunglasses. Fluorescein examination of the eyes in such cases reveals scattered, diffuse defects or frank erosion of the cornea. Corneal ulceration may occur if superficial corneal abrasions or infections are not aggressively treated. Such ulceration produces deeper defects, most commonly appearing as whitish spots on the cornea that light up with fluorescein only at the periphery. Most patients with keratoconjunctivitis should be treated with topical antibiotic drops or ointment as well as appropriate pain medication for their discomfort. They should be referred within 24 to 48 h to an ophthalmologist for follow-up and to assure that progression of the disease does not extend to corneal ulceration. Patients with corneal ulcers should be examined carefully for infection in the anterior chamber (hypopyon) as well as full ophthalmologic examination. Corneal ulcers should be treated aggressively with topical antibiotics, usually with a fluoroquinolone such as ciprofloxacin or ofloxacin, two drops every hour in the affected eye. Most patients also require a topical cycloplegic agent such as 1% cyclopentolate (Cyclogyl) to assist with pain control. Most ophthalmologists recommend that patients with corneal ulcers should not have their eye patched, because of the risk of secondary *Pseudomonas* infection. All patients with corneal ulcers should be seen by an ophthalmologist within 24 h from the time that they present.

Herpes simplex virus (HSV) is an uncommon but important cause of eye infections. While HSV can diffusely affect the eye, its effects on the cornea are most pronounced. Research indicates that many cases of herpes simplex keratitis can be mild and self-limited, although more dramatic symptoms can also occur. In addition, as in other areas of the body, HSV can become latent in the affected nerve area (the trigeminal ganglion), reactivating in response to stress. Patients typically complain of lacrimation, photophobia, a mild discharge, and a persistent foreign-body sensation. Herpetic vesicles can be seen in the conjunctiva or eyelid, but many patients have no overt vesicular lesions. Fluorescein staining of the cornea typically shows the dendrite ulcers, although most ophthalmologists have found that a diffuse corneal uptake of fluorescein is actually the more common finding. The "dendrite" of herpes keratitis is an epithelial defect consisting of a branching pattern, with or without terminal bulging or bulbing (Fig. 7-4).

Mild outbreaks of HSV on the lids and conjunctivae should be treated with oral acyclovir agents such as Zovirax or Famvir and topical antiviral drops (Viroptic). In most cases, erythromycin ophthalmic ointment should be added simply to prevent secondary infection. Because of the potential for permanent damage to the eye, the patient should be referred to the ophthalmologist within 24 h, and immediate consultation should be obtained via telephone whenever possible to help coordinate therapy.

More severe cases of herpes zoster involving the eye are referred to as *herpes zoster ophthalmicus* (HZO). This disease, which occurs in patients with shingles, involves ocular involvement of that condition in the trigeminal nerve distribution. These patients present with more dramatic symptoms, including both cutaneous lesions and eye involvement. In addition to having conjunctival and corneal symptoms, patients with

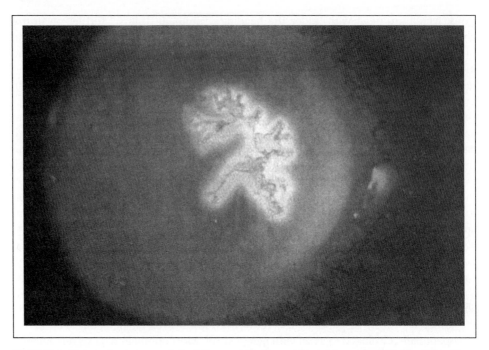

FIGURE 7-4   Herpes simplex corneal dendrite seen with fluorescein staining and cobalt-blue light. (From Tintinalli JE et al: *Emergency Medicine: A Comprehensive Study Guide,* 5th ed. New York: McGraw-Hill; 2000. With permission.)

HZO often present with symptoms of iritis as well. They should be referred to an ophthalmologist immediately, as most of them require hospital admission and intravenous acyclovir therapy, particularly if intracranial extension is a possibility.

Anterior Chamber, Posterior Chamber, and Uveal Tract

The anterior eye segment comprises structures in front of and including the lens, iris, anterior chamber, cornea, sclera, conjunctiva, eyelids, eyelashes, lacrimal gland, and its drainage system. The anterior chamber itself is a space between the anterior surface of the iris and the corneal endothelium. The posterior chamber is a small space between the posterior iris and suspensory ligaments of the lens. The ciliary body produces the clear aqueous humor and is the region for attachment of the suspensory ligaments. Contraction of the ciliary muscles releases the tension on the suspensory ligaments, allowing the lens to thicken and compensate for near vision (accommodation). The uveal tract comprises the iris, ciliary body, and choroid, with the iris separating the anterior and posterior chambers. The pupil is the center aperture of the iris and indeed of the eye itself. Constriction size is controlled by parasympathetic fibers innervated by the third nerve and dilation size through sympathetic fibers from the long ciliary nerves.

In cases where aqueous humor is formed but does not drain, as in angle-closure glaucoma, the intraocular pressure rises, with subsequent symptoms. *Acute angle-closure glaucoma* usually presents as a fairly sudden onset of photophobia accompanied by severe and deep pain as well as headache. Nausea and vomiting occur in a large number of patients as well. The classic presentation of glaucoma includes a cornea that is "hazy" or "steamy," which is noticeable both to the patient and to even the most casual of examiners. The anterior chamber of the eye is shallow, and the pupil is most commonly in midposition and poorly reactive to light. Vision is decreased in the affected eye to varying degrees.

Normal intraocular pressure (IOP) ranges from 10 to 21 mmHg and may be determined by three primary methods. The most accurate measurements are made by applanation tonometry, but considerable skill and experience are required with the slit lamp attachment for this procedure. Relatively few UCC and emergency physicians have sufficient experience with applanation tonometry to use it as an accurate estimate of the IOP. The more recent development of the Tonopen has been helpful in accurately determining intraocular pressures in that it is a hand-held instrument that rapidly and accurately determines IOP. The Tonopen uses a corneal contact area of only about 2.5 mm versus Schiotz tonometry (discussed below), which has a contact area of about 9 mm. If neither applanation tonometry nor a Tonopen is available, the Schiotz tonometer can be utilized. In all methods, the eye should be anesthetized with topical drops and the patient reassured with a detailed explanation of the procedure. The IOP should be measured in both eyes, and the measurement should be repeated at least once for accuracy. In addition, the method of measurement should be recorded and discussed with the ophthalmologist. Any discrepancy between the eyes of greater than 4 mmHg should be considered significant and referred to an ophthalmologist.

The acute treatment of acute angle-closure glaucoma (Fig. 7-5) includes 0.5% timolol drops (not to be used in asthmatics or patients intolerant of beta blockers),

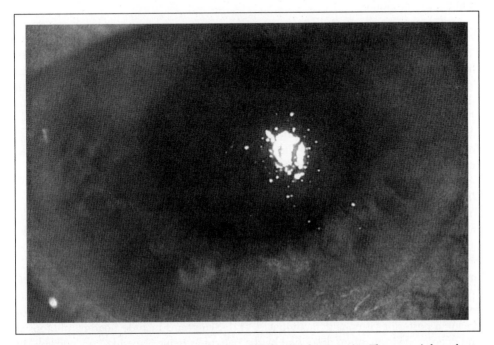

FIGURE 7-5   Acute angle-closure glaucoma. Pupil is middialated and nonreactive. The cornea is hazy due to stromal edema. (From Tintinalli JE et al: *Emergency Medicine: A Comprehensive Study Guide*, 5th ed. New York: McGraw-Hill; 2000. With permission.)

1% pilocarpine drops every 15 min as needed, 500 mg acetazolamide (not to be used if patient is allergic to sulfa) by mouth or intravenously, and 1 to 1.5 g/kg of mannitol intravenously as an osmotic diuretic agent. All such patients should be referred immediately to an ophthalmologist for definitive treatment, consisting of laser iridotomy or surgical peripheral iridectomy. In most cases, the prognosis is good, although prolonged elevations of IOP can result in blindness or decreased vision in the affected eye.

Uveitis is the most common uveal tract disease. Patients with anterior uveitis (which is also known as *iritis* or *iridocyclitis*) usually present with excessive lacrimation, photophobia, and eye pain, which may or may not be accompanied by blurred vision. Slit-lamp examination of such patients often shows white cells and pigment in the aqueous humor and "flare" from increased protein concentration. Patients with acute anterior uveitis or iritis have pain in the affected eye on accommodation because of the phenomenon of a consensual constriction. Most cases of anterior uveitis or iritis are due to inflammatory as opposed to infectious causes. Patients should be treated with adequate doses of oral nonsteroidal anti-inflammatory drugs (NSAIDs) and topical cycloplegic-mydriatic agents. Cycloplegic agents relax the ciliary body, thereby relieving ciliary spasm and much of the pain associated with the disease, while mydriatic agents dilate the pupil. Many agents (cyclopentolate 0.5, 1.0, or 2.0%; homatropine, 2 or 5%; and tropicamide 0.5 or 1.0%) have both cycloplegic and mydriatic properties. The most commonly used treatment is homatropine hydrobromide, with one to two drops given twice daily, particularly in severe cases or those with deeply pigmented eyes, which require the 5% solution, while milder cases and those with lightly pigmented eyes usually resolve with the 2% solution. The patient should be referred to an ophthalmologist within 24 to 48 h of initial presentation.

Ocular Lens

Problems involving the lens are relatively uncommon in the ED and urgent care setting, the most common being traumatic or spontaneous dislocation of the lens, presenting as double vision, blurred vision, or acute glaucoma. While many patients present with cataracts, rarely is this their primary reason for seeking medical care, nor do they usually have acute problems relating to the cataracts that require immediate treatment. The lens itself sits between the iris anteriorly and the vitreous posteriorly and is suspended from the ciliary body by zonules. The size and shape of the lens change in response to contraction and relaxation of the ciliary body.

Vitreous

The vitreous humor comprises the largest part of the eye, filling the globe with a clear mixture of collagen fibrils and hyaluronic acid. While it is attached to the retina throughout the eye, those attachments are particularly strong at the outer edge of the ciliary body, the optic disk, and the macula. The most common problems presenting to UCCs involving the vitreous humor are *vitreous hemorrhage, posterior vitreous detachment,* and, more rarely, *endophthalmitis.* There is a normal process of aging whereby the vitreous contracts and may actually separate from the retina or detach completely, producing a posterior vitreous detachment (PVD). Symptoms include floaters, photopsia, and decreased vision, often described by the patient as being "lace-like" or "cobweb" in nature. The diagnosis is usually made on the history alone, but examination of the fundus may reveal a vague opacity in the posterior segment. PVD requires no specific treatment but should be referred to an ophthalmologist for follow-up. Vitreous hemorrhage also presents with floaters and photopsia and some blurring of vision, but this blurring is usually more diffuse in nature. The diagnosis is usually made on funduscopy, where there is a more clearly delineated opacity in the area of the hemorrhage. Vitreous hemorrhage most commonly occurs in patients with either diabetic retinopathy or retinal tears, although it can also be seen in patients with sickle cell disease and macular degeneration. Patients with vitreous hemorrhage should be referred to an ophthalmologist and should be at bed rest with the head of the bed elevated until they are seen by the ophthalmologist.

The majority of cases of endophthalmitis follow either eye surgery or trauma, and these patients present with fever, pain, visual disturbances, discharge, and a clear history of either trauma or recent eye surgery. The slit-lamp examination usually shows a hypopyon (pus in the anterior chamber). These patients require urgent referral, intravenous antibiotics, and admission to the hospital.

Retina and Optic Nerve

The retina is in many respects the most active area of the eye, comprising an outer pigmented layer of retinal epithelium and an inner neural retina adjacent to the vitreous. The macula is the area of highest visual acuity (20/20) and is located approximately two disk diameters temporal to the optic nerve. The central avascular area of the macula, containing only cones, has a depression called the fovea. Visual acuity diminishes rapidly moving away from the fovea and in a normal person decreases to only 20/400 at 3 mm outside the fovea. The optic nerve, frequently referred to as the optic disk, enters the posterior aspect of the globe medial to the midline, accompanied by the central retinal artery and central retinal vein through a depressed area of the nerve called the optic cup. The ratio of the cup diameter to the nerve diameter is the cup:disk ratio and is important in evaluating patients for glaucoma. The central retinal artery and vein branch out to supply the retina in quadrants: superonasal, superotemporal, inferonasal, and inferotemporal. These are the landmarks utilized to describe optic pathology, particularly retinal landmarks. Only the posterior 40 to 50 percent of the retina can actually be visualized by the direct ophthalmoscope, and retinal tears and detachments are actually more common in the anterior portion. Experience with the ophthalmoscope should allow the physician to carefully inspect the retina for normal landmarks, hemorrhages, exudates, tearing, and detachment.

Patients suffering a retinal detachment often describe it as either a veil or a curtain falling across the visual field. They may also describe flashes of light or floaters, and almost all patients have some degree of visual loss, which is more marked if the macula is involved. Patients with retinal detachments should be referred immediately to the ophthalmologist, since some will have lesions amenable to surgical therapy.

One of the most important causes for urgent referral of patients in UCCs and EDs is *central retinal artery occlusion* (CRAO). Both CRAO and central retinal vein occlusion cause painless monocular vision loss, with arterial occlusion resulting in an ischemic stroke of the retina. On funduscopic examination, patients with CRAO show a paucity (or absence) of arterial vessels, normal retinal veins, a pale fundus, and a "cherry-red" macula (Fig. 7-6). Patients with hypertension, cardiac disease, collagen

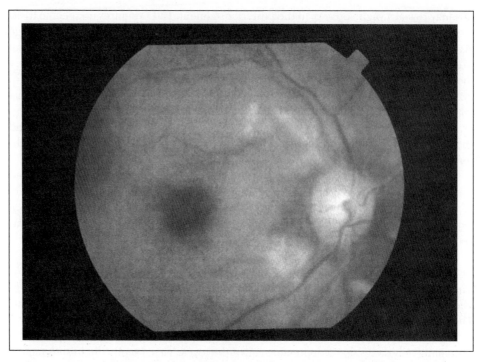

FIGURE 7-6 Central retinal artery occlusion. Note macular "cherry-red spot" and retinal pallor between macula and disk. The retinal veins appear normal in size, but the arteries are barely visible and attenuated. (From Tintinalli JE et al: *Emergency Medicine: A Comprehensive Study Guide*, 5th ed. New York: McGraw-Hill; 2000. With permission.)

vascular disease, vasculitis, sickle cell disease, and diabetes are particularly prone to CRAO. *Any patient with sudden, persistent, painless monocular vision loss should be assumed to have CRAO until proven otherwise, particularly since reestablishment of useful vision must be done as rapidly as possible.* Both clinical and bench research indicates that unless reperfusion is established within 80 to 120 min of the onset of illness, acceptable vision cannot be salvaged. When patients present with acute, persistent, painless monocular vision loss, the immediate therapy is gentle digital globe massage, followed by firm thumb pressure to the patient's closed lids for 5 s and then an abrupt release of this pressure, which should be repeated several times. An ophthalmologist should be called immediately and arrangements should be made for immediate transport to the nearest ED. Most authorities recommend breathing a mixture of 95% oxygen/and 5% carbon dioxide or rebreathing into a brown paper bag. These therapies are intended to direct or dislodge the embolus, dilate the artery to promote anterior blood flow, and reduce intraocular pressure to allow an increase in effusion gradient. Intraocular pressure can be manipulated by instilling timolol maleate 0.5% into the affected eye and administering acetazolamide 500 mg intravenously or by mouth.

Central retinal vein occlusion also causes painless monocular vision loss, with the severity of the symptoms depending upon the degree of venous obstruction. Vision loss ranges from minimal to quite dramatic. Thrombosis of the vein causes venous stasis, hemorrhage, and edema, producing a classic "blood and thunder" fundus (Fig. 7-7).

These patients often have a history of venous stasis disorders, hypertension, or vasculitis. Patients with central retinal vein occlusion should be referred to an ophthalmologist within 24 to 48 h for confirmation of the diagnosis. Unless contraindications are present, aspirin 325 mg daily should be started.

Immediate Ophthalmologic Referral of Nontraumatic Ocular Problems

There are four primary clinical presentations that require urgent ophthalmologic referral, three of which have already been discussed and one of which is discussed below (Table 7-3):

1. Central retinal artery occlusion
2. Orbital cellulitis/increase in retrobulbar pressure
3. Acute angle-closure glaucoma
4. Acute temporal arteritis

Patients with central retinal artery occlusion have an extremely limited period of time during which reperfusion must be established in order to save vision. These patients should receive the initial stabilizing therapy indicated above but should also have a telephone call placed immediately to the nearest ED and ophthalmologist to arrange for transfer and an attempt at a definitive therapy. Patients with CRAO should

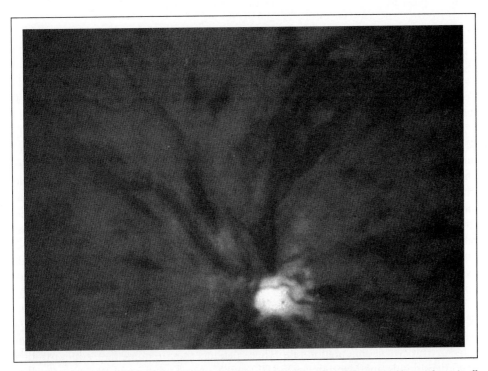

FIGURE 7-7   Central retinal vein occlusion "blood and thunder" fundus. Note diffuse retinal hemorrhages in all retinal quadrants and blurred disk margins. (From Tintinalli JE et al: *Emergency Medicine: A Comprehensive Study Guide*, 5th ed. New York: McGraw-Hill; 2000. With permission.)

TABLE 7-3

ACUTE NONTRAUMATIC OCULAR EMERGENCIES

Diagnosis	Treatment
Central retinal artery occlusion	Consult ophthalmology immediately Digital globe massage 95% O_2/5% CO_2 or paper bag breaths Timolol 0.5% one drop Acetazolamide 500 mg IV or PO Rapid transport to ED/ophthalmologist

Orbital cellutis/retrobulbar infection	Antibiotic therapy:
	    Adults: ticarcillin-clavulanate 3.1 g IV or
	    cefuroxime 1.5–3.0 g IV or
	    vancomycin 1–2 g IV <PCN alleg
	Children: cefuroxime 50 mg/kg IV
	CT scan of orbit
	Admission and ophthalmology consult

Acute angle-closure glaucoma	Timolol 0.5% one drop Pilocarpine 1–2%, 2 drops every 15 min Acetazolamide 500 mg IV or PO Mannitol 1 g/kg IV Consult ophthalmology immediately
Acute temporal arteritis	Prednisone 100 mg PO or methylprednisolone 250 mg IV Consult ophthalmology

be taken to the ED either by private vehicle or by ambulance, depending on which is faster. Patients with acute angle-closure glaucoma also require immediate ophthalmologic consultation, but a number of acute interventions can be taken at the UCC to help reduce intraocular pressure, including timolol (if not sensitive to beta blockers) and pilocarpine drops, acetazolamide, and mannitol. Consultation with the ophthalmologist and the ED must be immediate, but transfer can usually be effected by private vehicle rather than by ambulance. Patients with acute orbital cellulitis or other entities that increase retrobulbar pressure (retrobulbar hematoma, carotid cavernous fistula, and cavernous sinus thrombosis) also require urgent ophthalmologic consultation and hospital admission. In these patients, appropriate antibiotic therapy should be instituted if available, and most of them should be transported to the ED either by emergency medical services or by private vehicle, but only after consultation with the local ED and the ophthalmologist.

Temporal or giant cell arteritis often manifests itself as acute vision loss associated with eye pain, headache, and systemic symptoms of inflammatory arthritis, including a tender temporal artery, myalgia, and jaw pain. Most of the patients have a markedly elevated erythrocyte sedimentation rate. These patients require immediate administration of corticosteroids (methylprednisolone 250 mg IV or oral prednisone 100 mg) as well as urgent consultation and transfer to the ED for hospital admission.

TRAUMATIC OCULAR EMERGENCIES

Injuries to the eye and the surrounding structures are among the most common reasons for patients with eye problems to present to UCCs and EDs. The majority of these patients have fairly minor, often self-limited, and eminently treatable problems. However, patients with severe eye injuries may present to UCCs as well. This section describes the evaluation and treatment of these injuries.

Severe Eye Injuries

There are two eye injuries that require urgent evaluation and treatment: injuries penetrating the globe and chemical burns (particularly alkaline burns). Penetrating ocular trauma can result from quite dramatic sources, such as knife or gunshot wounds, but they are more commonly caused by metallic objects that penetrate the eye. Such wounds include carpentry injuries as well as those caused by lawn-mower projectiles, BB pellets, or other small metallic foreign bodies. Even the most seemingly innocuous projectiles can injure the eye and penetrate it. Therefore any patient who complains of a possibly projectile injury should be considered to have a penetrating injury to the globe until proven otherwise. For example, patients with lid lacerations from sharp objects should have both slit-lamp examination and, in most cases, radiographic examination to exclude penetrating foreign bodies. In all such cases, a detailed examination of the eye should be undertaken to search for a deep penetrating injury (traversing a single laceration of the cornea or sclera without an exit wound) or a perforating injury (involving two full-thickness lacerations). In particular, scleral rupture or penetration can often be missed if a careful examination is not performed, since the scleral layer is highly avascular. Scleral rupture or penetration should be suspected when there is diminished visual acuity, subconjunctival hemorrhage or chemosis, hyphema, or decreased intraocular pressure following ocular injury. Teardrop-shaped pupils usually indicate a laceration in the perilimbal region of the eye and can often result in prolapse of the ciliary body or iris. A shallow anterior chamber present on examination suggests the possibility of corneal penetration. Signs and symptoms of a ruptured globe include a shallow anterior chamber, an irregular pupil, hyphema, and change in visual acuity; on funduscopic examination, landmarks are often difficult or impossible to locate. Leakage of aqueous humor can be detected using the Seidel test. In a fluorescein-stained eye, leakage of aqueous humor from the anterior chamber will dilute the stain. Alternatively, the cobalt-blue setting on the slit lamp will show a lime-green color if aqueous humor is leaking from the eye. (Any time a metallic foreign body is a possibility, plain orbital radiographs should be obtained. These films alone cannot necessarily determine whether the foreign body is intraocular, but they may be helpful in determining the possibility of penetrating injury. In patients with a strong clinical suspicion or confirmation of a foreign body on plain radiography (even if the location is not fully known), such patients should be referred for CT scanning or ultrasonography of the eye. In most institutions, CT is the preferred methodology for localizing intraocular or potentially intraocular foreign bodies. When penetrating or perforating injuries of the globe have occurred, there should be no attempt to check the intraocular pressure; rather, a protective metal eye shield (Fox Shield) should be placed over the patient's injured eye without an eye patch.

Tetanus status should be quickly assessed and appropriate intravenous broad-spectrum antibiotics should be given while transport to the ED and consultation with the ophthalmologist are arranged.

Chemical injuries to the eye are true ocular emergencies and should be handled rapidly and aggressively. The eye should be irrigated copiously with at least 2 L of saline following rapid topical anesthesia and placement of a Morgan lens to allow for irrigation directly to the corneal surface. While acid and alkali burns are both serious, acid burns tend to coagulate the proteins on the surface of the eye, which often limits the depth of penetration. By contrast, alkali burns rapidly penetrate the cornea and cause substantial damage in a very brief period of time and may continue to cause damage until neutralized. The pH of the eye should be checked, the normal range being 7 to 8. Following copious irrigation, the eye should be carefully reexamined for current pH status, which should be carefully documented. A topical cycloplegic agent such as 1% cyclopentolate should be used for pain reduction in almost all cases. Topical ophthalmic ointment should be applied to the eye and the patient should be referred for immediate ophthalmologic evaluation.

Corneal Abrasions

Corneal abrasions are among the most common reasons for presenting to the ED or UCC and can be caused by foreign bodies, scratches (particularly in young children), gardening and carpentry accidents, sports injuries, etc. Regardless of the etiology of the corneal abrasion, the goal of the UCC physician should be to provide pain relief, prevent infection, facilitate healing, and provide for a rapid and thorough evaluation of the eye. The eye should be fully anesthetized and a complete examination, including slit-lamp examination and fluorescein staining, should be performed. In most cases, the diagnosis of corneal abrasion will be straightforward and the examination by an ophthalmoscope and slit lamp can be confirmed with fluorescein staining. Following fluorescein staining, the eye should be irrigated and the patient prepared for treatment. When the cornea has been damaged even to a mild degree, a prophylactic topical antimicrobial agent should be used for 2 to 5 days, either as ophthalmic drops or ointment. For patients wearing contact lenses, a fluoroquinolone agent should be utilized to provide antimicrobial coverage for *Pseudomonas* species. A cycloplegic agent should be administered to help relieve spasm. Cycloplegics that have an intermediate range of action are the most appropriate, since spasm persists for a number of hours. Either 1% cyclopentolate or 2% homatropine are reasonable choices. Significant controversy regarding the need for eye patching in patients with corneal abrasions continues to exist. While the literature supports either patching or no patching, it is largely a matter of personal preference. However, patches should not be used in contact lens wearers, diabetics, or immunocompromised patients, since secondary *Pseudomonas* infection frequently occurs.

Corneal Ulcers

Corneal ulcers most commonly result from posttraumatic infection that is allowed to set up superficially within the cornea and then invades more deeply. However, corneal ulcers can also develop from any break in the epithelial barrier; they are more common in contact lens wearers and patients with diabetes or other immunocompromised states. In addition, some patients have exposure keratitis due to an inability to close the lid completely (Bell's palsy, ectropion, etc.). The ensuing chronic exposure results in bacterial invasion of the cornea and the development of an ulcer.

Patients with corneal ulcers typically have a painful red eye with excessive tearing and photophobia. The discharge is rarely mucopurulent, but in severe infections it may progress to this state. Corneal examination shows an epithelial defect, which is often visible with the ophthalmoscope. However, during staining and examination with the slit lamp, the epithelial defect becomes much clearer and often has a white, somewhat hazy appearance underlying the defect and sometimes spreading into adjacent tissues (Fig. 7-8). If this condition is allowed to progress long enough, a hypopyon may also be present on slit-lamp examination. Because of their potential to progress to more serious infections, corneal ulcers should be treated aggressively with topical antibiotics, using a fluoroquinolone such as ofloxacin (Ocuflox) or ciprofloxacin (Ciloxan), utilizing one to two drops every hour in the involved eye. Cyclopentolate 1% (Cyclogyl), one drop three times a day, can be utilized as a topical cycloplegic agent to help with pain control. Under no circumstances should the eye be patched, since the risk of *Pseudomonas* infection is substantially higher following eye patching in patients with corneal ulcers. All corneal ulcers should be sent to the ophthalmologist within 12 to 24 h for further evaluation. In addition to the use of cycloplegic agents, oral narcotic pain medications may also be necessary for patient comfort.

Corneal Foreign Bodies

Patients with corneal foreign bodies are frequently seen in UCCs and EDs; such injuries may be caused by occupational, recreational, or home injuries. Patients typically present

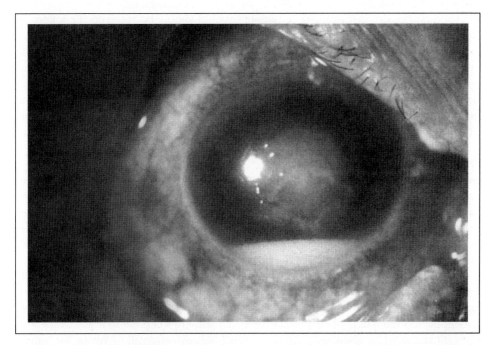

FIGURE 7-8   Corneal ulcer with hypopyon. The ulcer is seen as a shaggy white corneal infiltrate surrounding the borders of the epithelial defect. The hypopyon represents the accumulation of white cells layering out in the lower one-sixth of the anterior chamber. (From Tintinalli JE et al: *Emergency Medicine: A Comprehensive Study Guide,* 5th ed. New York: McGraw-Hill; 2000. With permission.)

with a clearly delineated history of a foreign object either being placed into or flying into the eye, followed by a consistent foreign-body sensation, pain, and variable degrees of photophobia, tearing, and discharge. Patients with such a history should be assumed to have a corneal foreign body and/or abrasion until proven otherwise.

The eye should be appropriately anesthetized with topical agents and a detailed examination of the eye undertaken, including everting both lids to assure that no foreign body is present. The slit-lamp examination is usually easily performed, although in some cases a retractor may be helpful to make sure that the upper lid is more easily everted during the examination. However, in most cases, a simple examination using the hand to retract the upper and lower lids can be performed and the cornea adequately visualized. The majority of corneal foreign bodies are superficial and can be removed easily and safely by using either an opthalmic spud, a small 25- to 30-gauge needle under slit-lamp magnification or a moistened cotton-tipped applicator. Prior to removal of the object, the slit-lamp examination should include an assessment for the depth of the injury.

Following removal of the foreign body, the slit-lamp examination should be repeated to make sure that the entire foreign body has been removed and that there are no other foreign bodies present. In addition, metallic foreign bodies can often create rust rings that are toxic to the corneal tissue. When rust rings are present, an ophthalmic burr should be utilized to remove as much of the rust as possible. In most cases, the entire rust ring can be polished off using the ophthalmic burr. However, even when rust has been thoroughly extracted on the initial examination, ongoing oxidation reveals additional rust on follow-up visits in some cases. All such patients should receive an ophthalmologic consultation or revisit within 24 to 48 h. Conversely, if all rust cannot be removed on the original evaluation, patients should simply be referred for follow-up within 24 h, since additional rust is likely to show up at that time as well.

All corneal foreign bodies involve some degree of corneal abrasion; therefore the eye should be treated with antibiotic ointment. As in the case of corneal abrasions, patching of the eye is a matter of personal preference and comfort and should be discussed openly with the patient, as either approach is acceptable. The patient should then be referred to an ophthalmologist to be seen within a 24- to 48-h period, with a strong preference toward a referral within 24 h.

Traumatic Hyphema

Blunt trauma to the eye can often result in bleeding in the anterior chamber. Hyphemas can also be spontaneous, but the majority seen in UCCs are due to blunt eye trauma. Most such bleeding occurs from blood vessels at the base of the iris, with the blood settling inferiorly due to gravity (Fig. 7-9). The hyphema can usually be easily visualized with the naked eye, the ophthalmoscope, or the slit lamp. Hyphemas are graded from I through IV based on the percentage of the anterior chamber occupied by blood (Table 7-4).

There is considerable controversy regarding the optimal management of patients with hyphema. In the past, all such patients were admitted to the hospital for bed rest and eye patching to help assure that spontaneous rebleeding did not occur. However, outpatient management of hyphema has become increasingly accepted, so that treatment of the patient should be discussed with the ophthalmologist who will be caring for him or her on an ongoing basis. Most ophthalmologists treat patients with class I injuries as outpatients, reserving inpatient therapy for injuries of class II and above. Regardless of whether inpatient or outpatient treatment is selected, the patient is put at bed rest and

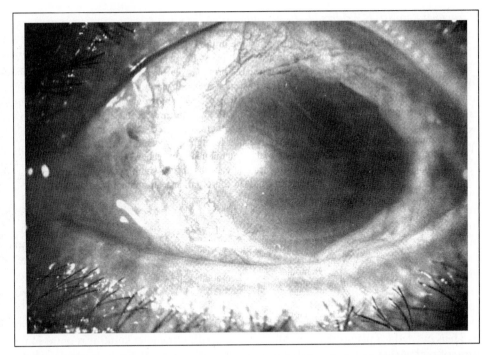

FIGURE 7-9 Hyphema secondary to blunt trauma. Note the blood filling the lower half of the anterior chamber and hazy appearance of the cornea, suggesting increased intraocular pressure. (From Tintinalli JE et al: *Emergency Medicine: A Comprehensive Study Guide*, 5th ed. New York: McGraw-Hill; 2000. With permission.)

eye rest with the head of the bed elevated to at least 45 degrees. In most cases, a protective eye shield is used and cycloplegia is instituted with topical drops. In some cases, children may require mild sedation to assure that their activity is appropriately decreased. Topical steroid drops such as prednisolone acetate 1% (PRED forte) one drop four times a day are also utilized. The IOP should be measured to assure that it is below 30 mmHg. If it exceeds this level, topical beta blockers such as timoptic 0.5% should be given and acetazolamide 500 mg should be given by mouth or intravenously. If the IOP does not drop quickly with this regimen, mannitol 1 to 2 g/kg IV may also have to be given.

TABLE 7-4

GRADING SYSTEM FOR TRAUMATIC HYPHEMA

GRADE	PHYSICAL FINDINGS IN ANTERIOR CHAMBER
Microscopic	RBCs in aqueous, no layering
Grade I	≤33% of anterior chamber
Grade II	33–50%
Grade III	50–95%
Grade IV	100%

Ultraviolet Keratitis ("Welders Flash" or "Sunburned Eyes")

As mentioned previously, one of the most common causes of keratitis or keratoconjunctivitis is exposure to ultraviolet or other forms of radiation. These patients are typically one of two types: those with a sudden acute flash of light such as "welder's flash" and those exposed to ultraviolet radiation without appropriate eyewear. Both etiologies result in similar clinical presentations of pain, tearing, photophobia, and a foreign-body sensation. These symptoms typically occur from 4 to 12 h following exposure to light. Slit-lamp examination and fluorescein staining show a classic superficial punctate keratitis, which appears as numerous small dots of staining on the corneal surface. A careful slit-lamp examination also shows these punctate dots even without fluorescein staining.

The primary goal in caring for patients with ultraviolet keratitis or keratoconjunctivitis is to provide pain relief, facilitate healing, and prevent infection while the epithelium replaces itself, usually within 24 to 48 h. As with corneal abrasions and corneal foreign bodies, the efficacy of patching the eyes remains controversial. In most cases the injury is bilateral, so the concept of patching both eyes is rarely utilized owing to patient discomfort with bilateral patching. Topical antimicrobials should be utilized for approximately 2 to 5 days, using ointments and/or drops as appropriate. Patients with contact lenses should be asked not to use them and antimicrobial coverage for *Pseudomonas* species with a fluoroquinolone should be utilized. Cycloplegic agents such as 1% cyclopentolate or 0.25% scopolamine should be used in each eye and repeated every 6 to 8 h as needed for pain reduction. Most patients with ultraviolet keratitis require some form of oral analgesia as well, including narcotic analgesics if the pain is severe. These patients should be referred to an ophthalmologist within 24 to 48 h.

Cyanoacrylate (Super Glue) Exposure

The most typical presentations of cyanoacrylate exposure occur at the extremes of age, in the elderly and young children. In the elderly, super-glue drops have been confused with therapeutic eye drops, resulting in eye exposure. Younger children, unless their house has been "poison proofed," may have access to super glue and accidentally instill it into the eye. Depending upon the amount of exposure, the eye may actually be glued closed in some cases. While the glue itself is not particularly toxic to the eye or the cornea, the hardness of the adhered glue may result in corneal abrasions. The eye should be irrigated copiously, and very gentle attempts at separating the adhered lids should be made. However, if the lids are tightly adherent even after adequate irrigation, the eye should be copiously covered with topical antibiotic ointment (erythromycin or other agents) and patched. Over 2 to 3 days, the glue typically loosens and becomes easier to remove. The patient should be referred to an ophthalmologist within 24 h and appropriate pain relief considered, particularly in those with presumed corneal abrasions. Patients should be instructed to repeat the erythromycin ointment application to the eye four to six times per day.

Traumatic Iritis and Iridodialysis

Following blunt trauma to the eye, inflammatory cells and exudate may enter the anterior chamber, causing acute iritis. Such patients usually present with a red eye (most common over the ciliary body) as well as photophobia and pain. Sports injuries quite commonly cause traumatic iritis, although any form of blunt trauma to the eye can cause these symptoms. The diagnosis of traumatic iritis is confirmed by slit-lamp examination, which shows red cells in the anterior chamber. Many of these patients also have traumatic iridodialysis, which is a tearing of the iris from its insertion site on the ciliary body and may be associated with hyphema. This often results in traumatic mydriasis, in which there is a dilated pupil that does not respond to either light or accommodation. Traumatic mydriasis is usually a transient phenomenon but can be permanent, depending on the degree of tearing of fibers. In any patient who is awake and alert but has posttraumatic anisocoria, traumatic mydriasis should be considered.

The treatment of traumatic iritis includes cycloplegic drops, appropriate oral pain medication, and referral to an ophthalmologist within 24 to 48 h. When traumatic mydriasis or iridodialysis is present, associated intraocular injuries should be excluded and the patient given the same treatment as for traumatic uveitis, with emphasis on adequate cycloplegia and pain medication. In some cases, the ophthalmologist may prefer to have patients placed on steroid ophthalmic drops as well, so the ophthalmologist should be consulted when this diagnosis is made.

CONTROVERSIES IN PATIENT MANAGEMENT

Topical Anesthetic Drops

Topical anesthetic drops form an important part of the adequate examination of the eye, since patients cannot tolerate a detailed examination of the eye without proper anesthesia, particularly when pain is a part of the initial presentation. Both proparacaine 0.5% and tetracaine 0.5% drops can be utilized; most patients find that proparacaine drops cause less discomfort. It is extremely common for patients with eye pain or other ocular complaints to request a prescription for topical anesthetic drops. Under *no* circumstances should these drops be prescribed to patients or given to them, since topical anesthetics alter the protective blink reflex, are toxic to corneal epithelium if administered for a prolonged time, and can lead the patient to further abrade or scratch the eye, since there is no sensation when the drops are in place. This should be carefully explained to the patient, and bottles of topical anesthetic drops should *never* be left in the patient's room, since there is a natural temptation to remove them.

Topical Antibiotic Drops versus Ointment

A large body of literature suggests that normal tearing mechanisms dilute topical antibiotic drops literally within seconds of the time that they are instilled within the eye. However, other literature suggests that the cornea and surrounding tissues may take up the antibiotic drops rapidly, even though they are present for only a short time. Because of the somewhat transient nature of topical drops, many authorities recommend the use of antibiotic ointments when topical agents must be utilized. However, the use of such ointments is somewhat messy, results in some discharge of the ointment from the eye, and may cause temporary blurring of vision because of the coating on the surface of the eye. While there are no clear-cut answers as to the best means to effect topical antibiotic therapy, some general principles do apply. First, in the case of both external and internal hordeola, the more prolonged contact with the tissue afforded by ointment suggests that it is the more effective therapy for these infections. Second, the more severe the infection or the greater the potential for secondary infection, the more ointments may be considered, since their contact with the eye does seem to last longer. Third, many ophthalmologists and emergency physicians use topical antibiotic drops during the day and ointments at night, when the problems with administration of ointment are less likely to present difficulties. However, both topical antibiotic drops and ointments are effective and undoubtedly have a place in the management of patients with eye infections and injuries.

Management of Patients with Hyphema

As indicated previously, considerable controversy exists regarding whether such patients should be handled as inpatients or outpatients, with a predominance of more recent literature suggesting that outpatient therapy is appropriate in most cases. However, because controversy still exists in the ophthalmology literature, virtually all cases of hyphema should prompt a telephone call to the treating ophthalmologist to determine his or her preference for the care of the patient.

Eye Patching

In the past, patients with corneal abrasions and other eye injuries routinely received eye patching, often with very careful instructions for how best to make sure that the eye remained closed until seen by the ophthalmologist in follow-up. However, more recent literature suggests that this may not be necessary. The primary reasons to patch the eye include patient comfort and the need to make sure that instilled ointments remain in contact with the eye for as long as possible. However, more recent studies indicate that pain and healing are no different in patients with corneal abrasions who are treated with or without eye patching. What is known is that eye patching does decrease corneal oxygen delivery and therefore might potentially decrease wound healing and reepithelialization. However, while oxygen saturations have been clearly documented to be decreased, no studies have indicated conclusively that wound healing and reepithelialization are markedly diminished in the presence of eye patching. What is quite clear is that eye patching should *never* be used in patients with corneal injuries secondary to the use of contact lenses or in diabetic patients, patients with corneal ulcers, or those with other immunocompromised states, since *Pseudomonas* superinfection is a substantial possibility when eye patching is used.

References

Barish RA, Naradzay JF: Ophthalmologic therapeutics. *Emerg Med Clin North Am* 13:649–667, 1995.

Berson FG (ed): *Ophthalmology Study Guide*, 5th ed. American Academy of Ophthalmology; 1987.

Hild WJ: *Revision and Translation of Sobotta/Figge—Atlas of Human Anatomy*, 10th English edition. Baltimore-Munich: Urban and Schwarzenberg; 1983.

Kirkpatrick J: No eye pad for corneal abrasion. *Eye* 17:468, 1993.

Knoop K, Trott A: Ophthalmologic procedures in the emergency department. Part I: Immediate sight-saving procedures. *Acad Emerg Med* 1:408–412, 1994.1

LaVene D, Halpern J, Jagoda A: Loss of vision. *Emerg Med Clin North Am* 13:539–560, 1995.

Newell FW: *Ophthalmology—Principles and Concepts*, 8th ed. St. Louis: Mosby; 1996.

Richard JM: *A Manual for the Beginning Ophthalmology Resident*, 3d ed. American Academy of Ophthalmology; 1980.

Stein HA, Slatt BJ, Stein RM: *The Ophthalmic Assistant—Fundamentals and Clinical Practice*, 7th ed. St. Louis: Mosby; 1999.

Tonsak RL: Visual recovery and combined central retinal artery and central retinal vein occlusion. *Am J Ophthalmol* 105:221, 1998.

Wilson FM II (ed): *Practical Ophthalmology—A Manual for Beginning Residents*, 4th ed. American Academy of Ophthalmology; 1996.

EAR, NOSE, AND THROAT

Deborah A. Loney / Jesse Wardlow

Ear, nose, and throat (ENT) complaints are among those that most frequently bring patients to the urgent care setting. Many of these disease processes are episodic, making the urgent care setting ideal for their evaluation and treatment, particularly when patients have no primary care physician or are unable to obtain an appointment with their private physician in a timely manner. It is important for all urgent care physicians to be well versed in the diagnosis and management of these entities. While many of these problems can be treated safely in the urgent care setting, it is incumbent upon urgent care physicians to know when emergent consultation and intervention is necessary.

THE ENT EXAMINATION

A thorough and detailed ENT evaluation often requires special equipment, setup, and supplies. Ideally an "ENT room" with an ENT chair, appropriate lighting, and all necessary equipment should be in place. Having all required materials easily accessible allows for an unencumbered examination—one that is more comfortable for both patient and physician. Use of the appropriate equipment will provide a better examination and ultimately better evaluation and treatment.

Examination of the ear requires an otoscope. There are two types of otoscope heads. The "closed" head is required to obtain a seal for pneumatic insufflation. The open head allows for magnification and the use of instruments for manipulation of cerumen, foreign bodies, etc. It is best to use the largest-diameter ear speculum that the ear canal will accommodate. This allows optimal visualization and room for manipulation. Other equipment that is useful for ear evaluation includes ear suction, irrigation equipment, curettes, ear wicks, and a tuning fork. Materials and medications that are useful include Calgiswab, Cortisporin-TC Otic Suspension and other otic antibiotic drops, tobramycin and dexamethasone (Tobradex) ophthalmic suspension, acetic acid/cortisone drops (Vosol HC), and cerumen-dissolving agents (i.e. hydrogen peroxide).

Examination of the nose and throat requires excellent lighting, usually via a properly functioning head lamp with or without a mirror. Nasal suction, nasal speculums, Gelfoam, packing material, bayonet forceps, and alligator forceps may also be required. Medications include 1% neosynephrine, cocaine, and 4% lidocaine.

OTITIS MEDIA

Otitis media is a descriptive term for inflammation of the middle ear cleft (mesotympanum). Numerous classification schemes have been devised, but it is easiest to classify them as follows:

1. Acute otitis media (AOM)
2. Otitis media with effusion (OME) (serous, mucoid, or purulent), and
3. Chronic otitis media with effusion (COME), or an effusion that persists for 3 months or longer after a diagnosis of AOM

AOM is common in the pediatric population. In infants less than 2 years old, it can present with fevers sometimes greater than 103°F. There may be irritability, otorrhea, lethargy, and otalgia of sudden onset. There may also be a history of ear tugging or antecedent symptoms of upper respiratory infection (URI). In older children and adults, the most common symptoms are ear pain, hearing loss, and tinnitus.

 Physical Examination

The normal tympanic membrane (TM) is described as pearly gray, neutral in position, and having the long process of the malleus (umbo) visualized with the short lateral process at its superior aspect. The TM is translucent and has a range of normal variation in color from blue to pink. On pneumatic otoscopy, mobility will be normal.

In AOM, the TM will be thickened. It may be bulging or retracted. The color may be red, white, or dark. In OME, air bubbles or air-fluid levels may be seen behind the TM. Sometimes frank pus can be seen in the middle ear space. The TM will have either decreased mobility or no movement with insufflation. If it is retracted, the TM may move only with negative pressure. It may also wrinkle with insufflation rather than move crisply in a lateral and medial direction.

- The "light reflex" may be absent in healthy ears and present in ears with effusions. Thus, it is not helpful in making the diagnosis.

Diagnosis of otitis media is made based on history and physical examination and should be documented based on the findings described above. The presence of fever should be noted. If the child is over 2 years of age, or has a negative examination, other sources of fever should be evaluated. Meningeal signs or swelling, erythema, or tenderness on the mastoid process (the bone behind the auricle) require immediate evaluation. If tympanometry is available, it can be used for confirmation of effusion.

Etiology

The most common organisms responsible have been well documented: *Streptococcus pneumoniae* (30 to 50 percent), nontypable *Haemophilus influenzae* (20 to 30 percent), *Moraxella catarrhalis* (10 to 20 percent), and group A streptococcus (1 to 5 percent). Other bacteria such as *Staphylococcus aureus* and gram-negative enteric organisms are rarely although consistently isolated in a few percent of patients. The number of beta-lactamase-producing bacteria has been on the rise over the last 10 to 15 years. Viruses also have recently been identified as causative or copathogenic organisms involved in otitis media.

Treatment

AOM has a 60 to 80 percent spontaneous resolution rate. Thus, some advocate no initial antibiotic therapy and treatment using only medications to address pain and fever as well as close observation. If the child is not better in a few days, then antibiotics are begun; several studies, however, suggest a higher rate of resolution and lower rate of complications if antimicrobials are given from the beginning.

The choice of antibiotic should be based on the presumed pathogen, local resistance patterns, patient age, disease duration, and history of antibiotic use.

Amoxicillin is still the antibiotic of choice to treat a first or infrequent episode; sulfa medications can be used in penicillin-allergic patients. Follow-up care is essential and should be with the primary care physician in 2 to 3 weeks.

Medications for the Treatment of Otitis Media*

1. Amoxicillin
2. Trimethoprim/sulfamethoxazole (TMP/SMX; Bactrim, Septra)
3. Erythromycin/sulfisoxazole (in the pediatric population)
4. Amoxicillin/clavulanate
5. Azithromycin
6. Cefuroxime axetil*

Bullous myringitis is an inflammatory/infectious condition of the TM which should be treated like AOM but may resolve more slowly. It is not well understood and may represent an atypical infection—e.g., due to *Chlamydia*.

Complications

Potential complications to be aware of can be divided into intratemporal and intracranial types. Intratemporal complications include hearing loss, TM perforation, subperiosteal abscess, cholesteatoma, acute or coalescent mastoiditis, petrositis, labyrinthitis, and facial paralysis. Postauricular pain, tenderness, swelling, and erythema; edema of the posterior superior canal skin; or protrusion of the pinna could be indicative of acute mastoiditis. Mental status changes and seizures are late complications of acute mastoiditis that may occasionally be seen.

Any patient with a draining ear and subtle signs such as headaches, fever, and nausea could possibly be exhibiting early presentation of intracranial complications. Intracranial complications include meningitis, intracranial abscess, sigmoid sinus thrombosis, otitic hydrocephalus, and epidural and subdural abscesses. Cranial neuropathies, vertigo, nystagmus, or disequilibrium can suggest impending intracranial complications.

*Adapted from Tintinalli J et al: *Emergency Medicine: A Study Guide.* New York: McGraw-Hill, 2000.

Other Causes of Ear Pain

If pain is present in an adult patient and there is only mild retraction or a normal examination, eustachian tube dysfunction may be present. Ask whether the patient experiences popping sounds with yawning or swallowing. In this case an oral decongestant and/or nasal spray may be of benefit.

Other potential etiologies for pain in a normal-appearing TM include referred pain from the temporomandibular joint, dental impaction, and infection. In patients who use alcohol and tobacco, malignant lesions of the hypopharynx, base of the tongue, or tonsil must be ruled out by an otolaryngology evaluation.

 Errors to Avoid

- Failure to recognize meningeal signs: vertigo, disequilibrium, and cranial neuropathies
- Misdiagnosis of Bezold's abscess (abscess over the zygoma or sternocleidomastoid muscle) representing acute mastoiditis
- Subtle signs of headache, fever, and nausea possibly indicating early presentation of intracranial complications

 Key Points of Documentation

- Presence or absence of otorrhea
- Temperature
- TM perforation
- History of recurrent episodes
- Appearance of tympanic membrane
- Hearing loss
- Facial nerve function
- Discharge instructions and follow-up care

Otitis Externa

Otitis externa (OE) is an infectious/inflammatory condition of the external ear, lateral to the tympanic membrane. It exhibits a range of severity from the mild form of "swimmer's ear" to a necrotizing otitis externa (formerly called malignant otitis externa), which is an osteomyelitis of the temporal bone.

Clinical Presentation

The chief complaint is ear pain. This can range from tenderness when laying the ear against a pillow to a sharp, continuous pain. There is often a complaint of muffled hearing or hearing loss. There may be drainage.

The history may include exposure to water in the ear (e.g., swimming, at the beauty parlor, after showering, etc.). Frequently there is a history of mild trauma to the ear canal a few days before onset of symptoms. Trauma may be caused by scratching or the use of Q-tips or hearing aids. Once the trauma and moisture have disrupted the normal layer of protective epithelium, the acute infective process may become self-perpetuating. Acute otitis externa is commonly caused by *S. aureus* or *Pseudomonas aeruginosa.* In some cases, however, there may be a history of prior treatment with eardrops containing antibiotics and steroid; when this is the case, a fungal OE is more likely.

 ## Physical Examination

On physical examination, inspect and document the appearance and color of the auricle, noting any erythema or edema. The ear canal may be extremely swollen and tender, to the point where the patient cannot tolerate the examination or no ear speculum will fit. This examination makes the diagnosis. If the ear canal *can* be visualized, it may be filled with watery exudate and desquamated skin cells.

1. Tenderness to gentle medial pressure on the tragus and/or gentle traction on the pinna is highly suggestive of OE, even in the absence of other symptoms.
2. Black specks of material that looks like pepper are suggestive of *Aspergillus* and a fungal OE.
3. If there is tenderness in the postauricular region or an asymmetrical lateralization of the pinna (particularly in children), a mastoiditis should be suspected and appropriate referral made.

For a thorough examination to be done, the ear canal should be cleaned of exudates and squamous debris. This is done under direct vision using the open-head otoscope and ear suction. Ideally, the patient is seated in a reclining position with the head supported and the chin up toward the ceiling. Even a straight-backed chair should be moved against the wall. The technique involves working from the center of the visualized portion of the canal and inserting the suction as far as you can see with the thumb hole uncovered. The thumb hole is then covered as you gently withdraw the suction, taking care to avoid/minimize contact with the ear canal. After each pass, debris is removed with a gauze and the suction cleaned by drawing saline through it. A narrowed meatus may be gently dilated with ear speculums of increasing sizes to facilitate visualization.

- Careful cleaning of the ear canal is important to permit penetration of topical antibiotics.

Treatment

Once the ear canal is clean, a wick should be inserted to help deliver the antibiotics to the infected site. Some commercially manufactured, preformed wicks are available. Otherwise, a ¼-in.-thick gauze strip (NuGauze) can be used. The wick is inserted less than ½ in. in length under direct vision. Drops should then be applied in the office and continued on an outpatient basis. The patient is advised that as the swelling goes down, the wick may fall out. Continued use of the prescribed drops until follow-up evaluation should be stressed, which should be in about 3 to 7 days, depending on the severity of the infection.

- It is important to instruct the patient to maintain strict dry-ear precautions during treatment and to avoid swimming or any further trauma to the ear.

Use of Topical Drops

Standard otologic drops are a combination of antibiotics and a steroid and are very effective in treating this condition. Most commonly used is Cortisporin-TC or Coly-Mycin S, which is a combination directed specifically toward the treatment of *Pseudomonas* and other gram-negative organisms.

- When treating otitis externa, the prescription should always specify "suspension," which is an aqueous preparation. The "solution" form is an oil-based preparation that floats above the edematous mucosa.

Ophthalmic drops containing tobramycin (Tobrex or Tobradex) or gentamicin (Garamycin) are sometimes used if a perforation is present or for individuals with a contact allergy. These drops have a more neutral pH and are less irritating to the mucosa of the middle ear. Recently, quinolone otic drops have been introduced to the market, which have excellent *Pseudomonas* coverage (Cipro-HC Otic). Acetic acid solutions (Vosol and Domeboro) acidify the external ear canal, creating a less favorable environment for fungal or bacterial growth; they may be effective in early management, but not for the more severe cases.

Patients who are elderly, diabetic (or with a family history of diabetes mellitus), debilitated, or immunosuppressed are at increased risk for *P. aeruginosa* infection of the ear canal. This is the principal etiologic agent for necrotizing OE. In patients who are high risk or have a discharge with a greenish tinge, it is best to treat with an oral quinolone and topical drops that cover *Pseudomonas*. Patients who are diabetic should have their blood sugar checked, and any patient who is ill-appearing should be considered for inpatient management.

Fungal otitis externa should be suspected when there is evidence for it on clinical examination ("black pepper specks" in the exudate), or if there is a history of abuse of previously prescribed antibiotic drops (which can lead to fungal superinfection). Sometimes the diagnosis is made with culture results. *Aspergillus nigrans* and *Candida* species are the common pathogens. The initial management requires careful cleaning of the ear canal to remove all fungal debris and then application of an antifungal cream or suspension directly to the ear canal.

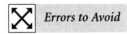 *Errors to Avoid*

- Failure to clean ear canal
- Failure to place wick
- Missing the presence of granulation tissue, which may indicate osteomyelitis (or malignancy)
- Failure to obtain temporal bone computed tomography (CT) scan if osteomyelitis is suspected
- Missing any cranial nerve palsies, as this is suggestive of skull-base involvement

Key Points of Documentation

- History of water exposure
- History of diabetes or immunocompromise
- Extent of edema
- Character of exudates
- Periauricular erythema or swelling
- Culture of the exudates if symptoms are persistent
- Stressing importance of water precautions
- Avoidance of trauma to ear
- Avoidance of wearing hearing aid until ear is completely clear

CERUMEN IMPACTION

Clinical Presentation

Cerumen impaction is a common problem seen in the urgent care setting. It often presents with complaints of hearing loss and pressure or discomfort in the ear canal. Less common presenting symptoms include tinnitus, vertigo, or headache.

The history should elicit any symptoms of ear pain, trauma, otorrhea, bleeding from the ear, perforation, acute or chronic otitis media, recurrent "swimmer's ear," or previous ear surgery.

On physical examination, the cerumen can range in color from light yellow to dark brown. It can be dry and hard or very moist and sticky. Cerumen can be mixed with hair or exfoliated skin cells from the external canal. These types of mixed impactions are much more tenacious and difficult to remove than the standard cerumen impaction.

Treatment

Irrigation

- If there has been a positive answer to any of the items in the history, this technique should not be performed due to the increased risk of infusing bacteria into the middle ear or predisposing the patient to otitis externa. Although this technique is frequently used without negative sequelae, the physician should be aware of this risk.

When irrigation is selected, a solution of 50:50 saline and hydrogen peroxide can be infused using a large metal ear irrigation syringe, which is commercially available. Alternatively, a large-volume syringe with a large-bore angiocatheter can be used. The patient should be draped for protection and an emesis basin or other receptacle used to catch the runoff. The auricle is grasped gently in the middle, posterior to the deepest portion of the concha, and gently retracted *laterally*. A gentle stream of irrigation solution should then be introduced against the posterior wall of the canal and directed medially. This is repeated until the impaction has come out, usually within about three syringes.

- If the patient has an adverse reaction (e.g., severe dizziness or pain) or if the impaction has not come out after persistent effort, alternative methods should be used.

Manual Removal

It is possible to remove cerumen using appropriate curettes and working through a large-bore ear speculum and an open-head otoscope. The ear canal is least sensitive superiorly and inferiorly; beginning in these areas, the examiner can mobilize the cerumen plug and remove it. This technique requires patience and practice. It is very easy to lacerate the skin of the external canal, which can lead to profuse bleeding. In these cases, the patient should be informed of the problem, started on eardrops, and referred for specialist follow-up.

Otic Drops

Alternatively, glycerite of peroxide can be used 2 to 3 days before further attempts at cleaning. Cerumen-dissolving agents should be used carefully, since their action is dependent on enzymes or chemicals that frequently irritate the canal and cause external otitis. These solutions may remove a mild to moderate impaction, but they will not remove an extensive one. When indicated, such patients should be referred to an otolaryngologist for follow-up.

- Patients should be counseled that if symptoms of tinnitus, vertigo, or headache persist after cerumen removal, further evaluation is necessary.

 Errors to Avoid

Do not perform irrigation if a history of otitis media, otitis externa, previous ear surgery, TM perforation, otorrhea, or otalgia is present.

- Failure to cease irrigation if increased pain, dizziness, or decreased hearing results
- Too vigorous irrigation resulting in perforation of TM

 Key Points of Documentation

- Prior history of cerumen impaction
- Prior history of otitis media or otitis externa
- History of otorrhea or otalgia
- Appearance of tympanic membrane and ear canals after cerumen removal

TRAUMATIC PERFORATION OF THE TYMPANIC MEMBRANE

 History

Traumatic perforation of the tympanic membrane (TM) is often caused by a stiff object (Q-tip, bobby pin, wooden match) used to scratch the ear canal. Through an unexpected bump, fall, or sudden movement, the object is pushed deep into the ear canal. The result is sharp pain, often accompanied by bleeding. A forceful slap with an open palm landing directly over the auricle, water sports (diving or water skiing), explosive injuries, or too forceful irrigation of the ear canal can also result in perforation. Welders, too, are prone to perforation when hot chips of metal fly into the ear canal. On history, patients with traumatic perforations may note severe but rapidly decreasing pain at the time of injury. Hearing loss—conductive, mixed, or sensorineural—is typical.

- Water-related injuries may become infected rapidly, resulting in a seropurulent discharge.

 Physical Examination

Blood will often be present in the ear canal. If it is fresh blood, it should be suctioned away using an appropriate suction and the open-head otoscope. Every effort should be made to visualize the entire tympanic membrane, including the circumference of the tympanic ring, to determine if there is a laceration of the canal wall's skin at the tympanic ring. Sometimes there will be a superficial laceration of the TM. The capillary circulation can cause enough bleeding to pose a significant problem in visualization. Topical application of a vasoconstrictive agent can be helpful (e.g., several drops of 1% lidocaine with epinephrine 1:100,000) for evaluation.

- Irrigation should never be used in an effort to clean the ear canal when a perforation is suspected.

In some cases, a blood clot will be present that cannot easily be suctioned away or removed with a curette, especially if it is lying against the tympanic membrane.

- Copious clear, watery drainage acutely may indicate a cerebrospinal fluid (CSF) leak. When this is noted, some fluid should be collected to evaluate for beta-lactamase. If a CSF leak is suspected, emergent consultation is required.

After clearing of the canal has been completed, the TM should be inspected with the closed-head otoscope, using the largest possible ear speculum. Insufflation should be performed. If there is movement of any visualized portion of the TM, the presence of a perforation is very unlikely. Nonetheless, these patients should still be referred for evaluation by an otolaryngologist, particularly when blood clots are present that have not been completely removed. If there is a partially obscured TM or if there is no movement of the TM when insufflating with a good seal, then a perforation is much more likely. When a perforation is visualized, always note the location of the perforation, which can have significant impact on treatment and patient management. Circumferential lacerations at the tympanic ring require more urgent ENT evaluation.

- A posterior superior perforation with symptoms of vertigo and nystagmus requires urgent otolaryngologic evaluation and possible operative exploration to rule out stapes dislocation and perilymphatic fistula.

The Weber examination with a tuning fork can be used to document the presence of a hearing loss.

- Remember that with a TM perforation (a conductive hearing loss), the patient should hear the sound in the injured ear!

Evaluation of the cranial nerves is also important, as well as notation of any nystagmus or vestibular symptoms, as these are indicative of inner ear damage. Also, since the energy of any traumatic force may be transmitted by the ossicular chain to the inner ear, an audiogram is essential. Last, if a severe force has caused the perforation, temporal bone and skull films should be obtained to determine whether a temporal bone fracture is present.

Treatment

Initial treatment consists of eardrops and dry-ear precautions. Many otolaryngologists will use antibiotic *ophthalmic* drops such as Blephamide (3 gtt., t.i.d. for 7 to 10 days). Ophthalmic drops are less irritating to the middle ear mucosa due to a pH that is generally closer to 7.4. (Avoid aminoglycoside drops, as these may be toxic to the inner ear.)

The patient should be instructed *in detail* not to let water get into the ear when bathing and to avoid swimming. The use of cotton coated with petroleum jelly (e.g., Vaseline) as an earplug while bathing will help to prevent water from getting into the ear. Depending on the mechanism of injury and the clinical setting, oral antibiotic prophylaxis may be indicated. Referral should be within a week.

Traumatic TM perforations often heal spontaneously with appropriate care; about 90 percent close spontaneously within 3 months. There is a risk, however, of implantation of external skin (keratinized epithelium) into the middle ear mucosal space. This phenomenon can lead to development of cholesteatoma, which requires otolaryngology evaluation and treatment.

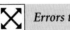 **Errors to Avoid**

- Failure to treat with otic drops
- Failure to instruct the patient to maintain dry-ear precautions
- Failure to instruct regarding the need for follow-up and audiogram
- Failure to note temporal bone fracture or evidence of inner-ear damage, which, if not caught early, might result in a "dead ear"
- Failure to recognize CSF leak

 Key Points of Documentation

- Cranial nerve function (especially the seventh cranial nerve)
- Presence or absence of vertigo/nystagmus
- Mechanism of injury
- Extent of bleeding
- Observations of the TM, especially canal obstruction, perforation, and the presence or absence of mobility
- Hearing loss with tuning fork evaluation
- Treatment plan

- Referral for audiogram and otolaryngologic evaluation
- Location, location, location of perforation

INFECTIOUS PERFORATION OF THE TYMPANIC MEMBRANE

 ## History

Infectious perforations occur as a complication of untreated acute otitis media. In this condition, pus is trapped in the middle ear space under pressure and eventually ruptures the TM, which is the weakest wall of that cavity. The patient typically gives a history of fever, pain, and hearing loss that is progressive over several days. The pain is relieved after the sudden onset of bleeding and discharge from the ear. Drainage may be intermittent or continuous and may be malodorous.

 ## Physical Examination

Findings of infectious perforations are ear canal drainage that is watery to purulent in color and a hole in the tympanic membrane. It may not always be possible to visualize the perforation initially due to purulent debris in the canal. Usually the opening will be pinhole-sized, located in the posterosuperior quadrant, with discharge that is pulsatile. The tympanic membrane will be inflamed and thickened.

Treatment

In most instances, local treatment with antibiotic eardrops (as discussed for traumatic perforation) combined with cleaning of the ear canal is the best initial therapy. Oral antibiotics may be added to the regimen if cellulitis and/or significant pain are present; however, they do not penetrate the pus well (which is like that in an abscess cavity) and are relatively ineffective. Goals of treatment are to eradicate the infection and drainage as well as decrease the likelihood of chronic disease. These goals are best realized by the direct application of medication to the infection.

 Errors to Avoid

- Treatment with oral antibiotics only
- Failure to clean ear canal to allow penetration of local antibiotic drops
- Failure to culture drainage if it has been of long standing
- Failure to stress the importance of follow-up, as a chronic process (i.e., cholesteatoma) may be present
- Missing signs of early mastoiditis (postauricular pain, tenderness, swelling, and erythema)

- Missing signs of early labyrinthitis (vertigo, nystagmus, disequilibrium, and hearing loss)
- Failure to recognize CSF otorrhea

 Key Points of Documentation

- Color, smell, and consistency of drainage
- Presence of pulsation
- Prior history of otitis media and ear drainage
- Vestibular symptoms

ACUTE TONSILLITIS

 History

This condition can present at any time from infancy to adulthood. The presentation consists of both systemic and localized signs and symptoms.

- Children with strep throat infections may complain of headache, fever, and vomiting initially, even prior to onset of throat pain

Systemic complaints include fever, chills, malaise, and loss of appetite. Localized symptoms include dysphagia, odynophagia, severe throat pain, otalgia, halitosis, and swelling and tenderness of the regional nodes. In severe cases, particularly when a peritonsillar abscess has developed, there may be a muffled quality of the voice ("hot-potato voice") and the patient may have dyspnea, particularly when lying down. The patient may be sleeping upright to avoid the prone position. These patients may also be unable to swallow their own saliva and present with drooling. There may be a history of prior sore throats or infections, raising the suspicion of an underlying chronic condition.

 Physical Examination

On physical examination, both the tonsils and the surrounding areas are generally swollen and erythematous. Yellow-white spots or follicles may be present on the tonsils, or, if severe, the spots may coalesce, resulting in a membranous or pseudomembranous tonsillitis. The tongue may be coated with a grayish covering and mucus thick and tenacious. Fetor oris may be present as well. Evaluation of the regional lymph nodes (cervical, occipital, and posterior cervical) may reveal marked tenderness and adenopathy. Fever is often present.

Laboratory Tests

A strep antigen test should be performed. If positive, the diagnosis is made. If negative, a follow-up throat culture should be obtained. In select patients, a Monospot test may be indicated to rule out mononucleosis, particularly if tonsillar hyperplasia is significant, a gray-white membrane is present on the tonsils, or tender cervical adenopathy in the posterior two-thirds of the chain is marked.

Treatment

The etiologic agent 5 to 20 percent of the time is group A streptococcus. Group B and C strep are also found, as are *Staphylococcus*, pneumococci, *H. influenzae*, *Escherichia coli*, *Clostridium difficile*, and *Mycoplasma pneumoniae*. First-line treatment is penicillin, amoxicillin, or erythromycin. Second-line treatments include cefuroxime, amoxicillin/clavulanate, azithromycin, and clarithromycin. Clindamycin should be given if halitosis is a prominent feature. Bed rest, hydration, analgesics, and antipyretic medications also play a role.

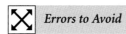 *Errors to Avoid*

- Failure to diagnose peritonsillar abscess (see "Peritonsillar Abscess," below)
- Failure to recognize infectious mononucleosis
- Failure to differentiate from
    Viral pharyngitis
    Diphtheria (firmly adherent grayish membrane, hoarseness, stridor, and croupy cough are additional symptoms)
    Scarlet fever (strawberry tongue and diffuse erythematous papular skin rash are added symptoms)
    Vincent's angina (gingiva or tonsillar bleeding and gangrenous stomatitis)

 Key Points of Documentation

- Presence or absence of dysphagia or dyspnea
- Throat culture or results of rapid strep test
- Symmetry of tonsil and oropharyngeal examination
- Ability to control secretions
- Presence or absence of trismus
- Voice quality
- Airway patency, including tonsillar size
- Examination of all regional nodes

PERITONSILLAR ABSCESS

Peritonsillar abscess is usually a complication of recurrent tonsillitis and occurs when infection penetrates the lateral capsule of the tonsil and spreads into the peritonsillar space. Patients complain of progressive throat pain with odynophagia, ipsilateral otalgia, dysphagia, and dyspnea when lying down. Often these patients are drooling because they cannot swallow their own saliva. Mild to moderate trismus may be present, as well as a "hot-potato voice."

 Physical Examination

The patient is often febrile, although fever may be low-grade. The oral cavity shows asymmetrical bulging of the soft palate. At times a pointing area of the abscess can be seen and pus may be draining from this site. The uvula may be pushed away from the midline. The tonsils are enlarged and may be asymmetrical in appearance due to the pressure of the abscess occupying the lateral peritonsillar space. The tonsils may be displaced medially, forward, and downward. Exudative tonsillitis may or may not be evident. Cervical lymphadenopathy may be present. Trismus, if present, suggests inflammation involving the muscles of mastication and possible spread of the infection beyond the peritonsillar region.

Laboratory Studies

The white blood cell count (WBC) is usually elevated, sometimes markedly so (greater than 20,000/µL).

Diagnosis

The diagnosis can often be made clinically, based on the history and physical examination, particularly if a pointing abscess is seen.

At times, the clinical picture can be unclear between a severe tonsillitis and peritonsillar abscess. Sometimes a phlegmon (extensive soft tissue edema without the formation of a loculated abscess) is present. In these cases, computed tomography (CT) of the neck with contrast is the most useful imaging study.

Treatment

If an abscess is identified either clinically or radiologically, it must be drained; when the diagnosis of peritonsillar abscess has been made, the patient should be transferred to the care of an otolaryngologist or surgical specialist for emergent treatment due to the risk of developing deep neck infection and airway compromise. The patient should receive intravenous antibiotic coverage immediately (clindamycin, ampicillin/sulbactam, or cefuroxime are good choices), as well as hydration, analgesia, and/or steroids (once the WBC has been checked).

The treatment for an abscess is incision and drainage, with antibiotic coverage as appropriate. In an older adolescent or adult, incision and drainage may be done in the clinic setting. Large-bore needle aspiration of peritonsillar abscess has been advocated; however, the inability to open loculated areas with this method may lead to undertreatment and subsequent recurrence. In a child or adult with a history of recurrent peritonsillar abscesses or recurrent acute tonsillitis, it should be done in the operating room with a concurrent tonsillectomy (quinsy tonsillectomy).

If, on computed tomography (CT) scan, a phlegmon is diagnosed (soft tissue edema without a specific fluid collection) and there is no clinically apparent abscess on examination and no airway compromise, the patient may be treated with intravenous antibiotics and observed.

 Errors to Avoid

- Failure to recognize and manage urgently, leading to spread to lateral pharyngeal space

 Key Points of Documentation

- Asymmetry of tonsils or soft palate
- Presence or absence of trismus
- Otalgia
- Dysphagia
- Dyspnea
- Drooling
- Cervical adenopathy

Postoperative Tonsillectomy Bleeding

Postoperative tonsillectomy bleeding is a condition that occurs after tonsillectomy reportedly about 0.1 to 9.3 percent of the time. Hemorrhage after tonsillectomy and adenoidectomy (T&A) has been divided into primary (bleeding that occurs in the first 24 h postop), and secondary (bleeding that occurs later on). Primary hemorrhage is more likely to be serious and require acute operative intervention due to the brisk bleeding and impaired airway protection. The reopening of small vessels in the surgical wound usually causes the hemorrhaging. Secondary bleeding generally occurs 7 to 10 days after surgery and is believed to be due to a blood vessel being uncovered when the postoperative eschar falls off. Other factors such as advancing the diet too quickly; smoking postoperatively; ingestion of aspirin, ketorolac, ibuprofen, or other products that would impair clotting function; and dehydration may also play a role.

 History

The patient may present with sudden onset of bleeding from the mouth and possibly airway compromise after tonsillectomy. More frequently, bloody stains on the bed linen or blood on lips or tongue caused by short-lived, self-limited episodes of bleeding are noted. There may be a history of excessive swallowing and nausea and vomiting prior to the incident. It is important to obtain estimates of the amount of blood lost and any history of drug use that would affect clotting.

Laboratory Studies

Hemoglobin and hematocrit values should be obtained as well as PT, PTT, and a platelet count. If the blood count is extremely low or the patient is symptomatic, in-house observation may be required, since the values will drop with intravenous hydration. In some cases, transfusion may be necessary.

 Physical Examination and Treatment

- In unstable patients, an in-depth evaluation should be forgone and the patient stabilized for emergency transport.
- The operating surgeon should always be contacted and informed of the problem as early as possible in the evaluation. Secondary to the potential for serious rebleeding, patients with a primary hemorrhage will often require transfer to the operating room for evaluation in a more controlled setting and in the presence of a larger support staff.
- Blood pressure readings must always be checked and documented in adult patients, and for evaluating both for hypotension and for uncontrolled hypertension.

The following recommendations for evaluation and treatment are guidelines to be used only if the operating surgeon is not available.

The examination should be carried out bimanually, using a headlight. Necessary equipment includes topical anesthetic spray (lidocaine, Ponticaine), several tongue blades, long curved tonsil clamps, round tonsil sponges, 1% lidocaine with 1:100,000 epinephrine, long silver nitrate cautery sticks, bite blocks (for young children), and Yankauer suction.

For a thorough examination, topical anesthesia must be applied and allowed to take effect in order to suppress the gag reflex. In children under 8 years of age, it may be necessary to use a bite block.

Bleeding usually occurs from the inferior aspect of the tonsillar fossa. Two tongue blades should be used along with the suction to remove saliva and exudates. The inferior aspect of both tonsillar fossae should be inspected. In some cases, as soon as the patient's mouth is open, a large blood clot may be seen. This is indicative of a severe bleed, which should be immediately referred to the operating surgeon or other appropriate specialist. The clot should not be dislodged, as this may lead to active hemorrhage. These patients should be stabilized as needed and transferred without delay to the emergency department.

Sometimes only granulation tissue will be seen. In these cases, a tonsil sponge soaked in 1% lidocaine with 1:100,000 epinephrine can be grasped on a long tonsil clamp and pressed into the area with the granulation tissue. Firm pressure should be placed on the area for 15 min. Initially, the patient will have some discomfort, but he or she soon adjusts to the presence of the clamp. The suction is used to remove excess saliva.

After 15 min, the area is reinspected. Any visible granulation tissue is cauterized with silver nitrate cautery, using two sticks at a time. The patient is then observed for another 30 min.

If the hemoglobin and hematocrit levels are normal and there is no evidence of active bleeding, these patients may be discharged with referral for specialist follow-up within 24 h.

The patient should be instructed to be on a liquid diet, avoid all heavy lifting, and follow up with the operating surgeon. He or she should also be warned that rebleeding may occur, in which case surgical intervention could be necessary. The patient is instructed to take only acetaminophen or acetaminophen with codeine elixir, avoiding aspirin and other nonsteroidal anti-inflammatory drugs (NSAIDs).

 Errors to Avoid

- Failure to contact operating surgeon
- Failure to refer appropriately
- Dislodgement of clot during examination, leading to recurrence of acute bleeding
- Failure to obtain family history of bleeding abnormalities
- Failure to discover and address elevated blood pressure
- Failure to identify ingestion of products that affect clotting function (this includes Gingko biloba and garlic pills)

 Key Points of Documentation

- Physical findings
- Hemoglobin and hematocrit
- Efforts to contact and recommendations of operating surgeon
- Blood pressure

LUDWIG'S ANGINA

Ludwig's angina is a bilateral submandibular and lingual space infection characterized by rapid spread via direct extension. In this condition, there is generalized induration of the submandibular space, which is not limited to the submandibular gland. Oro-dental disease, particularly of the second and third lower molars, frequently gives rise to this infection. *Streptococcus* and bacterial anaerobes including *Bacteroides* are usually the cause.

- Ludwig's angina often develops as a complication of a molar tooth abscess.

Clinical Presentation

The site of the infection dictates the symptoms. If it is above the mylohyoid muscles, brawny edema may displace the tongue upward and posteriorly, thus threatening the airway and resulting in difficulty breathing, especially when the patient is supine. If the submandibular spaces are involved, difficulty swallowing, neck pain, odynophagia, or referred otalgia may result. Often systemic symptoms such as fever, chills, and malaise may be present as well.

On physical examination, there is generalized inflammation with erythema and tenderness of the overlying skin; a diffuse, tense, brawny submandibular swelling is present that may spread into the neck. A purulent mouth odor (halitosis) may be noted. Though significant trismus, which often is present, may limit evaluation, the floor of the mouth should be examined. It may be firm to palpation and the tongue may be elevated and pushed posteriorly. Careful inspection of the lower molars may reveal dental disease. Generally, diffuse tender lymphadenopathy, which may be significant, is associated. Any stridor, hoarseness, or shortness of breath suggests that the infection may have spread into the neck, leading to airway compromise.

Diagnosis

The diagnosis is made based on the history and physical examination. The condition may be due to dental infection, sialoadenitis, or tonsillitis. In severe cases, it may be difficult to determine the extent of the infection. If there is any significant trismus or suspicion of airway compromise, a CT scan of the neck with contrast is indicated to determine the extent of the infection and identify possible abscess formation.

Treatment

- All patients presenting with Ludwig's angina require an emergent otolaryngology referral with transfer for inpatient treatment.

Treatment consists of intravenous antibiotics and surgical drainage when necessary. Antibiotic coverage, which can be started in the urgent care center if it will not delay definitive treatment, should be directed at streptococcal species and other oral pathogens. In early, limited cases—without evidence of airway compromise, trismus, or dysphagia—antibiotic therapy alone may be adequate. There is, however, a high risk of airway compromise due to spread of the infection into the neck; airway compromise is the major cause of death. Urgent intubation or even tracheotomy may be required.

Surgical intervention is usually indicated to relieve tissue pressure even if an abscess has not yet formed. Immediate otolaryngology consultation is indicated, particularly if there are any symptoms indicating progression of disease beyond a very localized area.

- At times, an infected tooth must be extracted and any abscesses must be drained.

 Errors to Avoid

- Underestimation of the rapidity with which the infection can spread
- Failure to rapidly diagnose and treat, leading to extension of the infection to the lateral pharyngeal and retropharyngeal spaces or the mediastinum
- Failure to address orodental disease that represents the source of infection

Key Points of Documentation

- Prior history of dental or oral infection
- Imaging study to identify the presence of abscess
- Status of airway
- Condition of dentition, with close attention to lower molars

RHINOSINUSITIS

Sinusitis is now being classified as rhinosinusitis by the Academy of Otolaryngology Head and Neck Surgery since it is usually associated with nasal symptoms; this classification also distinguishes sinusitis from other headache symptoms of a different etiology. Sinusitis is typically caused by aerobic organisms including *Streptococcus pneumoniae, H. influenzae, Branhamella catarrhalis*, and *Streptococcus pyogenes*. Other organisms may also contribute, including viruses, which may initiate an acute mucosal reaction. Once the sinus is obstructed, growth of pathogens ensues.

 History

Often the symptoms of sinusitis are little different from those of URI. Unless localizing pain or physical findings indicate purulent pyogenic infection, a diagnosis of sinusitis should be considered only if the symptoms have been present beyond 7 to 10 days. Facial pain, nasal obstruction, purulent discharge, and hyposmia are classified as major symptoms of sinusitis. Minor symptoms include fever, halitosis, dental pain, fatigue, and cough.

 Physical Examination

On examination, the patient has edematous, inflamed nasal mucosa with yellow-green exudates visible in the nose. Percussion of the sinus areas (maxillary, ethmoid, frontal) may elicit tenderness. The patient may be febrile. Periorbital swelling or erythema, anisocoria, chemosis, proptosis, ocular dysmotility, meningismus, and diplopia are all indications of complications that require emergent referral.

The diagnosis of rhinosinusitis is primarily made on the basis of history and physical examination. Confirmatory studies include a white count (which may be normal or elevated) and plain sinus films. If a maxillary or frontal sinus is opacified on x-ray, a diagnosis may be made. (Plain films, however, frequently do not provide sufficient detail, and there is a high false-negative rate for sphenoid and ethmoid sinuses.) If complications are suspected, a CT scan of the sinuses (not the head or brain) should be ordered. Bone window images in axial and coronal sections provide the most useful information. Contrast can be helpful to distinguish periorbital cellulitis from subperiosteal abscess. Magnetic resonance imaging (MRI) may be used in conjunction with CT to localize abscesses or define the extent of an infraorbital inflammatory process. Uncomplicated cases of sinusitis do not require CT scanning, since they will almost invariably have positive findings.

Nasal cultures have been found to be very inaccurate unless performed at the sinus outflow tract under direct endoscopic vision. It is generally not useful to swab the nose due to the routine colonization of S. *aureus* in the nares and nasal vestibules of many individuals. The primary organisms that cause sinusitis are well known. Thus, in the routine assessment of any uncomplicated acute sinusitis, antibiotic therapy need not be culture-based.

Treatment

The treatment must be directed at the most common organisms for the upper respiratory tract, taking into account regional rates of resistant organisms and the patient's prior therapy. For first-line therapy, amoxicillin in areas of low resistance and amoxicillin with clavulanic acid in areas of high resistance are appropriate. The penetration of the sinus mucosa and sinus fluid contents should be adequate with the penicillins, cephalosporins, sulfonamides, macrolides, and quinolones.

Additionally, it is necessary to treat the inflammatory/obstructive component of the problem in order to promote sinus drainage. Oxymetazoline or neosynephrine (over the counter), two sprays each nostril two to three three times a day for 3 to 4 days will help to maximize the opening into which the purulent secretions can be drained. Nasal cilia can be paralyzed by oxymetazoline; thus, it is important to limit the duration of therapy. In nonbacterial cases or after several days of decongestant spray usage, the patient should begin one of the anti-inflammatory steroidal nasal sprays or a saline nasal spray. If the drainage is very thick, guaifenesin (600 to 1200 mg b.i.d.) will help to thin it, thus promoting sinus drainage. Inhalation of steam may also be helpful. One regimen for management includes installation of over-the-counter decongestant spray followed by inhalation of a saline nasal solution and 20 min of steam inhalation. This regimen can be repeated with each use of the decongestant spray. If allergic symptoms are present (such as sneezing or itching), steroid spray will help control many allergic symptoms. Promoting drainage rather than drying up of secretions is the main objective, so antihistamines and/or oral decongestants should be used only after the acute episode has resolved.

Complications

Sinusitis that is undertreated or untreated may give rise to serious complications involving the orbital, periorbital, and intracranial spaces. Orbital and periorbital complications have a reported incidence of anywhere from 0.05 to 3.9 percent. Orbital extensions of sinusitis are predominantly of ethmoid origin and occur most frequently in pediatric and adolescent patients who are anatomically predisposed. Orbital involvement ranges from periorbital cellulitis to subperiosteal abscess to orbital cellulitis or abscess. Periorbital cellulitis presents as sinusitis with predominant findings of eyelid edema, tenderness, and erythema; visual acuity is normal.

Direct extension of ethmoid or frontal sinusitis results in formation of a subperiosteal abscess. In addition to the findings of periorbital cellulitis, these patients may have proptosis with either lateral or downward globe displacement. Orbital cellulitis due to an inflammatory reaction with the globe results in proptosis, chemosis, and possible ulcerations of the globe. Erosion of a subperiosteal abscess or coalescence of orbital cellulitis may give rise to an orbital abscess with severe proptosis, chemosis, pain, optic neuritis, and partial or complete ophthalmoplegia; blindness may result.

Intracranial infections due to sinusitis have a reported incidence of 3.7 to 5.9 percent. The frontal sinus is the most frequent cause, followed by the ethmoids, sphenoids, and infrequently the maxillary sinuses. Adolescents and young adults are at highest risk. Frontal lobe cerebral abscess, meningitis, epidermal abscess, subdural abscess, and cavernous sinus thrombosis are the intracranial infections that result from sinusitis in descending order of frequency. In addition to the usual symptoms of sinusitis, persistent headache and spiking fevers should raise one's suspicion. Once meningeal signs appear, mental status changes and neurologic deficits may rapidly follow. Cavernous sinus thrombophlebitis additionally may present with proptosis, anisocoria, ophthalmoplegia, V_1 and V_2 anesthesia, as well as decreasing visual acuity. Many of these potential complications have a high morbidity and mortality rate. Thus, once there is a suspicion of extrasinus extension of disease, an imaging study and specialist consultation should urgently be obtained.

 Errors to Avoid

- Prescribing oral decongestants inappropriately
- Failure to stress need to limit use of decongestant nasal sprays (as "rebound" effect may result)
- Missing signs or symptoms of extrasinus extension: eyelid changes, proptosis, chemosis, ophthalmoplegia, decreasing visual acuity, spiking fevers, etc.
- Failure to obtain the correct imaging studies when indicated
- Failure to use adjunctive treatments (e.g., mucolytics, steroid nasal sprays, saline nasal sprays as indicated) to facilitate drainage
- Performing a lumbar puncture without ensuring absence of an intracranial abscess first (as brain herniation may result)

 Key Points of Documentation

- The presence of drainage: color, location, and viscosity
- Orbital description, including presence or absence of lid edema, erythema, tenderness, or globe mobility
- Appearance of nasal mucosa, with attention to any gross structural abnormalities, growths, or lesions
- Any sinus tenderness to palpation
- Instructions for follow-up care

EPISTAXIS

Epistaxis is a common problem, which can progress to a life-threatening situation. Patients may present actively bleeding or with a history of previous or intermittent epistaxis but no active bleeding at time of presentation.

History

The history should include questions regarding any recent nasal trauma, surgery, or unusual bleeding tendency—e.g., frequent nose bleeds, bleeding from the gums, prolonged bleeding after injuries or surgery, family history of bleeding abnormalities, or easy bruisability. Details of the immediate epistaxis history should be taken, including frequency, duration, on which side the bleeding occurred, and whether blood came from the mouth. Vital signs may detect uncontrolled hypertension, which should be brought under control. Medication history may include usage of aspirin or other NSAIDs or anticoagulants. Many patients take aspirin daily based on recommendations of the popular press. All medically prescribed anticoagulation or antiplatelet therapy should be discontinued (unless absolutely contraindicated) with appropriate consultation with the prescribing/primary care physician. Patients who are on anticoagulants will require a stat PT/PTT. Laboratory tests (CBC, PT/PTT, platelet count) may also be indicated if there is suspicion of significant blood loss, underlying bleeding disorder (including iatrogenic causes), or aspiration.

 Physical Examination

- Universal precautions should be observed, with the examiner covered in a body suit or gown, a fluid-shield mask, and gloves. The patient should also be appropriately covered and gowned.
- An emesis basin is held by the patient at chin level for expectoration and/or a working area for the examiner to place instruments.

Equipment
Headlight (or head mirror), bayonet forceps, nasal suction, nasal speculum. Consumable materials include 50:50 mixture of 1% neosynephrine (or cocaine) and 4% lidocaine (or cocaine), cotton balls, Gelfoam.

The nasal cavity extends directly posterior into the head. To minimize patient discomfort and cooperation, it is very important to put in the time and effort to achieve topical anesthesia. Although the patient will feel you working, pain sensation should be significantly decreased.

- Anatomic obstacles to working in the nose include septal deviation, turbinate hypertrophy, and maxillary crest hypertrophy.

Patients Who Are Not Actively Bleeding
Initially, a topical decongestant/anesthetic (solution) should be sprayed into the nose with a hand-held or powered atomizer. Cotton pledgets soaked in topical solution can then be placed in the nose using the bayonet forceps under direct illumination provided by the headlight. These are placed along the septum as far posteriorly as possible along the floor of the nose and higher to the region of the middle turbinate. They should be left in place for approximately 10 minutes, then removed with the forceps. Suction is used to remove excess mucus and blood clots, taking care to note which side the bleeding appears to be

on and any mucosal lesions. The region of Kiesselbach's vascular plexus on the nasal septum (the site of many nosebleeds) should specifically be examined.

Silver nitrate sticks should be used to cauterize any suspicious areas including visible blood vessels, granulation tissue, or mucosal excoriation. Sometimes two sticks at once should be used. They should be applied for several minutes at a time. Check the posterior oropharyngeal wall for any continued bleeding.

Even if the bleeding is controlled, patients who are at high risk for rebleeding (the elderly, patients who are anticoagulated, those with a coagulopathy) should have the involved side of the nose packed with Gelfoam coated with antibiotic ointment. Fairly long pieces of Gelfoam (4 to 6 cm) should be used, which are pressed down manually and folded over into a "V." These are then coated with antibiotic ointment and inserted with the bayonet forceps using firm, gentle, continuous pressure. The forceps may have to be repositioned several times as they pass through the Gelfoam. This step creates a hemostatic compression packing. The nasal mucus breaks down the Gelfoam; within 48 h, it will slide out atraumatically. The patient should be counseled that this will occur and should be instructed to begin using a nasal saline spray (OTC product, three sprays t.i.d.) after 48 h. Patients should also be instructed not to attempt any lifting heavier than a book, not to bend over, and if they have to sneeze, to do so with an open mouth. Follow-up should be in 1 week with the primary care physician.

Patients Who Are Actively Bleeding

The principles of control are similar, particularly with regard to thorough preparation of the patient and examiner and with all of the materials mentioned above readily at hand.

- With active bleeding, there will be more need for suction.

Initial efforts to control bleeding should take the form of direct pressure applied to the entire soft part of the nose, which is pinched between the thumb and forefinger of the patient or examiner for 10 min (20 min if anticoagulation or antiplatelet activity is involved). Topical solution is applied as described above. Using the nasal speculum and the headlight, a thorough examination is performed to check for specific bleeding points. These are then cauterized with silver nitrate. When bleeding is controlled anteriorly, the oropharynx is checked for posterior bleeding.

In some cases, the examiner will not be able to visualize and/or control the bleeding site. Sometimes the site will be hidden behind a septal deviation or bony spur. Sometimes there will be multiple bleeding sites, particularly if the patient has had recent packing and this is a recurrent episode. After a systematic effort has been made to control the bleeding, nasal packing should be inserted. This is a pressure type of packing which remains in place for at least 48 h. One or both sides are packed as indicated by the clinical situation. If both sides are packed, antibiotic prophylaxis is required with coverage for *S. aureus*, the causative agent for toxic shock syndrome.

The classic packing technique that is often used and described is the layering technique using Vaseline gauze ribbon (½ by 72 in.). In this technique, working in the anesthetized nose and using the headlight and bayonet forceps, the gauze strip is laid along the floor of the nose as far posteriorly as possible in a continuous strip. The ribbon is laid down in a layered fashion until the nose is completely packed. Excess ribbon is trimmed.

The first layer should be grasped about 6 in. from the end. This allows the free end to hang out of the front of the nose, thereby minimizing the chance of its falling back and stimulating the gag reflex when the patient gets home.

Another technique involves the use of inflatable surgical sponges. These are available in a commercially prepackaged form; the loose ones are larger and provide more pressure. They can be trimmed with a scalpel blade as appropriate. Lengths of 8 or 10 cm should be used. The sponge is placed inside the longest finger of a powder-free glove, from which it has been cut. This is then coated with antibiotic ointment. If there is no drawstring on the sponge, one can be created by placing a surgical stitch through the free end of the sponge, tying it in position, cutting off the needle, and leaving the ends long. This is then inserted with firm, gentle pressure directly posterior with the inferior edge along the floor of the nose. (Insertion will be uncomfortable for the patient.) The sponge can then be inflated with saline injected into the glove's finger through an angiocatheter. Subsequent management is the same as for ribbon packing.

Posterior Epistaxis

If there is persistent bleeding in the oropharynx despite these maneuvers or if the bleeding cannot initially be controlled via the anterior approach, a posterior bleed may be present. Patients with posterior bleeds require posterior packing and/or surgical intervention. These patients require hospital admission for observation, antibiotic coverage, sedation, continuous pulse oximetry, and supplemental oxygen.

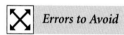 **Errors to Avoid**

- Inadequate preparation of needed materials to permit the examiner to work with two hands and with adequate light
- Inadequate nasal decongestion and inadequate topical anesthesia
- Antibiotic prophylaxis if both nostrils are packed
- Alar notching by poor positioning of packing
- Failure to ambulate patient prior to discharge to check for rebleeding
- Failure to check chest x-ray if aspiration is suspected

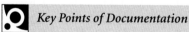 **Key Points of Documentation**

- Blood pressure
- History of epistaxis
- Medications that may affect coagulation
- Dominant side of bleeding
- Identification of bleeding site
- Cessation of active bleeding anteriorly and posteriorly after treatment
- Family history of bleeding abnormalities
- Home care instructions given to patient (no nose blowing, straining, bending over, heavy lifting, etc.)

Nasal trauma and facial fractures

 History

Patients who sustain trauma to the nose often experience acute epistaxis as well as nasal fractures. There are many mechanisms of impact, including athletic injuries, physical assault, and motor vehicle accidents. It is important to diagnose other facial fractures if present, particularly in the case of high-velocity or heavy-impact trauma, since other serious, possibly life-threatening injuries may coexist. In these cases, the cervical spine must be cleared and the patient should have a neurologic evaluation before the nasofacial fractures are treated.

 Physical Examination

Initially bleeding is controlled by direct pressure to the nose between the thumb and index finger over the soft tissue portion of the nose (lower half of the nostrils) for 10 to 15 min by the clock—longer if the patient takes aspirin regularly or uses anticoagulants. Pressure is usually adequate to control bleeding in these cases. Ice is applied to the nasal dorsum every 2 h for the first 24 h to minimize swelling.

After control of epistaxis, a headlight and nasal speculum are used to examine the nose. Alternatively, an otoscope with a speculum can be used for the intranasal examination. The presence of blood clots, active bleeding, septal deviation (along with its direction), and any septal hematoma should be noted. Next, the nasal dorsum is evaluated externally; swelling, dorsal deviation (with its direction), and any ecchymosis are documented. The nasal dorsal bones should also be grasped and palpated. The presence of crepitus, "step-off," or mobility makes the diagnosis of nasal fracture; x-ray is not typically necessary.

If there has been a high-velocity or high-impact injury or if subperiorbital ecchymosis is present, the orbital rims should be palpated bilaterally to determine whether an orbital rim fracture is present. In many cases, a step-off will be palpable. Particular care should be given to evaluation of the inferior orbital rim as well as the zygomatic-frontal suture line (the superolateral quadrant of the orbit). Extraocular motion should be evaluated; the presence of diplopia suggests entrapment and a possible blowout fracture.

If there is clinical suspicion that an orbital floor fracture may be present, a CT scan of the facial bones (no contrast) should be done, with thin cuts through the orbits to evaluate this.

Examination of the oral cavity should document evidence of bleeding, if present, on the posterior oropharyngeal wall.

Treatment

- Treatment requires appropriate lighting and equipment for intranasal examination.

Septal Hematoma

If a septal hematoma is present, it should be drained. After obtaining informed consent, topical anesthesia is applied and the overlying mucosa is injected using 1% lidocaine with 1:100,000 epinephrine until blanched. A stab incision is made at the inferior margin of the hematoma with a #15 or #11 blade. Any blood clot present is evacuated using a small curved clamp. The nares are then loosely packed with the edge of a strip of ¼-in. NuGauze packing, which is left in place for 24 h. The packing can generally be removed by the patient, but ENT follow up is mandatory.

- Untreated septal hematomas can lead to saddle deformities of the nose due to cartilage necrosis.

Nasal Fracture

The nose is the most commonly fractured facial bone, with 39% of facial fractures involving nasal bones. If a bony dorsal fracture has been diagnosed by examination or imaging study, the extent of the deformity must be evaluated. There is usually edema, and this will obscure subtle deformities, which cannot be evaluated until the swelling has resolved. The patient should be told to decrease his or her activity, apply ice packs as frequently as possible for the first 24 h, and sleep in a reclining position (or at least with the head elevated), to minimize swelling. Analgesics should be given, with the avoidance of aspirin and other NSAIDs if possible, due to possible platelet inactivation and the potential for bleeding. The patient should be referred for evaluation within 72 h.

If there is grossly visible dorsal deformity, it should be reduced and set with a cast/splint as soon as possible by an ENT specialist.

Orbital Rim Fracture

If there is a palpable orbital rim step-off, if the patient complains of double vision on examination of extraocular motion, if periorbital ecchymosis is present, or if there is any suspicion of facial trauma, facial films should be ordered.

Any patient with a finding suspicious for orbital rim or floor fracture should be referred to an otolaryngologist for evaluation within 24 to 48 h. If entrapment is present, there should be an immediate evaluation by both an otolaryngologist and an ophthalmologist.

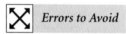 *Errors to Avoid*

- Failure to obtain a head and facial CT scan with open nasal fracture (due to force involved in injury) to rule out facial and brain injuries
- Missing a frontal sinus fracture and/or CSF rhinorrhea
- Failure to note and address a septal hematoma, which can ultimately lead to saddle-nose deformity

Key Points of Documentation

- The presence or absence of a septal hematoma
- The presence or absence of diplopia
- Periorbital ecchymosis
- Extent of nasal dorsal deformity
- Orbital step-off
- Appropriate follow-up and/or referral where indicated
- Time from injury to presentation
- History of previous nasal or facial surgery
- Preinjury olfaction
- Facial nerve function and hypoesthesia of the nasal and surrounding skin

SALIVARY GLAND DISEASE

Sialoadenitis

Infections of the major salivary glands affect elderly adults most often. Dehydration, chronic medical conditions, and immune compromise increase the risk. Retrograde transmission of bacteria from the oral cavity via the salivary duct is the mechanism believed to be responsible for this infection. The organism most commonly causing acute sialoadenitis is penicillin-resistant *S. aureus*, but *Streptococcus*, anaerobic, and rarely gram-negative organisms have also been responsible.

 History

The history can be one of progressive swelling over several days; or a rapid onset of pain and swelling, induration, and fever may be reported. The swelling that occurs may be associated with situations that stimulate saliva production—e.g., before or after eating. A foul taste in the mouth is sometimes described. At times, there may be a history of previous episodes that have resolved spontaneously.

 Physical Examination

The inflammation and tenderness present are localized to the gland itself and felt on palpation, although there may be some associated cervical adenopathy and erythema of the overlying skin. The diagnosis can be made by expressing pus from the associated duct (Stensen's duct for the parotid gland, Wharton's duct for the submandibular gland). The duct may be erythematous or inflamed and purulence may not be visualized.

- The mucous membranes of the oral cavity may appear dry, indicating reduced salivary flow.

Saliva can be expressed from the parotid gland by applying pressure to the tail of parotid area from behind, pressing anteriorly. The fingers are then drawn along the lateral aspect of the cheek, applying continuous pressure at the level of Stensen's duct. The corner of the mouth is turned outward, so that liquid coming from the duct orifice can be visualized. The patient will experience some discomfort from this maneuver, particularly if infection is present.

Alternatively, a tongue depressor can be used inside of the mouth. Beginning posteriorly at the level of Stensen's duct, behind the last molar tooth, the depressor is pressed laterally and drawn forward to the duct orifice. Fluid expressed from the duct ranges from clear to turbid and milky to frank pus. Normal saliva is clear and may be difficult to see. Wiping the orifice with the edge of a tongue depressor several times helps the examiner to establish its presence by causing the reaccumulation of fluid. Any discoloration of the fluid indicates infection.

- If no fluid is expressed and the examination is otherwise consistent with the diagnosis, an obstruction may be present. These patients are most likely to experience sudden onset of swelling and should be referred to an otolaryngologist for duct dilation. They should be treated for acute sialoadenitis as indicated below.

The submandibular gland can be examined in a similar manner as outlined above, expressing fluid with digital pressure applied either externally in the submandibular region or intraorally on the floor of mouth.

If the physical examination is positive, no imaging study is required unless there is a concern regarding dysphagia, airway compromise, or abscess formation. Infection of the salivary glands typically involves the gland parenchyma diffusely rather than presenting as a discrete abscess. On occasion, however, the infection may coalesce and form an abscess.

- Fluctuance is rarely palpable, even if an abscess is present, due to the dense fibrous nature of the glandular tissue and fascia. If clinically an abscess is suspected due to pitting edema over the affected gland or poor response to systemic antibiotics, then a CT scan or ultrasound may be helpful.

Treatment

The goal of treatment is to reverse salivary stasis and stimulate salivary flow as well as address the acute infection. Warm compresses should be applied to the affected area; oral hygiene should be maximized, aggressive hydration initiated, and use of sialagogues such as lemon drops or citrus juices encouraged to promote salivary flow. The patient should be instructed to massage the gland every few hours as tolerated. Antibiotic coverage targeting *S. aureus* with a beta-lactamase-resistant penicillin or cephalosporin should be prescribed for 10 to 14 days. If the patient does not improve within 48 to 72 h of therapy, an abscess should be considered. Incision and drainage of the abscessed gland by an ENT specialist may then be necessary.

A *ranula* is a cyst of the submandibular gland or duct that presents as a fullness of the floor of mouth that is painful and may be of sudden onset. This should be treated as above and referred to an otolaryngologist.

SIALOLITHIASIS

 History

Sialolithiasis involves the formation of hardened deposits in the ductal salivary gland system. Factors contributing to the development of this condition include salivary stagnation, ductal injury, and glandular inflammation. The submandibular (Wharton's) duct is where 80 percent of duct stones develop, with 19 and 1 percent occurring in the parotid and sublingual ducts, respectively.

Typical symptoms consist of colicky postprandial pain and swelling with variable degrees of resolution between attacks. Recurrent gland infections give rise to ductal strictures and atrophy of the gland parenchyma.

 Physical Examination

Physical examination is carried out as described above for evaluation of sialoadenitis. At times, small crystals may be seen in the saliva expressed from the duct. Occasionally, a large stone may be visible trapped in the puncta of the duct or may be palpated. Calculi are often identified along the course of the involved duct by bimanual palpation of the floor of the mouth. Sometimes there are no physical findings. If there is a strong suspicion of stone, plain lateral neck films may be positive, although the stones may not be radiopaque. Contrast studies are helpful for the visualization of radiolucent stones associated with proximal duct dilatation and slowed emptying. If purulent material is draining, the patient may have a sialoadenitis as well.

Treatment

Treatment of an acute episode consists of antibiotic coverage for *S. aureus*, analgesics (NSAIDs are usually adequate), warm compresses, and increased oral fluid intake. If this is the first episode, the patient should be counseled that the problem may recur. If it does, he or she should seek treatment by a specialist. If the patient has had previous episodes, more immediate specialist referral is indicated, as stone extraction or incision of the ductal orifice may be necessary.

 Errors to Avoid

- Failure to note signs of glandular abscess (pitting edema, fluctuance, or refractoriness to appropriate antibiotic therapy)
- Failure to stress importance of hydration and sialagogues
- Failure to identify signs of glandular neoplasm (painless, slow-growing masses)
- Missing salivary gland involvement as the initial manifestation of HIV (gradual nontender enlargement of one or more salivary glands with xerostomia)

Key Points of Documentation

- Presence of erythema or cervical adenopathy
- Presence or absence of saliva draining from duct orifice
- Presence or absence of pus draining from duct orifice
- Culture of pus if present
- Glandular fluctuance or lack thereof
- Instructions for follow-up care
- Facial nerve function if parotid gland is involved

DEEP-SPACE NECK INFECTIONS

Deep-space neck infections are relatively common despite the progress of antibiotic therapy. The neck has many potential spaces bordered by well-defined fascial planes; an abscess can occur within any of these areas. Therefore, submandibular, sublingual, parapharyngeal, retropharyngeal, prevertebral, carotid sheath, visceral, and the "danger" spaces can all be involved. The peritonsillar space is not a true deep-neck space but is in this category due to the similar presentation and potential complications of infections there.

Typical infections involving the submandibular, sublingual, and parapharyngeal spaces are odontogenic and thus of polymicrobial (aerobic and anaerobic) origin, made up of the bacteria found in oral flora. Other deep-space neck infections are of nonodotogenic origin—i.e., peritonsillar abscesses. Direct extension traumatic injuries, foreign bodies, or even tuberculosis of the spine all may cause deep-space neck infections.

Clinical Presentation

These infections typically present with both localized and systemic signs and symptoms. Fever, chills, malaise, and decreased appetite may be present. Local symptoms that may be signs of deep-space infection include trismus, odynophagia, dysphagia, voice changes, dyspnea, and otalgia; there may be a history of neck edema, erythema, fluctuance, tenderness, and drooling as well as cervical rigidity.

Knowledge of the specific combinations of signs and symptoms facilitates the diagnosis. For instance, a peritonsillar abscess presents with dysphagia, odynophagia, otalgia, and "hot-potato" voice. On examination, uvular deviation, palatal bulging, and erythematous exudative tonsils are often evident. Prompt management is necessary to prevent the spread of infection to the parapharyngeal space (see "Peritonsillar Abscess," above).

A sublingual space abscess presents with the floor of mouth bulging; patients will complain of pain and/or dysphagia. A submandibular space abscess is characterized by unilateral submandibular fluctuance and tenderness; the patient will have dysphagia and trismus. Often, infection involves both of these spaces, as they are contiguous posterior to the mylohyoid muscle (see "Ludwig's Angina," above).

Severe dysphagia, odynophagia, and marked trismus, as well as a unilateral tonsillar or lateral pharyngeal wall fullness, are evident with a parapharyngeal (or lateral pharyngeal) space abscess. These same symptoms with minimal trismus plus or minus dyspnea, hoarseness, and crepitance indicate a visceral space infection. Involvement of the carotid sheath space is evident when torticollis and pitting edema over the sternocleidomastoid muscle are present. Retropharyngeal abscesses occur most commonly in infants and young children. Sore throat and dysphagia are the most common symptoms. Fever, drooling, torticollis, and neck swelling are typical signs. If the process has progressed, symptoms of airway obstruction may also be evident. Infections of the prevertebral space exhibit few findings due to the restricted nature of this compartment. These infections can extend anywhere from the skull base to the coccyx. Therefore, signs and symptoms vary based on the abscess's vertical position.

Ancillary Studies

A WBC, which should be elevated, may be helpful if the diagnosis is unclear. A CT scan is critical to define the presence and position of an abscess with the exception of a peritonsillar abscess. Peritonsillar abscess is solely a clinical diagnosis unless extension is suspected.

Treatment

First and foremost, it is important to ensure that the airway is clear. A large abscess may compress the airway. Posterior tongue displacement or swollen soft tissue may obstruct it directly. Urgent evaluation by an ENT specialist with flexible fiberoptic laryngoscopy is key, particularly when there is any suspicion of compromise. Nasotracheal intubation or emergent tracheotomy may be necessary due to distortion of landmarks and associated airway edema. Intravenous antibiotic therapy should be initiated once the airway is deemed stable. In the past, penicillin was the drug of choice, but due to the increasing emergence of beta-lactamase–producing organisms, clavulanic acid or metronidazole must be added to any penicillin regimen. Alternatively, clindamycin in conjunction with a second-generation cephalosporin (e.g., cefoxitin or cefuroxime) is an effective regimen. The next priority is abscess drainage. CT imaging is useful prior to this in order to identify the exact location and size of the abscess.

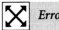 *Errors to Avoid*

- Failure to monitor patient throughout entire evaluation process, since status of airway can change rapidly
- Failure to be prepared for emergency airway intervention

 Key Points of Documentation

- Airway assessment
- Condition of dentition and gingiva
- Previous history of neck or oral cavity surgery

FOREIGN BODY OF THE NOSE

In most cases, a nasal foreign body does not constitute an emergency. However, small batteries (which can cause necrosis of the mucosa within hours), a food item (which may swell), or bilateral nasal foreign bodies in an infant do require emergent treatment. Additionally, certain patients are at increased risk for aspiration—i.e., those with neurologic or pulmonary diseases—and therefore require urgent removal.

 History

The patients at highest risk of having a nasal foreign body, such as young children or institutionalized adults, are the least likely to provide a history. Therefore it is important to be aware of the symptoms generally associated with the presence of a nasal foreign body. Unilateral purulent or malodorous nasal discharge, halitosis, nasal pain, recurrent rhinosinusitis, epistaxis, nasal whistling, excessive sneezing, and nasal airway obstruction may all point to the diagnosis.

 Physical Examination

A complete head and neck examination should be performed, since the presence of one foreign body indicates a high risk of additional foreign bodies. Examination of the nasal passage is performed using the wide, shortened speculums found with some otoscope sets, or the widest-bore ear speculum available. A pediatric-size nasal speculum may be used if the child is old enough to cooperate. In some cases, a foreign body will clearly be seen. In other cases, there will be unilateral purulent drainage that can be suctioned away using a small ear suction to better identify the object. Intranasal examination should rule out edema, erythema, ulceration of the nasal mucosa, granulation tissue, septal perforation, and epistaxis. If the foreign body has been long-standing, a rhinolith may have formed by the deposit of layers of calcium on the foreign body.

It is also very important to examine the chest and larynx in anyone with a suspected foreign body of the aerodigestive tract. Disastrous consequences can result if a second object or piece of the original object is missed. Laboratory studies generally are not necessary, although imaging studies of the nasopharynx and nose can be helpful in identifying radiopaque foreign bodies.

Treatment

Nasal foreign body is primarily a diagnosis in young children. The ability to perform procedures on children is based on their age, ability to cooperate, and level of fear and anxiety. It is important to be fully prepared with all necessary equipment and assistance before beginning. In some cases, it may be helpful to enlist the aid of the parents.

- As a general rule, the first effort will most likely be the best opportunity. If inexperience, limited availability of the proper equipment, or other circumstances indicate that successful retrieval is unlikely, it is often best to refer the patient directly for removal. Astute early referral may ultimately make retrieval easier for both the patient *and* the referral doctor. Young children may require general anesthesia for removal.

The application of a topical anesthetic and decongestant will facilitate the removal process. It is important to try to identify the shape and material involved. An object with a leading edge (e.g., a pistachio nut shell) may be grasped with an alligator forceps and removed. Multifaceted objects may be grasped, but removal may be traumatic. Organic material (e.g., food) may break easily if grasped and can be better removed with suction. Round objects are extremely difficult to remove, since there is no leading edge to grasp. Removal requires reaching *past* the object with a blunt, angled instrument and pulling it out. Unless the object is very close to the opening of the nares and can be gently pried out, round objects should be referred to a specialist for removal. Repeated efforts at removal using grasping instruments may simply push the object farther into the nose and may result in epistaxis or aspiration. A Fogarty catheter removal may be attempted by insertion along the floor of the nose and past the object. The balloon can then be inflated and the catheter advanced anteriorly, presumably pushing the foreign body out in front of itself.

If the object cannot be removed, the patient should be started on a first-line antibiotic that covers *S. pneumoniae* and on a decongestant nasal spray (three sprays in each nostril t.i.d.). These patients must be referred to a specialist as soon as possible.

If the object is removed and there has been purulent drainage, the patient should be treated as above and referred for follow-up to the primary care physician. If there is no evidence of infection, several days of nasal saline spray should be recommended.

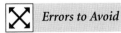

Errors to Avoid

- Attempting to remove any object without the proper equipment
- Posterior displacement of foreign body
- Failure to inspect foreign body for evidence of incomplete removal
- Failure to make sure that object in nose is a foreign body and not an encephalocele, carcinoma, arteriovenous malformation, etc.
- Persisting in futile attempts at removal, resulting in intranasal trauma
- Not obtaining a chest x-ray for any suspicion of aspiration

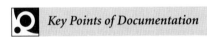

Key Points of Documentation

- Intranasal examination after foreign-body removal
- Disorders pertaining to differential diagnosis (e.g., nasal polyposis, choanal atresia, etc.)
- Absence of other foreign bodies
- Anatomic abnormalities related to foreign body

FOREIGN BODY OF THE EAR

Foreign body of the external ear canal (EAC) is usually a presenting complaint in the pediatric population. It is often not an emergency, but prompt attention can prevent infection and facilitate removal. Certain foreign bodies—such as insects and batteries—require urgent intervention to prevent further injury; other foreign bodies are associated with middle ear trauma and can lead to complications including hearing loss, vertigo, and facial nerve injury.

- Removal of these objects is a difficult task due to the sensitivity and anatomy of the ear canal.

 History

The patient frequently has a history of playing with a small object or inserting items into the ear canal to scratch an itching canal. Most objects will lodge at the isthmus (narrowest portion) of the EAC or the bony cartilaginous junction. Purulent drainage or a conductive hearing loss due to complete obstruction may be the presenting symptom. Foreign bodies that have penetrated typically present with otalgia, otorrhagia, and decreased hearing. More severe injury involving the middle ear can present with facial nerve weakness and vertigo.

 Physical Examination

A full head and neck examination is essential to rule out foreign bodies in other sites. When the patient is a small child, the child is placed in the parent's lap with its back against the adult's chest. The parent holds the child's legs between his or her legs and holds the child's hands crossed in front of its chest. The nurse then holds the child's head by pressing it firmly but gently against the adult's chest.

- Pressure should always be applied above the ear, never on the mandible.

For evaluation, the largest-bore speculum is used with the open-head otoscope. Microscopic otoscopy is indicated when there is incomplete visualization, contact with the tympanic membrane, or evidence of middle ear trauma.

Treatment

The child's cooperation is very important in this task, and the opportunity to remove a foreign body will depend on the child's ability to cooperate. All necessary materials should be on hand before beginning.

- Lacerations of the external ear canal can bleed quite a bit. If a laceration occurs during manipulation of the object, have the patient use otic drops (4 gtt., t.i.d.), keep the ear dry, and refer to a specialist immediately.

If an insect is present and alive, infuse 4% lidocaine liquid into the ear with an angiocatheter and leave it in place for 15 min. This will serve to paralyze the bug and topically anesthetize the ear canal. Excess fluid can be removed with ear suction.

A hearing aid battery requires immediate removal to prevent destruction of local tissue by three possible mechanisms: pressure necrosis, low-voltage burn, and direct corrosion by the battery's electrolytes. Administration of drops prior to removal of the battery has been shown to increase the depth of the burn and therefore should never be done.

If the object has a leading edge, it may be grasped with the alligator forceps and removed. Care must be taken when introducing the forceps to keep them closed and not touch the skin of the external ear canal, which is very sensitive. The forceps are opened when the tips reach the foreign body. For most objects, the ball-end right-angle hook is the instrument of choice, particularly if the foreign body has a smooth surface.

If the object is round, a special technique must be used (see "Foreign Body of the Nose," above). Attempts to remove the object with a grasping instrument like a forceps will only push it farther into the ear canal, with the potential to damage the tympanic membrane (TM). Irrigation with room-temperature water works well when the TM is intact. The irrigation stream should be directed to the posterosuperior aspect of the canal if possible. This technique is contraindicated, however, if the foreign body is hygroscopic, since it could then lead to swelling and further impaction as well as otitis externa. Additionally, irrigation should be avoided if there is a preexisting hearing loss. These patients should be treated with otic drops, told to maintain dry-ear precautions, and referred for follow-up evaluation to a specialist.

- If there is purulent drainage present, the patient should be treated with oral antibiotics as well as otic drops and referred to a specialist. No attempts should be made at removal in this case since the limited visualization and canal inflammation makes a poor outcome likely.

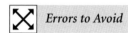 *Errors to Avoid*

- Any manipulation of a foreign body lodged in an only-hearing ear
- Prescribing use of eardrops if a battery is the foreign body, as this will increase the depth of the low-voltage tissue burn
- Manipulation of any foreign body medial to the bony canal isthmus, which can result in middle ear trauma (these should immediately be referred to a specialist)
- Failure to refer for hearing evaluation as indicated (any subjective hearing loss or evidence of middle ear trauma)
- Irrigation if the foreign body is hygroscopic or there is a preexisting hearing loss

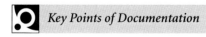 *Key Points of Documentation*

- Any history of TM perforation
- Patient's description of his or her premorbid hearing level

- Examination of ear canal after foreign-body removal to note injury to canal skin, tympanic membrane, or ossicles
- Facial nerve function
- Presence or absence of vertigo
- Results of hearing check after removal of foreign body

ESOPHAGEAL FOREIGN BODY

Foreign bodies of the esophagus are common in children under 3 years of age and in the older age group, particularly denture wearers who have diminished oral sensation. An impacted foreign body may cause few symptoms or severe symptoms and can lead to fatal complications. Since the muscular activity of the upper esophagus is weak in comparison to the pharyngeal musculature, foreign bodies propelled into the hypopharynx are most likely to lodge immediately below the cricopharyngeus.

 History

The history is very important: when, how, and a description of the object and associated symptoms can prove to be critical information. Symptoms typically vary with size, position, and composition of the foreign body (10 percent of patients are asymptomatic). Objects in the upper esophagus can produce suprasternal pain and dysphagia. Larger objects will cause obstructive symptoms, including a globus sensation, excessive salivation and regurgitation, cough due to aspiration, and dyspnea if the trachea is compressed by the object's bulk. Rough objects may cause a superficial abrasion of the mucosa en route to the stomach, resulting in pain that subsides within 24 h. Persistent pain suggests that the foreign body has remained lodged. Disk batteries may become lodged and react with the esophageal mucosa, resulting in esophageal burn with resultant perforation and mediastinitis.

 Physical Examination

Radiopaque objects are usually readily identified with plain chest x-rays or neck films. An increase in the distance between the cervical vertebrae and larynx and trachea or air in the cervical esophagus can represent evidence of nonradiopaque objects. If the foreign body cannot be located in this fashion, a barium swallow may demonstrate it. However, it is better to avoid contrast material, if feasible, since it can obscure the foreign body on endoscopy and delay retrieval. At times, very small, radiodense objects can be demonstrated on CT. A contrast esophagogram or CT scan can identify a perforation.

Treatment

The great majority of esophageal foreign bodies can be removed endoscopically using either rigid or flexible esophagoscopy. Objects that have traversed the esophagus generally pass through the GI tract without event. The patient's stool can be examined for 5 to 7 days until the foreign body is recovered.

Errors to Avoid

- Failure to recognize how rapidly an esophageal foreign body can be regurgitated into the trachea
- Failure to obtain urgent specialist attention for sharp or pointed foreign bodies or disk batteries. (Mucosal injury occurs within 1 h, muscular layer injury within 4 h, and possible perforation within 8 to 12 h.)

 Key Points of Documentation

- Any history of preexisting esophageal disease, particularly strictures
- Description of the foreign body
- Status of the airway

VERTIGO

Patients who present with dizziness can be severely disabled and may pose great diagnostic challenges. There can be numerous etiologies to the perception of imbalance, including cardiovascular disease, volume depletion, cerebellar infarction, or central neurologic disease (neoplastic or due to hemorrhage). If signs or symptoms of other organ system pathology are present (chest pain, focal neurologic deficits, headache, orthostatic hypotension), these must be evaluated. Underlying systemic disorders as seen in metabolic imbalances (e.g., uncontrolled diabetes mellitus) or neurosyphilis may present "silently," initially manifesting only as "dizziness." Any history of alcohol or drug use should be elicited and verified with testing, as appropriate.

Vertigo is often episodic, and the patient may present when the disease is not active. These patients, especially the elderly, can be very anxious owing to their fear of sudden, disabling attacks of vertigo or fear of falling. Such episodes can occur randomly—for example, while driving or working with machinery, which can add to the patient's fear. The objective of the history and physical is to identify a pattern of attacks and to evoke the symptoms if possible. While making a diagnosis can be challenging for the physician, it is important to take the necessary time with these patients, counseling them that dizziness can be a difficult medical problem which may require repeated evaluation, but that help is available for acute symptoms in many cases, even before a specific diagnosis is made.

 History

People have varying definitions for the term *dizziness*. These include feeling faint, visual changes, feeling flushed, disequilibrium, a spinning sensation, etc. A careful, detailed history of the onset, duration, characteristics, and precursors of the vertigo can be of great help in determining the correct diagnosis.

Vertigo of labyrinthine origin can be best defined by the term "hallucination of motion." The patient feels that he or she is spinning or that the environment is spinning. When symptoms are current and short-lived, elicited by rolling over in bed or changes in head position, this is suggestive of benign paroxysmal positional vertigo (BPPV). A history of prior URI or GI disease in the preceding 4 to 6 weeks is suggestive of a viral etiology (viral labyrinthitis or vestibular neuritis), particularly if the vertigo is prolonged and slowly improves over several days. Any history of prior head trauma (especially with loss of consciousness) should be elicited, as this would suggest the possibility of dislodged calcium particles irritating the vestibular nerve endings (cupulolithiasis). Fluctuating tinnitus or hearing loss temporarily associated with episodic vertigo may suggest Ménière's disease. Any history of ear pain, otorrhea, hearing loss, ear surgery, or chronic otitis media should be noted.

On history, it is important to ask about the first time that the patient ever experienced dizziness or vertigo. It is often necessary to repeat this question multiple times in order to emphasize the importance of knowing when the patient had this experience for the *first* time. Next, the patient should characterize the onset, duration, intensity, etc., of the first episode, followed by details of the most recent event. This often gives a picture of whether this is an acute problem or has been episodic and progressive for many years, with this episode finally being severe enough to require medical attention.

Physical Examination

The ears are examined for evidence of an acute infectious inflammatory process. If otitis media is present, it can cause symptoms of imbalance and should be treated. A cholesteatoma also may be responsible and should be readily identifiable. Fistula testing by pneumatic otoscopy should be performed. Tuning-fork testing may reveal a conductive or sensorineural hearing loss, which, if present, respectively suggest a peripheral or retrocochlear pathology. A neurologic examination should be performed, with close attention to cranial nerve function, cerebellar function, and cognition. The presence or absence of nystagmus should be noted. Nystagmus of central origin is generally vertical and persistent, unlike that of peripheral origin, which is usually torsional and of short duration. The Romberg, modified Romberg, finger-to-nose, and Fukada stepping tests as well as tandem gait evaluation and the Hallpike maneuver can be performed to elicit signs of vestibular dysfunction. It is important to note, with the Hallpike maneuver, whether the patient reports vertigo as well as the presence or absence of nystagmus. Should central pathology be unlikely, infection (WBC, syphilis screen) or autoimmune disease (ESR) must be ruled out. If, however, a central etiology is possible, imaging studies (magnetic resonance imaging) should be obtained immediately.

Treatment

Initial treatment of the vertiginous dizzy patient involves the use of vestibular suppressants. These treatments do provide the patient with relief of symptoms but do not establish the diagnosis or treat underlying disease processes. If the problem has been a chronic one or if there is no clear diagnosis, the patient should be referred to a specialist. This referral should be to an otolaryngologist and/or neurologist, based on the findings of the evaluation. Also, the patient should be counseled that if the symptoms are refractory or recurrent, a specialist should be consulted.

Antihistamines and benzodiazepines are the mainstays of pharmocotherapy for vestibular suppression. Anticholinergics, sympathomimetics, and sedatives have been used as well.

- Patients should be counseled about the sedative effects of many of these medications as well as risks of combining them with alcohol or operating heavy machinery.

Mild to moderate cases that are not severely disabling can be treated with oral medications. Meclizine 25 to 50 mg can be given t.i.d. up to the patient's tolerance for the sedative effects. When the sedative effect is too strong, patients may be counseled to take a full tablet at bedtime and half a tablet during the day. Oxazepam, 10 mg up to three times a day, can be used for moderate cases. Diazepam, 5 mg two to three times a day, can be used for moderate to severe cases; patients who are refractory to this dose should be admitted to the hospital for management. Nausea and vomiting can be treated on an outpatient basis with prochlorperazine (Compazine) or trimethobenzamide (Tigan) suppositories. The suppositories can be used in conjunction with the oral medications.

To control severe symptoms of vertigo with evident nystagmus of a presumed vestibular origin on initial presentation, intravenous diazepam 5 to 10 mg by slow push can be very effective. Ondansetron (Zofran) 4 mg IV can be used to control nausea and vomiting. An intravenous steroid bolus (dexamethasone 6 to 10 mg) can be used to reduce inflammation in the vestibular system if viral labyrinthitis is suspected. These patients should be monitored for control of symptoms and referred for specialist evaluation.

Pediatric Patients

Any child who presents with new onset of vertigo or nystagmus should be referred for evaluation to an otolaryngologist as well as a neurologist. It is, however, important to rule out otitis media as an etiology.

- There are certain congenital syndromes which include congenital nystagmus. While the appearance of these patients is striking, they do not report any dizziness or vertigo.

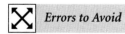 *Errors to Avoid*

- Failure to diagnose underlying systemic complaint
- Failure to elicit associated symptoms, e.g., headache, tinnitus, otalgia, otorrhea
- Failure to examine the ear
- Failure to identify life-threatening causes of vertigo, i.e., central nervous system abnormalities, infarcts and hemorrhages, brainstem neoplasms
- Failure to identify associated hearing loss
- Failure to discuss needed behavioral limitations, e.g., refraining from driving, care on stairs, etc.

Key Points of Documentation

- Prior history of viral illness (upper respiratory or gastrointestinal)
- Prior history of vertigo or head trauma
- Presence or absence of nystagmus
- Examination of the ear
- Results of Hallpike maneuver and neurologic testing
- Other central nervous system symptoms
- Presence or absence of hearing loss

IDIOPATHIC SUDDEN HEARING LOSS

 History

Patients with idiopathic sudden hearing loss typically present with the complaint of waking up deaf, having decreased hearing or a muffled sensation in one ear, or acute onset of loud ringing or buzzing. There is no prior history of ototoxin exposure, otitis media, otalgia, otorrhea, vertigo, tinnitus, barotrauma, or head trauma. By definition, it is a loss of 30 dB or more across three contiguous frequencies within a 24-h period. The incidence is estimated to be 1 in 10,000 to 15,000 persons.

- The diagnosis of idiopathic sudden hearing loss can only be made when other potential causes of hearing loss have been ruled out.

 Physical Examination

Physical examination of the ear is unremarkable. There are normal landmarks as well as mobility of the tympanic membrane. No effusion, erythema, or vesicles are found on the tympanic membrane.

Tests

If sudden hearing loss is suspected, the patient requires an audiometric evaluation prior to treatment in order to establish baseline hearing thresholds. If this is not practical, hearing can be documented with tuning forks of different frequencies. Blood work should include CBC, thyroid function tests, fluorescent treponemal antibody absorption, ESR, antineutrophilic cytoplasmic antibodies, (to rule out Wegener's granulomatosis), antinuclear antibody, rheumatoid factor, chemistry panel, lipid profile, Lyme disease titers, HIV testing (if risk factors are present), and MRI to evaluate the cerebellopontine angle.

Treatment

There are many causes of asymmetrical sensorineural hearing loss that require extensive investigation, including tumors of the cerebellopontine angle, trauma, Ménière's disease, presbycusis, etc. The key to the diagnosis of this idiopathic condition is its sudden onset without any preceding symptoms or findings. In these situations, the treatment is high-dose steroids (80 to 120 mg PO per day) for 4 to 7 days with a taper over 2 to 3 weeks. The patient should be questioned for medical contraindications to steroid therapy (history of diabetes; history of peptic, duodenal, or bleeding ulcers; pregnancy; HTN), and given appropriate instructions and warnings.

A sudden hearing loss constitutes an otologic emergency, since the sooner treatment is initiated, the better the prognosis is for recovery. These patients, therefore, require referral to an otolaryngologist, with a telephone consultation prior to discharge for any further direction of care that should be started while awaiting specialty evaluation. For instance, antivirals such as acyclovir (Zovirax) or valacyclovir (Valtrex) are advocated by some, as these medications have minimal adverse effects and may be helpful in cases of persistent loss. Some more experimental treatments—including dextran (to improve blood flow), histamine and carbogen (to cause vasodilation and increase O_2 delivery to the cochlea), diuretics (for hearing losses due to endolymphatic hydrops), or heparin (to address embolic causes)—are utilized typically in association with university-based protocols.

 Errors to Avoid

- Inadequate history of prior or associated symptoms
- Failure to document contraindications to steroid treatment
- Failure to refer to an otolaryngologist for prompt evaluation
- Failure to identify and discontinue ototoxic medications
- Failure to elicit a history of previous ear surgery or trauma

 Key Points of Documentation

- Documentation of the absence of any prior history or associated symptoms
- Documentation of the hearing at time of presentation as a baseline
- Establishment of the presence or absence of vertigo, as this is a key prognostic factor

TEMPOROMANDIBULAR JOINT SYNDROMES

Temporomandibular joint (TMJ) syndromes encompass a range of pathologies. The types that are addressed here include TMJ dislocation and uncomplicated TMJ syndrome.

TMJ Dislocation

 History

Patients with TMJ dislocations present with a sudden "lockjaw"—i.e., the inability to move the mandible freely. This is sudden in onset and may have occurred when opening the mouth very wide while yawning or biting into an overstuffed sandwich. There may be a prior history of similar episodes or problems with the TMJ.

Physical Examination

On physical examination, the mouth will be partially open and the patient will complain of mild to severe pain, be unable to fully open or close the mouth, and experience pain upon any effort to do so. The mandibular condyle will be palpable anterior to the inferior aspect of the mastoid process. X-ray examination can document the deformity at the TMJ, although these films may be difficult to read.

Treatment

The treatment of TMJ disease is closed reduction. Performing the reduction requires working against the masseter muscle, which is one of the stronger muscles of the body. The patient should be given narcotics intravenously or by mouth and muscle relaxants in age- and weight-appropriate doses.

Once adequate relaxation has been achieved, the patient's mandible is grasped in both hands with the thumbs on the lower molars. The examiner should stand facing the seated patient in order to have the advantage of leverage. Firm, continuous pressure is applied downward with the thumbs. Pressure should continue until the mandibular condyle is felt to slide into place. The patient should experience immediate relief and return of nearly normal mandibular excursion. A repeat x-ray should be obtained documenting the reduction.

The patient should be treated with NSAIDs and given a referral for ENT follow-up. Patients should be warned to avoid wide opening of the mouth for 6 to 8 weeks and instructed to adhere to a soft diet, which will allow the ligaments of the joint to heal.

 Errors to Avoid

- Attempting to reduce without appropriate muscle relaxation

 Key Points of Documentation

- Physical findings, including extent of mouth closing and opening in centimeters, degree of final excursion in centimeters
- Postreduction physical findings and x-ray results
- Discharge instructions not to drive while under the influence of the pain medications and muscle relaxants used for reduction
- Discharge instructions regarding a soft diet and limited mouth excursion

TMJ Syndrome

 History

These patients often present with the complaint of ear pain and a normal otologic evaluation. The pain may be felt in the preauricular region, anterior to the tragus. It may radiate into the jaw. The patient should be questioned regarding pain with opening the mouth wide when yawning or while chewing hard or crunchy foods. The differential diagnosis includes eustachian tube dysfunction, tonsillitis, pharyngitis, and parotitis.

 Physical Examination

On physical examination, the tympanic membrane has normal landmarks and no evidence of active disease. The examiner places the fingers over the TMJ bilaterally while the patient repeatedly opens and closes his or her mouth. Crepitus elicited by palpation, locking or clicking of the joint with motion, and/or tenderness to intraoral palpation should be documented. The symmetry of the mandibular motion should also be evaluated. (Does the jaw move to one side or the other?) The masseter muscles bilaterally are palpated for tenderness. The tonsils and parotid gland should be evaluated as described in the previous section. Positive physical findings on the examination and the ruling out of an infectious source makes the diagnosis.

Treatment

Uncomplicated TMJ syndrome is often due to soft tissue injury to the ligaments of the joint. The treatment is anti-inflammatory medications and avoidance of reinjury for 8 to 12 weeks. If there are no contraindications, long-term NSAID treatment for 1 month should be initiated, a soft diet is adhered to, and warm compresses as needed are used for 2 months. The patient should avoid any food that requires hard chewing or wide opening of the mouth. If the joint is reinjured prior to healing, the healing process has to start over again.

Patients with TMJ syndrome should be referred to an otolaryngologist or oral surgeon who specializes in the treatment of this condition.

REFERENCES

Ballenger JJ, Snow JB: *Otolaryngology Head and Neck Surgery*, 15th ed. Baltimore: Williams & Wilkins; 1996.

Brook I: Diagnosis and management of parotitis. *Arch Otolaryngol Head Neck Surg* 118:469–471, 1992.

Brook I: Diagnosis and management of anaerobic infections of the head and neck. *Ann Otol Rhinol Laryngol*; 101:9–15, 1992.

Cotton RP, Myers CM III: *Practical Pediatric Otolaryngology*. Philadelphia: Lippincott-Raven; 1999.

Clayman GL et al: Intracranial complications of paranasal sinusitis: a combined institutional review. *Laryngoscope*; 101:234–239, 1991.

Cummings CW et al, eds: *Otolaryngology: Head and Neck Surgery*. St. Louis: Mosby-Year Book; 1993.

Ferrera PC, Busino LJ, Snyder HS: Uncommon complications of odontogenic infections. *Am J Emerg Med* 14:317–322, 1996.

Gates G: *Current Therapy in Otolaryngology Head and Neck Surgery*, 6th ed. St. Louis: Mosby-Year Book; 1998

Gidley PW, Ghorayeb BY, Stiernberg CM: Contemporary management of deep neck space infections. *Otolaryngol Head Neck Surg* 116:16–22, 1997.

Heimdahl A, Nord CE: Treatment of orofacial infections of odontogenic origin. *Scand J Infect Dis* 45:101, 1985.

Holinger LD: *Pediatric Laryngology and Bronchoesophagology*. Baltimore: Williams & Wilkins; 1996.

Karlin RJ, Robinson WA: Septic cavernous sinus thrombosis. *Ann Emerg Med* 13:449–455, 1984.

Maniglia et al: Intracranial abscesses secondary to nasal, sinus and orbital infections in adults and children. *Arch Otolaryngol Head Neck Surg* 115:1424–1429, 1989.

Mann W, Amedee RG, Maurer J: Orbital complications of pediatric sinusitis: treatment of periorbital abscess. *Am J Rhinol* 11:149–153, 1997.

Marra S, Hotaling AJ: Deep neck infections. *Am J Otolaryngol* 17:287–298, 1996.

Maves MD, Carithers JS, Birck HG: Esophageal burns secondary to disc battery ingestion. *Ann Otol Rhinol Laryngol* 93:364, 1984.

Myers E, ed: *Advances in Otolaryngology Head and Neck Surgery*. Vol 6. St. Louis: Mosby; 1992.

Spires JR et al: Treatment of peritonsillar abscess: a prospective study of aspiration vs incision and drainage. *Arch Otolaryngol* 113:984–986, 1987.

Wald ER et al: Sinusitis and its complications in the pediatric patient. *Pediatr Clin North Am* 28:777–796, 1981.

CARDIOLOGY

Louis Kofi Essandoh

CHEST PAIN SYNDROMES

The diagnosis and treatment of chest pain syndromes (Table 9-1) in an urgent care setting is often quite challenging due to the heterogeneity of conditions likely to be encountered. These conditions span the entire spectrum of disease, including true cardiac emergencies requiring the facilities of a fully equipped emergency department. The urgent care physician must therefore be proficient in formulating a differential diagnosis that will allow for the appropriate evaluation, treatment, and triage of patients presenting with a complaint of chest pain. The practice of referring nearly every patient for expensive tests or consultations should be discouraged, as should the reckless approach of not obtaining appropriate studies needed to assess potentially serious conditions. Of prime importance is the need to distinguish between various chest pain syndromes. Key points that should be elicited on history include character of the pain, location and duration of the pain, aggravating or alleviating factors, reproduction of the pain on palpation, history of trauma, previous similar episodes, and any associated symptoms (e.g., shortness of breath, coughing, orthopnea, paroxysmal nocturnal dyspnea, dyspnea on exertion, and fever). It is also important to obtain a full cardiac history, including any family history of cardiac disease and any personal history of diabetes, hypertension, smoking, hyperlipidemia, or previous cardiac conditions. The physical examination should include a full cardiac and pulmonary evaluation, including documented blood pressure and peripheral pulses, inspection and palpation of the chest wall, abdominal examination, and the evaluation of the extremities for deep venous thrombosis. Acute evaluation of the patient presenting with chest pain may also include an electrocardiogram and/or chest x-rays as dictated by patient history, clinical presentation, physical examination, and associated risk factors for cardiac, pulmonary, or aortic disease. Echocardiography may be useful in the evaluation of chest pain, since a normal echocardiogram (no left ventricular wall motion abnormalities) in a patient with ongoing chest pain reduces the likelihood that the pain is due to myocardial ischemia. Valvular heart disease and pericardial effusion can also be readily diagnosed by the echocardiographic examination. Similarly, exercise stress testing can be very helpful in

TABLE 9-1

DIFFERENTIAL DIAGNOSIS: CHEST PAIN SYNDROMES

CAUSES	DISTINGUISHING FEATURES
Noncardiac	
Gastrointestinal	
Esophageal reflux	Exacerbated by food intake
Esophageal spasm	Nonexertional; may be relieved by nitroglycerin
Peptic ulcer disease	Epigastric location; relieved by antacids; food may relieve pain immediately; worsens 2 h later
Gallbladder disease	Right-sided pain, but may be referred to left chest
Pulmonary	
Pulmonary embolism	Dyspnea, tachycardia, tachypnea, pleuritic chest pain
Pneumothorax	Pleuritic pain and dyspnea of sudden onset
Pleuritis	Sharp pain, may be positional
Neuromuscular	
Shoulder joint inflammation	Pain, tenderness, reduced range of motion
Costochondritis	Reproducible chest wall tenderness on palpation; may worsen with inspiration
Herpes zoster	Radicular distribution; typical rash; rash may follow rather than precede onset of pain
Cardiac	
Ischemic heart disease	
Coronary atherosclerosis	Exacerbated by exertion, risk factors often present
Vasospastic angina	Rest angina. ST-segment elevation, transient or relieved with nitroglycerin
Nonischemic heart disease	
Aortic stenosis	Typical murmur of AS on exam
Mitral valve prolapse	May have typical murmur or click
Pericarditis	Sharp, pleuritic; changes with position; tachycardia; friction rub
Proximal aortic dissection	Sharp, interscapular pain, pulse deficits

excluding coronary artery disease, though extreme care should be taken to avoid exercising patients with unstable angina or atypical presentations of myocardial infarction. Unfortunately, these diagnostic modalities are generally not readily available to the urgent care physician.

Noncardiac Chest Pain

Patients with noncardiovascular causes of chest pain most commonly have musculoskeletal or gastrointestinal disorders. The pain associated with musculoskeletal conditions such as costochondritis is often reproduced or aggravated by deep inspiration, isometric stress, or direct palpation of the involved area. There is often a history of increased or new activity, a history of recent trauma, or symptoms of other noncardiac illnesses causing chest wall irritation (e.g., acute bronchitis with frequent coughing).

Differentiation of gastrointestinal disorders from cardiac disease is often a more difficult task. Patients with peptic ulcer disease may present with symptoms that are temporarily ameliorated by antacids or various "GI cocktails." Chest pain due to esophageal spasm, however, may be indistinguishable from angina, since either may be relieved by rest or nitroglycerin and respond favorably to calcium antagonists. When differentiation is difficult, further evaluation or admission for additional testing may be required.

A frequently overlooked noncardiac cause of chest pain is herpes zoster infection, in which the characteristic rash and dermatomal location of the pain are often diagnostic.

Unstable Angina Pectoris

Unstable angina is generally defined as angina that occurs at rest, occurs with minimal exertion, is of new onset (within a few weeks), or is increasing in frequency or intensity from a stable anginal pattern. If untreated, unstable angina carries a high rate of progression to acute myocardial infarction or other cardiovascular complications.

Clinical Presentation
The classic presentation of unstable angina is that of substernal chest pain described as heavy, tight, or squeezing. The pain may radiate to either upper extremity or to the neck or jaw area. There may be associated symptoms of diaphoresis, nausea, palpitations, light-headedness, or shortness of breath. The pain is likely to start quickly and become progressively more severe, lasting between 5 and 15 min. The pain may increase with exertion and respond favorably to rest. Generally, chest pain that is either constant over hours to days or fleeting (i.e., lasting only seconds) is not consistent with anginal type pain.

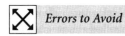 *Errors to Avoid*

- Failure to diagnose angina secondary to an "atypical" description of chest pain—i.e., pain that is described as "sharp." *Patients will often consider "sharp" to mean severe and not as a description of the character of the pain.*
- Failure to diagnose angina secondary to a history of pain that has been present for an extended period of time. (Further questioning of patients with a history of ongoing pain will often reveal that the pain has actually been intermittent since onset and not constant. The patient should be asked whether the pain has been continuous or if it waxes and wanes.)

Patients with a history of stable angina can also present with unstable or crescendo angina. These patients may present with changes in their typical anginal pattern including increasing frequency and/or severity of attacks, pain at rest or with less exertion than with prior episodes, or increased need for medications. These symptoms will typically have increased over the preceding weeks prior to presentation.

Errors to Avoid

- Attributing decreased potency of nitroglycerin (NTG) to unstable angina. Check for associated symptoms of headache and burning on NTG use to help assess potency of the medication. Tablets retain potency for several months only; sublingual spray may retain potency for several years

 Physical Examination

On physical examination there is no unique presentation that will establish the diagnosis of ischemic heart disease. The physical exam may be completely normal or may show findings of underlying hypertension or diabetes. On auscultation, an S4 may be heard or the murmur of mitral regurgitation may be noted.

 Errors to Avoid

- Assuming that palpable chest pain excludes angina—Always ask if the pain produced on palpation is the *same* type of pain that brought the patient in for evaluation.

Laboratory and Ancillary Aids in Evaluation

The electrocardiogram (ECG) in the patient with unstable angina may be normal, show ST-segment shifts (usually ST depressions) or have T-wave inversions. If present, the ECG changes of unstable angina usually resolve spontaneously or with appropriate anti-ischemic therapy. Persistence of ST or T-wave changes may imply progression to a non-Q-wave myocardial infarction, necessitating different diagnostic and therapeutic measures.

 Management (Table 9-2)

The first step in the management of any patient initially suspected of having unstable angina should be the initiation of oxygen (administer at a rate of 2 to 4 L/min via nasal cannula), intravenous access, and continuous cardiac monitoring. Once the diagnosis is more clearly established, arrangements for hospital transfer and admission should be made and patients should immediately be treated with aspirin, 325 to 650 mg. The aspirin should be chewed, not swallowed, and coated aspirin should not be used, since its absorption is delayed. Although experience with "broad-spectrum" antiplatelet agents such as ticlopidine or clopidogrel in unstable coronary syndromes is still evolving, it appears that these medications will have a role in treatment and may be considered for patients in whom aspirin therapy is contradicted.

- Clopidogrel has nearly completely replaced ticlopidine because of a lower incidence of hematologic complications when compared to ticlopidine.

Of note, clopidogrel may be added to aspirin in high-risk patients or in patients undergoing percutaneous coronary intervention, but it is not, as yet, a replacement for

TABLE 9-2

ACUTE TREATMENT OF UNSTABLE ANGINA

Oxygen: 2 to 4 L/min
IV access
Continuous cardiac monitoring
Aspirin: 325 to 650 mg (chewed)
Nitroglycerin
   Sublingual (1 tablet or 1 to 3 puffs of spray)
   Intravenous (5 to 10 μg/min titrated up by 5 to 10 μg/min q 3 to 5 min)
   Transdermal (1 to 2 in. to the chest wall; not to be used to treat active/ongoing pain)
Heparin
   Subcutaneous (7500 to 10,000 U q 12 h) or
   Intravenous (bolus: 75 U/kg with maximum of 5000 U, followed by continuous weight-based infusion.) Low-molecular-weight heparin preparations (given subcutaneously) may be superior to unfractionated heparin.

aspirin in patients who can tolerate the latter. The dose for clopidogrel (Plavix) is 75 mg once daily. In unstable angina, administration of an initial loading dose of 300 mg of clopidogrel has been shown to be beneficial.

 Errors to Avoid

- Administration of 81 mg of aspirin. While this may be adequate for chronic maintenance of antiplatelet activity, it is not an appropriate dosage for the acutely ill patient.

Nitrates, heparin, and beta blockers should be considered for all patients requiring hospital admission. Nitroglycerin, given sublingually, may be useful acutely and can be given in tablet (0.3 to 0.6 mg) or in spray form (1 to 3 puffs). Similarly, topical nitroglycerin may also be used, but it is more appropriate in the patient who is not currently experiencing pain. For the patient with ongoing symptoms, especially at rest, intravenous nitroglycerin should be given at a dose of 5 to 10 μg/min initially and titrated up by 10 μg/min every 3 to 5 min, with an endpoint being resolution of pain or hypotension. Heparin, when administered, can be given as a subcutaneous injection at a dose of 7500 to 10,000 U every 12 h or intravenously as a bolus of 75 U/kg but not exceeding 5000 U. When intravenous heparin is used, the initial bolus should be followed by a continuous infusion of 15 U/kg/h.

- It is likely that low-molecular-weight heparins (which can be conveniently given subcutaneously) and nonaspirin platelet inhibitors (such as intravenous glycoprotein IIb–IIIa inhibitors) will have a therapeutic role in the management of acute ischemic syndromes in the near future.

Of note, while intravenous beta-adrenergic antagonists may be helpful in reducing myocardial oxygen demand, they must be administered under continuous electrocardiographic and blood pressure monitoring, which is usually best initiated after the patient has arrived at the emergency department or coronary care unit.

Acute Myocardial Infarction

Clinical Presentation

The classic presentation of patients with acute myocardial infarction (MI) may be similar to that described for the patient with unstable angina, though the symptoms are usually of longer duration (generally greater than 15 to 30 min) and of greater severity. While the physical examination may be entirely normal, many patients acutely experiencing infarction may exhibit an uneasy restlessness as well as an ashen appearance. There may be slight elevation in blood pressure and pulse rate, except in patients with inferior infarctions, in whom bradycardia, which can be profound, may be seen. If there is involvement of the papillary muscles, new murmurs of mitral regurgitation may be present; in the setting of pericarditis, a friction rub may be noted.

Patients who have sustained an infarction several hours to days prior to evaluation may present only with symptoms suggestive of an acute MI, such as new congestive heart failure, weakness, fatigue, light-headedness, heartburn, or symptoms caused by conduction disorders. Certain patient subgroups—such as women, diabetics, and the elderly—may present with atypical or unimpressive symptoms. In these patients, it is important to maintain a high index of suspicion in order to avoid misdiagnosis.

Laboratory and Ancillary Tests

- While electrocardiographic (ECG) evaluation is thought of as the classic approach to diagnosing an acute MI, only about half of patients with MIs will have a diagnostic ECG at the time of presentation (Table 9-3). Therefore, while an abnormal ECG is helpful, a normal ECG does not rule out MI, and disposition decisions should not be based solely on ECG tracings.

In the setting of an acute MI, the initial ECG will vary depending on the location of the infarct, time of presentation, and patient's underlying cardiac status. The ECG may be normal, may show nonspecific ST-T-segment changes, or may show one of several classic infarction patterns (see Table 9-4).

Nondiagnostic ECGs may occur due to left bundle branch block, left ventricular hypertrophy, or pacemaker rhythms, all of which can produce bizarre QRS complexes and repolarization abnormalities that make the diagnosis of acute MI by ECG difficult or impossible. Uncommon ECG patterns of infarction—such as posterior wall infarc-

TABLE 9-3

ELECTROCARDIOGRAPHIC CHANGES ASSOCIATED WITH INFARCTION

ST-segment depression of at least 1 mm (subendocardial infarction)
ST-segment elevation of at least 1 mm (epicardial injury or infarction)
Deep and symmetrical T-wave inversion
Presence of Q wave (requires several hours to develop)

TABLE 9-4

LOCALIZATION OF INFARCTION BY CHANGES ON ELECTROCARDIOGRAM

Anteroseptal	Leads V_1 to V_3
Anterolateral	Leads V_4 to V_6; I and aV_L (may involve V_1 to V_3)
Anterior	V_2 to V_4; I and aV_L
Lateral	I, AV_L, may involve V_4 to V_6
Inferior	Leads II, III, and aV_F
Posterior	V_1 to V_2 with tall R wave and ST-segment depression

tion, repeat infarction, infarction associated with minimal ECG changes, or infarction in the diabetic patient who may present without pain—may also be seen, and in such cases a high index of suspicion should be maintained in order to avoid missing the diagnosis.

- Given the often difficult diagnosis of ischemic cardiac disease, it is prudent to have a low threshold for transfer and/or hospitalization of patients with chest pain and nondiagnostic ECGs.

See Figs. 9-1 through 9-4 for various types of ECG tracings in acute MI.

 Errors to Avoid in ECG Interpretation

- *Mistaking the ST-segment elevation of coronary spasm for acute myocardial injury.* These changes usually resolve after the administration of nitroglycerin (NTG) and should be suspected in the setting of cold- or emotion-induced symptoms.
- *Failure to note the ST-segment elevation of pericarditis (see Fig. 9-5), which may not involve all ECG leads.* Acute pericarditis usually causes very typical symptoms consisting of sharp, pleuritic chest pains, which are exacerbated when the patient is in the recumbent position. In a minority of patients, acute pericarditis will present with symptoms indistinguishable from those of acute MI. Furthermore, pericarditis can itself occur as a complication of acute MI.
- *Failure to distinguish repolarization abnormalities due to left bundle branch block, left ventricular hypertrophy, and pacemaker rhythms.* These repolarization abnormalities make the diagnosis of acute MI by ECG difficult.

Some clinical conditions in which ECG interpretation can be difficult are listed in Table 9-5.

Myocardial Markers
Myocardial markers are another useful adjunct in helping in the diagnosis of MI. It is important, however, to interpret the level of elevation (if present) in relation to the onset of infarction (see Table 9-6). As with ECGs, myocardial markers should not be used as the sole basis of disposition. Results of serum markers are generally not readily available in the urgent care setting and patients should never have blood drawn for cardiac enzymes and then be discharged from the facility prior to obtaining the results.

(text continued in page 162)

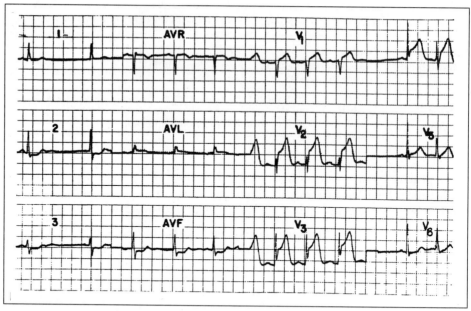

FIGURE 9-1 Anterior myocardial infarction. (From Tintinalli J et al: *Emergency Medicine,* 4th ed. New York: McGraw-Hill; 1996:330, with permission.)

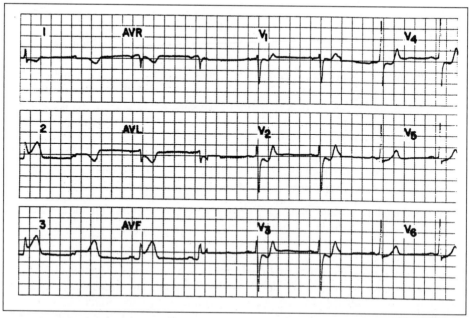

FIGURE 9-2 Inferior myocardial infarction. (From Tintinalli J et al: *Emergency Medicine,* 4th ed. New York: McGraw-Hill; 1996:330, with permission.)

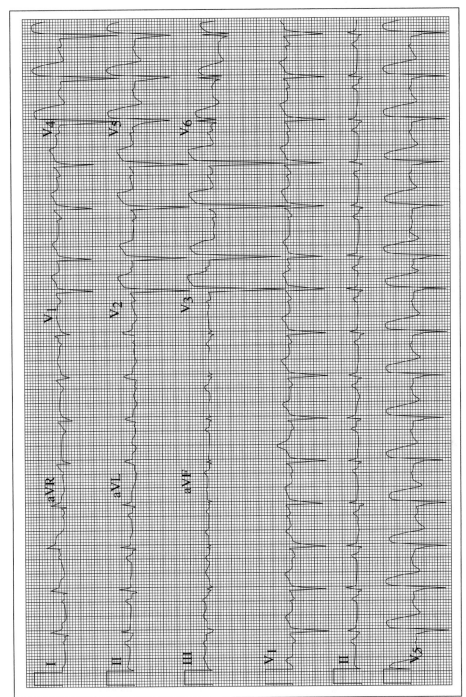

FIGURE 9-3   Lateral wall myocardial infarction. (From Ferry DR: *Basic Electrocardiography in Ten Days*. New York: McGraw-Hill; 2001:105, with permission.)

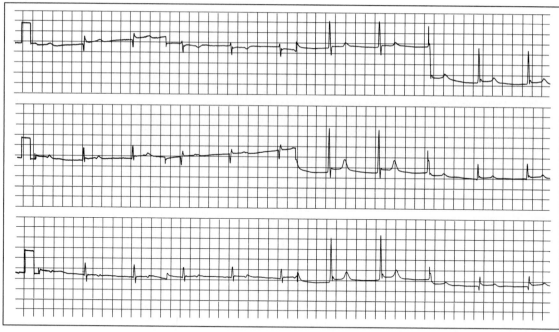

FIGURE 9-4   Posterior myocardial infarction. (From Tintinalli J et al: *Emergency Medicine,* 4th ed. New York; McGraw-Hill: 1996:331, with permission.)

TABLE 9-5

CLINICAL CONDITIONS WHERE ELECTROCARDIOGRAPHIC INTEPRETATIONS CAN BE DIFFICULT

May have ST-segment elevation in the absence of acute myocardial infarction	Paced rhythms
Early repolarization	Left bundle branch block
Left ventricular hypertrophy	May have T-wave inversions in the absence of ischemia
Pericarditis	Persistent juvenile pattern
Myocarditis	Stokes-Adams syncope or seizures
Left ventricular aneurysms	Post-tachycardia T-wave inversion
Idiopathic hypertrophic subaortic stenosis	Post-pacemaker T-wave inversion
Hypothermia	Intracranial pathology (CNS bleeds)
Paced rhythms	Mitral valve prolapse
Left bundle branch block	Pericarditis
May have ST-segment depressions in the absence of ischemia	Primary or secondary myocardial diseases
Hypokalemia	Pulmonary embolism or cor pulmonale from other causes
Digoxin effect	Spontaneous pneumothorax
Cor pulmonale and right heart strain	Myocardial contusion
Early repolarization	Left ventricular hypertrophy
Left ventricular hypertrophy	Paced rhythms
	Left bundle branch block

SOURCE: Tintinalli J et al: *Emergency Medicine: A Study Guide,* 5th ed. New York: McGraw-Hill, 2000:360, with permission.

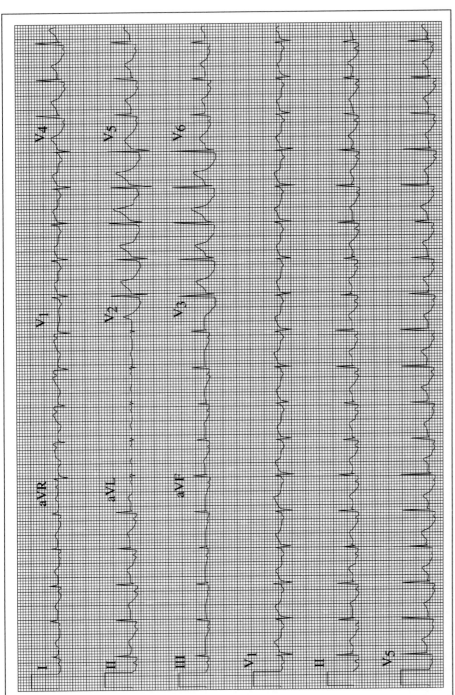

FIGURE 9-5   Acute pericarditis with sinus tachycardia. (From Ferry DR: *Basic Electrocardiography in Ten Days*. New York: McGraw-Hill; 2001:228, with permission.)

TABLE 9-6

CARDIAC MARKERS

Marker	Initial Elevation	Peak Elevation	Duration of Elevation
Myoglobin	1 to 4 h	6 h	24 h
Cardiac troponin I	3 to 12 h	18 h	5 to 10 days
Cardiac troponin T	3 to 12 h	12 h	5 to 14 days
CK-MB	3 to 12 h	18 to 24 h	2 days
LDH	10 h	1 to 2 days	10 to 14 days

 Management (Table 9-7)

The initial therapy for non-Q-wave or non-ST-segment elevation MI is similar to that for unstable angina. Whenever possible, therapy should be initiated at the urgent care facility prior to transfer to an inpatient facility. Cardiac monitoring is mandatory while awaiting emergency transfer and must be continued throughout transport.

In addition to oxygen, aspirin, nitrates, heparin, and beta-blockers, thrombolytic therapy should be considered in patients presenting with acute ST-segment elevations (Table 9-8). Certain thrombolytic agents such as tenecteplase (TNKase), anistreplase (Eminase), and reteplase (Retavase) can be administered as a single or double intravenous bolus over 2 to 3 min and may be particularly useful in the urgent care setting. It is imperative that any initiation of thrombolytic therapy be done in concert with the receiving facility, emergency medical services (EMS) transport, and the admitting

TABLE 9-7

TREATMENT OF ACUTE MYOCARDIAL INFARCTION

Oxygen 2 to 4 L/min
IV access
Continuous cardiac monitoring
Beta blocker: metoprolol 2.5 to 5 mg IV; 12.5 to 50 mg PO
Aspirin: 325 to 650 mg (chewed)
Nitroglycerin
   Sublingual (0.4 mg q 5 min × 3)
   Intravenous (5 to 10 µg titrated up by 10 µg q 3 to 5 min)
   Transdermal (1 to 2 in. to the chest wall; not to be used to treat active/ongoing pain)
Morphine: 2 to 5 mg IV q 5 to 10 min
Heparin:
   Subcutaneous (7500 to 10,000 units) or
   Intravenous (bolus: 75 U/kg with maximum of 5000 U)
Thrombolytic agents (as indicated)
Hospital transport

TABLE 9-8

INDICATIONS FOR THROMBOLYTIC THERAPY

Symptoms of myocardial infarction with:
  Symptoms present less than 6 to 12 h
  ECG with ST-segment elevation of at least 1 mm in two contiguous leads

cardiologist and that protocols be firmly established in the urgent care facility, with all providers being fully knowledgeable in the administration of thrombolytic agents.

While the greatest benefits of thrombolytic therapy are seen in the highest-risk patients (e.g., elderly patients or those with acute anterior infarction and cardiogenic shock), benefit also occurs in low-risk patients, such as the young patient with inferior wall infarction and no electrical or hemodynamic complications. In patients with relative contraindications to thrombolytic therapy (Table 9-9), the decision to use this therapy should be made in concert with the receiving cardiologist based on a careful risk/benefit analysis, with particular attention paid to the desires of the patient.

TABLE 9-9

CONTRAINDICATIONS TO THROMBOLYTIC THERAPY

Absolute contraindications
  Previous hemorrhagic stroke at any time
  Bland strokes or cardiovascular accident in past year
  Known intracranial neoplasm
  Active internal bleeding (excluding menses)
  Suspected aortic dissection
  Diabetic retinopathy
Relative contraindications
  Severe uncontrolled blood pressure (>180/100 mmHg)
  History of prior cerebrovascular accident or known intracranial pathology not covered
    in contraindications
  Current use of anticoagulants with international normalized ratio > 2 to 3
  Known bleeding diathesis
  Recent trauma (past 2 weeks)
  Prolonged cardiopulmonary resuscitation > 10 min
  Major surgery < 3 weeks
  Noncompressible vascular punctures
  Recent internal bleeding (2–4 weeks)
  Prior allergic reaction to streptokinase (should not receive streptokinase)
  Pregnancy
  Active peptic ulcer disease
  History of chronic severe hypertension

SOURCE: Tintinalli J et al: *Emergency Medicine: A Study Guide*, 5th ed. New York: McGraw-Hill; 2000:367, with permission.

Complications of Acute MIs

Complications that can be seen in the setting of an acute MI include dysrhythmias, congestive heart failure, acute pulmonary edema, neurologic events, syncope, and cardiac arrest. It is imperative to be prepared to treat any of these entities in patients presenting with an acute MI, even if they are initially stable.

Disposition of Patients with Stable Angina

Patients who have no new ECG changes and who have stable angina responsive to nitrates may be appropriate for home discharge from the urgent care setting. Discharge instructions should include early follow-up with the primary care physician, instructions regarding activity level, and criteria for returning to an emergency department should the symptoms recur or worsen.

Similarly, patients whose history and examination suggest a likelihood of previously undiagnosed *stable* ischemic heart disease do not require hospital admission for workup and can be referred for subsequent cardiology evaluation and stress testing. A typical example would be a patient who presents for the first time with a long-standing history of exertional angina that occurs only at a relatively high exercise workload, is responsive to rest, and has been stable over time. For these patients, discharge instructions should also include a prescription for sublingual NTG and specific criteria for its use.

Disposition of Patients with Noncardiac Chest Pain (Table 9-10)

In those patients whose history and examination strongly suggest a noncardiac cause, cardiac testing should be avoided. This is especially pertinent for exercise stress testing, in which minor, falsely positive abnormalities may lead to unnecessary anxiety, difficulty in obtaining insurance coverage, and occasionally the performance of unnecessary and potentially risky invasive tests. Treatment should be aimed at the underlying condition and follow-up should be with the primary care physician for any ongoing care or further evaluation, as indicated.

TABLE 9-10

CHEST PAIN: CRITERIA FOR DISCHARGE HOME

Stable vital signs
Ischemic heart disease excluded or, if present, determined not to be acute or unstable
Resolution of symptoms or the diagnosis of a specific noncardiac condition prior to discharge
Appropriate follow-up arrangements made

Aortic Dissection

Patients with acute aortic dissection often present with symptoms of chest pain. Dissection of the aorta results from a transverse tear in the intima and inner layer of the media of the aortic wall, separating this layer of the media and adventitia of the aorta. Following this initial tear, a longitudinal tearing of the aortic wall along the media occurs, with propagation of the tear proximally, distally, or in both directions along the length of the aorta.

Classification

Several classification systems are used to define types of aortic dissection. The simplest classification divides aortic dissection into proximal and distal dissection, with the tear originating in the ascending and descending aorta, respectively. Another classification emphasizes the affected portion of the aorta rather than the segment in which the dissection originates. In this classification system, type A dissection refers to the situation in which the tear originates in the descending aorta (distal dissection) but propagates retrogradely to involve the ascending aorta (proximal dissection). In yet a third classification system used in the literature, emphasis is placed on the location of the dissection. In this system, type I dissection refers to a primary tear in the ascending aorta, type II dissection involves only the descending aorta, and type III dissection originates from the subclavian artery and extends distally.

 History

- A useful approach that minimizes the likelihood of missing an aortic dissection is to consider aortic dissection in the differential diagnosis of any patient presenting with chest pain; patients presenting with acute MI should be assumed to have aortic dissection until proven otherwise.

The typical patient with aortic dissection is a middle-aged male presenting with sudden, severe anterior or posterior chest pain. The pain may be described as "tearing," "ripping," or feeling as though something were "bursting" in the chest or back. There is radiation of the pain caudally (to the hips, buttocks, and legs) or rostrally (to the head, neck, and arms), depending on the presence or absence of distal extension of the dissection. Certain features of the clinical presentation may suggest the location of the dissection, but these signs may be variable and their absence does not rule out the diagnosis. For example, dissection in the ascending aorta tends to present with substernal pain, whereas dissection of the descending aorta is more likely to cause interscapular or epigastric pain.

 Physical Examination

Physical examination often reveals an ill-appearing patient with diaphoresis and pallor, resembling the appearance of a patient in cardiogenic shock. With aortic dissection, however, the blood pressure is usually elevated, especially if the dissection originates in the proximal descending aorta. Additionally, new cardiac murmurs, systolic and diastolic, may be heard and arterial pulse deficits, which are common in dissections involving the aortic arch or arch vessels, may also be noted. Chest x-ray may show a widening of the mediastinum, separation of intimal calcium from the aortic wall, tracheal deviation to the right, downward depression of the left mainstem bronchus, a left pleural effusion, or changes in shape and size of the aorta from previous films.

Diagnosis

Confirmatory tests for diagnosing an aortic dissection include contrast-enhanced computed tomography (CT) scan or magnetic resonance imaging (MRI) of the chest and/or abdomen. In patients who are hemodynamically unstable, bedside transesophageal echocardiography is preferred. This procedure has comparable sensitivity and specificity to CT scanning or MRI. The above tests have decreased the need for aortography, although this may still be necessary to plan surgical treatment.

 Management

If the diagnosis of aortic dissection is made or suspected in the urgent care setting, immediate transfer to the intensive care unit is mandatory. The goal of initial therapy of aortic dissection is to maintain hemodynamic stability while reducing the aortic pressure sufficiently to reduce the risk of rupture.

Most patients will be normotensive or hypertensive and should be treated with an intravenous beta blocker—e.g., propranolol 1.0 to 2.0 mg IV or metoprolol 5 to 10 mg IV every 2 to 4 h. The goal is to maintain systolic blood pressure between 100 and 110 mmHg. If additional blood pressure reduction is desired, intravenous nitroprusside may be added and titrated to a systolic pressure of 100 to 110 mmHg. Pain and anxiety should be relieved with morphine and benzodiazepines. A urinary catheter should be inserted to monitor urine flow volume, and a higher blood pressure should be maintained if there is a decrease in the urine output or evidence of renal compromise due to involvement of the renal arteries. Surgical consultation should be initiated while preparing the patient for emergency transport.

Chest Pain

 Key Points of Documentation

- Location of pain
- Character of pain
- Duration of pain
- Precipitating factors
- Factors aggravating/relieving symptoms (including medications)
- Relationship to exertion/rest
- Presence or absence of associated
    dyspnea
    nausea/vomiting
    diaphoresis
- Presence or absence of cardiac risk factors:
    diabetes
    hypertension
    smoking
    family history or past cardiac history
    hyperlipidemia
- Blood pressure
- Distal pulses
- Respiratory rate and character
- Cardiac auscultation
- Pulmonary auscultation

- Reproducibility of pain on palpation if present
- ECG findings
- Response to treatment

 Errors to Avoid

- Missing the presentation of an aortic aneurysm. Dissection of the proximal aorta involving the epicardial coronary arteries can produce ST-segment elevations that simulate acute MI. Patients will classically have sharp, interscapular pain, often associated with pulse deficits, unequal pulses, or new murmurs. *This distinction is crucial, since thrombolytic therapy is contraindicated in aortic dissection.*
- Missing the presentation of pulmonary embolism.
- Missing the "silent" MI.
- Missing atypical anginal equivalents (nausea, dizziness, dyspnea). Ischemic heart disease can often present very atypically, especially in patients with diabetes mellitus. Dyspnea is often an anginal equivalent. Nonspecific symptoms such as epigastric discomfort or nausea may be the sole presenting complaint. The diabetic patient with acute ischemia may also have few or no ECG abnormalities. A high index of suspicion is necessary to avoid misdiagnosis in diabetic patients.
- Missing cardiac illness in a patient who is young (male or female) or without apparent risk factors.
- Attributing cardiac symptoms to other chronic, underlying illnesses such as esophageal spasms. A history of other underlying illnesses such as esophageal spasms does not rule out new cardiac illness

CARDIAC DYSRHYTHMIAS

Symptoms of cardiac dysrhythmias may be the primary reason for an urgent care visit or may be detected only as incidental findings in a patient seen for other complaints. When patients present with hemodynamic compromise (Table 9-11), emergent treatment is required. In those circumstances when a dysrhythmia presents only as an incidental finding, the urgent care physician must determine what potential the arrhythmia has to cause hemodynamic instability and whether it is a sign of an increased risk of sudden cardiac death. Once this decision has been made, it is possible to decide whether the arrhythmia needs to be treated urgently, electively, or not at all.

TABLE 9-11

SYMPTOMS OF HEMODYNAMIC COMPROMISE

Shock	Altered mental status
Cardiac/anginal chest pain	Signs of cerebrovascular compromise/stroke
Congestive heart failure/pulmonary edema	

Extrasystoles

Premature beats (ventricular or supraventricular) occur commonly in the general population. While these usually do not cause symptoms, such cases may be seen in the urgent care setting when they result in palpitations or when premature beats are noted as an incidental finding in patients presenting for other complaints. In these patients, the history may be remarkable for exogenous cardiac stimulants such as caffeine, nicotine, or over-the-counter cardioactive medications. The patient may also give a history of an illness or condition (e.g., vomiting, diarrhea) resulting in hypokalemia or other electrolyte disturbance. The physical examination is generally unremarkable except for auscultation or palpation of the premature beats or possible evidence of dehydration if gastrointestinal losses are present. In the absence of structural heart disease, pharmacologic treatment should be optional and should be started only in consultation with the primary care physician. Often, removal of exogenous cardiac stimulants may be helpful in mitigating symptoms and may be all that is needed. If hypokalemia exists, it should be corrected with appropriate supplementation, and the culprit condition (e.g., gastroenteritis) causing the electrolyte disturbance should be treated. When treatment is considered for premature atrial beats, a beta blocker or an anxiolytic (such as a benzodiazepine) is the medication of choice. Antiarrhythmic medications should be avoided, since the risk of proarrhythmia usually outweighs the benefits of symptom relief. In unusual cases, patients with persistently bothersome premature ventricular contractions who fail to respond to the above measures may be treated with antiarrhythmic agents. The initiation of these medications, however, falls outside the scope of the urgent care department, particularly given that antiarrhythmic therapy will not, in general, improve patient survival.

Sinus Tachycardia

Sinus tachycardia is arbitrarily defined as a sinus rate exceeding 100 beats per minute. Common causes include hypovolemia, exertion, stress, anemia, and febrile illnesses. Less common causes are thyroid excess, drug effects (sympathomimetics, alcohol, caffeine), pericarditis, or cardiomyopathy. Many acute cardiopulmonary conditions—including MI, pulmonary embolism, and aortic dissection—may cause sinus tachycardia. Not infrequently, sinus tachycardia is idiopathic ("inappropriate sinus tachycardia"). Treatment of sinus tachycardia should be directed at correcting the underlying condition—e.g., by hydration or correction of hypoxemia.

- Carotid sinus massage usually slows the sinus rate and may permit the differentiation of sinus tachycardia in the presence of bundle branch block from other widecomplex tachycardias such as ventricular tachycardia.

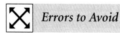 *Errors to Avoid*

Failure to diagnose atrial flutter. Apparent sinus tachycardia occurring at a rate of 150 beats per minute should raise the suspicion of atrial flutter at 300 beats per minute, with a 2:1 atrioventricular conduction block.

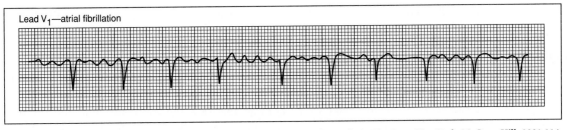

FIGURE 9-6 Atrial fibrillation, lead V$_1$. (From Ferry DR: *Basic Electrocardiography in Ten Days.* New York: McGraw-Hill; 2001:114, with permission.)

Atrial Fibrillation (Fig. 9-6)

Atrial fibrillation is the most common supraventricular tachyarrhythmia encountered in the urgent care setting. It is usually associated with structural heart disease but may occur in the absence of any discernible abnormality of heart structure or function (lone atrial fibrillation). See Table 9-12 for the differential diagnosis of atrial fibrillation. In the usual scenario, the patient with atrial fibrillation will present with tachycardia, palpitations, chest pain, dyspnea, and/or dizziness. In patients with preexisting coronary artery disease, the rapid ventricular response to atrial fibrillation may cause the patient to present with an acute ischemic syndrome, such as unstable angina or acute MI. In the elderly and in patients already taking heart-rate-slowing drugs for other purposes, atrial fibrillation may be asymptomatic and may only be detected when the patient presents for an unrelated complaint. Initial diagnostic testing should include a complete blood count, chemistry profile, thyroid function tests, chest x-ray, and ECG. Tests to exclude MI should be performed only when the clinical picture suggests this possibility. Other causes of atrial fibrillation that should also be considered are valvular heart disease (mitral regurgitation, mitral valve prolapse, aortic stenosis), hypertensive heart disease, cardiomyopathy, and acute ingestion of recreational drugs and/or alcohol (the "holiday heart" syndrome).

 Management

- Treatment of atrial fibrillation with hemodynamic compromise: synchronized cardioversion starting at 100 J

TABLE 9-12

CAUSES OF ATRIAL FIBRILLATION

Hyperthyroidism	Rheumatic heart disease
Ischemic heart disease (including acute myocardial infarction)	Alcohol/illicit drug use
	Pericarditis
Hypertension	Acute lung disease, e.g., pulmonary embolism
Valvular heart disease	Electrolyte abnormalities
Cardiomyopathy	Chronic lung disease

Patients presenting with hemodynamic compromise secondary to atrial fibrillation should be treated with electrical cardioversion. These patients will require hospital admission; therefore simultaneous arrangements should be made for emergency transfer to an acute care facility.

Pharmacologic therapy may be used to treat rapid atrial fibrillation in stable patients without hemodynamic compromise or chest pain.Medications for this purpose can be viewed in two broad categories: (1) drugs that slow the ventricular rate and (2) antiarrhythmic agents, which may be used after the ventricular rate has been controlled to effect conversion to sinus rhythm.

Drugs That Slow the Ventricular Rate   Beta-adrenergic blocking drugs (such as metoprolol, propranolol, and esmolol) are useful for rate control in atrial fibrillation. Either the oral or intravenous route may be used, depending on the urgency of the situation. The use of a beta blocker is especially logical when atrial fibrillation presents in the setting of thyroid excess, hypertensive heart disease, or ischemic heart disease. Beta blockers, however, should be avoided in situations where the atrial fibrillation is the result of a disease process (such as cardiomyopathy or obstructive lung disease) in which the negative inotropic properties are a contraindication to their use.

Rate-limiting calcium channel antagonists are an alternative to the use of beta blockers for rate control in atrial fibrillation. Both diltiazem and verapamil may be administered by the intravenous route. Diltiazem may be preferred because it is slightly less negatively inotropic (see caution for beta blockers previously discussed) and can be continued as an intravenous infusion after the initial bolus. Intravenous verapamil is given as a bolus of 5 mg. Intravenous diltiazem is given as an initial bolus of 0.25 mg/kg over 2 min, followed by a maintenance infusion of 5 to 15 mg/h.

Digoxin is an alternative medication for rate control in atrial fibrillation. Its major advantages are the absence of any negative inotropic effects, ease of administration, and low cost. In a patient who is not already taking digoxin, beta blockers, or rate-limiting calcium antagonists, digoxin loading may be accomplished with intravenous doses of 0.25 mg given at 20- to 30-min intervals to a total dose of approximately 1 g. The loading dose can then be followed by additional oral or intravenous maintenance doses. The loading dose may be unnecessary if the patient is already on digoxin, a beta blocker, or a rate-slowing calcium antagonist.

Of note, digoxin is relatively ineffective in controlling exercise heart rates due to vagal withdrawal and the increased sympathetic tone that occurs during exercise. Therefore, a beta blocker or calcium antagonist is preferred for active patients. Combinations of digoxin with a beta blocker or calcium antagonist are also very effective in ventricular rate control in atrial fibrillation and may minimize the side effects seen with larger doses of a single drug.

- Patients, such as the elderly, who have preexisting conduction system disease may present with a slow ventricular response to atrial fibrillation and will not require any rate-controlling therapy.

Once adequate ventricular rate control has been achieved, the patient may be discharged home (Table 9-13) or transferred, as indicated, to an inpatient facility for further evaluation and treatment. For patients with new-onset atrial fibrillation (i.e., less

TABLE 9-13

ATRIAL FIBRILLATION: CRITERIA FOR DISCHARGE

Adequate control of the ventricular rate
Stable vital signs
Correct maintenance dosage of rate-slowing drug prescribed
Appropriate follow-up arrangements made
Potentially serious causes of atrial fibrillation (e.g., pulmonary embolism, acute myocardial infarction) have been excluded
Initiation of anticoagulation if atrial fibrillation persists

than 24 h in duration), the risk of embolic events with cardioversion is low. Intravenous anticoagulation should be started and arrangement for cardioversion made. Patients with atrial fibrillation of longer duration (greater than 24 h) generally require anticoagulation for 3 to 4 weeks before cardioversion is attempted. As an alternative to this approach, transesophageal echocardiography may be performed to exclude intracardiac thrombi; cardioversion can then be performed immediately if no thrombi are found.

For those high-risk patients who require hospitalization, it may be reasonable to begin intravenous heparin in the urgent care setting. For low-risk patients who are to be followed as outpatients, warfarin or aspirin can be initiated in consultation with the cardiologist or primary care physician.

Atrial Flutter (Fig. 9-7)

As with most dysrhythmias, the presentation of patients with atrial flutter will depend on the ventricular rate. Patients therefore generally present with either symptoms of hemodynamic compromise or complaints of palpitations. Most episodes of atrial flutter are due to a reentrant mechanism involving pathways confined to the atrium. The result is typical atrial sawtooth flutter waves, which occur at a rate of approximately 250 to 350 beats per minute. Often, a 2:1 (or higher) atrioventricular block is present, resulting in a ventricular rate between 125 and 200 beats per minute (most typically at 150 beats per minute).

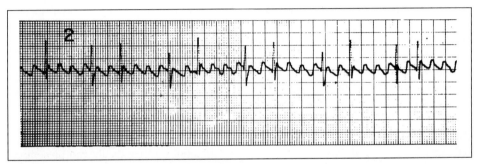

FIGURE 9-7   Atrial flutter. (From Tintinalli J, et al: *Emergency Medicine*, 5th ed. New York: **McGraw-Hill; 2000:174**, with permission.)

TABLE 9-14

CAUSES OF ATRIAL FLUTTER

Ischemic heart disease or myocardial infarction	Cardiomyopathy
	Myocarditis
Pulmonary embolism	Digoxin toxicity

- Since atrial flutter can masquerade as sinus tachycardia, any regular, narrow complex tachycardia must be assumed to represent atrial flutter until proven otherwise.

 Management

- Atrial flutter with hemodynamic compromise; synchronized cardioversion starting at 25 to 50 J

Acute atrial flutter is often difficult to treat pharmacologically. The goal of treatment is to reduce the ventricular rate by using a beta blocker (esmolol or propranolol), verapamil, diltiazem, or digoxin (see "Management" under "Atrial Fibrillation"). Once rate control is achieved, conversion to sinus rhythm can be attempted electively by the cardiologist, using electrical cardioversion or pharmacologic agents such as procainamide or quinidine. Although atrial activity is preserved in atrial flutter, there is still a significant thromboembolic risk from cardioversion. Anticoagulation, therefore, is required prior to cardioversion if the atrial flutter is of long standing. Oral anticoagulation should be started at the urgent care facility in consultation with the cardiologist who will follow the patient. Potential acute causes of atrial flutter, particularly pulmonary embolism or acute MI, must be ruled out prior to discharge (Table 9-14).

Paroxysmal Supraventricular Tachycardia (Fig. 9-8)

Paroxysmal supraventricular tachycardia (PSVT) is commonly seen in the urgent care setting and frequently results from valvular heart disease (e.g., mitral valve prolapse) or preexcitation syndromes (e.g., Wolff-Parkinson-White syndrome). Two mechanisms of PSVT are recognized: (1) increased automaticity and (2) atrioventricular (AV) reentry. In PSVT due to increased automaticity, atrial tachycardia originates from an atrial site other than the sinus node and usually has a rate exceeding 200 beats per minute. The ECG will show a nonsinus P wave that precedes each QRS complex.

Atrioventricular reentry SVT may be divided into AV node–dependent circuits and AV node–independent circuits. Vagal maneuvers and adenosine administration are therapeutic for the former and diagnostic for the latter (i.e., absence of effect in the AV node–independent tachycardias).

Clinical Presentation

Patients with PSVT will typically present with palpitations. Occasionally, the presenting complaints may include dizziness, syncope, chest pain, dyspnea, fatigue, or exercise intolerance. In general, the severity of the symptoms depends on the rate of the arrhythmia, the underlying condition, and the presence or absence of concomitant cardiopulmonary diseases.

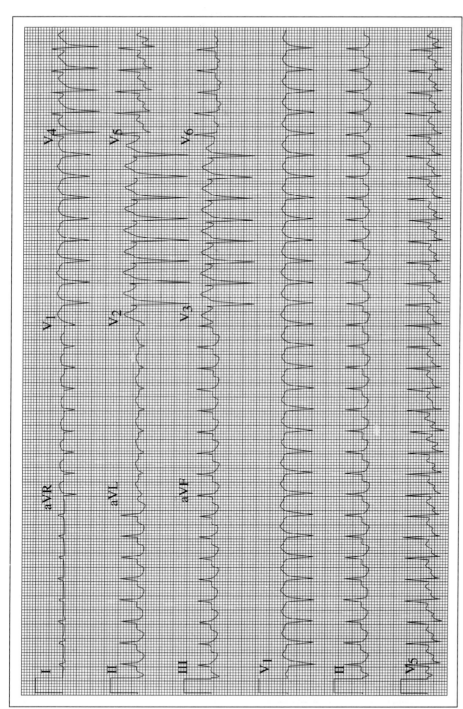

FIGURE 9-8 Supraventricular tachycardia. (From Ferry DR: *Basic Electrocardiography in Ten Days*. New York: McGraw-Hill; 2001:158, with permission.)

Management

Treatment for PSVT depends on the clinical situation in which it occurs. Unless the clinical situation is urgent due to hemodynamic compromise, the first step in treatment should be application of vagal maneuvers (Valsalva, carotid massage, ice immersion, etc.). The presence of severe conduction system disease (e.g., in the elderly) is a contraindication to carotid sinus massage. Pharmacologically, intravenous adenosine is the drug of choice for terminating most episodes of acute sustained supraventricular tachycardia. It is given as a 6-mg rapid intravenous bolus. If that is unsuccessful, a 12-mg dose should be tried. Intravenous verapamil (5- to 10-mg bolus) or diltiazem (20 mg over 2 min, followed by continuous infusion as necessary) may be used if the patient's history is unclear or if the patient is suspected of having underlying bradycardia. Similarly, intravenous beta blockers (propranolol or metoprolol) may be used if they are not contraindicated because of congestive heart failure or bronchospasm.

- Supraventricular tachycardia occurring in the presence of preexcitation (e.g., Wolff-Parkinson-White syndrome) may present a therapeutic problem. Many varieties of supraventricular tachycardia, including atrial flutter or fibrillation, can result in acceleration of antegrade conduction over the accessory pathway to cause ventricular tachycardia or fibrillation. Drugs such as digoxin and verapamil, which shorten the refractory period of the accessory pathway, may enhance conduction over the antegrade pathway and should be avoided.

Multifocal Atrial Tachycardia (Fig. 9-9)

The development of multifocal atrial tachycardia is often associated with advanced pulmonary disease or use of medications prescribed in the treatment of advanced pulmonary disease, including bronchodilators. In multifocal atrial tachycardia (MAT), in addition to an atrial rate exceeding 100 beats per minute, the ECG will show at least three distinct morphologies of the P waves. The atrial and ventricular rates are often irregular, thus simulating atrial fibrillation. Treatment of MAT consists of treating the underlying pulmonary disorder. Drug therapy with verapamil has been used to treat MAT with some success, but digoxin should be avoided, as it can aggravate the dysrhythmia. In fact, digoxin is known to cause MAT in some circumstances.

As in the case of other cardiac arrhythmias, serum electrolytes and magnesium should be checked and appropriate treatment, including replenishing the magnesium, initiated.

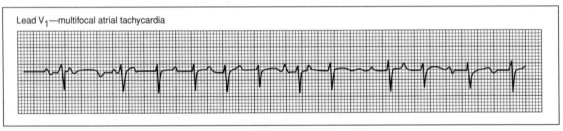

FIGURE 9-9 Multiatrial tachycardia, lead V_1. (From Ferry DR: *Basic Electrocardiography in Ten Days*. New York: McGraw-Hill; 2001:125, with permission.)

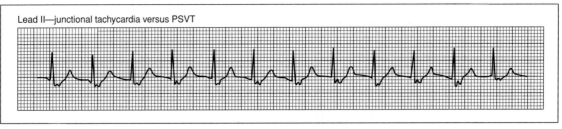

FIGURE 9-10   Nonparoxsymal junctional tachycardia. (From Ferry DR: *Basic Electrocardiography in Ten Days.* New York: McGraw-Hill; 2001:126, with permission.)

Nonparoxysmal Junctional Tachycardia (Fig. 9-10)

Nonparoxysmal junctional tachycardia is a rhythm that can be seen in (1) digoxin toxicity, (2) the early phase of (inferior) MI, (3) myocarditis or severe mitral valve disease, (4) following cardiac surgery, and (5) as a consequence of treatment with class 1a antiarrhythmic agents such as quinidine and procainamide. The mechanism for nonparoxysmal junctional tachycardia involves enhanced automaticity of the AV junction. The ventricular rate is usually between 70 and 130 beats per minute. When the tachycardia is irregular, as it often is, it may be confused with ventricular tachycardia—especially if the QRS complexes are widened due to aberrant conduction or in the presence of a bundle branch block. Treatment of nonparoxysmal junctional tachycardia consists of correcting the underlying cause.

Ventricular Tachycardia (Fig. 9-11)

Ventricular tachycardia, which may be sustained or nonsustained, is defined as three or more ventricular premature complexes occurring in tandem at a rate exceeding 100 beats per minute. Nonsustained ventricular tachycardia lasts 3 to 15 beats and terminates spontaneously. Sustained ventricular tachycardia lasts more than 30 beats and generally requires antiarrhythmic treatment, pacing, or cardioversion for termination. Ventricular tachycardia nearly always implies the existence of cardiopulmonary disease or another systemic condition such as electrolyte disturbance or drug toxicity. Rare instances of ventricular tachycardia in apparently normal hearts have been described.

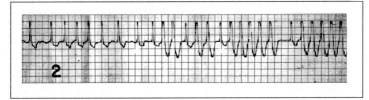

FIGURE 9-11   Ventricular tachycardia. (From Tintinalli J et al: *Emergency Medicine,* 5th ed. New York: McGraw-Hill; 2000:180, with permission.)

Clinical Presentation

The rate of ventricular tachycardia is generally between 100 and 250 beats per minute, and presenting symptoms will often reflect the rate at the time of presentation. Patients with slow, nonsustained ventricular tachycardia may be asymptomatic or minimally symptomatic (e.g., palpitations). In contrast, patients with rapid, sustained tachycardia will usually show signs of hemodynamic compromise. By history or physical examination, patients will usually have evidence of underlying heart disease. This is typically coronary artery disease, although other disease entities, such as cardiomyopathy or valvular heart disease, may also be seen. In general, ability to tolerate the arrhythmia depends on the prior cardiovascular state. In patients with poor myocardial function, the ventricular tachycardia may degenerate into ventricular fibrillation and cardiovascular collapse, requiring cardiopulmonary resuscitation.

Differential Diagnosis

If possible, ventricular tachycardia should be differentiated from supraventricular tachycardia with aberration. This differentiation may be difficult at times, since both conditions produce a wide complex tachycardia. Many ECG criteria have been developed to distinguish between the two, including the width of the QRS complex (greater than 140 ms favors ventricular tachycardia) and the presence of AV dissociation, fusion beats, or concordance across the precordium, all of which favor ventricular tachycardia. It should be noted that the vast majority (greater than 90 percent) of the wide-complex tachycardia seen in patients with structural heart disease (coronary artery disease, cardiomyopathy, valvular heart disease, etc.) represent ventricular tachycardia.

 Management

Treatment of ventricular tachycardia should be individualized. In the presence of hemodynamic compromise, immediate synchronized cardioversion should be performed, starting with 100 J. Arrangements should be made simultaneously for immediate emergency department transfer via an advanced life support (ALS) transport unit. Pharmacologic treatment with lidocaine, procainamide, or amiodarone may be indicated.

- Pharmacologic treatment can cause other, more unstable arrhythmia that may require immediate cardioversion or antitachycardia pacing

Bradycardias and AV Block

Definitions

Sinus bradycardia is defined as sinus rhythm at a rate of less than 60 beats per minute. It may signify the presence of conduction system disease or, as in the trained athlete, merely reflect cardiovascular fitness.

First-degree AV block (Fig. 9-12) is defined as prolongation of the PR interval beyond 200 ms. First-degree block is usually an indication of conduction system disease, most commonly due to aging. The length of the PR interval is also related to the heart rate; extreme bradycardia, such as that due to drug effect, may cause first-degree AV block.

In *second-degree AV block*, there is intermittent failure of AV conduction. Two types of second-degree AV block are recognized: in type I (Wenckebach) block, the PR inter-

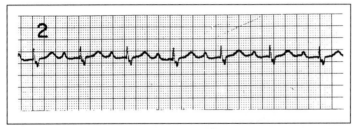

FIGURE 9-12 First-degree AV block. (From Tintinalli J et al: *Emergency Medicine*, 5th ed. New York: McGraw-Hill; 2000:183, with permission.)

val preceding the dropped beat is different from the interval following it (Fig. 9-13). In type II block, the PR interval stays the same before and following the dropped beat— that is, the AV conduction time stays constant (Fig. 9-14).

In *third-degree AV block* (complete heart block), there is complete dissociation of atrial and ventricular activity (Fig. 9-15). The atrial impulses are not conducted to the ventricle, and ventricular electrical activity originates from an "ectopic" focus within or below the AV node.

Clinical Presentation
Bradyarrhythmia may occur as the result of intrinsic cardiac conduction system disease or myocardial damage (e.g., in MI), or as a side effect of drug therapy. First-degree AV block does not produce any hemodynamic effects and patients with this bradyarrhythmia are typically asymptomatic. Similarly, type I AV block, like first-degree AV block, usually causes no symptoms except in situations of extreme bradycardia, where dizziness or syncope may result. Type II AV block frequently causes symptoms of hypoperfusion, including syncope or fatigue. With type II AV block, there is a high risk of progression to third-degree AV block. Third-degree (complete) heart block nearly always causes symptoms, although some patients with a stable escape rhythm may remain asymptomatic. Symptoms—which may include angina, dyspnea, or syncope—depend on the rate of the resulting bradycardia and whether the complete heart block is intermittent or sustained.

 Management
First-degree AV block rarely if ever requires permanent pacing. Type I heart block requires pacing only if it is associated with severe bradycardia resulting in symptoms such as chest pain, shortness of breath, hypotension, or congestive heart failure. Type II

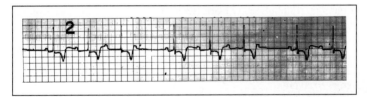

FIGURE 9-13 Second-degree AV block, Mobitz I. (From Tintinalli J et al: *Emergency Medicine*, 5th ed. New York: McGraw-Hill; 2000:184, with permission.)

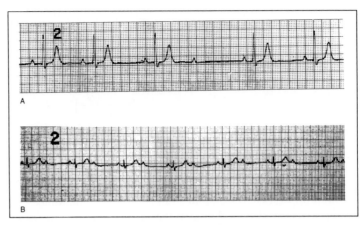

FIGURE 9-14   Second-degree AV block, Mobitz II. (From Tintinalli J et al: *Emergency Medicine*, 5th ed. New York: McGraw-Hill; 2000:184, with permission.)

second-degree heart block and third-degree block, however, require treatment with a permanent pacemaker unless the reason for the bradyarrhythmia is potentially reversible, as in ischemia involving the conduction system.

In the urgent care setting, patients with symptomatic bradycardia may be treated with intravenous atropine (0.5- to 1.0-mg doses). Repeat bolus injections up to a total of 0.03 mg/kg may be given every 20 to 30 min (or sooner for severe or unresponsive symptoms), while awaiting hospital transport. An external pacer may be useful for short-term treatment. For severe symptoms requiring additional treatment, dopamine for hypotension may be initiated at a rate of 5 to 20 μg/kg per minute or epinephrine at a rate of 2 to 10 μg/min if needed.

- Multiple doses of atropine may result in cholinergic side effects, including dry mouth, bladder dysfunction, mydriasis, etc.

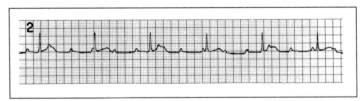

FIGURE 9-15   Third-degree AV block. (From Tintinalli J et al: *Emergency Medicine*, 5th ed. New York: McGraw-Hill; 2000:185, with permission.)

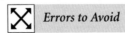 *Errors to Avoid*

- Use of lidocaine in third-degree AV block with ventricular escape beats

HYPERTENSIVE CRISES

Hypertension can present in the urgent care setting in a variety of ways, ranging from transient, anxiety-associated hypertension to the true hypertensive emergency. Hypertensive urgencies and emergencies are the two presentations of hypertension requiring treatment in the urgent care setting.

Definitions

- *Hypertensive urgencies* are situations in which blood pressure reduction is desirable over a period of several hours in order to reduce the risk of progression to pressure-related symptoms or target-organ damage. While the blood pressure seen with *hypertensive urgencies* usually exceeds 180/110 mmHg, it is not the blood pressure elevation per se but rather the potential for developing or aggravating target-organ damage that defines the existence of the urgency. *Hypertensive emergencies*, in contrast, are situations that require immediate blood pressure reduction in order to forestall or limit target-organ damage.

Clinical Presentation

Most patients with hypertensive urgencies will already have a diagnosis of hypertension and may give a history of inadequate or poor control of their blood pressure. These patients are usually seen in the urgent care setting for other problems, and an elevated blood pressure is noted when routine vital signs are taken. On questioning, the patient may give a history of noncompliance with medication, of having run out of medication, or of taking over-the-counter medicines that can elevate the blood pressure. Patients with hypertensive urgencies are generally asymptomatic. In contrast, patients presenting with hypertensive emergencies may exhibit any number of symptoms related to end-organ involvement, including headaches, blurred vision, nausea or vomiting, chest pain, congestive heart failure, confusion, and/or other neurologic defects.

- Examples of hypertensive emergencies include extremely high blood pressures (usually exceeding 200/120 mmHg) in the setting of acute MI, pulmonary edema, or intracranial hemorrhage.

 ## Physical Examination

Physical examination of all patients presenting with elevated blood pressures should focus on the presence of target-organ damage. Fundoscopic, cardiovascular, and neurologic examinations must be performed, as well as auscultation for abdominal bruits, which may be indicative of renovascular hypertension.

- A careful evaluation for neurologic findings is extremely important in order to document existing abnormalities as well as to establish a baseline should any new abnormalities develop.

Laboratory Tests

Useful laboratory tests for the evaluation and management of patients with hypertensive crises include a complete blood count, serum electrolytes, urinalysis, chest x-ray, and ECG. The chest x-ray should be evaluated carefully for evidence of cardiomegaly or pulmonary congestion. The ECG, which may show evidence of left ventricular hypertrophy, may also show changes indicative of cardiac ischemia.

- Side-by-side comparisons with previous chest x-rays and ECGs are preferred, if possible, over comparisons with reports of those examinations.

When the clinical situation so dictates, toxicologic screening may be needed, since ingestion of cardiac stimulants, as in cocaine intoxication, can result in extreme hypertension.

- It is important to note that small increases in the serum creatinine or the presence of mild abnormalities on the urinalysis may indicate the onset of renal dysfunction, which can progress rapidly unless adequate blood pressure reduction is achieved.

Hypertensive Crises

 Key Points of Documentation

- The presence or absence of
    chest pain
    visual changes
    headaches
    dyspnea
    papilledema and retinopathy
    rales or pulmonary congestion
    abdominal bruits
    neurologic symptoms
- ECG findings
- Results of urinalysis
- Response to treatment

 Management

Again, while the blood pressure in hypertensive episodes requiring immediate treatment usually exceeds 200/120 mmHg, the absolute level of blood pressure elevation is less important than the nature of the associated condition. The blood pressure in hypertensive emergencies should be reduced, within minutes to an hour, by up to 25 percent, making sure to avoid excessive or erratic drops. Blood pressure reduction in hypertensive emergencies is best accomplished using parenteral therapy and calls for continuous monitoring. Thus, these patients require hospital transfer and admission for treatment of the elevated pressures or end-organ involvement. A list of parenteral medications appropriate for treating hypertensive emergencies is listed in Table 9-15. Intravenous nitroglycerin is a particularly good choice for treatment in the urgent care setting while awaiting hospital transport.

TABLE 9-15

PARENTERAL DRUGS FOR TREATMENT OF HYPERTENSIVE EMERGENCIES[a]

Drug	Dose[b]	Onset of Action	Duration of Action	Adverse Effects[c]	Special Indications
Vasodilators					
Sodium nitroprusside	0.25–10 μg/kg per min as IV infusion[d] (maximal dose for 10 min only)	Immediate	1–2 min	Nausea, vomiting, muscle twitching, sweating, thiocyanate and cyanide intoxication	Most hypertensive emergencies; caution with high intracranial pressure or azotemia
Nicardipine hydrochloride	5–15 mg/h IV	5–10 min	1–4 h	Tachycardia, headache, flushing, local phlebitis	Most hypertensive emergencies except acute heart failure; caution with coronary ischemia
Fenoldopam mesylate	0.1–0.3 μg/kg per min as IV infusion	< 5 min	30 min	Tachycardia, headache, nausea, flushing	Most hypertensive emergencies; caution with glaucoma
Nitroglycerin	5–100 μg/min as IV infusion[d]	2–5 min	3–5 min	Headache, vomiting, methemoglobinemia, tolerance with prolonged use	Coronary ischemia
Enalaprilat	1.25–5 mg q 6 h IV	15–30 min	6 h	Precipitous fall in pressure in high-renin states; response variable	Acute left ventricular failure; avoid in acute myocardial infarction
Hydralazine hydrochloride	10–20 mg IV 10–50 mg IM	10–20 min 20–30 min	3–8 h	Tachycardia, flushing, headache, vomiting, aggravation of angina	Eclampsia
Diazoxide	50–100 mg IV bolus repeated, or 15–30 mg/min infusion	2–4 min	6–12 h	Nausea, flushing, tachycardia, chest pain	Now obsolete; when no intensive monitoring available
Adrenergic inhibitors					
Labetalol hydrochloride	20–80 mg IV bolus q 10 min 0.5–2.0 mg/min IV infusion	5–10 min	3–6 h	Vomiting, scalp tingling, burning in throat, dizziness, nausea, heart block, orthostatic hypotension	Most hypertensive emergencies except acute heart failure
Esmolol hydrochloride	250–500 μg/kg/min for 1 min, then 50–100 μg/kg/min for 4 min; may repeat sequence	1–2 min	10–20 min	Hypotension, nausea	Aortic dissection, perioperative
Phentolamine	5–15 mg IV	1–2 min	3–10 min	Tachycardia, flushing, headache	Catecholamine excess

[a]These doses may vary from those in the Physicians' Desk Reference (51st edition).
[b]IV indicates intravenous; IM, intramuscular.
[c]Hypotension may occur with all agents.
[d]Require special delivery system.

Most patients with hypertensive urgencies may be adequately treated with rapid-acting oral medications, such as angiotensin-converting enzyme (ACE) inhibitors, alpha-$_2$ agonists, loop diuretics, or calcium channel blockers (Table 9-16). Captopril, in doses of 25 to 50 mg orally, and clonidine, 0.1 to 0.3 mg orally, are examples of oral antihypertensive medications that may be used in the outpatient management of hypertensive urgencies.

- The use of sublingual nifedipine should be discouraged, inasmuch as it has been associated with severe and unpredictable blood pressure drops, which can cause cerebral, cardiac, or renal ischemia.

All patients should be monitored after the administration of antihypertensive medication; if the blood pressure can be reduced to acceptable levels with oral therapy, the

TABLE 9-16

ORAL MEDICATIONS FOR USE IN HYPERTENSIVE URGENCIES

	USUAL DOSAGE	ONSET OF ACTION/ PEAK BP LOWERING	SIDE EFFECTS	COMMENTS
Captopril (Capoten)	12.5–50 mg chewed	15–30 min/ 1–2 h	Renal failure in bilateral renal artery stenosis. ACE inhibitor–induced angioedema	Risk of excessive BP reduction in volume-depleted patients.
Clonidine (Catapres)	0.1 mg PO initial dose 0.1–0.2 mg PO q 1–2 h to max. 0.7 mg/24 h	30–60 min/ 2–4 h	Dry mouth, sedation. Avoid abrupt discontinuation	Excessive BP reduction in elderly/volume depletion. May be continued in oral and transdermal form.
Labetalol (Trandate, Normodyne)	400 mg PO initial dose 200 mg PO q 6 h	1–2 h after oral dose/2–4 h after oral dose	Postural hypotension, bradycardia, syncope, bronchospasm, aggravation of AV block, CHF	Rebound hyper-tension, exacerbation of angina after abrupt discontinuation. Combined alpha and beta blocker
Nifedipine (Adalat, Procardia capsules)	5–10 mg PO initially; repeat in 30–60 min to max. 20 mg	15–30 min/ 1–2 h	Reflex tachycardia; headache; peripheral edema; palpitations; syncope (rare)	Sublingual administration may cause angina or cerebrovascular insufficiency and should be avoided

KEY: ACE, angiotensin-converting enzyme; AV, atrioventricular; CHF, congestive heart failure; BP, blood pressure.

TABLE 9-17

ANTIHYPERTENSIVE TREATMENT REGIMENS FOR SPECIFIC POPULATIONS

Coexisting Condition	Diuretic	β Blocker	Angiotensin-Converting Enzyme Inhibitor	α Blocker	Ca²⁺-Channel Blocker
Older age	++	+/−	−	+	+
Black race	++	+/−	+/−	+	++
Angina pectoris	+	++	−	+	++
Postmyocardial infarction	+	++	+	+	−
Congestive heart failure with systolic dysfunction	++	−	++	+	−
Cerebrovascular disease	+	+	+	+/−	+
Renal disease (Cr > 200 μmol/L)	++	+/−	−	+	+
Diabetes mellitus with nephropathy	+	+/−	+	+	+
Migraine	+	++	−	+	+
Atrial fibrillation (with rapid ventricular response)	+	++	+	+	+
Paroxysmal supraventricular tachycardia	+	++	−	+	+
Senile tremor	+	++	+	+	+

KEY: ++, preferred; +, suitable; +/−, usually not preferred; −, usually contraindicated.
Tintinalli J et al: *Emergency Medicine: A Study Guide*, 5th ed. New York: McGraw-Hill; 2000:407, with permission)

patient may be discharged home on chronic antihypertensive therapy. The selection of antihypertensive therapy should be guided by issues such as the cost of medications and associated medical conditions (Tables 9-16 and 9-17). It is crucial that the patient be followed within days in order to reduce the risk of rebound hypertension and recurrence of a hypertensive crisis (Table 9-18).

• Many patients treated in the urgent care setting for a hypertensive urgency have poorly controlled chronic hypertension for which acute blood pressure reduction is unnecessary and may in fact be hazardous.

TABLE 9-18

HYPERTENSIVE URGENCIES: CRITERIA FOR DISCHARGE

Absence of acute or progressing end-organ damage
Blood pressure reduction to an acceptable range in response to treatment
Absence of acute ECG changes suggestive of ischemia
Scheduled follow-up
Ability to comprehend discharge instructions regarding medication, blood pressure monitoring, and criteria for reevaluation

Congestive heart failure

In patients with acute heart failure, it its useful to distinguish between symptoms of right heart failure and left heart failure. In chronic heart failure, however, this distinction becomes less important, since the two conditions frequently overlap, leading to significant overlap in presentation. When pure left-sided heart failure is present, symptoms will include dyspnea (at rest or with exertion), orthopnea, paroxysmal nocturnal dyspnea, fatigue, and various other signs of cerebral or systemic hypoperfusion. Pure right-sided failure, on the other hand, typically presents with symptoms secondary to the backing up of blood in the venous system, including peripheral edema, ascites, and hepatomegaly. Ultimately, the reduced venous return to the left heart will result in symptoms of cerebral hypoperfusion, such as confusion, weakness, and fatigue.

- Left heart failure of long duration may eventually result in concomitant signs of right heart failure.

In addition to being classified as right- or left-sided, congestive heart failure can be determined to be cardiac or noncardiac in etiology. Cardiac causes of congestive heart failure can further be categorized into those that directly affect the myocardium (e.g., cardiomyopathy, acute or chronic myocardial ischemia or infarction) or those that are extrinsic to the myocardium (e.g., valvular and pericardial heart disease).

For any patient presenting with signs or symptoms of congestive heart failure, a quick differential diagnosis must first be formulated. Many patients who present in congestive heart failure will have an acute exacerbation of previously diagnosed chronic heart failure. Often, a specific precipitating cause can be identified. These precipitating conditions may include infections, medication noncompliance, myocardial ischemia, and/or dietary (especially salt) indiscretion. One of the most common causes of an acute exacerbation of heart failure is inadvertent or inappropriate reduction in heart failure therapy. This may occur through noncompliance on the part of the patient with compensated heart failure and mild symptoms or through changes in medications made by other physicians. Poor control of hypertension, especially abrupt elevation of blood pressure, often results in acute decompensation of heart failure. Another common precipitating event is an acute dysrhythmia, frequently atrial fibrillation. Sometimes, however, it is difficult to determine whether an event such as atrial fibrillation was the cause or the result of the exacerbation of heart failure. For patients with renal disease, acute decompensation may be due to worsening of renal function, resulting in fluid overload.

- Patients with renal failure may become refractory to loop diuretics and may then require dialysis to restore fluid homeostasis.

For many patients, the differential diagnosis for congestive heart failure is between cardiac and pulmonary diseases such as chronic obstructive lung disease, asthma, or pulmonary embolism. Pulmonary and cardiac conditions often coexist, making it difficult to determine the relative contributions of the two conditions. For example, patients with severe congestive heart failure who are sedentary or confined to bed are predisposed to the development of pulmonary embolism.

Other causes for the development of congestive heart failure that are noncardiac in nature include anemia, thyroid excess, pregnancy, or any condition causing a high-output state. Additionally, medications may lead to failure, particularly medications such as beta and calcium antagonists, which are direct cardiac depressants. Others, such as steroids and nonsteroidal anti-inflammatory medications, may also precipitate heart failure by causing sodium and water retention.

Clinical Presentation

Breathlessness, the most common presenting complaint of patients with left heart failure, may occur only with exertion if the heart failure is mild. With increasing severity of heart failure, the patient may develop orthopnea, paroxysmal nocturnal dyspnea, and eventually dyspnea at rest. There may also be complaints of weight gain, ankle swelling, and right-upper-quadrant tenderness. On physical examination, patients may present with tachycardia and tachypnea. Lung examination will reveal rales and possibly wheezing (cardiac asthma). An S3 gallop may also be noted. Additionally, peripheral edema, jugular venous distention, hepatomegaly, and hepatojugular reflux may be present.

Laboratory Tests

Laboratory tests useful in the urgent care setting for the evaluation of the patient with congestive heart failure include a complete blood count, serum electrolytes, liver enzymes, and thyroid function tests. Chest x-ray may show the typical pattern of failure with cephalization, vascular congestion, Kerley B lines, and cardiac enlargement. An ECG should be obtained in order to exclude ischemia as either a cause or a result of the failure. In most cases, pulse oximetry suffices as a surrogate for arterial blood gases in the assessment of the adequacy of oxygenation of peripheral tissues. For acutely ill patients, measurement of arterial blood gases (if available) may be useful in excluding pulmonary disease as the cause of the patient's symptoms.

 Management

- If possible, correctable precipitating causes must be addressed first. For example, if the acute exacerbation of heart failure is due to myocardial ischemia, the latter must be relieved with appropriate anti-ischemic therapy before therapy for congestive heart failure or concomitant with it.

Pulmonary Edema

Patients presenting with acute pulmonary edema require immediate stabilization and transfer to an inpatient facility (Table 9-19). The goal of therapy is to improve oxygenation and reduce left heart filling pressure. The patient should be placed in a sitting position to reduce the central venous pressure. *Oxygen* should be administered by face mask. *Morphine* (5 to 10 mg IV) should be given to reduce preload as well as patient anxiety. The possibility of morphine-induced respiratory depression should be considered, but this risk is quite low and, in any case, can be easily managed with morphine antagonists, such as naloxone.

In addition to their diuretic properties, *loop diuretics* (typically furosemide) also produce venodilation, thereby reducing left ventricular preload, and should be administered as an intravenous bolus.

TABLE 9-19

ACUTE MANAGEMENT OF PULMONARY EDEMA

1. Place patient in the sitting position
2. Administer supplemental oxygen by face mask
3. Morphine 5 to 10 mg IV (watch for respiratory depression)
4. Furosemide: 40 to 80 mg IV
5. Nitroglycerin: sublingual (0.4 mg) or IV (10 μg and titrated by response of symptoms and pressure)
6. Intubation (nasal if possible) and mechanical ventilation for respiratory failure
7. Continuous pulse oximetry monitoring
8. Continuous cardiac monitoring
9. EMS transport to inpatient facility
10. ECG tracing while awaiting EMS transport, if feasible

Nitroglycerin reduces both preload and afterload and is especially useful in the presence of hypertension or myocardial ischemia. Nitroglycerin may be given sublingually (0.3 or 0.4 mg) if the intravenous form is not available. If it is available, the dose should typically begin at 10 μg/min and be titrated up by 5 μg/min every 3 to 5 min until symptoms are relieved, mean blood pressure is decreased by 30 percent, or hypo-tension develops.

- *Intravenous nitroprusside* is the most effective agent for the acute reduction of left ventricular afterload, but its use is usually not feasible in the urgent care setting because of the difficulty of titrating the dose and the need for continuous monitoring.

Congestive Heart Failure

In contrast to patients with pulmonary edema, the majority of patients who present to urgent care facilities with congestive heart failure will have a mild exacerbation of chronic heart failure and can be managed as outpatients. The mainstay of outpatient therapy is loop diuretics, ACE inhibitors, digoxin, and vasodilators. Intravenous furosemide may be given to accelerate therapy. The patient can then be observed over several hours (including the monitoring of urine output) and discharged on an augmented maintenance dosage of oral furosemide or bumetanide.

- One mg of bumetanide is approximately equivalent to 40 mg of furosemide. Bumetanide probably has slightly greater renal toxicity and slightly less ototoxicity than furosemide; otherwise the side-effect profiles are similar.

Many studies have confirmed the reduction in mortality in patients with heart failure treated with ACE inhibitors in adequate doses. Unless a specific contraindication exists, the goal of therapy should be to maximize the dosage of ACE inhibitor (e.g., 150 mg of captopril or 40 mg of enalapril or lisinopril per day). Hypotension should not be an absolute contraindication to the use of an ACE inhibitor unless the hypotension causes symptoms or is aggravated by the ACE inhibitor. Similarly, renal insufficiency

TABLE 9-20

CRITERIA FOR OUTPATIENT TREATMENT OF CONGESTIVE HEART FAILURE

Patient with a documented history of congestive heart failure who has had a mild exacerbation
Patient has returned to baseline functional status posttreatment in the urgent care facility
No evidence of dysrhythmia or infarction as a precipitating event

should not be a contraindication to ACE inhibitor therapy unless it was caused or aggravated by such therapy.

- The most common error in ACE inhibitor therapy is the use of inadequate doses.

Preliminary data suggest that angiotensin receptor blockers (losartan, valsartan, irbesartan, etc.) may be used instead of ACE inhibitors when the latter are contraindicated due to cough.

Digoxin continues to be a useful drug for the treatment of congestive heart failure, particularly in the presence of atrial fibrillation. Digoxin, however, should be avoided in heart failure due to left ventricular diastolic dysfunction, as seen in patients with left ventricular hypertrophy and normal left ventricular systolic function. This is especially true if there is obstruction of the left ventricular outflow tract, as in hypertrophic cardiomyopathy, where the increased left ventricular contractility can worsen the outflow tract gradient.

- While digoxin probably has no beneficial effects on cardiac mortality in patients with congestive heart failure, its withdrawal from a patient who has been taking digoxin chronically may result in exacerbation of heart failure.

Disposition and Follow-up Care

Patients successfully treated in the urgent care center who have a mild exacerbation of chronic heart failure can be discharged home with the consultation and input of their primary care physician (Table 9-20). Patients and their family members should be educated about congestive heart failure and measures to prevent acute exacerbations. Daily weights should be charted and preemptive measures such as avoidance of alcohol or excessive dietary sodium consumption should be taken. An increase in diuretic dosage as well as changes in antihypertensive regimens may be warranted. Such changes should be made in concert with the primary care physician. A follow-up visit with the primary physician should be arranged prior to discharge.

SYNCOPE

The terms *syncope* and *fainting* are used synonymously to describe the condition of a brief disturbance of consciousness with spontaneous recovery. Transient loss of consciousness is one of the most common presenting complaints to urgent care centers and emergency departments. Owing to the large number of potential causes, the inexperienced physician often resorts to a "cookbook" approach that results in unnecessary testing and/or hospitalization.

Clinical Presentation

Arguably there is no other area of cardiology where the history is more vital to making the correct diagnosis or at least excluding enough possible causes that cost-effective testing can be done. The history should focus on possible triggering events, such as pain, exposure to a noxious environment, or standing in line for long periods. The presence or absence of a prodrome and the duration of prodromal signs or symptoms should be ascertained. For example, the young patient with vasovagal syncope may describe a typical prolonged prodrome consisting of fatigue, nausea, and yawning; in the older patient with carotid sinus hypersensitivity, there may be spells associated with shaving, moving the neck, or wearing a tight neck collar. A detailed history of the patient's medications and the time of use is often helpful. A family history of sudden cardiac death or congenital deafness should be ascertained in all patients presenting with syncope.

- Virtually all cardiac medications are capable of causing syncope, but the most common culprits are nitroglycerin, diuretics, and adrenergic inhibitors.

It is particularly important to interview family members, friends, or other witnesses, since many patients will have no recall of the events preceding or following the syncopal spell. The physical examination should be detailed but should emphasize the cardiovascular and neurologic systems. A good cardiovascular examination can exclude most cases of valvular heart disease (murmurs, abnormal pulses), orthostatic hypotension, carotid sinus hypersensitivity, and/or subclavian steal syndrome (unequal pulses).

Laboratory Tests

Unless there is clear-cut evidence of neurologic dysfunction (e.g., epilepsy), routine neurologic tests—such as CT of the head, electroencephalogram (EEG), or carotid ultrasound—should not be performed, since the yield is low (see "Syncope" in Chap. 19). An ECG should always be performed, looking for evidence of conduction abnormalities (e.g., preexcitation), bradyarrhythmias, tachyarrhythmias, or a prolonged QT interval. (The latter can be a marker for the existence of syndromes that predispose to polymorphic ventricular tachycardia and secondary syncope.) Other tests—such as echocardiography, ambulatory ECG monitoring (Holter monitor or loop recordings), tilt-table testing, and cardiac electrophysiology testing—may be useful but can be obtained on an elective basis through the patient's primary care physician or a cardiologist.

Differential Diagnosis

Table 9-21 outlines the more common causes of loss of consciousness. By far the most common cause is neurocardiogenic syncope, of which vasovagal syncope is the prototype (the terms are often used synonymously). Vasovagal syncope is a phenomenon of dysfunctional autonomic control of the heart rate and vascular tone. Strictly speaking, it is not a disease, since everyone is capable of experiencing this type of syncope when the

TABLE 9-21

CAUSES OF LOSS OF CONSCIOUSNESS

Cardiac
- *Neurocardiogenic*
  Vasovagal
  Micturition
  Postprandial
  Postdefecation
  Orthostatic
- *Hemodynamic derangements*
  Hypovolemia (dehydration, blood loss, ectopic pregnancy, etc.)
  Aortic stenosis
  Mitral regurgitation
  Hypertrophic cardiomyopathy
  Subclavian steal syndrome
  Left atrial myxoma
  Pulmonary embolism
- *Arrhythmia*
  Bradyarrhythmia
  Tachyarrhythmia
- *Cardiac medication*
  Vasodilators
  Antiarrhythmic agents (proarrhythmia)

Neurologic
- *Seizures*

Miscellaneous
- *Hypoglycemia*
- *Hyperventilation*

right conditions exist. It has been estimated that 50 to 75 percent of individuals will have vasovagal syncope at some point in their lives. It is often triggered by stimuli as diverse as pain and prolonged standing, causing paradoxical responses of bradycardia and hypotension. The history is usually diagnostic, and tilt-table testing may confirm the diagnosis. Other variants of reflex-mediated syncope are carotid sinus hypersensitivity, micturition syncope, and postprandial and postdefecation syncope.

 Management and Follow-up Care

Since 50 to 80 percent of patients presenting with their first syncopal episode will never have a recurrence or will have a long prodrome that limits the likelihood of injury, it is often sufficient to reassure the patient who has no evidence of structural cardiac or neurologic disease. The young patient with rare episodes who has typical, prolonged prodromal symptoms needs nothing more than education on appropriate evasive action (e.g., sitting down or leaving a noxious environment), which can abort an attack (see Table 9-22 for criteria for safe discharge). The decision to admit a

TABLE 9-22

SYNCOPE: CRITERIA FOR DISCHARGE

First episode of syncope
No evidence of structural heart disease
Low risk of injury—e.g., due to falls—if symptoms recur
Presence of prodromal signs
Appropriate follow-up arrangements made

TABLE 9-23

MANAGEMENT OF SYNCOPE REQUIRING HOSPITAL ADMISSION

1. Continuous cardiac or neurologic monitoring
2. IV placement for access
3. Supplemental oxygen as indicated
4. Administration of appropriate cardiac medications, as indicated (e.g., atropine for profound bradycardia)
5. EMS transport

patient with syncope should be individualized. In general, patients with abnormal ECGs, physical injury resulting from the syncopal episode, history of coronary artery disease, or other structural heart disease will need hospital admission for further observation, work-up, and treatment (see Table 9-23 for management in the urgent care center). More specific therapies may include the use of vasoconstrictor drugs, intravascular volume enhancers (such as increased salt consumption or the use of mineralocorticoids), beta blockers, and, in appropriate cases, implantation of a permanent pacemaker.

- Apparent abnormalities on examination or testing should not always be assumed to be responsible for the patient's symptoms. For example, many elderly patients may have evidence of conduction system disease, such as sinus bradycardia or pauses of up to 2.0 s, especially at night, when vagal tone is increased. Similarly, small drops in orthostatic blood pressure (less than 15 mmHg) or bradycardia on carotid sinus massage are common findings in the elderly and are not necessarily etiologic for the particular patient. Unless these findings correlate with symptoms, they should not lead to treatment (such as the placement of a pacemaker), since such treatment may not relieve the symptoms.

Deep venous thrombosis

Background

Venous thrombosis refers to the presence of thrombus within a vein. When the development of venous thrombosis is accompanied by varying degrees of inflammation of the venous wall, this combination is referred to as *thrombophlebitis.*

In the venous system of the extremities, veins may be classified as superficial or deep. Deep veins run in close proximity to the arteries and connect to the superficial veins via perforating veins. Thrombosis occurring in the superficial veins generally carries little risk of distal embolic complications, whereas deep venous thrombosis (DVT) represents a greater risk for pulmonary embolism.

- The superficial femoral vein (a misnomer) was so-named because of its anatomic relationship to the deep femoral vein. Thrombosis in this "deep" vein does pose a risk for pulmonary embolism.

History

The patient who has developed a deep venous thrombosis typically will give an antecedent history of recent surgery, trauma, prolonged immobilization, underlying illness, or the use of estrogen. Orthopedic, thoracic, abdominal or pelvic interventions increase the risk of developing deep venous thrombosis. Traumatic injuries, especially fractures of the spine, pelvis, or femur, also predispose to deep venous thrombosis, as do certain malignancies, particularly cancer of the pancreas. A history of prolonged immobilization (due to illness, long trips, or casting) and prior history of deep venous thrombosis are other risk factors associated with developing this condition. Of note, deep venous thrombosis is most common in women, possibly reflecting the increased risk from pregnancy and the use of estrogen for contraception and postmenopausal hormone replacement.

 Physical Examination

On examination, the affected extremity is often warm, with varying degrees of swelling, erythema, or tenderness. Rarely, a cord is palpable along the course of the culprit vein, but this is more commonly a feature of superficial thrombophlebitis. There may be pain noted in the region of the thrombosed vein; this pain can occur at rest or with exercise. Increased pain or resistance during voluntary dorsiflexion of the foot (the so-called Homans' sign) is not reliable in the diagnosis of calf vein thrombosis; nonetheless, Homans' sign should be evaluated and documented appropriately during examination, inasmuch as its presence may correlate with venous thrombosis elsewhere in that extremity. Any evidence of distended collateral veins should be sought, and bilateral calf circumferences should be checked and documented.

- Absence of any or all of these signs does not exclude deep venous thrombosis because there is redundancy in the venous drainage of the extremities by other, patent, collateral veins.
- Slight differences in the maximal circumference of the extremities do not necessarily indicate venous thrombosis of the larger extremity. For example, differences of up to 1.0 cm in the maximal calf diameter may be a normal finding. In the absence of other confirmatory signs, the diagnosis of deep venous thrombosis should not be based on small differences in size between the two extremities.

Venous thrombosis involving the axillary vein, the subclavian vein, or the superior vena cava is often missed. Prominent collateral veins are usually present but may be missed on physical examination. Often there will be a history of impeded venous return, such as that caused by the use of crutches.

Laboratory and Radiographic Evaluation

Basic laboratory tests—such as a complete blood count, serum electrolytes, or chest x-ray—are rarely diagnostic but should be obtained because of the high probability of the existence of associated medical conditions. Since hypercoagulable states predispose to deep venous thrombosis, blood for basic coagulation testing, prothrombin time/international normalized ratio (INR), and activated partial thromboplastin time (APTT) should also be drawn. Venous duplex ultrasonography and impedance plethysmography are both highly sensitive and specific for the diagnosis of proximal deep venous thrombosis. These tests can often be ordered emergently on an outpatient basis.

• Owing to the small size of calf veins, the sensitivity of duplex ultrasonography and impedance plethysmography for the detection of calf vein thrombosis is poor (50 to 60 percent), although the specificity is quite high (90 to 95 percent).

If the clinical suspicion of calf vein thrombosis is high in a patient with a negative ultrasound or plethysmographic study, additional testing, as by iodine-125 (^{125}I) fibrinogen scanning or contrast venography, should be performed. Fibrinogen scanning has a sensitivity exceeding 90 percent for the detection of calf vein thrombosis but is relatively insensitive for detection of thrombi in proximal veins owing to high background pelvic radioactivity.

• The uptake and incorporation of radioactive iodine into the propagating thrombus may take up to 72 h after administration of the radioisotope. Therefore, if the index of suspicion is high, the patient will require appropriate anticoagulation therapy until a firm diagnosis is established.

In many radiology departments, contrast venography remains the "gold standard" for the diagnosis of deep venous thrombosis, and this should be obtained if clinical suspicion is high in a patient with a negative or equivocal ultrasound, plethysmographic, or ^{125}I fibrinogen study.

Differential Diagnosis

Many conditions causing unilateral pain, inflammation, or swelling of the extremity may be confused with deep venous thrombosis. Diverse conditions such as trauma or severe muscle cramps may result in localized swelling of the extremity. Superficial thrombophlebitis can present with unilateral swelling and pain, but it can usually can be distinguished from deep venous thrombosis by the presence of redness, tenderness, and a palpable cord corresponding to the inflamed vein. A ruptured popliteal synovial cyst (Baker's cyst) may also present with symptoms resembling those of calf vein thrombosis. This diagnosis should be suspected if there is a history of arthritis of the knees. An arthrogram of the knee joint can help make the diagnosis. Acute inflammatory exacerbations of certain chronic conditions, such as lymphedema, may also be confused with deep venous thrombosis. Making the correct diagnosis is crucial, since anticoagulation is usually contraindicated for these other conditions.

 Management

The patient with suspected deep venous thrombosis should be hospitalized for treatment with parenteral anticoagulation using heparin. Recent studies show that subcutaneous low-molecular-weight heparin may be as effective as intravenous unfractionated heparin. In most cases, oral anticoagulation can be initiated immediately, but the heparin will have to be continued for 4 to 5 days even when the INR is in the "therapeutic range."

Deep venous thrombosis involving a proximal vein (ileofemoral thrombosis) carries a high risk of pulmonary embolism. Isolated calf vein thrombosis, in contrast, carries a low risk of pulmonary embolism and, under certain circumstances, may be treated at home with intravenous or subcutaneous heparin. The recent introduction of low-molecular-weight heparin has made this option a viable alternative to hospitalization. It must be noted, however, that calf vein thrombosis may propagate proximally, thereby substantially increasing the risk of pulmonary embolism. The potential for propagation of isolated calf vein thrombosis requires that the patient receive oral anticoagulation for 6 to 12 weeks, unless serial ultrasound or plethysmographic examination has documented the absence of proximal propagation. Those patients with contraindications to anticoagulation should be hospitalized and considered for the placement of mechanical filters in the inferior vena cava (for lower extremity venous thrombosis) or thrombectomy. Patients who appear on clinical grounds to have a large clot burden should be considered for the use of thrombolytic therapy, such as urokinase, streptokinase, or tissue plasminogen activator.

- All patients with deep vein thrombosis should be treated with bed rest for at least 1 to 2 weeks in order to reduce the inflammation and possibly the risk of proximal embolization of the thrombus.

Deep Venous Thrombosis

 Key Points of Documentation

- The presence or absence of chest pain by history
- The presence or absence of risk factors for DVT:
    recent immobilization (casting, long trips, prolonged bed rest)
    recent surgery
    recent long bone fracture
    estrogen use (oral contraceptives, hormone replacement)
    recent delivery
    history of malignancy
- Tachycardia
- Tachypnea or increased respiratory rate
- The presence or absence of Homans' sign
- The presence or absence of Moses's sign
- Calf dimensions (bilateral)
- The presence or absence of a palpable cord

 Errors to Avoid

- Assuming that radiologic findings of thrombosis in the *superficial femoral vein* indicate a thrombosis of the superficial venous system. Its name notwithstanding, the superficial femoral vein is a *deep* vein and as such is a source of emboli.

INFECTIVE ENDOCARDITIS

Infective endocarditis is an infection of the endocardial surfaces of the heart and heart valves due to microorganisms. The valvular endocardium is most commonly affected, but the term *infective endocarditis* encompasses infection involving any endocardial surface, including septal defects and extracardiac structures such as arteriovenous shunts. Causative microorganisms include bacteria, fungi, chlamydia, and viruses.

Historically, endocarditis has been classified as acute or subacute. Acute endocarditis involves normal cardiac valves, has a more fulminant course, and is associated with a higher prevalence of infection caused by *Staphylococcus aureus, Streptococcus pneumoniae,* and *Neisseria gonorrhoeae.* In contrast, subacute endocarditis usually occurs in patients with prior valvular heart disease, presents with a more indolent course, and has a higher prevalence of infection caused by *Streptococcus viridans* or enterococci. From the standpoint of the urgent care physician, however, the relevant classification should be based on the etiologic agent (bacterial, fungal, viral, etc.), the valves affected (native or prosthetic; right- or left-sided) and patient-specific characteristics such as the presence of an immunocompromised status, a history of intravenous drug abuse, and/or underlying illnesses.

Clinical Presentation

See Table 9-24 for signs and symptoms that may be associated with infective endocarditis.

The typical patient with infective endocarditis gives a history of an antecedent event, usually 2 to 4 weeks before the onset of symptoms, that results in bacteremia. Examples of such events include dental procedures, urinary tract infections, genitourinary instrumentation, or gastrointestinal procedures. Except for patients who have been treated with antibiotics, fever is almost invariably present. In the subacute presentation, patients will generally report a history of a low-grade fever and vague systemic symptoms, such as weight loss, fatigue, chills, and diaphoresis. In contrast, patients with acute endocarditis generally give a history of high fever and appear gravely ill, with signs and symptoms of sepsis. The physical examination can be quite variable and is dependent on the duration of illness, the microorganism involved, and the affected organ or organ system. As previously indicated, virtually all patients have at least a mild fever. A new heart murmur or a change in an existing murmur is nearly always present in endocarditis involving a left heart valve but may be absent in nonvalvular endocarditis or right heart

TABLE 9-24

SIGNS AND SYMPTOMS THAT MAY BE SEEN WITH INFECTIVE ENDOCARDITIS

Fever (mild to high grade)	Janeway lesions
Cardiac murmur (new or change in previous murmur)	Roth spots
	Mild anemia
Petechiae (skin, conjunctiva, or mouth)	Left shift on CBC differential
Subungual splinter hemorrhages	Microscopic hematuria or proteinuria
Osler's nodes	

endocarditis. One or more peripheral findings of endocarditis are often present, but these are nonspecific and can occur in other disease states. Peripheral findings include conjunctival, skin, or oral cavity petechiae, subungual splinter hemorrhages, and clubbing. Less common but more specific manifestations include Osler's nodes, Janeway lesions, and Roth spots.

Laboratory Tests

A complete blood count, chemistry profile (including liver panel), chest x-ray, and ECG should be obtained on any patient suspected of having infective endocarditis. At least three sets of blood cultures should be drawn, and more if the patient has been taking antibiotics since the onset of symptoms. The blood cultures should be obtained from different sites. Binding resins may be used to remove antibiotics in situations where prior therapy renders the cultures negative. On the complete blood count, a mild anemia will often be present and is usually characterized by normocytic normochromic indices, as seen in anemia of chronic disease. The leukocyte count may be normal or mildly elevated, and a left shift of the differential is common. Urinalysis frequently shows microscopic hematuria and proteinuria. Echocardiography (transthoracic or transesophageal) is useful for the detection of valvular or endocardial vegetations and for the characterization of complications of endocarditis, such as valvular regurgitation and abscess formation.

 Management

In the urgent care setting, the primary goal is recognition of the disease. Treatment requires hospital admission for administration of intravenous antibiotic therapy and treatment of any complicating or underlying disorders. Venous access should be secured and blood cultures drawn prior to transport. Empiric antibiotic therapy can be started immediately after blood for culture has been drawn if the appropriate antibiotics are at hand in the urgent care facility.

- A high index of suspicion must be maintained for this diagnosis. Infective endocarditis should be included in the differential diagnosis of any patient presenting with a fever of unknown origin, a history of persistent fever, or a new or changed cardiac murmur in the presence of a febrile illness.

BIBLIOGRAPHY

Aquilar D, Goldhaber S: Clinical uses of low-molecular-weight heparins. *Chest* 115:1418–1423, 1999.

Autore C, Agati L, Piccininno M, et al: Role of echocardiology. *Am J Cardiol* 200; 86(suppl): 41G–42G, 2000.

Bales A: Hypertensive crisis: how to tell if it's an emergency or an urgency. *Postgrad Med* 105(5): 119–126, 130, 1999.

Barton CW, Manning JE: Cardiopulmonary resuscitation. *Emerg Med Clin North Am* 13:811–829, 1995.

Bayer A, Bolger A, Taubert K, et al: Diagnosis and management of infective endocarditis and its complications. *Circulation* 98:2936–2948, 1998.

Benditt D, Fahy G, Lurie K, et al: Pharmacotherapy of neurally mediated syncope. *Circulation* 100:1242–1248, 1999.

Bloomfield D, Sheldon R, Grubb B, et al: Panel consensus: putting it together: a new treatment algorithm for vasovagal syncope and related disorders. *Am J Cardiol* 84:33Q–39Q, 1999.

Borzak S, McCord J: Multifocal atrial tachycardia. *Chest* 113:203–209, 1998.

Brodsky MA, Hwang C, Hunter D, et al: Life-threatening alterations in heart rate after the use of adenosine in atrial flutter. *Am Heart J* 130:564–571, 1995.

Calkins H. Pharmacologic approaches to therapy for vasovagal syncope. *Am J Cardiol* 84: 20Q–25Q, 1999.

Carman TL, Fernandez BB Jr: Issues and controversies in venous thromboembolism. *Cleve Clin J Med* 66(2):113–123, 1999.

Carson P: Rationale for the use of combination angiotensin-converting enzyme inhibitor/ angiotensin II receptor blocker therapy in heart failure. *Am Heart J* 140:361–366, 2000.

Connors S, Dorian P: Management of supraventricular tachycardia in the emergency department. *Can J Cardiol* 13(suppl A):19A–24A, 1997.

Dajani A, Taubert K, Wilson W, et al: Prevention of bacterial endocarditis: recommendations by the American Heart Association. *JAMA* 227:1794–1801, 1997. (*Circulation* 96:358–366, 1997.)

Davidson B. Controversies in pulmonary embolism and deep venous thrombosis. *Am Fam Physician* 60:1969–1980, 1999.

Eagle K: Update in cardiology. *Ann Intern Med* 133:439–446, 2000.

Fontaine G, Fontaliran F, Frank R: Arrhythmogenic right ventricular cardiomyopathies: clinical forms and main diffferential diagnoses. *Circulation* 97:1532–1535, 1998.

Frantz RP: Beta blockade in patients with congestive heart failure: why, who and how. *Postgrad Med* 108(3):103–106, 109–110, 116–118, 2000.

Freudenberger RS, Gottlieb SS, Robinson SW, Fisher ML: A four-part regimen for clinical heart failure. *Hosp Pract* 34(9):51–56, 59–64, 1999.

Gold MR, Josephson ME: Cardiac arrhythmia: current therapy. *Hosp Pract* 34(9):27–28, 31–32, 35–38, 1999.

Gorton ME: Current trends in peripheral vascular surgery: when is surgical intervention the best option? *Postgrad Med* 106(3):87–94, 1999.

Grubb B: Pathophysiology and differential diagnosis of neurocardiogenic syncope. *Am J Cardiol* 84:3Q–9Q, 1999.

Haji S, Movahed A: Update on digoxin therapy in congestive heart failure. *Am Fam Physician* 62:409–416, 2000.

Hoesly C, Cobbs G: Endocarditis at the millennium. *J Infect Dis* 179(suppl 2):S360–S365, 1999.

Janeira LF: Wide-complex tachycardias: the importance of identifying the mechanism. *Postgrad Med* 100:(3)259–262, 265–266, 269–272, 1996.

Jones J, Geninatti M: Cardiology. *Emerg Med Clin North Am* 15:341–363, 1997.

Keys TF: Infective endocarditis: prevention, diagnosis, treatment, referral. *Cleve Clin J Med* 67(5): 353–360, 2000.

Lensing A, Prandoni P, Prins M, Büller H: Deep-vein thrombosis. *Lancet* 353:479–485, 1999.

Lewis W, Amsterdam E: Evaluation of the patient with "rule out myocardial infarction." *Arch Intern Med* 156:41–45, 1996.

Lip GY, Watson RD: ABC of atrial fibrillation: differential diagnosis of atrial fibrillation. *Br Med J* 311:1495–1498, 1995.

Morelli V, Zoorob R: Alternative therapies: part II: Congestive heart failure and hypercholesterolemia. *Am Fam Physician* 62:1325–1330, 2000.

National Institutes of Health: *The Sixth Report of the Joint National Committee on Prevention, Detection, Evaluation, and Treatment of High Blood Pressure.* NIH Publication No. 98–4080. Bethesda, MD: National Institutes of Health; 1997.

Rosendaal F: Venous thrombosis: a multicausal disease. *Lancet* 353:1167–1173, 1993.

Rubins JB, Rice K: Diagnosis of venous thromboembolism: step-by-step appoach to a still lethal disease. *Postgrad Med* 108(1):175–180, 2000.

Rydberg EJ, Westfall JM, Nicholas RA: Low-molecular-weight heparin in outpatient treatment of DVT. *Am Fam Physician* 59(6):1607–1612, 1999.

Sarko J, Pollack CV Jr: Beyond the twelve-lead electrocardiogram: diagnostic tests in the evaluation for suspected acute myocardial infarction in the emergency department. *J Emerg Med* 15:839–847, 1997.

Schamberger MS: Cardiac emergencies in children. *Pediatr Ann* 25:339–344, 1996.

Schattner A, Klepfish A, Caspi A: Chronic aortic dissection presenting as a prolonged febrile disease and arterial embolization. *Chest* 110(4):1111–1114, 1996.

Sheldon R: Role of pacing in the treatment of vasovagal syncope. *Am J Cardiol* 84:26Q–32Q, 1999.

Varon J, Fromm RE Jr.: Hypertensive crises: the need for urgent management. *Postgrad Med* 99(1):189–191, 195–196, 199–200, 1996.

Varon J, Marik P: The diagnosis and management of hypertensive crises. *Chest* 118:214–227, 2000.

Vaughan CJ, Delanty N: Hypertensive emergencies. *Lancet* 356:411–417, 2000.

Weir MR: Indicators and treatment of hypertensive heart disease. *Hosp Pract* 34(9):93–94, 99–100, 103–104, 1999.

Yeager BF, Matheny SC: Low-molecular-weight heparin in outpatient treatment of DVT. *Am Fam Physician* 59(4):945–952, 1999.

PULMONARY MEDICINE

Lynn M. Schnapp / Safy John /
Susan Gregory / Tanise I. Edwards

Cough

Cough is one of the most common reasons patients seek medical attention. Cough, by definition, is an explosive expiration that provides a means of clearing the tracheobronchial tree of secretions and foreign bodies. It protects the lungs against aspiration and may be initiated voluntarily or reflexively. Coughing is produced by stimulation of the cough receptors, which are located in the large bronchi, trachea, and larynx. The stimulus may be inflammatory, mechanical, chemical, or thermal.

Acute Cough

An acute cough, by definition, lasts less than 3 weeks and is generally symptomatic of a benign disease process. However, an acute cough may, on occasion, represent a serious underlying disorder such as pulmonary embolism, congestive heart failure, or pneumonia. (This concern is particularly relevant in the elderly population, where other signs and symptoms may be absent.)

The most common cause of an acute, transient cough is an upper respiratory infection (URI). Coryza, sore throat, malaise, sweating, and fever will frequently accompany the cough associated with a URI.

Other common causes of acute cough include:

- Acute bacterial sinusitis
- Pertussis
- Exacerbations of chronic obstructive pulmonary disease (COPD)
- Allergic and irritant rhinitis

Less common causes include asthma, pneumonia, congestive heart failure, aspiration syndromes, pulmonary embolism, and exacerbations of bronchiectasis.

Chronic Cough

Chronic cough lasts more than 3 weeks and can be persistently troublesome. The most common causes of a chronic cough include:

- Postnasal drip syndrome
- Asthma
- Gastroesophageal reflux disease
- Chronic bronchitis
- Bronchiectasis
- Use of an angiotensin-converting enzyme inhibitor

Less frequent causes of chronic cough include bronchogenic carcinoma, chronic interstitial pneumonia, sarcoidosis, left ventricular failure, and aspiration secondary to pharyngeal dysfunction.

 History

In the evaluation of cough, a detailed history and a thorough physical examination are essential and will usually help to establish a diagnosis. On history taking, certain questions should be addressed, including character of the cough, chronicity, and associated symptoms. Distinguishing between a productive cough and a dry cough is a useful first step. A productive cough generally indicates infection in the tracheobronchial tree or lungs. A dry cough, in contrast, has an extensive differential, which includes interstitial lung diseases, bronchogenic carcinoma, benign tumors, and foreign bodies.

The character of the cough may also help to suggest the anatomic site of involvement. Examples include a "barking" cough heard with epiglottal involvement (i.e., whooping cough or croup in children), the loud, "brassy" cough heard with tracheal or major upper airway involvement, and the cough associated with wheezing, which generally occurs in bronchospasm of the lower airways. Other helpful characteristics of a cough include the timing [nocturnal in congestive heart failure, association with meals in gastroesophageal reflux disease (GERD), recumbency with postnasal drip] and the type of sputum expectorated. A medication history may reveal use of drugs such as angiotensin-converting enzyme (ACE) inhibitors or beta blockers, which have a noted association with cough. An occupational history may reveal exposures that result in pneumoconiosis. Factors such as intermittent wheezing and exercise or a cold-induced cough suggest the presence of hyperreactive airways. Smoke-induced inflammation is another important cause of a chronic cough and can be caused by all tobacco products.

 Key Points of Documentation

1. Chronicity: acute vs. chronic
2. Character of cough: brassy, croupy, productive (color of sputum) vs. nonproductive; relationship, if any, to respiratory cycle
3. Time of day cough occurs
4. Relationship to activities (occurs on exertion, when in certain locations, when recumbent, in relationship to meals, etc.)

5. Associated symptoms (fever, postnasal drip, etc.)
6. Comorbidities
7. The presence or absence of sinus tenderness
8. The presence or absence of allergic findings (cobblestoning, boggy nasal mucosa, postnasal drip)
9. The presence or absence of wheezing, rales, rhonchi, rubs

 Physical Examination

The physical examination can further help to delineate the cause of a patient's cough. A detailed head and neck exam should look for nonpulmonary causes such as allergies, sinusitis, or postnasal drip (PND). The exam should include evidence of pale or boggy mucous membranes (allergies), acute sinus tenderness (sinusitis), or posterior pharyngeal cobblestoning (as in PND). Auscultatory findings may help localize the site of a pulmonary lesion, particularly wheezing (lower airway disease), consolidation (pneumonia), friction rubs, or the presence of rales (as in congestive heart failure).

A chest radiograph should be considered in all patients presenting with acute cough and should definitely be obtained in all patients being evaluated for chronic cough. Sinus films should also be considered if the history and physical examination are suggestive of sinusitis or PND syndrome.

 Management

Specific therapy is aimed at the underlying disease and is generally the most effective means of eliminating cough. When the history, physical examination, and radiographic studies are nondiagnostic, the patient should be referred to his or her primary care physician (PCP) for further follow-up and evaluation. In current smokers or patients on ACE inhibitors, no additional diagnostic tests may have to be performed until at least 4 weeks after smoking cessation or drug discontinuation. Because asthma and esophageal reflux are among the most common causes of cough, with cough being the only presenting symptom in over half of these patients, a methacholine challenge may be appropriate. If this is negative, esophageal pH monitoring may be indicated. In the absence of an abnormal chest radiograph, bronchoscopy has an extremely low diagnostic yield.

Listed below are recommendations for specific therapy of the most common causes of cough not related to infectious etiologies. Avoidance of obvious environmental irritants (e.g., smoke) and discontinuation of ACE inhibitors in consultation with the patient's PCP should, however, always be performed first.

Allergy/Postnasal Drip Syndrome.   Useful therapeutic regimens to treat sinusitis include an oral antihistamine-decongestant (for at least 3 weeks) and a decongestant nasal spray (for a maximum of 5 days). A 3-week course of antibiotics (to treat upper respiratory tract organisms) is often beneficial. Intranasal corticosteroids are indicated for the treatment of allergic rhinitis. The avoidance of known irritant or allergic precipitating factors is also important.

TABLE 10-1

THERAPY FOR CHRONIC COUGH

Increase latency or threshold of cough center:
  Codeine   15 mg qid
  Dextromethorphan   15 mg qid
Expectorants:
  Guaifenesin   100 mg tid
  Iodinated glycerol   30 mg qid
Alteration of mucociliary clearance:
  Ipratropium
Protussive:
  Hypertonic aerosolized saline

Asthma. Treatment with inhaled beta agonists and inhaled corticosteroids is generally effective for cough from hyperreactive airways. If components of the aerosol are causing airway irritation, oral beta agonists can be used instead.

Gastroesophageal Reflux Disease. Resolution of cough due to GERD may require prolonged therapy (3 to 6 months). The most effective regimen is use of H_2 blockers or metoclopramide, combined with strategies aimed at decreasing reflux: elevation of the head of the bed at night, no food or drink 2 to 3 h prior to sleep, and a high-protein, low-fat diet.

Nonspecific therapy is aimed at treating the symptoms of cough. If the cause of the cough is not known or treatment of the underlying disease is not practical or has not begun to be effective, then control of the cough through pharmacotherapy may be indicated (Table 10-1). Antitussive medications suppress cough by increasing the latency or threshold of the cough center. Hydration, expectorants, or humidification of the air using an ultrasonic nebulizer with ipratropium bromide may be helpful when secretions are thick and tenacious. Protussive (cough-enhancing) treatment is used to increase the effectiveness of useful but inadequate cough; in cystic fibrosis, however, only aerosolized hypertonic saline appears to be of benefit.

Dyspnea

Definition

Dyspnea is defined as an abnormally uncomfortable awareness of breathing or respiratory effort and results from a complex interplay of physiologic and psychological factors (Table 10-2). The physiology of dyspnea remains unclear, but it is thought that multiple stimuli, receptors, nerves, and neural pathways mediate the sensation. The differential diagnosis is extensive and includes any disease process that involves the respiratory system. A systematic approach is therefore recommended in evaluating dyspnea.

In assessing complaints of dyspnea, it is important first to determine what symptoms the patient is describing, since the sensation of dyspnea is subjective and may be

TABLE 10-2

COMMON CAUSES OF DYSPNEA

• Asthma	• Deconditioning
• Interstitial lung disease	• Psychogenic/hyperventilation
• Cardiomyopathy	• Neuromuscular disease
• Gastroesophageal reflux disease	• Anemia

poorly or vaguely defined. Patients will often describe a feeling of choking, tightness, lack of air, air hunger, inability to take in air, and chest tiredness. In certain situations (hyperventilation associated with metabolic acidosis), breathing is labored but dyspnea does not occur. In other circumstances, patients may have apparently normal breathing patterns but still complain of a sense of shortness of breath. Of note, the awareness of breathing that occurs in normal people after mild to moderate exertion usually presents no discomfort or distress and therefore should not be considered true dyspnea.

Evaluation

A detailed history and physical examination is essential to determine the etiology of dyspnea. Questions that address the onset, duration, intensity, frequency, and precipitating factors are helpful in establishing a diagnosis.

Intermittent dyspnea is suggestive of reversible processes such as asthma or congestive heart failure, while *persistent or progressive* dyspnea is associated with chronic underlying pulmonary diseases. The relationship of dyspnea to body position or the time of day may also give clues to etiology. For example, nocturnal dyspnea may be seen with CHF, asthma, GERD, or PND syndrome. Potentially life-threatening conditions (pulmonary embolism, cardiac abnormalities, asthma, etc.) as the cause of dyspnea must always be considered in the differential and ruled out by history, physical examination, and diagnostic evaluation.

- It is important to determine degree of disability, if any, since many patients will modify their behaviors to avoid activities that induce dyspnea.

 History

 Key Points of Documentation on History

1. Onset of symptoms
2. Frequency
3. Relationship to activity or position
4. Precipitating factors
5. Associated symptoms: wheezing, chest pain, syncope, palpitations, fevers, choking episodes

6. Past medical history: previously diagnosed pulmonary disease (asthma, COPD), cardiac or valve disease, risk factors for pulmonary embolism [immobilization (including casting or long trips), recent surgery, oral contraceptive use], malignancy, renal disease, high use of aspirin, recent delivery, occupational exposure history
7. Smoking history

 ## Physical Examination

Since a wide spectrum of disease can contribute to dyspnea, a thorough physical examination is important. Vital signs including respiratory rate should be recorded, as well as any degree of respiratory distress. The pattern of breathing and the patient's ability to speak in full sentences should be noted, as should the patient's stance and positioning. To minimize dyspnea, some patients may exhibit pursed-lip breathing; rapid, shallow breathing; or use of accessory muscles of respiration. Any agitation or undue somnolence, which can be an indication of hypoxemia, should be noted, as should any cyanosis, which may be seen with severe hypoxemia. Depending on the etiology of the dyspnea, adventitious lung sounds or decreased breath sounds may be observed. Any fever or purulent sputum should be noted. On cardiac examination, evidence of dysrhythmia, pulmonary hypertension, or ventricular dysfunction should be looked for (right or left ventricular heave, increased pulmonic sound, jugular venous distention, pedal edema). Clubbing may be noted if an underlying malignancy is present. Additionally, the lower extremities should be checked for any evidence of deep venous thrombosis, including asymmetrical calf swelling, palpable cords, or a positive Homans' sign.

 Key Points of Documentation of Physical Examination

1. Cyanosis
2. Body habitus
3. Respiratory rate and quality of respirations
4. Use of accessory muscles/retractions
5. Presence or absence of:
   - Rales
   - Rhonchi
   - Wheezing
   - Decreased breath sounds
   - Dullness to percussion
6. Murmurs, rubs, gallops
7. Jugular venous distention
8. Peripheral edema, asymmetrical calf swelling or tenderness, Homans' sign

Ancillary Studies

A chest radiograph is an essential part of the evaluation of all patients with dyspnea, looking for evidence of parenchymal abnormalities such as infiltrates, a mass, or evidence of congestive heart failure. Pulse oximetry, if available, should be obtained in all patients presenting with dyspnea. It is important to remember, however, that potentially serious conditions can exist even in the face of normal oxygen saturations and that a normal pulse oximetry does not rule out a significant underlying pulmonary abnormality. If available, arterial blood gas analysis and pulmonary function testing are extremely useful in the diagnosis of dyspnea.

 Management

Treatment of dyspnea is initially aimed at diagnosing and treating underlying lung or cardiac disease. Information from the patient's history, physical examination, and ancillary studies must all be used to determine the patient's diagnosis and his or her stability for discharge. If a potentially life-threatening condition cannot be ruled out or if any doubt exists, the patient should be referred directly for further evaluation including arterial blood gases, a ventilation/perfusion scan, or cardiac evaluation, as indicated. Unstable patients, patients exhibiting hypoxia, or those with the potential for rapid deterioration should be transferred via ambulance to an emergency facility. Other patients, depending on the working diagnosis, may be referred directly for further lab or radiographic evaluations or to their PCP's office.

Hiccups

Hiccups are a common entity whose mechanism and function remain unknown. Hiccups (or singultus) are the sudden contraction of inspiratory muscles accompanied by the sudden closure of the glottis to produce the characteristic sound. *Acute hiccups* are usually transient and benign and do not require medical attention. Common causes of acute hiccups include gastric distention (secondary to the ingestion of carbonated beverages, air, food, and alcohol). Acute cases of hiccups do not require laboratory evaluation; treatment usually consists of a home remedy aimed at interrupting the hiccup reflex. Reported home remedies include:

- Breath holding
- Swallowing granulated sugar
- Drinking water without breathing
- Sudden fright
- Valsalva maneuver
- Drinking water without turning the glass
- Pulling hard on the tongue

In contrast, *persistent hiccups* can be severely debilitating and result in weight loss, sleep deprivation, and fatigue. The associated causes of persistent hiccups are protean, ranging from the benign to more serious underlying disorders (Table 10-3). A foreign body in the external auditory canal lying against the tympanic membrane is another notable cause of persistent hiccups that occur secondary to the stimulation of the auricular branch of the vagus nerve.

Patients presenting with persistent, intractable hiccups should undergo evaluation aimed at ruling out potential causes. Physical examination should include careful

TABLE 10-3

ASSOCIATED CAUSES OF PERSISTENT HICCUPS

Metabolic disorders

- Uremia
- Diabetes
- Alcohol intoxication
- Gout
- Hyperventilation
- Electrolyte abnormalities

Drugs

- Steroids
- Benzodiazepines
- Barbiturates
- Antibiotics

Central nervous system pathology

- Structural lesions (i.e., tumor, ventriculoperitoneal shunt)
- Vascular lesions (arteriovenous malformation, hemorrhage)
- Trauma
- Infections (encephalitis, meningitis)

Gastrointestinal pathology

- Esophageal reflux
- Esophagitis
- Hiatal hernia
- Gastric distention
- Gastritis
- Peptic ulcer disease
- Hepatitis
- Peritonitis

Thoracic pathology

- Pericarditis
- Myocardial infarction
- Open-heart surgery
- Pleurisy
- Pneumonia
- Subdiaphragmatic irritation

Recent intraabdominal or thoracic surgery

Tympanic membrane irritation

Psychogenic disease

- Stress
- Excitement
- Anorexia nervosa

inspection of the oral pharynx and external auditory canal and a chest x-ray to rule out intrathoracic disease.

If the cause of persistent hiccups is unknown or untreatable, control of symptoms becomes important. Chlorpromazine is currently the only drug approved by the U.S. Food and Drug Administration (FDA) for the treatment of hiccups. The usual starting dose is 25 to 50 mg intravenously followed by a maintenance dose of 25 mg qid if necessary. Recently, a randomized, placebo-controlled trial showed that baclofen was efficacious for the treatment of hiccups. Atropine and quinidine have been reported to have limited success. Phenytoin and carbamazepine may be useful in patients with central nervous system (CNS) pathology.

All patients with intractable, recurrent, or persistent hiccups should be referred for full workup and evaluation.

HEMOPTYSIS

Patients with a history of hemoptysis can present with symptoms ranging anywhere from occasional blood-streaked sputum to massive bleeding with respiratory compromise. The presentation of the patient with hemoptysis will vary, depending on the etiology. Historically, the most common causes of hemoptysis are pulmonary infections (including tuberculosis, bronchitis, and pneumonia), bronchiectasis, and lung cancer (Table 10-4).

Definitions

Gross hemoptysis: The definition of gross hemoptysis is not universally agreed upon but is often stated as the expectoration of "several tablespoons" of blood.

Massive hemoptysis: Expectoration of greater than 100 ml of blood in 24 h.

 History

In a stable patient presenting with mild hemoptysis, a detailed history and physical can be performed in the urgent care setting; this may elicit clues as to the etiology of the hemoptysis. The most important first step in considering this diagnosis is to determine whether the blood is actually coming from the lower respiratory tract and not the nasopharynx or gastrointestinal (GI) tract. Historical features that point to an ear-nose-

TABLE 10-4

CAUSES OF HEMOPTYSIS

Infectious	**Drugs**
Tuberculosis	Aspirin
Pneumonia (*S. aureus, Klebsiella*)	Anticoagulants
Mycetoma	Crack cocaine
Fungal	**Vascular**
Viral	Arteriovenous malformation
Pulmonary	Aortic aneurysm
Bronchitis	Primary pulmonary
Bronchiectasis	Hypertension
Pulmonary embolism	**Systemic Disease**
Cystic fibrosis	Vasculitis
Neoplastic	Systemic lupus erythematosus
Bronchial adenoma (carcinoid)	Wegener's granulomatosis
Lung cancer	Goodpasture's syndrome
Metastatic cancer	**Cardiac**
Kaposi's sarcoma	Mitral stenosis
Hematologic	Congenital heart disease
Platelet dysfunction	**Miscellaneous**
Thrombocytopenia	Trauma
Coagulopathy	Endometriosis
	Foreign body

throat (ENT) source of bleeding include an antecedent history of epistaxis, sinus symptoms, or throat and pharyngeal complaints. A history of nausea, vomiting, and abdominal pain or of peptic ulcer disease or GI bleeding may indicate a GI source of blood. Additionally, blood originating from the GI tract will often be dark red or brown in color. In contrast, bleeding from the respiratory system will usually present with frothy, bright red blood.

Once it has been established that the bleeding is indeed from the respiratory tract, the onset, duration, and amount of hemoptysis should be determined.

Symptoms of an infectious etiology should be sought, particularly any history of an acute cough, antecedent cold, fever, and/or purulent sputum. The patient should be questioned regarding symptoms suggestive of tuberculosis (TB), including weight loss, malaise, night sweats, or exposure to TB. Any medication use, including aspirin and anticoagulants, should be obtained. History of illicit drug use—such as crack cocaine, which can cause diffuse alveolar hemorrhage—should also be sought. A positive history of cigarette smoking and chronic cough, particularly with blood-streaked sputum, may suggest a primary pulmonary malignancy. Any risk factors for pulmonary embolism—including shortness of breath, history of immobilization, malignancy, or contraceptive use—should be documented. The patient should also be asked about any symptoms that may indicate a coagulopathy, such as easy bruising, spontaneous bleeding, or gingival bleeding or hematuria. Last, a history of childhood rheumatic fever could indicate mitral stenosis, while symptoms of systemic disease could indicate pulmonary vasculitis.

 Physical Examination

On physical examination of the patient with hemoptysis, careful monitoring of the blood pressure and heart rate is warranted to assess hemodynamic stability. Once a patient is determined to be stable, the physical examination should, as with the history, help to distinguish between respiratory and nonrespiratory bleeding as well as narrow the working differential. The patient's overall appearance should be noted for any cachexia, pallor, bruising, or petechiae. A thorough head, ear, nose, and throat examination should be performed looking for signs of nasal pathology (epistaxis or nasal lesions), sinusitis (sinus percussion tenderness, purulent or bloody nasal drainage), or oropharyngeal disorders (pharyngeal erythema, edema or lesions, or gingival bleeding). The neck and supraclavicular fossa should be examined for adenopathy. A cardiac evaluation should include careful auscultation of the heart for gallops, rubs, and murmurs as well as any evidence of CHF or peripheral edema. The respiratory exam should document the rate and quality of respirations along with any observed or perceived dyspnea. The lungs should be auscultated for wheezes, rales, rubs, and E-to-A changes consistent with consolidation.

Ancillary Studies

A chest radiograph should be obtained in any patient with hemoptysis and usually provides important diagnostic information. Findings of pneumonia, metastatic disease, aortic aneurysms, pulmonary hypertension, or pulmonary embolism may be evident. The presence of a cavitary lung mass is suggestive of malignancy, lung abscess, or tuberculosis. In patients with underlying disease or if there is any concern regarding the patient's oxygenation status, oxygen saturation should be checked. Also, when the amount of blood expectorated is more than streaks of blood in the sputum or if there is any indication to suggest a coagulopathy, a complete blood count (CBC) and coagulation profile should be obtained.

 Key Points of Documentation

1. Onset, duration, amount of expectorated blood
2. Vital signs
3. Smoking history
4. Presence or absence of cough and sputum production
5. Medical and drug history
6. Pertinent positives and negatives on ENT and cardiac history and physicals
7. Findings on pulmonary exam
8. Chest x-ray findings

 Management

- The clinical course of hemoptysis is unpredictable and short-term mortality secondary to hemoptysis is directly related to the amount of blood expectorated and the *rate* of bleeding, regardless of cause.

In cases of massive hemoptysis, careful evaluation of blood pressure and heart rate is warranted to assess hemodynamic stability. Maintenance of an adequate airway and control of bleeding are the immediate therapeutic goals. Brisk bleeding from the airways obviously requires hospitalization for further evaluation and management. Supplemental oxygen should be started and endotracheal intubation performed for airway protection and hemorrhage control as indicated. Two large-bore intravenous lines for fluid resuscitation should be started, along with cardiac monitoring. Immediate emergency transport should be arranged. The patient should be placed in the Trendelenburg position; if the site of bleeding can be identified, the patient should be positioned such that the side of bleeding is dependent.

For patients presenting only with blood-streaked sputum without active bleeding, a rigorous attempt at making a definitive diagnosis is warranted. Patients who are thought to require immediate further evaluation or treatment (i.e., patients with active TB, a pulmonary abscess or cavitary lung lesions, or possible pulmonary embolism) will require hospital transfer. The more difficult diagnostic dilemma is hemoptysis in the patient with a normal chest radiograph. Generally, once life-threatening diagnoses have been excluded, evaluation and treatment can be instituted on an outpatient basis. Close follow-up with a PCP is mandatory, and the patient should be instructed to seek immediate medical attention if the amount of expectorated blood increases. Evaluation on an outpatient basis may include observation by the PCP or bronchoscopy to exclude an endobronchial lesion. (It is generally accepted that bronchoscopy is warranted in a patient with a history of cigarette smoking and hemoptysis even if the chest radiograph is normal.)

Errors to Avoid

- Underestimation of the rate of bleeding
- Failure to diagnose nonpulmonary causes of bleeding
- Failure to diagnose pulmonary embolism
- Failure to obtain a chest radiograph
- Failure to arrange adequate follow-up

Asthma in adults

Definition

Asthma is a chronic inflammatory disorder of the airways characterized by bronchial hyperresponsiveness and reversible airflow obstruction that remits spontaneously or with therapy. During an acute episode, mucus production and edema of the bronchial mucosa additionally contribute to the narrowing and obstruction of the airways. While asthma has features that overlap with other chronic obstructive disorders such as chronic bronchitis, emphysema, and cystic fibrosis, asthma typically occurs in younger individuals and exhibits a tremendous heterogeneity in clinical features and severity.

Although asthma has traditionally been classified as extrinsic or intrinsic, there is a large overlap between the two groups. Extrinsic asthma typically occurs in atopic individuals with a strong family history of asthma. Attacks are often seasonal and specific precipitating stimuli are identifiable. Peripheral blood eosinophilia and elevated serum IgE levels are common. Intrinsic asthma, by contrast, generally occurs in older individuals who have attacks throughout the year and may or may not have a history of atopy. In spite of this classification system, acute management does not vary with the asthma type.

Epidemiology

In the United States, asthma affects approximately 15 million people, resulting in 100 million days of restricted activity, half a million hospitalizations, and more than 5000 deaths annually. It is the most common chronic disease of childhood. African Americans and children have the highest hospitalization rates, with death rates remaining the highest in African Americans 15 to 24 years of age.

Clinical Features

While many patients presenting to the urgent care setting have a known diagnosis of asthma, it is important to keep in mind that other disease entities may mimic asthma and should be considered in evaluating a patient for the first time. Additionally, when an asthmatic patient with an acute exacerbation is being evaluated, it is important to elicit not only information on current symptoms but also facts that will help to predict the severity and outcome of an acute attack.

History

The typical patient presenting with an acute exacerbation of asthma will give a history of progressive dyspnea, chest tightness, wheezing, and cough. Patients with cough-variant asthma, however, may present with atypical symptoms, complaining only of a persistent, nonproductive cough. When any patient with asthma is being evaluated, in addition to the patient's specific symptoms, information of particular importance that should be obtained includes the duration of the current episode, use of medication prior to arrival (especially heavy use of a beta agonist), recent or current use of steroids, smoking habits, and previous history of hospitalizations and intubations. It is also important to try to determine precipitating or contributing factors. Factors to specifically ask for include effects of exercise, occupational exposures, exposure to animals, exposure to inhalant allergens or irritants (pollution or cigarette smoke), any history of rhinitis or sinusitis, gastroesophageal reflux, medication use (aspirin or other nonsteroidal anti-inflammatory medications, sulfites, beta blockers), and preceding viral infections.

 Physical Examination

On presentation, patients are usually in varying degrees of respiratory distress, exhibiting rapid, noisy breathing. They may be anxious and diaphoretic and may prefer to stay in an upright position.

- Recumbency may signal exhaustion or an impaired sensorium.

On chest examination, there will be hyperresonance to percussion, decreased intensity of breath sounds, prolongation of the expiratory phase, and wheezing. The intensity of the wheeze is not reliable in assessing the severity of airflow obstruction, since the absence of wheezing may actually indicate markedly decreased airflow. Clinical findings that do indicate a severe exacerbation are agitation or altered mental status, breathlessness at rest, an inability to speak in full sentences, the use of accessory muscles, a respiratory rate >30/min, tachycardia (>120/min), paradoxical respirations, decreased air movement or loud wheezing throughout inspiration and expiration, pulsus paradoxus above 25 mmHg, and a peak expiratory flow rate (PEFR) that is 50 percent of the predicted value. Patients with impending respiratory failure may present with drowsiness, absent breath sounds, and bradycardia.

Laboratory Evaluation

- Laboratory evaluation should not delay the initiation of therapy.

Pulmonary function tests during an acute asthma attack typically demonstrate airflow obstruction, as indicated by a decreased PEFR and decreased forced expiratory volume in 1 s (FEV_1). The PEFR can be measured with a peak flow meter at the bedside and correlates well with the FEV_1. Serial PEFR measurements are useful to determine response to therapy. Severe obstruction is indicated by a PEFR less than

120 L/min or less than 50 percent of the predicted value. Serial PEFR measurements are an excellent way to monitor response to therapy.

Although severe hypoxemia during an acute asthma attack is rare, measurements of oxygen saturation by pulse oximetry should be obtained in all patients with moderate to severe exacerbations. Studies have shown that patients with severe hypoxemia (PaO_2 <60 mmHg) and/or a $PaCO_2$ greater than 42 mmHg had PEFRs below 200 L/min or FEV_1s less than 1 L. PEFR measurements, therefore, may be useful as a guide to determine whether further oxygenation studies should be performed. In patients with a PEFR <30 percent predicted value, an arterial blood gas (ABG) measurement should be considered. If ABGs are not available, emergency room transfer may be needed.

- When ABGs are available, it is important to realize that during the early phases of an asthma attack, hyperventilation generally occurs, with a resultant low $PaCO_2$. With progressive worsening of airflow obstruction, the $PaCO_2$ normalizes at approximately 40 mmHg. Thus, a "normal" ABG should be interpreted in the context of the patient's physical examination. In a patient who appears in extremis, a normal $PaCO_2$ value should be viewed with concern and may indicate the need for more aggressive intervention, including intubation.

Chest radiographs in an acute asthma attack are not routinely recommended but may be used to rule out other conditions that mimic asthma and to help exclude other complicating conditions, such as pneumonia or a pneumothorax. The most common radiographic finding is hyperinflation. Chest radiographs, however, will not assist in estimating the severity of asthma.

The High-Risk Asthmatic

There are several circumstances associated with poor outcomes in caring for a patient with an acute asthma exacerbation, as indicated in Table 10-5. In addition to those listed, advanced age, smoking history, and heavy use of bronchodilators also correlate with poor outcome. Because of the increased incidence of poor outcomes including death, transfer to an emergency department should be considered in this subgroup of patients.

TABLE 10-5

FACTORS INDICATING HIGH RISK FOR POOR OUTCOME IN ASTHMA

Prior intubation and mechanical ventilation
PEFR or FEV_1 less than 33% of predicted or of the patient's personal best
Pneumonia
Severe hypoxemia (PaO_2 < 60 mmHg) or unequivocal central cyanosis
Diminished or absent breath sounds on auscultation
Bradycardia (heart rate < 45/min)
Arterial hypotension (systolic BP < 90 mmHg)
Pulsus paradoxus greater than 12 mmHg

SOURCE: Based on The National Heart, Lung, and Blood Institute, World Health Organization, and British Thoracic Society recommendations.

TABLE 10-6

DIFFERENTIAL DIAGNOSIS OF WHEEZING	
• Cardiogenic pulmonary edema ("cardiac asthma")	• Upper airway obstruction
• Chronic bronchitis	• Pulmonary embolism
• Emphysema	• Psychogenic vocal cord dysfunction

Differential Diagnosis

Most patients give a prior history of asthma. Therefore the new onset of wheezing in an adult should prompt consideration of other causes of wheezing. Table 10-6 lists the diseases most commonly confused with asthma.

Chronic bronchitis and *emphysema* are often difficult to distinguish from asthma. In general, these patients are older at initial presentation, have a significant smoking history, and, in the case of chronic bronchitis, have a history of a chronic productive cough.

Upper airway obstruction is often initially misdiagnosed as asthma. Months to years may elapse before the correct diagnosis is made. The obstruction may involve the larynx, trachea, or main bronchi and can be caused by tumors, laryngeal spasm, aspirated foreign bodies, tracheal stenosis, or vocal cord dysfunction. The clinical hallmarks of upper airway obstruction are stridor (a continuous low-pitched sound, often heard in inspiration) or a localized wheeze. Chest radiographs may demonstrate partial atelectasis or obstructive emphysema, or they may show mediastinal or thyroid masses.

Patients with *acute pulmonary emboli* may present with diffuse wheezing. The clinical setting of a patient at risk for pulmonary emboli includes cardiac disease, pregnancy, postoperative state, and debilitating disease; the absence of a prior history of asthma should alert the physician to consider this diagnosis.

Psychogenic vocal cord dysfunction is an entity most commonly seen in young adults (ages 20 to 40) with psychological disorders. In this disorder, audible wheezes are produced when the patient exhales against constricted laryngeal muscles. The diagnosis may be difficult to make, and these patients are often intubated for acute exacerbations. Direct visualization with a laryngoscope during an acute attack reveals paradoxical motion of the vocal cords. Treatment involves a multidisciplinary approach that includes speech therapists, psychologists, and internists.

A variety of other conditions can present with wheezing, including bacterial and viral pneumonias, toxic fume inhalations, carcinoid syndrome, the pulmonary vasculitides (especially Churg-Strauss syndrome), hypereosinophilic syndrome, and tropical eosinophilia.

 Management

Treatment of the Acute Attack

• Supplemental oxygen should be administerd if oxygen saturation is <90 percent.

Treatment of an acute asthma attack should be initiated as soon as possible (Table 10-7). The main goals of treatment are reversal of airway obstruction and correction of hypoxemia. *Beta-adrenergic agonists* are the bronchodilators of choice for acute asthma attacks, and short-acting inhaled beta$_2$ agonists are the mainstay of therapy. Beta$_2$ agonists can be administered by nebulizers or via metered dose inhaler (MDI) using a spacer device. The standard adult dose of nebulized albuterol is 2.5 to 5 mg, which can be repeated every 20 min for three doses. Continuous administration of albuterol in doses up to 10 mg/h has also been documented to be safe, though patients should be closely monitored during treatment, including frequent checking of vital signs and continuous cardiac monitoring.

The standard dose for a MDI is albuterol 4 to 8 puffs, which can be repeated every 20 min up to 4 h. When used correctly, MDIs are as effective as nebulizers. However, nebulized therapy is less dependent on patient coordination and cooperation and is preferred in patients with moderate to severe exacerbations. Selective beta$_2$ agonists (albuterol, terbutaline, pirbuterol, bitolterol) are the preferred agents because of their decreased risk of cardiac toxicity. Systemic beta$_2$ agonists (i.e., subcutaneous epinephrine or terbutaline) offer no benefit over inhaled administration of beta$_2$ agonists. Additionally, epinephrine is contraindicated in the elderly and those with preexisting cardiac disease.

Corticosteroids are also an essential component of therapy for acute asthma. Corticosteroids should be administered to all patients with moderate to severe exacerbations, patients who do not respond to initial beta-agonist therapy, and those who take oral steroids as part of their regular medical regimen. An initial dose of 30 to 60 mg of prednisone orally, or 125 mg of methylprednisolone intravenously, should be administered. Oral prednisone is as effective as intravenous methylprednisolone and is generally preferred.

- Early administration of corticosteroids may reduce the need for subsequent hospitalization; benefit from corticosteroids is usually seen 6 h after administration.

Anticholinergics are less potent bronchodilators than beta agonists in acute asthma. Studies have shown variable benefit of the use of ipratropium in acute asthma. However, when the initial response to a beta agonist is suboptimal, the addition of ipratropium can be considered. Ipratropium bromide solution (0.5 mg every 30 min for three doses, then every 2 to 4 h as needed) can be combined with an albuterol solution for administration.

TABLE 10-7		
MEDICATIONS USED TO TREAT ASTHMA		
Short-acting beta agonists	Albuterol, metaproterenol, bitolterol, pirbuterol, terbutaline	
Corticosteroids (inhaled)	Beclomethasone dipropionate, flunisolide, fluticasone propionate, triamcinolone acetonide, budesonide	
Corticosteroids (oral)	Prednisone, methylpredisolone, prednisolone	
Leukotriene modifiers	Zafirlukast, montelukast, zileuton	
Long-acting bronchodilators	Long-acting beta agonists (salmeterol), long-acting oral beta agonist (sustained-release oral albuterol), sustained-release theophylline	

Aminophylline does not appear to add any benefit over bronchodilation achieved by nebulized beta agonists and may increase side effects. Therefore its routine use in acute asthma is not indicated.

Although improvement in expiratory flow has been reported in acute asthma, the benefit of administration of intravenous magnesium sulfate in mild and moderate asthma exacerbations has not been proven. Current data, while unclear, suggest that magnesium adds little benefit to intensive therapy with inhaled beta agonists and corticosteroids.

The routine use of antibiotics in acute asthma is not recommended unless there is evidence of pneumonia or the presence of fever and purulent sputum. Chest physical therapy, mucolytic agents, and sedation are also not recommended for asthma exacerbations.

- All patients should be reassessed after each bronchodilator treatment. Documentation of patients' subjective response, physical examination, and PEFR should be noted. The response to initial therapy is a good predictor of the need for hospitalization.

 Management

1. Immediate triage to treatment area
2. Check peak expiratory flow rate (PEFR)
3. Check oxygen saturation in case of more than a mild attack
4. Initiate supplemental O_2 for saturations < 90%
5. Simultaneously initiate beta-agonist inhalation therapy
6. Reassess postinhalation treatment by physical examination and PEFR measurement
7. Repeat inhalation therapy as indicated with reassessment of response to each treatment
8. Initiate corticosteroid use for moderate or severe attacks

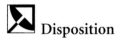 Disposition

Criteria for Discharge to Home with Outpatient Management

The following criteria should all be met:

1. PEFR is > 250 L/min
2. Response is sustained 60 min after last treatment
3. Patient is in no respiratory distress
4. Physical examination is normal

Before discharge, the medications and action plan should be reviewed and patients should be instructed on the correct usage of MDIs. In general, all patients should be discharged on short-acting $beta_2$ agonists. If patients have received systemic corticosteroids, they should continue oral corticosteroids at 40 to 60 mg/day for 3 to 10 days or until the PEFR is >70 percent of the predicted value. A follow-up visit should be made with their PCP or asthma specialist to reassess the need for continued oral corticosteroid therapy. Classification of asthma severity and step therapy (Table 10-8) can

TABLE 10-8

CLASSIFICATION OF ASTHMA SEVERITY AND STEP THERAPY

1. **Mild intermittent**
   - Symptoms occur less than or equal to two times per week
   - Nighttime symptoms occur less than or equal to two times per month
   - Lung function greater than or equal to 80% predicted
   - Peak flow variability less than 20%

   Step 1 therapy: Short-acting bronchodilator (inhaled beta agonist) as needed.

2. **Mild persistent**
   - Symptoms occur more than two times per week
   - Nighttime symptoms occur more than two times per month
   - Lung function greater than or equal to 80% predicted
   - Peak flow variability 20 to 30%

   Step 2 therapy: Short-acting bronchodilator as needed and single anti-inflammatory agent (low-dose inhaled corticosteroids or cromolyn, or nedocromil)

3. **Moderate persistent**
   - Daily symptoms
   - Nighttime symptoms occur more than once a week
   - Lung function greater than 60% but less than 80% predicted
   - Peak flow variability more than 30%

   Step 3 therapy: Short-acting bronchodilator as needed and medium- to high-dose inhaled corticosteroids. Long-acting bronchodilator if needed for nighttime symptoms

4. **Severe persistent**
   - Continual symptoms
   - Frequent nighttime symptoms
   - Lung function less than or equal to 60%
   - Peak flow variability more than 30%

   Step 4 therapy: Short-acting bronchodilator as needed, high-dose inhaled corticosteroids, long-acting bronchodilator; oral corticosteroids added if needed.

SOURCE: Based on Expert Panel Report II, National Institutes of Health (NIH), May 1997.

also be used as a guideline for discharge medications. Additional medication should be considered according to the guidelines of step therapy. Patients should receive a peak flow meter and be instructed to use it in the morning and evening, recording best of three tries each time. They should be encouraged to keep a diary for recording their results and should contact their PCP for any decrease in their readings.

CHRONIC OBSTRUCTIVE PULMONARY DISEASE

Definitions

Chronic obstructive pulmonary disease (COPD) is characterized by the presence of airflow obstruction, which may be due to two pathologically distinct entities: chronic bronchitis or emphysema. The obstruction seen in COPD is generally progressive, may be accompanied by airway reactivity, and may be *partially* reversible. The last of these differentiates COPD from asthma, in which the airflow obstruction is completely reversible. *Chronic bronchitis* is defined clinically by excessive secretion of mucus with chronic or recurrent productive cough, which is present on most days for at least 3 months of the year and for not less than 2 successive years. *Emphysema* is defined anatomically as abnormal, permanent enlargement of the airspaces distal to the terminal bronchioles, accompanied by destruction of their walls but without obvious fibrosis. Both entities may coexist in the same patient; "pure" forms are the exception rather than the rule.

Epidemiology

It is estimated that approximately 14 million people in the United States suffer from COPD. Most of these individuals have predominantly chronic bronchitis. The prevalence and morbidity (and mortality) appears to be rising, which can partly be explained by the increasing number of people who are living longer.

Risk Factors

COPD is more common in men than in women. The highest incidence occurs after age 40, and the single most important risk factor for the development of COPD is exposure to tobacco smoke, particularly in the form of cigarette smoking. The only known genetic abnormality that leads to COPD is alpha$_1$ antitrypsin deficiency (which accounts for less than 1 percent of COPD in the United States).

Clinical Presentation

In the past, patients with COPD were divided into "pink puffers" and "blue bloaters." This distinction no longer holds true, as patients can present with features of both syndromes as well as features of asthma. Chronic symptoms for both entities include dyspnea, cough, and wheezing.

- Patients with predominantly chronic bronchitis tend to be younger and present with mild dyspnea and a chronic productive cough. During exacerbations, the cough may become copious and purulent in appearance. These patients are prone to repeated episodes of bronchial infections and respiratory insufficiency.
- In contrast, patients with predominantly emphysema tend to be older (in their sixties) and to have a history of severe dyspnea.

In the urgent care setting, patients with decompensated COPD will generally present with an exacerbation of their chronic disease, primarily complaining of increased dyspnea and orthopnea. The history obtained in such patients should be targeted toward helping determine the precipitating factors. Acute exacerbations (or decompensation) of COPD can be provoked by viral and bacterial infections, inhalation of environmental irritants, gastroesophageal reflux, aspiration, pulmonary emboli, or cardiac events such as heart failure or arrhythmias. Other precipitating factors include active smoking, noncompliance with medication, or use of medications that alter ventilatory drive, such as hypnotics or tranquilizers.

On physical examination, most of these patients appear to be in respiratory distress. They generally present sitting up and leaning forward. There is accessory muscle use, pursed-lip breathing, and often marked diaphoresis. A pulsus paradoxus may be noted. Most symptoms are related to worsening hypoxemia and hypercapnia. Hypoxemia is manifest by tachypnea, cyanosis, tachycardia, hypertension, agitation, and anxiety. Hypercapnia will result in confusion, tremor, stupor, and eventually apnea.

Findings on auscultation of the chest depend on the severity of airway obstruction and the presence of large bullae. Breath sounds may be diminished, with a prolonged expiratory phase. Wheezing, which may be prominent, is usually diffuse and polyphonic. However, it is not a reliable indicator of reversibility or the degree of obstruction. With long-standing hypoxemia, features of right heart failure—such as neck vein distention, an early diastolic gallop, functional tricuspid regurgitation, and peripheral edema—may also be present. Digital clubbing is not a feature of COPD and if present should prompt a search for a comorbid condition. Additional physical findings depend on the stage of disease.

- Late in emphysema, patients are thin, tachypneic, and often barrel-chested; they present using accessory muscles of respiration and pursed-lip breathing.
- Chronic bronchitics are more heavy-set and usually appear to be in less respiratory distress; they may, however, be cyanotic and may have evidence of right heart failure.

A pulse oximetry measurement, which may show varying degrees of hypoxia, should be obtained in most patients presenting with exacerbation. The PEFR, which correlates well with the FEV_1, should be measured with a peak flow meter. When the PEFR is < 250 L/min, an ABG should be obtained to determine the possible presence of hypercapnia. Other laboratory findings may include polycythemia, hypercapnia, and metabolic alkalosis.

Chest radiographs are useful during acute exacerbations to detect complicating disorders such as pneumonia, pneumothorax, and coexisting pathology. Chest radiographs in patients with emphysema will show overdistention of the lungs, hyperlucency, and bullae. The findings in chronic bronchitis are less specific. Cardiomegaly, pulmonary hypertension, and right ventricular hypertrophy may be noted.

The ECG may be abnormal in COPD. The most frequent abnormalities are a rightward P and QRS axis, which is due to right ventricular hypertrophy. Other changes include low voltage in the limb leads, evidence of P pulmonale, right ventricular hypertrophy, and right bundle branch block. ECGs are indicated depending on the precipitating factors, comorbid disease, and severity of the attack.

 ## Management of Acute Exacerbations

Bronchodilators

The goals of therapy during an acute exacerbation are the correction of hypoxemia and the treatment of airflow obstruction.

Selective beta$_2$ agonists are the bronchodilators of choice to treat airflow obstruction. In general, they should be administered by inhalation through a nebulizer or MDI to reduce toxicity. If the response to the initial dose is not adequate, repeat therapy at frequent intervals should be considered, e.g., 2.5 mg of albuterol every 1 to 2 h.

Continuous nebulization can be used (10 mg of albuterol over 1 h); however, advanced age and coexisting cardiac disease must be taken into consideration. The addition of ipratropium may be beneficial in conjunction with beta$_2$ agonists. Corticosteroids can be useful if there is an asthmatic component in patients who show responsiveness to beta-agonist therapy. Steroids may be given orally or intravenously (initial bolus dose). It is vital, however, to avoid prolonged high-dose steroid therapy, especially in those patients who show little improvement on steroids.

Oxygen Supplementation

Severe hypoxemia is the most immediate life-threatening feature of COPD, and its correction is mandatory. Pulse oximetry, therefore, should be checked initially on all patients presenting with an exacerbation of COPD and should be monitored throughout the course of treatment. Oxygen should never be withheld because of fear of respiratory drive depression, though patients placed on supplemental oxygen should be observed closely for evidence of hypercapnia (altered mental status, sleepiness, apnea). While hypoxemia can be detected by pulse oximetry measurements, an arterial blood gas measurement is often necessary to detect hypercapnia.

- Hypercapnia is unusual when the FEV$_1$ is greater than 1 L (PEFR > 250 L/min), and severe hypoxemia is generally not seen when the FEV$_1$ is greater than 50 percent of predicted.

Role of Antibiotics in Acute Exacerbations of COPD

The most commonly identified cause of a chronic bronchitis exacerbation is an URI. The use of antibiotics has been shown to produce a small but statistically significant improvement, especially in patients with low baseline flow rates. The most common organisms isolated are *Streptococcus pneumoniae*, *Haemophilus influenzae*, and *Moraxella catarrhalis*. Empiric antibiotic use, therefore, should be considered, and antibiotic selection should be guided by local experience and severity of illness. Commonly used antibiotics include doxycycline, trimethoprim/sulfamethoxazole, amoxicillin/clavulanate, oral cephalosporins, one of the new-generation macrolides (clarithromycin, azithromycin), or a quinolone (levofloxacin, ofloxacin, trovafloxacin). Duration of therapy is usually for 10 days (except for azithromycin, for which it is 5 days). Viral etiologies resulting in exacerbations, however, should not be forgotten.

Assisted Ventilation

Despite aggressive pharmacologic support, some patients progress to respiratory insufficiency that requires assisted ventilation. These patients should immediately be transferred to an emergency department. Indications for assisted ventilation include worsening respiratory acidosis, altered mental status, and uncorrectable severe hypoxemia.

 Criteria for Discharge to Home with Outpatient Management

1. Inhaled beta-agonist treatments not required more frequently than every 4 h.
2. A noted response to treatment with return to baseline status.
3. Patient fully understands correct use of medications.
4. No evidence of severe or progressing hypoxia; ABG measurement is not required.

5. No requirement for parenteral therapy.
6. Respiratory distress has been minimized (i.e., no accessory muscle use, patient is able to ambulate, respiratory rate has returned to baseline).

If these criteria are not met or there is any doubt regarding the patient's stability or potential for acute decompensation, hospital transfer should be initiated. Patients with poor oxygen saturations, underlying processes such as pneumonia, evidence of tiring, persistent increase in respiratory rate, poor response to treatment, or a significant decrease in exercise tolerance should also be transferred for inpatient treatment.

Acute bronchitis and pneumonia

Acute Bronchitis

Acute bronchitis is an infection and inflammation of the respiratory tree affecting the upper and lower airways. The vast majority of cases of acute bronchitis are caused by viruses, particularly adenovirus, parainfluenza virus, influenza A and B, coxsackievirus, respiratory syncytial virus (RSV) (from exposure to infected children), and rhinovirus. Of note, herpes simplex viruses and measles can also cause bronchitis and tend to result in severe cases of the illness. Bacterial causes include *Chlamydia pneumoniae*, *Mycoplasma pneumoniae*, *Bordetella pertussis*, and perhaps *S. pneumoniae* and *H. influenzae*.

 History

Patients with bronchitis typically will present with a history of an antecedent URI, including symptoms of rhinorrhea, myalgias, fatigue, and, at times, fever and chills. A dry, nonproductive cough that progressively becomes productive of clear to discolored phlegm then follows. Patients may also complain of a history of associated wheezing, shortness of breath (secondary to bronchospasm), burning in the chest on breathing, and possibly the development of blood-tinged sputum.

 Physical Examination

On physical examination, vital signs may be remarkable for fever as well as an increased respiratory rate (particularly if bronchospasm is present). A full head, ear, nose, and throat (HEENT) examination should be performed looking for any signs of associated pharyngitits, otitis, or sinusitis. A detailed lung examination is essential, though it may be entirely normal or there may be wheezing, scattered rhonchi, and/or rales. Lung examination, however, should not reveal any dullness to percussion, frankly diminished breath sounds (except as related to bronchospasm), or E-to-A changes. Any signs of consolidation indicate a possible progression to pneumonia.

As the diagnosis of acute bronchitis is purely clinical, ancillary studies should be used primarily as a means of assessing severity, and, if indicated, ruling out other diagnoses. To that end, a pulse oximetry should be checked on patients exhibiting signs of shortness of breath or hypoxia, or who appear markedly ill. If a bacterial infection is considered (i.e., patients presenting with high fever or with protracted cases and severe symptoms), a CBC may be indicated. Generally, however, in routine cases, a CBC is not needed.

Chest x-rays generally do not need to be ordered on a routine basis but can be helpful in supporting the diagnosis as well as in ruling out other diagnoses. Patients who present with protracted symptoms, shortness of breath, abnormal pulse oximetry, or chest pain, who are acutely ill, or who have any indication of a possible pneumonia do require x-ray evaluation.

 Management

The treatment of acute bronchitis is primarily supportive and directed at alleviating the symptoms associated with the patient's presentation. Patients should be instructed to increase fluids (but with caution with those patients at risk for fluid overload) and rest as needed. Antipyretics can be used to control fever if present. Avoidance of smoke and irritants and use of humidified air and cough preparations may help with the cough, which may persist for 3 to 4 weeks. Cough suppressants can be prescribed for patients with a dry, nonproductive cough; productive coughs, however, should not be suppressed, and expectorants may be more beneficial in those circumstances. If wheezing is a factor, bronchodilators such as albuterol should be prescribed.

- For patients who are unfamiliar with the use of inhalers, detailed instructions should be reviewed prior to discharge.

Antibiotics are indicated only if a bacterial component is thought to be present, if the patient has a protracted illness without improvement, or if the patient develops fever or worsening after an initial improvement. If the bronchitis is thought to be caused by influenza A, amantidine 100 mg PO bid should be prescribed.

- Patients requiring supplemental O_2 for hypoxia or who have debilitating underlying disease should be transferred for hospital admission.

Pneumonia

Definition

Community-acquired pneumonia (CAP) is an acute infection of the pulmonary parenchyma. It is estimated that there are 3 to 4 million cases of CAP per year in the United States, with approximately 500,000 hospitalizations and 45,000 deaths. Pneumonia is the sixth most common cause of death and the number one cause of death due to infection in the United States. The presence of chronic illness has been shown to increase both the morbidity and the mortality associated with pneumonia. Advanced age (>60 years), and/or coexisting illnesses are important host factors that determine the presentation and outcome of CAP.

Etiologic Agents

Pneumonia may be caused by many infectious agents (see Table 10-9) and much has been written about "classic" presentations of pneumonia as a clue to infectious etiology. In reality, a definitive microbiologic diagnosis is made with the tools of the microbiology laboratory, including but not limited to sputum Gram stain and culture, blood cultures, urinary antigen for *Legionella pneumophila* (serogroup type I), serology, and polymerase chain reaction. In the outpatient setting, however, many of these tests are

TABLE 10-9

ORGANISMS THAT CAUSE COMMUNITY-ACQUIRED PNEUMONIA (CAP)

Streptococcus pneumoniae
Mycoplasma pneumoniae
Chlamydia pneumoniae
Legionella pneumophila
Haemophilus influenzae
Respiratory viruses (influenza, adenovirus)
Aerobic gram-negative bacilli (in patients with comorbid illnesses or age > 60)
Polymicrobial with anaerobes (in patients with predisposition to aspiration)
Staphylococcus aureus (< 5% of CAP)
Mycobacterium tuberculosis
Endemic fungi (depending on geographic area)

impractical and treatment is usually prescribed empirically, based on characteristics of the patient rather than the infecting organism.

Clinical Features

Patients presenting with symptoms of pneumonia will often complain of cough (with or without sputum production), fever, chills, sweats, rigors, chest pain (which may be pleuritic in nature), and shortness of breath. Patients with chronic cough frequently will note an increase in sputum quantity or a change in sputum color. Nonspecific symptoms such as anorexia, fatigue, myalgias, or headache may be present. In some patients, a cough may not be a prominent complaint; the symptoms in these patients may be vague, including only malaise and fever.

- The elderly and those with underlying chronic illnesses may not present with clinical features typically suggestive of pneumonia.

A thorough history of chronic coexistent illness must be obtained, since the presence of COPD, bronchiectasis, diabetes mellitus, chronic renal failure, CHF, chronic liver disease, cerebrovascular disease, alcoholism, malignancy, and altered immune status has been clearly shown to increase the severity of community-acquired pneumonia. Additionally, other important historical points should be documented, including any contact with infected persons, recent travel, and a history of pets in the home.

The physical examination in patients with pneumonia is important not only for detecting the presence of pneumonia but also for assessing its severity. Vital signs—including temperature, blood pressure, heart rate, and respiratory rate—must be obtained and documented (Table 10-10).

TABLE 10-10

FACTORS ASSOCIATED WITH INCREASED MORTALITY IN THE PRESENCE OF PNEUMONIA

- Temperature < 35 or ≥ 40°C
- Pulse ≥ 125/min
- Respiratory rate ≥ 30/min
- Systolic blood pressure < 90 mmHg

Evaluation of the ears, sinuses, and oropharynx should be performed. The presence of localized rales on auscultation of the lungs is an important finding, as is the presence of rhonchi and egophony.

- The absence of rales does not exclude the diagnosis of pneumonia.

Other findings that may be present on lung examination include diminished breath sounds and/or dullness to percussion, which indicate the presence of a parapneumonic pleural effusion; a pericardial friction rub suggests an associated pericarditis.

- Alteration in mental status is a significant finding and has been shown to predict increased risk of mortality in patients with pneumonia.

Laboratory Evaluation

In a patient less than 60 years of age without coexistent illnesses, extensive laboratory studies are not warranted in the outpatient evaluation of pneumonia. However, the Infectious Disease Society of America (IDSA) recommends obtaining a Gram stain, when logistically feasible, of expectorated sputum for patients who will be treated on an outpatient basis. Addtionally, patients greater than 60 years of age or with comorbid illnesses should have a CBC and evaluation of electrolytes and renal function, and pulse oximetry. If significant abnormality is found on the pulse oximetry or if there is concern regarding the patient's oxygenation, ABGs should be obtained.

Blood cultures should be obtained if there is a history of shaking chills or concern for possible risk of bacteremia.

Radiographic Evaluation

The American Thoracic Society (ATS) and the IDSA recommend obtaining a radiograph of the chest in any patient with suspected pneumonia. Radiographic findings may present anywhere from localized consolidations or diffuse interstitial patterns to complete lobar "white-out." Of note, radiographic findings often lag behind the clinical picture.

- Radiographic findings in patients with pneumonia may be minimal initially, particularly in the elderly or in persons who are dehydrated.

Owing to the delay in radiographic findings and the lag time between radiographic changes and clinical improvement, chest radiographs should not be used to follow response to therapy. Follow-up chest radiographs to document resolution of infiltrates should, however, be obtained in patients greater than 40 years of age and in smokers. The recommended time for subsequent radiographs is 7 to 12 weeks after beginning antibiotic treatment.

Laboratory and radiographic findings associated with severe community-acquired pneumonia are given in Table 10-11.

 Management

Treatment of the otherwise healthy outpatient with community-acquired pneumonia is largely empiric. The most common infectious etiologies are *S. pneumoniae*, *M. pneumoniae*, *Chlamydia pneumoniae*, *H. influenzae*, *L. pneumophila*, and respiratory viruses.

TABLE 10-11

LABORATORY AND RADIOGRAPHIC FINDINGS ASSOCIATED WITH SEVERE
COMMUNITY-ACQUIRED PNEUMONIA[a]

- WBC < 4000 or $> 30,000/mm^3$
- Absolute neutrophil count $< 1,000$
- $PaO_2 < 60$ mmHg or $PaCO_2 > 50$ mmHg
- Serum sodium < 130 meq/L
- Serum creatinine > 1.2 mg/dL or BUN > 20 mg/dL
- Hematocrit $< 30\%$ or hemoglobin < 9 g/dL
- Metabolic acidosis
- Chest radiograph with bilateral involvement or greater than one lobe involvement
- Pleural effusion on chest radiograph

[a]These findings are associated with increased risk of morbidity and mortality.

The IDSA recommends a macrolide (erythromycin, azithromycin, or clarithromycin), fluoroquinolone (levofloxacin, grepafloxacin, or trovafloxacin), or doxycycline in the majority of outpatients with community-acquired pneumonia. Ciprofloxacin should be avoided, since it does not have enhanced antimicrobial activity against *S. pneumoniae*. Alternatives include amoxicillin/clavulanate or some second-generation cephalosporins. However, it is important to realize that penicillins and cephalosporins are not active against *Mycoplasma*, *Chlamydia*, or *Legionella* species.

- The incidence of intermediate and high-level penicillin-resistant *S. pneumoniae* has increased in the United States over the past decade and varies by geographic region. Knowledge of local susceptibility patterns is important in treating known or suspected pneumococcal infection.

Duration of treatment of community-acquired pneumonia is not well studied. It is generally recommended that bacterial infections such as those due to *S. pneumoniae* and *H. influenzae* be treated for 72 h after the patient becomes afebrile. The IDSA recommends that pneumonia caused by *Mycoplasma*, *Chlamydia*, and *Legionella* species be treated for at least 14 days. Response to therapy is often subjective and usually occurs within 3 to 5 days of initiation of treatment. Fever may persist for 2 to 5 days after initiation of antibiotics. The absence of response to treatment or clinical deterioration in the patient's condition should prompt reevaluation of the patient (Table 10-12). Considerations include an incorrect diagnosis, a resistant or unusual organism, improper choice of antibiotic, or an underlying host disease that prevents resolution of infection, such as an obstructing pulmonary malignancy.

TABLE 10-12

DIFFERENTIAL DIAGNOSIS OF PNEUMONIA

- Tracheobronchitis
- Reactive airways
- Congestive heart failure
- Pulmonary embolism
- Vasculitis
- Bronchiolitis obliterans with organizing pneumonia
- Hypersensitivity pneumonitis
- Pulmonary malignancy

Assessment of the severity of community-acquired pneumonia and the need for hospitalization is extremely important. Special attention should be paid to patients greater than 60 years of age and/or those with one or more comorbid illnesses that have been shown to contribute to the morbidity and mortality.

Key Points of Documentation

- Presenting symptoms
- The presence or absence of comorbid illnesses
- Drug allergies
- Complete vital signs (including presence or absence of physical findings indicating respiratory distress)
- Examination of the upper and lower respiratory tract
- Chest radiograph findings
- Laboratory findings (including pulse oximetry, if indicated)
- Treatment plan (antibiotic therapy and adjunct treatment)
- Follow-up care (specific follow-up appointment, instructions for signs/symptoms of worsening)

PNEUMOTHORAX

Definition

Pneumothorax is defined as the presence of air or gas in the pleural space. It may occur spontaneously, as a result of trauma, or secondary to iatrogenic causes. Spontaneous pneumothorax may be either primary or secondary. Primary spontaneous pneumothorax occurs in patients without underlying lung disease, usually as a result of rupture of sub-pleural blebs. Affected individuals tend to be tall, thin men between the ages of 20 and 40 years. Secondary spontaneous pneumothorax occurs in patients with underlying lung disease. COPD is the most commonly associated condition. Other associated pulmonary diseases include asthma, necrotizing infections, *Pneumocystis carinii* pneumonia, sarcoidosis, pulmonary fibrosis, and lung cancer. Disorders associated with secondary spontaneous pneumothorax are listed in Table 10-13.

A tension pneumothorax occurs when the opening in the visceral pleura acts as a one-way valve, allowing air to enter the pleural space during inspiration and not letting it escape during expiration. The pneumothorax increases in size, causing compression of the ipsilateral lung and shift of the mediastinum to the contralateral side. Ventilation is severely compromised, leading to hypoxemia and hypercapnia. Venous return is reduced, which leads to decreased cardiac output and subsequent hypotension.

Clinical Features

The most common presenting symptoms in patients with spontaneous pneumothorax are dyspnea and the abrupt onset of unilateral chest pain, which is pleuritic in nature. In patients with underlying lung disease, the degree of dyspnea may be severe, since

TABLE 10-13

DISORDERS ASSOCIATED WITH SECONDARY SPONTANEOUS PNEUMOTHORAX

Pulmonary infections	**Interstitial lung diseases**
Pneumocystis carinii pneumonia	Sarcoidosis
Tuberculosis	Idiopathic pulmonary fibrosis
Lung abscess	Eosinophilic granuloma
Necrotizing pneumonia	Lymphangiomyomatosis
Airway diseases	**Neoplasms**
Asthma	Primary lung cancer
Chronic obstructive pulmonary disease (COPD)	Pleural metastases
Cystic fibrosis	**Miscellaneous**
	Marfan's syndrome
	Ehlers-Danlos syndrome

these patients have less pulmonary reserve than those with primary spontaneous pneumothorax. Findings on physical examination vary depending on the size of the pneumothorax, the degree of respiratory compromise, and the presence or absence of a tension pneumothorax.

Patients with spontaneous pneumothorax usually have normal blood pressure and sinus tachycardia (generally < 140 beats per minute). A pulse greater than 140 beats per minute, hypotension, tracheal deviation, or cyanosis should alert the physician to the possibility of tension physiology.

- Deviation of the trachea will always be toward the contralateral side of the pneumothorax.

Examination of the chest often reveals decreased breath sounds on the side of the pneumothorax, hyperresonance to percussion, and decreased or absent tactile fremitus. These findings may be more difficult to elicit in patients with underlying COPD, who may have diminished breath sounds secondary to underlying lung disease.

A chest radiograph is the most important diagnostic tool in a patient with suspected pneumothorax. This should be obtained with the patient in the erect position for optimal visualization. Expiratory films may be helpful for the detection of small pneumothoraces. A pneumothorax appears as a distinct visceral pleural line, with the absence of lung markings peripheral to the pleural line. While radiologists will often attempt to quantify the size of the pneumothorax as a percent of the hemithorax, most estimates tend to underestimate the true size. If pulse oximetry is obtained, evidence of hypoxia may be noted.

Differential Diagnosis

The differential diagnosis of a spontaneous pneumothorax includes other causes of chest pain and dyspnea, such as pulmonary embolism, myocardial infarction, pneumonia, pleural effusion, pneumomediastinum, dissecting aortic aneurysm, and esophageal spasm. The chest radiograph is usually diagnostic in patients with pneumothorax. In patients with bullous emphysema, a large peripheral bulla can be mistaken for a pneumothorax.

Computed tomography of the chest can reliably distinguish a large bulla from a pneumothorax. This is an important distinction, since mistaken placement of a chest tube into a peripheral bulla will *create* a pneumothorax and a bronchopleural fistula.

 Management

A tension pneumothorax is a medical emergency and requires immediate treatment to decompress the increasing intrapleural pressure. Treatment should be initiated on the basis of physical examination and should *not* be delayed in an attempt to obtain a chest x-ray for confirmation. Supplemental oxygen should be administered and a large-bore angiocatheter placed in the second intercostal interspace, in the midclavicular line. This should be left in place until a definitive chest tube can be placed.

Treatment of a Simple Pneumothorax
Patients with primary spontaneous pneumothorax who are otherwise healthy, have minimal symptoms, and have pneumothoraces estimated at less than 15 percent can often be observed without placement of a chest tube. Under these circumstances, a chest radiograph should be repeated within 2 to 4 h after initial presentation to assess for increase in size of the pneumothorax. Worsening dyspnea or increasing size of the pneumothorax are indications for either simple aspiration of intrapleural air or placement of a chest tube. Since these patients require several hours of observation and the development of respiratory and/or hemodynamic compromise is unpredictable, it is generally prudent to arrange transfer by ambulance to an acute care facility. Supplemental oxygen should be administered while awaiting transfer to increase the rate of absorption of pleural air. Placement of an intravenous line should be considered, and the patient should have continual monitoring for any change in status.

Patients with spontaneous pneumothorax and underlying lung disease require tube thoracostomy for treatment. It is generally recommended that these patients undergo definitive therapy for prevention of subsequent pneumothoraces, although there is some controversy as to whether they should undergo bedside pleurodesis with a sclerosing agent (doxycycline or talc) or surgical pleurodesis.

 Key Points of Documentation

- Presence or absence of underlying lung disease
- Whether the pneumothorax is the patient's first episode or a recurrence
- Vital signs
- Signs or symptoms of respiratory distress
- Oxygen saturation
- Chest radiograph findings

It is important not to underestimate the patient's symptoms or the degree of respiratory and/or hemodynamic compromise.

Foreign-body aspiration

Definition

Aspiration of foreign material into the tracheobronchial tree occurs most commonly in children. Although a wide variety of aspirated substances have been described, the most commonly reported is the peanut. Aspiration does occasionally occur in adults. Risk factors that predispose to aspiration in adults include advanced age, altered level of consciousness, alcoholism, poor dentition, diseases that impair swallowing function (e.g., Parkinson's disease), and institutionalization. Poorly chewed meat is the most commonly aspirated material in adults.

Clinical Evaluation

The symptoms and clinical manifestations of foreign-body aspiration vary with the size of the aspirated material. Large pieces of meat may lodge in the larynx or trachea, resulting in acute upper airway obstruction. This presentation is often referred to as the "cafe coronary" syndrome and consists of the sudden onset of respiratory distress, cyanosis, and inability to speak. The symptoms may be mistaken for a myocardial infarction; however, the patient's inability to speak should alert bystanders to the likelihood that the patient is choking. Immediate removal of the aspirated material is required or unconsciousness and death will rapidly ensue. In the United States, the Heimlich maneuver (subdiaphragmatic abdominal thrusts) is the recommended method for dislodging aspirated foreign material from the upper airway in an adult. The maneuver elevates the diaphragm, forcing air out of the lungs and resulting in expulsion of the material. Complications of the Heimlich maneuver include rib fractures, ruptured abdominal viscera, and pneumomediastinum.

When smaller foreign bodies are aspirated, the material will descend farther down the tracheobronchial tree. Cough, secondary to bronchial wall irritation, is the most common clinical manifestation. Other symptoms may include dyspnea, chest pain, wheezing, or vomiting. Many patients are able to recall the precise moment of aspiration; however, a patient with an altered level of consciousness (including persons intoxicated at the time of aspiration) may have no recollection of the aspiration event.

Physical Findings

Vital signs may reveal tachypnea and tachycardia. If material is partially obstructing the trachea, stridor may be present. If the material is lodged in a more distal airway, a localized wheeze may be heard on auscultation of the chest. Lobar atelectasis due to airway obstruction may result in diminished breath sounds over the area of collapsed lung.

Radiographic Evaluation

A chest radiograph should be obtained in any patient with known or suspected foreign-body aspiration. The chest radiograph is usually abnormal, although several radiographic patterns may be seen. The lower lobes are involved more often than the upper lobes and, in adults, the right lower lobe is more commonly affected than the left lower lobe.

If the foreign body is radiopaque, it may be visualized in the airway on the chest film. In the majority of cases, changes on the chest radiograph reflect partial or complete airway obstruction. These changes may include obstructive hyperinflation, segmental or lobar collapse, or an infiltrate. Pneumomediastinum and pneumothorax have also been reported but are less common radiographic findings. If a foreign body causes complete obstruction of a lobar bronchus and insufficient time has elapsed for distal resorption of air to occur, an inspiratory chest radiograph may appear normal. An expiratory film, however, may show hyperinflation of the affected lobe, since air will be trapped behind the obstructing foreign body.

When the patient or observers give a history of foreign-body aspiration or severe coughing during eating, the diagnosis is obvious. In the patient with a poor mental status whose aspiration is not witnessed, findings may be more subtle. The patient may present with postobstructive pneumonia, bronchiectasis, or a history of recurrent pneumonia. In fact, any patient who presents with recurrent pneumonia in the same lobe of the lung requires further evaluation. Bronchoscopy may reveal the presence of a foreign body and/or excessive granulation tissue in the airway from long-standing obstruction and airway irritation or an endobronchial malignancy.

 ## Management

Foreign bodies in the airways should be removed as soon as possible after the diagnosis is made. A patient who is initially evaluated in an urgent care center will likely require transfer to a hospital with facilities available for bronchoscopy. If the foreign body has moved distally and there is no evidence of respiratory compromise, the patient can safely be transported in private vehicle. If there is any evidence of respiratory compromise, the patient should be transported via ambulance. In those patients requiring ambulance transport, oxygen saturation should be checked (and monitored if abnormal) and supplemental oxygen initiated as indicated; an intravenous line should also be started while awaiting transport. The receiving facility should be contacted as well as the pulmonologist.

Ultimate removal of the foreign body may be accomplished with a rigid or fiberoptic bronchoscope; however, rigid bronchoscopy is generally more successful. Occasionally, surgery is required to remove a foreign body that cannot be removed bronchoscopically.

 Key Points of Documentation

- Timing of the aspiration event
- The degree of respiratory compromise
- Chest radiograph findings
- The subsequent removal of the foreign body

- A high index of suspicion should be maintained for patients with altered mental status who may not be able to give a history of aspiration but who present with recurrent pneumonia or localized bronchiectasis.

ACUTE PULMONARY EMBOLISM

Definition

The estimated incidence of pulmonary emboli in the United States is greater than 300,000 cases per year. The majority of acute pulmonary emboli (>90 percent) arise from blood clots in the deep veins of the lower extremities that travel to the lungs and lodge in the pulmonary arterial circulation. Large thrombi can lodge in the proximal pulmonary arteries and cause significant hemodynamic compromise. In contrast, smaller thrombi travel distally within the pulmonary arterial bed and are more likely to cause dyspnea and pleuritic chest pain. If untreated, the mortality rate from pulmonary embolism is approximately 30 percent. Most patients who die of pulmonary embolism do so in the first few hours after the embolic event. For those patients who survive the initial event, death is usually related to recurrent embolic events. In these patients, diagnosis of pulmonary embolism and institution of therapy significantly decrease the mortality rate to 2 to 8 percent.

Clinical Evaluation

The diagnosis of pulmonary embolism is often difficult. Findings on history and physical examination may be suggestive of pulmonary embolism but are nonspecific. There are many risk factors for the development of venous thromboembolism and therefore pulmonary embolism (Table 10-14). Most patients who develop pulmonary emboli will have diagnosable risk factors.

Differential Diagnosis

The differential diagnosis of pulmonary embolism is extensive and includes pneumonia, bronchitis, pneumothorax, CHF, myocardial infarction, pericarditis, pleurisy, atelectasis, and upper gastrointestinal disorders.

TABLE 10-14

RISK FACTORS FOR VENOUS THROMBOEMBOLIC DISEASE

Hypercoagulable States	**Predisposing Medical Conditions**
Factor V Leiden	Congestive heart failure
Antiphospholipid antibody syndrome	Paralysis/stroke
Hyperhomocysteinemia	Prior deep venous thrombosis
Antithrombin III deficiency	Nephrotic syndrome
Protein C deficiency	Obesity
Protein S deficiency	Immobilization
Malignancy	
	Postoperative
Pregnancy	Hip fracture
Oral contraceptive use	Knee or hip replacement
Major trauma	Abdominal/pelvic surgery

History

A detailed history and physical examination, along with a search for diagnoses, must be undertaken when patients present with symptoms consistent with a pulmonary embolus. The Prospective Investigation of Pulmonary Embolism Diagnosis (PIOPED, 1990) found that the most common presenting symptoms were dyspnea, pleuritic chest pain, cough, and hemoptysis (presenting as blood-tinged or streaked sputum).

- When syncope—an uncommon symptom of pulmonary embolus—occurs, it is suggestive of hemodynamic compromise and acute pulmonary hypertension.

On physical examination, the most common findings from the PIOPED included tachypnea, rales, tachycardia, the presence of an S_4 gallop, and accentuation of the pulmonic component of the second heart sound. Other clinical findings included fever and new-onset wheezing. Evidence of deep venous thrombosis (DVT) should be sought during the examination, looking for unilateral calf pain, edema, and a Homans' sign. Of note, less than 30 percent of patients in the PIOPED had symptoms or signs of DVT.

Laboratory Studies

Given the nonspecific nature of the history and physical in patients with pulmonary embolism, further diagnostic testing is generally needed when the diagnosis is suspected. In all patients in whom the diagnosis of pulmonary embolus is considered, a pulse oximetry should be checked, which may show evidence of hypoxia. ABG studies, while generally not readily available in the urgent care setting, may be helpful in the evaluation of these patients. ABGs usually reveal hypoxemia and an elevated alveolar-arterial oxygen gradient. Hypocapnia and respiratory alkalosis are also common.

- Up to 10 percent of patients with pulmonary embolism may have either a normal alveolar-arterial oxygen gradient or a normal Pa_{O_2}.

Laboratory studies beyond oxygenation analysis, while generally nonspecific, are nonetheless useful in evaluating other potential diagnoses.

- CBC findings in pulmonary embolism may include a mild leukocytosis.

Recently, the measurement of serum D-dimer levels has been studied as a method of diagnosing deep venous thrombosis and pulmonary embolism. D-dimer levels may be assayed by two methods: a rapid latex agglutination assay or the more time-consuming enzyme-linked immunosorbent assay (ELISA). Nearly all patients with DVT and/or pulmonary emboli have D-dimer levels above 500 ng/mL by ELISA. However, elevated D-dimer levels are nonspecific and are commonly present in patients with malignancy or those who have had recent surgery. On the other hand, D-dimer levels less than 500 ng/mL may be useful in eliminating the diagnosis of pulmonary embolism. Studies to date have not found the rapid latex agglutination assay to be a reliable and reproducible means of measuring D-dimer levels when compared to the ELISA method. If one is using the measurement of D-dimer levels less than 500 ng/mL as supportive evidence against the diagnosis of pulmonary embolism, it is important to know which assay method the laboratory is using.

Ancillary Studies

The chest radiograph and ECG are other important studies that can readily be obtained in the evaluation of pulmonary embolism, not because they provide specific findings diagnostic of pulmonary embolism, but because they may confirm other diagnoses, such as pneumonia, pneumothorax, or acute myocardial infarction. The most common radiographic abnormality in patients with pulmonary embolism is atelectasis or a pulmonary parenchymal abnormality. Other abnormalities that may be noted include a pleural effusion (which may be seen in approximately half of patients with pulmonary embolism), an elevated hemidiaphragm, "Hamptom hump" (a pleural-based density with a rounded border facing the hilum), and Westermark's sign (dilated pulmonary vasculature proximal to the embolus).

- Some 10 to 15 percent of chest radiographs in patients with a pulmonary embolism may be entirely normal.

Although it is nonspecific, the ECG, like the chest x-ray, is often abnormal in patients with pulmonary embolism. Sinus tachycardia and nonspecific ST-segment and T-wave changes are found in more than 50 percent of patients. Right axis deviation, right bundle branch block, and atrial dysrhythmias are less commonly seen. Other ECG signs of pulmonary embolism include an S_1, Q_3 pattern, or P pulmonale with tall, peaked P waves.

Diagnostic Studies

Diagnostic studies designed to specifically evaluate for pulmonary embolism include ventilation/perfusion lung scanning, pulmonary angiography, and, more recently, helical (spiral) computed tomography of the chest, but even with these diagnostic studies, the definitive diagnosis of pulmonary embolism can still be difficult. An important and often quoted aspect of the PIOPED was the assignment of clinical pretest probability of pulmonary embolism and the correlation of clinical suspicion with findings on ventilation/perfusion lung scanning and pulmonary angiography. These data are summarized in Table 10-15.

These data show that a normal lung scan excludes the diagnosis of pulmonary embolism regardless of clinical suspicion. A very small number of patients with "near

TABLE 10-15

PROBABILITY OF PULMONARY EMBOLISM ACCORDING TO LUNG SCAN CATEGORY AND CLINICAL SUSPICION

	CLINICAL SUSPICION OF PULMONARY EMBOLISM		
SCAN CATEGORY	HIGH	INTERMEDIATE	LOW
High	95	86	56
Intermediate	66	28	15
Low	40	15	4
Normal/near normal	0	6	2

SOURCE: Data from PIOPED Investigators. *JAMA* 263:2753, 1990, with permission.

normal" scans, however, did have small pulmonary emboli confirmed by angiography. A high clinical suspicion of pulmonary embolism combined with a high-probability lung scan had a 95 percent chance of angiographic confirmation of pulmonary embolism.

- It is important to note that close to 60 percent of patients from the PIOPED with pulmonary embolism did not have high-probability ventilation/perfusion scans.

Patients with high or intermediate clinical suspicion for pulmonary embolism who do not have high-probability ventilation/perfusion scans require further evaluation. Evaluation for DVT may be helpful, the rationale being that if a DVT is found, treatment with anticoagulation is warranted whether or not there has been a pulmonary embolism. Compression ultrasound with color-flow Doppler of the lower extremities has a high sensitivity and specificity for the diagnosis of proximal DVT. Impedance plethysmography (IPG) is also highly sensitive, although slightly less specific than venous ultrasound. *Negative studies for DVT do not exclude the diagnosis of pulmonary embolism.*

Pulmonary angiography, in which intravenous contrast is injected into the pulmonary arterial circulation, remains the "gold standard" test for the diagnosis of pulmonary embolism and is therefore the definitive diagnostic study in its evaluation. The presence of a filling defect or a cutoff of vessels indicates a positive study. The morbidity associated with pulmonary angiography is approximately 5 percent. The mortality rate is 0.5 percent. Adverse events are usually secondary to intravenous contrast reactions or complications related to catheter insertion.

Helical CT is currently being studied as another imaging study for diagnosis of pulmonary embolism. As in pulmonary angiography, injection of intravenous contrast is required. While helical CT can identify pulmonary emboli in the proximal pulmonary vasculature, its ability to detect emboli in subsegmental pulmonary arteries is limited. In fact, the sensitivity of this test varies from 65 to greater than 90 percent, with a specificity of >90 percent. At this time, the role of helical CT in the evaluation for pulmonary embolism is still being defined. Magnetic resonance imaging is also under study but does not currently have an accepted role in the diagnosis of pulmonary emboli.

 Management

Patients who present to an urgent care center with signs and symptoms suggestive of pulmonary embolism and in whom an alternative diagnosis cannot be firmly established should be transferred to a facility capable of more extensive and specialized evaluation. Any patient with high suspicion of pulmonary embolism should have an intravenous line established and should be placed on supplemental oxygen while awaiting ambulance transfer to an acute care facility.

The majority of patients with pulmonary emboli are treated with anticoagulation using heparin, followed by oral warfarin. Low-molecular-weight (LMW) heparin, administered subcutaneously, is as efficacious as intravenous unfractionated heparin. LMW heparin has a more predictable dose-response curve than unfractionated heparin, thus eliminating the need to monitor the PTT. The goal of anticoagulation is to prevent recurrent emboli. Other treatment options include inferior vena caval filters and thrombolytic therapy.

Placement of an inferior vena cava (IVC) filter is indicated in patients with DVT/ pulmonary emboli in whom anticoagulation is contraindicated. Patients with massive pulmonary emboli in whom the next embolism may be fatal and those with documented thromboemboli while therapeutically anticoagulated may also benefit from IVC filter placement.

Thrombolytic therapy should be considered in patients with acute massive pulmonary embolism and hypotension. This group of patients has a mortality rate of 20 percent, even when treated with intravenous heparin and supportive measures. Studies have evaluated the use of streptokinase, urokinase, and tissue plasminogen activator. All have shown more rapid dissolution of thromboemboli; however, the use of thrombolytic therapy remains somewhat controversial. The risk of bleeding is higher with thrombolytic therapy than with heparin, although shorter infusion times with newer agents may decrease this risk.

 Key Points of Documentation

Key documentation points include a careful history, especially for the presence or absence of risk factors for thromboembolism. Documentation of vital signs, including respiratory rate, is important, as is the record of studies obtained. A normal oxygen saturation by pulse oximetry in a patient with dyspnea should not exclude blood gas sampling, since pulse oximetry cannot reflect the degree of hypocapnia or an increased alveolar-arterial oxygen gradient. Patients with low- or intermediate-probability ventilation perfusion scans and high or intermediate clinical suspicion for pulmonary emboli warrant further evaluation.

BIBLIOGRAPHY

American Thoracic Society: Standards for the diagnosis and care of patients with chronic obstructive pulmonary disease. *Am J Respir Crit Care Med* S77–S121, 1995.

Bartlett JG, Breiman RF, Mandell LA, et al: Community-acquired pneumonia in adults: guidelines for management. *Clin Infect Dis* 26:811–838, 1998.

Braman SS, Corrao WM: Cough: differential diagnosis and treatment. *Clin Chest Med* 8:177–188, 1987.

Cahill BC, Ingbar DH: Massive hemoptysis: assessment and management. *Clin Chest Med* 15:147–168, 1994.

Celli BR: Pulmonary rehabilitation in patients with COPD. *Am J Respir Crit Care Med* 152:861–864, 1995.

Cherniack NS, Altose MD: Mechanisms of dyspnea. *Clin Chest Med* 8:207–214, 1987.

Colacone A, Wolkove N, Stern E, et al: Continuous nebulization of albuterol (salbutamol) in acute asthma. *Chest* 97:693–697, 1990.

Curley FJ, Irwin RS, Pratter MR, et al: Cough and the common cold. *Am Rev Respir Dis* 138:305–311, 1988.

Depaso WJ: Aspiration pneumonia. *Clin Chest Med* 12:269, 1991.

Dyspnea: mechanisms, assessment, and management: a consensus statement. *Am J Respir Crit Care Med* 159:321–340, 1999.

Fine MJ, Auble TE, Yealy DM, et al: A prediction rule to identify low-risk patients with community-acquired pneumonia. *N Engl J Med* 336:243–250, 1997.

Fine MJ, Smith MA, Carson CA, et al: Prognosis and outcomes of patients with community-acquired pneumonia: a meta-analysis. *JAMA* 275:134–141, 1996.

Fraser RG, Pare JA, Pare PD, et al: Pulmonary disease caused by aspiration of solid foreign material and liquids, in *Diagnosis of Diseases of the Chest,* 3rd ed. Philadelphia: Saunders; 1989:2382.

Friedman NL: Hiccups: a treatment review. *Pharmacotherapy* 16:986, 1996.

Ginsberg JS: Management of venous thromboembolism. *N Engl J Med* 335:1816, 1996.

Goldhaber SZ: Pulmonary embolism. *N Engl J Med* 339:93, 1998.

Gonzales R, Steiner JF, Sande MA: Antibiotic prescribing for adults with colds, upper respiratory tract infections, and bronchitis by ambulatory care physicians. *JAMA* 278:901–904, 1997.

Guidelines for the diagnosis and management of asthma: Expert Panel Report II. Publication No. 97:4051A. Bethesda, MD: National Institutes of Health; 1997.

Harding SM, Richter JE: The role of gastroesophageal reflux in chronic cough and asthma (see comments). *Chest* 111:1389–1402, 1997.

Heimlich HJ: The Heimlich maneuver: best technique for saving any choking victim's life. *Postgrad Med* 87:38, 1990.

Ing AJ: Cough and gastroesophageal reflux. *Am J Med* 103:91S–96S, 1997.

Ingbar DH: A systematic workup for hemoptysis. *Contemp Intern Med* 1:60–70, 1989.

Irwin RS, Boulet LP, Cloutier MM, et al: Managing cough as a defense mechanism and as a symptom: a consensus panel report of the American College of Chest Physicians. *Chest 114:* 133S–181S, 1998.

Irwin RS, Curley FJ: The treatment of cough: a comprehensive review. *Chest* 99:1477–1484, 1991.

Irwin RS, French CL, Curley FJ, et al: Chronic cough due to gastroesophageal reflux: clinical, diagnostic, and pathogenetic aspects (see comments). *Chest* 104:1511–1517, 1993.

Irwin RS, Widdicombe J: Cough, in Murray JF, Nadel JA (eds.): *Textbook of Respiratory Medicine.* Vol. 1. Philadelphia: Saunders; 1994:529–544.

Jantz MA, Person DJ: Pneumothorax and barotrauma. *Clin Chest Med* 15:75, 1994.

Johnston J, Reisz G: Changing spectrum of hemoptysis: underlying causes in 148 patients undergoing diagnostic flexible fiberoptic bronchoscopy. *Arch Intern Med* 149:1666–1668, 1989.

Kane GC, Salazar A, Israel HL: Aspergillosis: expanding spectrum of pulmonary disease. *Clin Pulm Med* 5:151–157, 1998.

Karpel JP, Schacter EN, Fanta C, et al: A comparison of ipratropium and albuterol vs albuterol alone for the treatment of acute asthma. *Chest* 110:611–616, 1996.

Kelley MA, Abbuhl SA: Massive pulmonary embolism. *Clin Chest Med* 15:547, 1994.

Kolodzik PW, Eilers MA: Hiccups (singultus): review and approach to management. *Ann Emerg Med* 20:565, 1991.

Leatherman J: Life-threatening asthma. *Clin Chest Med* 15:453–479, 1994.

Light RW: Pneumothorax, in *Pleural Diseases.* Baltimore: Williams & Wilkins; 1995:242–277.

Limper AH, Prakash UBS: Tracheobronchial foreign bodies in adults. *Ann Intern Med* 112:604, 1990.

Mahler DA: Dyspnea: diagnosis and management. *Clin Chest Med* 8:215–230, 1987.

Mahler DA, Jones PW: Measurement of dyspnea and quality of life in advanced lung disease. *Clin Chest Med* 18:457–469, 1997.

Manning HL, Schwartzstein RM: Pathophysiology of dyspnea. *N Engl J Med* 333:1547–1553, 1995.

McFadden EJ: Dosages of corticosteroids in asthma (see comments). *Am Rev Respir Dis* 147:1306–1310, 1993.

Nelson HS: Beta-adrenergic bronchodilators. *N Engl J Med* 333:499–506, 1995.

Niederman MS et al: Guidelines for the initial management of adults with community-acquired pneumonia: diagnosis, assessment of severity, and initial antimicrobial therapy. *Am Rev Respir Dis* 148:1418–1426, 1993.

Nocturnal Oxygen Therapy Trial Group: Continuous or nocturnal oxygen therapy in hypoxemic chronic obstructive lung disease: a clinical trial. *Ann Intern Med* 93:391–398, 1980.

Nocturnal Oxygen Therapy Trial (NOTT): Is 12-hour oxygen as effective as 24-hour oxygen in advanced chronic obstructive pulmonary disease with hypoxemia? (editorial). *Chest* 78: 419–420, 1980.

O'Donnell DE, McGuire M, Samis L, Webb KA: The impact of exercise reconditioning on breathlessness in severe chronic airflow limitation. *Am J Respir Crit Care Med* 152: 2005–2013, 1995.

O'Neil KM, Lazarus AA: Hemoptysis: indications for bronchoscopy. *Arch Intern Med* 151: 171–174, 1991.

Patrick H, Patrick F: Chronic cough. *Med Clin North Am* 79:361–372, 1995.

Perrier A, Bounameaux H, Morabia A, et al: Diagnosis of pulmonary embolism by a decision analysis–based strategy including clinical probability, D-dimer levels, and ultrasonography: a management study. *Arch Intern Med*, 156:531, 1996.

The PIOPED Investigators: Value of the ventilation/perfusion scan in acute pulmonary embolism: results of the prospective investigation of pulmonary embolism diagnosis (PIOPED). *JAMA* 263:2753, 1990.

Rogers, RM, Donahoe M, Costantino J: Physiologic effects of oral supplemental feeding in malnourished patients with chronic obstructive pulmonary disease: a randomized control study. *Am Rev Respir Dis* 146:1511–1517, 1992.

Reardon J, Awad E, Normandin E, et al: The effect of comprehensive outpatient pulmonary rehabilitation on dyspnea. *Chest* 105:1046–1052, 1994.

Saint S, Bent S, Vittinghoff E, Grady D: Antibiotics in chronic obstructive pulmonary disease exacerbations: a meta-analysis (see comments). *JAMA* 273:957–960, 1995.

Schechter MS, Rubin BK: Viral pneumonia: not just a childhood disease. *Clin Pulm Med* 5: 282–289, 1998.

Seaman ME: Barotrauma related to inhalational drug abuse. *J Emerg Med* 8:141–149, 1990.

Silvestri GA, Mahler DA: Evaluation of dyspnea in the elderly patient. *Clin Chest Med* 14: 393–404, 1993.

Smoller JW, Pollack MH, Otto MW, et al: Panic anxiety, dyspnea, and respiratory disease: theoretical and clinical considerations. *Am J Respir Crit Care Med* 154:6–17, 1996.

Smyrnios NA, Irwin RS, Curley FJ, French CL: From a prospective study of chronic cough: diagnostic and therapeutic aspects in older adults. *Arch Intern Med* 158:1222–1228, 1998.

Stulbarg MS, Adams L: Dyspnea, in Murray JF, Nadel JA (eds.): *Textbook of Respiratory Medicine*. Vol. 1. Philadelphia: Saunders; 1994:511–528.

Sweer L, Zwillich CW: Dyspnea in the patient with chronic obstructive pulmonary disease: etiology and management. *Clin Chest Med* 11:417–445, 1990.

Tapson VF, Hull RD: Management of venous thromboembolic disease: the impact of low-molecular-weight heparin. *Clin Chest Med* 16:281, 1995.

Tietjen PA, Kaner RJ, Quinn CE: Aspiration emergencies. *Clin Chest Med* 15:117–135, 1994.

Urschel JD: Thoracoscopic treatment of spontaneous pneumothorax: a review. *J Cardiovasc Surg* 34:535–537, 1993.

Wait MA, Dal Nogare AR: Treatment of AIDS-related spontaneous pneumothorax. *Chest* 106:693–696, 1994.

Wait MA, Estrere A: Changing clinical spectrum of spontaneous pneumothorax. *Am J Surg* 164:528–531, 1992.

Weinmann EE, Salzman EW: Deep-vein thrombosis. *N Engl J Med* 331:1630, 1994.

Woolcock AJ: Asthma, in Murray JF, Nadel JA (eds.): *Textbook of Respiratory Medicine*. Vol. 1. Philadelphia: Saunders; 1994:511–528.

11

GYNECOLOGY

Tanise I. Edwards

OVERVIEW

Gynecologic problems are among the most frequent complaints that bring women to the urgent care setting. The evaluation of such problems requires a full knowledge of gynecologic diseases and their presentation. It is important for the urgent care physician to be fully versed in gynecologic treatment, including a knowledge of which entities can appropriately be managed in an urgent care setting, which require emergent gynecologic consultation, and which can safely be referred for specialty evaluation and ongoing care at a later time.

A thorough and accurate history followed by a comprehensive gynecologic examination are the cornerstones of a gynecologic evaluation. A comprehensive history should include the following:

1. Menstrual history
2. Obstetric history
3. Contraceptive history
4. Gynecologic history
5. History of the present illness
6. Pertinent past medical history

A detailed *menstrual history* will include the date of the last menstrual period, the date of the last *normal* menstrual period, and the regularity of menses. Depending on the presenting complaint, information may also include history of the duration of menstruation, amount of blood loss with menstruation, passage of clots, type of sanitary products used, dysmenorrhea, age of menarche, and/or age of menopause.

- The easiest way to assess amount of blood loss is by the number of pads or tampons used over a certain period of time, including the extent of saturation.

The *obstetric history* will include gravid status (the number of times the patient has been pregnant), the date of the last pregnancy, parity (the number of births), spontaneous abortions (i.e., miscarriages) with dates, elective abortions with dates, ectopic pregnancies, complicated pregnancies, and use of fertility medications or difficulties in conception.

The *contraceptive history* will include the type of contraceptives used (none, oral, barrier, rhythm, withdrawal, IUD, etc.), consistency of use (including history of missed pills, broken condoms, etc.), and the length of time the method has been in use.

The *gynecologic history* will include past gynecologic surgeries or procedures, history of pelvic inflammatory disease (PID) or sexually transmitted diseases (STDs), any known STD exposures, ovarian cysts, uterine fibroids, endometriosis, number of sexual partners (if any), use of vaginal products (i.e., feminine sprays, douches), and last Pap smear examination.

The *history of present illness* should include, in addition to in-depth information on the presenting complaints and relevant past medical history, any complaints of abnormal vaginal discharge, fever, nausea, vomiting, diarrhea, or urinary symptoms.

THE PHYSICAL EXAMINATION

The basic gynecologic examination comprises two primary components:

- *Visual examination*, which includes both external and speculum examination
- *Palpation*, which includes the bimanual and rectovaginal examination

Visual examination includes inspection of the vulva, perineum, vaginal canal, and portio vaginalis cervicis. The examination should note the presence or absence of any lesions (type of lesion and location), lacerations or tears, foreign bodies, swelling or masses, and character of the cervix (including color, shape of os, and discharge). Any vaginal discharge should be noted for character (thin, frothy, cottage cheese–like, etc.), quantity, color, odor, and source (i.e., vaginal or endocervical). The palpation portion of the examination should begin with evaluation of the abdomen for any evidence of abdominal tenderness (and its location), palpable masses, organomegaly, or any signs of peritoneal irritation (guarding, rebound, or rigidity). Next is the bimanual examination evaluating (1) the uterus for size, shape, location, tenderness, and consistency; (2) the adnexa (fallopian tubes and ovaries) for tenderness, masses, or fullness; (3) the cervix for cervical motion tenderness (CMT) and, if indicated, the state of the internal os (i.e., open or closed); and (4) the cul de sac for masses, fullness, or distention. The rectovaginal examination will provide information on gastrointestinal (GI) or rectal pathology as well as on the status of the posterior uterine wall.

Additionally, the physical examination should include the patient's general appearance, evidence of abnormal vital signs (particularly fever, tachycardia, or orthostatic changes), generalized rashes, and costovertebral angle tenderness. A breast examination—along with general cardiac, pulmonary, and lymphatic examination—may also be warranted depending on the presenting illness.

The key to performing a thorough and accurate examination is cooperation and relaxation of the patient. Comfortable positioning of the patient (to the extent that this is possible), while affording the patient as much privacy as possible, will aid in achieving compliance with the examination. All adjuncts to evaluation should be readily available, including adequate lighting, varying speculum sizes, and easy access to any diagnostic equipment (cultures, swabs, slides, etc.) that may be needed. A warmed speculum will also increase the patient's comfort. It is helpful to have an assistant to aid in the examination; while it is mandatory for all male examiners to have a female chaperone, this is strongly recommended for female examiners as well. It is also generally helpful to explain to the patient what she can expect as the examination is performed.

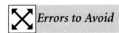 *Errors to Avoid*

- Attempting a bimanual examination on a patient with a full bladder
- Using a cold speculum
- Allowing interruptions during the examination
- Not ensuring complete patient privacy

EMERGENCY CONTRACEPTION

Some patients will present in the urgent care setting requesting evaluation for emergency contraception (Table 11-1). This request may be as a result of failed prophylaxis (i.e., broken condom, displaced diaphragm, displaced cervical cap) or of unprotected intercourse. To be effective, emergency contraception should be instituted within 72 h of intercourse. Under these circumstances, use of emergency contraception leads to a 75 percent reduction in pregnancy compared to no emergency contraception.[1]

With the Yuzpe method of emergency contraception, based on the use of ethinyl estradiol and DL norgestrel, the patient takes 2 tablets containing 0.5 mg of ethinyl estradiol and 0.5 mg DL norgestrel within 72 h of the unprotected intercourse. This is followed by a second dose 12 h later. The major side effect of this regimen is marked nausea and vomiting, such that an antiemetic should also be prescribed and taken 1 h prior to the hormone pills.

TABLE 11-1

EMERGENCY CONTRACEPTION

PROGESTERIN-ESTROGEN COMBINATIONS	
Ovral	2 tablets within 72 hours of unprotected intercourse followed by 2 tablets 12 h after the first dose
Lo-Ovral	4 tablets within 72 hours of unprotected intercourse followed by 4 tablets 12 h after the first dose
Levlen	4 tablets within 72 hours of unprotected intercourse followed by 4 tablets 12 h after the first dose
PROGESTERIN ONLY	
Plan B	One 0.75 mg tablet of levonorgestrel within 72 hours of unprotected intercourse followed by a second pill 12 hours after the first dose

An initial pregnancy test should be checked before prescribing emergency contraception in order to rule out the possibility of an existing pregnancy. Patients should also be counseled regarding the possibility of pregnancy due to treatment failure. They should be told to expect a menstrual period within 21 days after treatment; should menstruation not begin as expected, they would have to follow up with pregnancy testing. Last, patients should be counseled regarding the potential for STD exposure related to unprotected intercourse.

Of note, it is not known whether patients who have contraindications to daily oral contraceptive use have the same contraindications to this type of treatment.

PREGNANCY TESTING IN THE URGENT CARE SETTING

Pregnancy tests detect levels of beta human chorionic gonadotropin (HCG) in the serum or the urine. While serum tests can be either quantitative or qualitative, urine tests provide only qualitative results. In the urgent care setting, urine pregnancy testing is the more efficient and practical test, since it can be run in the urgent care center with immediate results. (Serum testing generally requires outside laboratory evaluation.) The lowest levels of HCG detectable by urine pregnancy tests are in the range of 10 to 20 IU/mL, which is present at about 1 week after implantation. It is important to remember that at these levels, diluted urine can lead to false-negative results; this should be taken into consideration if test results are negative, since serum testing may be required. At the time of a missed menses, levels are usually at approximately 100 IU/mL.

In a normal pregnancy, beta-HCG levels should double every 1.4 to 2 days during the first 2½ months, after which levels decline. Beta-HCG remains detectable, however, throughout pregnancy until approximately 2 weeks after delivery or termination (elective or spontaneous). In addition to the confirmation of pregnancy, pregnancy tests are also used in monitoring threatened abortions or as an indicator of the effectiveness of medical treatment of an ectopic pregnancy. (A persistently rising level would indicate treatment failure.)

- While not reliable for the diagnosis of an ectopic pregnancy, the beta-HCG level may rise more slowly than the normal 1.4- to 2-day doubling seen in an intrauterine pregnancy.
- An extremely elevated beta-HCG that does not correlate with pregnancy dates may be indicative of a molar pregnancy.

COMMON GYNECOLOGIC PROBLEMS SEEN IN THE URGENT CARE SETTING

The most common gynecologic complaints seen in the urgent care setting generally fall within the categories of abdominal pain, abnormal vaginal bleeding, vaginal discharge, or STD exposure. Women who present with any of these complaints must be evaluated for gynecologic as well as nongynecologic causes of their symptoms. Focusing solely on gynecologic concerns can lead to missed or delayed diagnosis and inappropriate treatment. A systematic approach should be developed in evaluating patients with any of these complaints. The possibility of pregnancy and the concerns associated with a confirmed pregnancy must also be considered, particularly given the expanded differential that accompanies a diagnosis of pregnancy.

Gynecologic Causes of Abdominal Pain (Fig. 11-1)

- Ectopic pregnancy
- PID
- Dysmenorrhea
- Mittelschmerz
- Ovarian cysts
- Adnexal torsion
- Endometriosis
- Leiomyomas
- Conditions not related to ectopic pregnancy

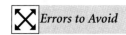 **Errors to Avoid**

- Failure to diagnose an ectopic pregnancy
- Failure to diagnose a ruptured hemorrhagic cyst
- Failure to diagnose PID
- Failure to diagnose a ruptured tuboovarian abscess
- Failure to diagnose adnexal torsion
- Failure to diagnose acute nongynecologic surgical pathology

Dysmenorrhea

Dysmenorrhea is a type of abdominal pain associated with menstruation; it is estimated that up to 10 percent of women suffer from severe dysmenorrhea at some time during their reproductive lives. Dysmenorrhea can be classified as primary or secondary. *Primary dysmenorrhea* refers to painful menstrual cramps not caused by underlying pathology and is thought to be due to uterine contractions mediated by prostaglandins. Patients with primary dysmenorrhea are often nulliparous and tend to be younger in age. *Secondary dysmenorrhea*, in contrast, is caused by an underlying disorder such as endometriosis, adenomyosis, use of an intrauterine device (IUD), fibroid tumors, pelvic infections, and cervical stenosis.

Patients who present with dysmenorrhea often have a previous history of similar symptoms occurring at the time of their menstrual cycle. These symptoms may precede or occur with the onset of menstruation and may last from 1 to 3 days, usually tapering after the first 24 h. Often patients will present complaining of an exacerbation of their usual symptoms, which, in addition to abdominal pain, may include nausea and vomiting, headache, and diarrhea; some patients may also complain of radiation of the pain to the back and/or legs.

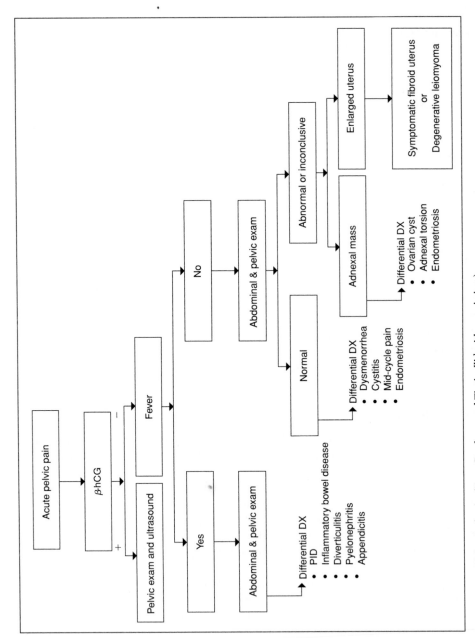

FIGURE 11-1   Abdominal pain. (From Pearlman and Tintinalli,[1] with permission.)

Evaluation

Evaluation of patients presenting with symptoms of dysmenorrhea (or a previous history of dysmenorrhea) must include the evaluation and exclusion of other disorders with more serious implications. The differential includes any condition associated with abdominal pain in a female patient, particularly ectopic pregnancy, PID, ovarian cysts, or spontaneous abortion. On history, detailed information regarding the last menstrual period, last *normal* menstrual period, history of abnormal vaginal discharge, history of sexual activity, and the potential for pregnancy is key. Examination should include blood pressure, pulse, and temperature as well as a detailed abdominal and pelvic examination (both speculum and bimanual). The approach to the examination should focus on eliminating any other causes for the patient's symptoms. Laboratory evaluation should include a pregnancy test, a complete blood count (CBC), and urinalysis as indicated to rule out other diagnosis.

 Management

Treatment of dysmenorrhea is geared toward alleviating the pain and any associated symptoms. Patients with nausea and vomiting may need antiemetic medications and intravenous hydration. Pain relief can usually be achieved with nonsteroidal anti-inflammatory drugs (NSAIDs) such as ibuprofen or naproxen. All patients with a discharge diagnosis of dysmenorrhea should receive a gynecologic referral for evaluation of possible secondary dysmenorrhea as well as possible prophylactic treatment with NSAIDs or oral birth control pills.

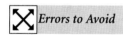 *Errors to Avoid*

- Failure to consider other diagnoses in a patient with a history of dysmenorrhea
- Failure to obtain a pregnancy test, thereby misdiagnosing vaginal bleeding in pregnancy
- Failure to evaluate for infection

Mittelschmerz

Mittelschmerz is abdominal pain associated with the menstrual cycle in which symptoms develop around the time of ovulation as a result of follicular rupture and resultant irritation of the peritoneum. Physical examination is remarkable for sharp, localized tenderness and, at times, a mildly enlarged ovary on the involved side.

To a certain extent, the diagnosis of mittelschmerz is a diagnosis of exclusion, which can be considered when the more serious diagnoses have been ruled out. The presenting clinical picture, therefore, will determine the evaluation needed. A pregnancy test, however, should be checked on all patients as indicated by the gynecologic history (i.e., all sexually active individuals of child-bearing age without a history of hysterectomy). The pain associated with mittelschmerz is self-limiting and can generally be treated using a NSAID. Abdominal pain discharge instructions should be reviewed with the patient prior to discharge, including strict criteria for reevaluation.

Ovarian Cysts

Abdominal pain is the predominant symptom for which women with ovarian cysts will seek treatment in the urgent care setting. These patients, who are typically in their childbearing years, may or may not have previously diagnosed cysts. The key to the evaluation of patients who present with abdominal pain and in whom an ovarian cyst is suspected is to rule out the possibility of pregnancy (particularly ectopic pregnancy) or other life-threatening or serious conditions (such as torsion, PID with tuboovarian abscess, and acute surgical intestinal disorders). Of note, pain secondary to ovarian cysts may simply be due to distention of the cyst's capsule or it may be caused by torsion, rupture, infarction, or secondary peritonitis.

On history, in addition to complaints of abdominal pain (typically unilateral), other symptoms seen include nausea, vomiting, vaginal spotting, or irregular menses. In patients in whom rupture has occurred, there may be a history of sudden onset of severe abdominal pain as well as of light-headedness, fever, and peritoneal symptoms. On physical examination, vital signs are typically normal if rupture has not occurred. (A low-grade fever or mild tachycardia may sometimes be present, or dehydration may be noted if nausea and vomiting accompany the presentation.) Reproducible tenderness will usually be noted on palpation of the abdomen and is generally localized to the side of the cyst. If a cyst has ruptured, diffuse tenderness, including peritoneal signs, may be present. The results of bimanual examination are variable. Depending on the size of the cyst, the patient's body habitus, patient cooperation, and skill of the examiner, an adnexal mass may be appreciated. Associated adnexal tenderness is typically present and cervical motion tenderness may be elicited.

- An adnexal mass in a postmenopausal woman is abnormal and should raise the suspicion of possible malignancy. All postmenopausal women with palpable ovaries, even without a mass, require gynecologic follow-up.

Laboratory
Laboratory evaluation must include a beta-HCG to rule out the possibility of pregnancy. A CBC with differential should also be checked, as well as a urinalysis.

In patients who present with significant discomfort or if the diagnosis is unclear, an urgent ultrasound may be required. This group of patients will include those who have difficult examinations (i.e., patients who are overweight, uncooperative with the examination, and those in extreme pain) as well as patients in whom ectopic pregnancy, torsion, or an abscess is of concern.

 Management
Management will vary with the patient's presentation. Patients who are experiencing mild pain, have stable vital signs, and show no indications of pregnancy or infection may be treated with NSAIDs and discharged with strict criteria for reevaluation. It is good medical practice to speak with the gynecologist who will follow the patient in case rupture or torsion develops and to establish a treatment plan (including possible follow-up ultrasound).

Patients with severe pain or those in whom torsion, infarction, or rupture is suspected will require transport for emergency gynecologic evaluation. Vascular access should be obtained and fluid resuscitation initiated as indicated.

Adnexal Torsion

Adnexal torsion is a gynecologic emergency requiring acute surgical intervention. Symptoms include sudden onset of unilateral lower abdominal pain, often with associated nausea and vomiting. The pain, which may be noted to occur after a sudden position change, may radiate to the back or pelvis. Other clinical findings that may be present include a low-grade fever, a tender adnexal mass (seen in over 90 percent of patients), or signs of peritonitis. On laboratory evaluation a CBC may show a mild to moderate leukocytosis. Emergency gynecologic consultation is required and the patient should be transferred via ambulance for definitive treatment.

Vaginitis and Vaginal Discharge

Of all gynecologic complaints, vaginal discharge is among those for which women most often seek medical care. Many of these women either lack a primary care physician or have been unable to arrange an appointment in a timely fashion. Often evaluation is sought not only for treatment of uncomfortable symptoms but also because of a pressing underlying concern of possible STD exposure. Under these circumstances, it is as important to address the underlying concerns as it is to treat the symptoms themselves.

Vulvovaginitis can be categorized as either infectious or noninfectious. The three most common etiologic agents are (1) *Candida*, (2) *Trichomonas*, and (3) bacterial vaginosis. These three entities account for over 90 percent of all vaginal infections. Other less common causes of vaginitis include herpesvirus, streptococcus, contact or chemical agents, atrophy, and retained foreign bodies. While each etiology has its own particular characteristics, there is considerable overlap in the presentation of each. Color and consistency, pH, odor, microscopic characteristics, and ultimately culture can all aid in the differentiation of the various organisms.

Candidiasis

While *Candida* species can be isolated from the vagina of up to 50 percent of asymptomatic women, they become a common cause of vaginal discharge and irritation when there is overgrowth or alteration of the vaginal flora. Predisposing factors for symptomatic infection include:

- Antibiotic use (especially ampicillin, cephalosporins, and tetracycline)
- Oral contraceptive use
- Diabetes
- HIV disease
- Pregnancy
- Corticosteroid use
- Frequent douching
- Stress

The most frequent candidal species seen in vaginitis is *Candida albicans*, with *Candida glabrata* and *Candida tropicalis* composing the majority of the remaining species. Symptoms, by history, may include prominent vulvovaginal itching and burning (which may increase at night or after bathing), dyspareunia, and dysuria. On physical examination, a nonodorous, white "cottage cheese" type of discharge is noted, which is generally adherent to the vaginal wall (the classic presentation); vulvar erythema and edema may be noted as well. There may also be associated pustulopapular lesions. Although the classic white discharge will generally be seen, there may be little or no discharge in some patients, a thin discharge, or only the patient's normal discharge. Wet-mount evaluation with a 10% KOH solution will help to isolate the fungal elements, pseudohyphae, spores, and mycelia, which may be readily identified on microscopic examination.

Management   *Candida* can be treated by a variety of topical antifungal regimens or by oral therapy (Table 11-2).

Topical Treatment   Topical or intravaginal agents in the treatment of candidal vaginitis include miconcazole, clotrimazole, and terconazole. These medications should not be used in patients with a history of allergy or hypersensitivity to "azole" products.

Oral Treatment   A single dose of oral fluconazole is also an effective means of treating candidal vaginitis. Immunocompromised women should receive a full 7-day course of treatment. This group includes diabetics, women with HIV disease, and those on steroid therapy. Recurrent or recalcitrant candidiasis should be referred to a gynecologist for ongoing suppression/prophylactic therapy.

TABLE 11-2

TREATMENT REGIMENS FOR VULVOVAGINAL CANDIDIASIS

AGENT	FORMULATION	DOSAGE REGIMEN
UNCOMPLICATED VVC		
Butoconazole	2% cream	5 g/d for 3 d
Clotrimazole	100-mg vaginal tablet	2 tablets/d for 3 d
Miconazole	200-mg vaginal suppository	1 suppository/d for 3 d
Nystatin	100,000-U vaginal tablet	1 tablet/d for 14 d
Tioconazole	6.5% ointment	5 g intravaginally in a single dose
Fluconazole	150-mg tablet PO	1 tablet as a single dose
COMPLICATED VVC		
Fluconazole	100-mg tablet PO	1 tablet weekly
Ketoconazole	200-mg tablet PO	1 tablet/d for 1–2 weeks
Clotrimazole	500-mg vaginal suppository or tablet	1 suppository or tablet weekly

SOURCE: Tintinalli et al,[4] with permission.

Bacterial Vaginitis

Bacterial vaginitis, also known as nonspecific vaginitis or *Gardnerella* vaginitis, is the most common etiology of vaginal discharge. *Gardnerella*, like *Candida*, is part of the normal vaginal flora. Bacterial vaginosis, however, is the result of an overgrowth of the normal bacterial flora and therefore is not considered a true "infection." Generally, there is no inflammatory response or vulval/vaginal itching. Symptoms for which women seek treatment usually relate to a profuse vaginal discharge with a notable "fishy" odor. Specific requirements for the diagnosis of bacterial vaginosis are evidence of at least three of the following findings:

- The typical thin, off-white vaginal discharge (which is generally homogeneous in nature and adherent to the vaginal walls)
- pH of the discharge >4.5
- Clue cells on microscopic examination
- A positive "whiff" test (a fishy odor to the discharge when 10% KOH is added; this reflects the presence of amine)

Of note, women with a diagnosis of bacterial vaginosis have an increased association with PID and postabortion infections. Pregnant women with bacterial vaginosis have an increased incidence of preterm labor and preterm rupture of membranes. There is also an increased incidence of chorioamnionitis and postpartum endometritis. While bacterial vaginosis is not considered a STD, there is an association between bacterial vaginosis and sexual activity. Treatment of partners, however, is not routinely performed.

 Treatment Options

- Oral metronidazole 500 mg bid for 7 days
- Oral metronidazole 2 g PO in a single dose
- Metronidazole vaginal gel (0.75%) intravaginally bid for 5 days
- Oral clindamycin 300 mg PO bid for 7 days
- Clindamycin vaginal cream (2%) 5 g intravaginally once daily for 7 days

- Metronidazole can cause an Antabuse type of reaction when mixed with alcohol; therefore patients should be cautioned to abstain while on this medication.

Trichomonas Vaginitis

Infection with *Trichomonas*, unlike that due to *Candida* or *Gardnerella*, is considered a sexually transmitted disease. Up to 40 percent of partners of women diagnosed with *Trichomonas* vaginitis will be positive for *Trichomonas*. Additionally, women may be infected with *Trichomonas* for years before manifesting symptoms of the infection. Symptoms, when present, include a profuse, generally malodorous discharge and associated vaginal irritation and itching. There may also be concomitant complaints of dysuria and dyspareunia. On physical examination, a profuse yellow-to-green frothy discharge with an offensive odor is typically noted. The manifestations of infection with *Trichomonas*, unlike that due to *Candida* or *Gardnerella*, may include more extensive local involvement of the endocervix, Skene's glands, and the urethra or trigone of the bladder. Vulvar erythema may be noted, along with vaginal erythema, labial edema, and punctate hemorrhages (a "strawberry appearance") of the cervix. Vaginal pH is generally > 5.0; on microscopic examination, motile trichomonads may be present.

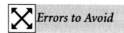 *Errors to Avoid*

- Using old saline for wet prep. Old saline can kill the trichomonads, thereby giving false results.

 Treatment Options

- Metronidazole 2 g PO for one dose
- Metronidazole 500 mg PO bid for 7 days

Partners should be treated simultaneously to prevent reinfection. In the urgent care setting, the partners should be registered and examined prior to initiating therapy.

Genital Herpes

Patients with a diagnosis of genital herpes may present with symptoms of localized infection or complaints of a more systemic nature. When symptoms are localized, patients will typically complain of painful lesions in the vaginal area. There may be urinary complaints, including dysuria or urinary retention, if involvement of the urethra has occurred; groin tenderness may also be noted secondary to inguinal adenopathy. Systemic symptoms will include fever, malaise, headache, and myalgias. Primary infections tend to be more severe than recurrent infections, and are more likely to be accompanied by systemic symptoms. Recurrences may be triggered by trauma or various stresses (either emotional or physical) and tend to erupt in the same locations. A prodrome of tingling or burning may be noted in patients with recurrences, signaling the onset of an active infection.

On examination, fluid-filled vesicles or shallow ulcers may be noted on the vulva, vagina, or cervix. The lesions may be isolated or in groups, and there may be an associated inflammation of the involved area. At times, the initial presentation may be that of only one or two isolated lesions. Laboratory evaluation may provide or confirm the diagnosis via culture of the vesical fluid or via culture of the base of a wet ulcer. A Tzanck prep will be positive for multinucleated giant cells in approximately 50 percent of cases.

Multiple treatment options are available for nonpregnant patients to help accelerate healing and decrease the severity of symptoms (Table 11-3). Suppressive therapy should be discussed with patients with frequent recurrences but generally should be instituted by the patient's primary physician. Patients with disseminated or severe disease require inpatient care and intravenous antiviral treatment. Oral acyclovir may be used to treat pregnant patients with a primary episode of genital herpes, but it should be started *only* in consultation with the patient's obstetrician; treatment with oral acyclovir is not recommended for the treatment of recurrent infections in the pregnant patient.

TABLE 11-3

TREATMENT OF GENITAL HERPES[a]

Primary Infection	Recurrent Infection
Acyclovir 400 mg PO tid for 7 to 10 days	Acyclovir 800 mg PO bid for 5 days
OR	OR
Famciclovir 250 mg PO tid for 7 to 10 days	Acyclovir 400 mg PO tid for 5 days
OR	OR
Valacyclovir 1 g PO bid for 7 to 10 days	Famciclovir 125 mg PO bid for 5 days
OR	OR
Acyclovir 200 mg PO five times daily for 7 to 10 days	Valacyclovir 500 mg PO bid for 5 days
	OR
	Acyclovir 200 mg PO five times daily for 5 days

[a]Topical treatment is not effective.

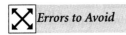 *Errors to Avoid*

- Failure to consider the diagnosis when only one or two isolated lesions are noted on examination
- Failure to counsel patients on the recurrent nature of the disease
- Failure to counsel patients on the need for condom use and to abstain from sexual contact during active infection or the onset of prodromal symptoms
- Failure to counsel and evaluate for other STDs (including gonorrhea, chlamydial infection, HIV disease, and syphilis)

Bartholin's Abscess

Bartholin glands can become infected if obstruction of the ducts occurs, leading to cyst formation, retention of secretions, and subsequent infection. These glands are located inferiorly, at the 5 o'clock and 7 o'clock positions of the vaginal vestibule. The organisms involved are polymicrobial, including both aerobes and anaerobes. *Bacteroides* species and gram-negative organisms are common. Infrequently, *Neisseria gonorrhoeae* and *Chlamydia trachomatis* may be isolated.

On clinical presentation, patients will give a history of swelling or a mass in the vaginal region and severe pain. Physical examination will typically show a painful, fluctuant mass; however, depending on the timing, there may be evidence of spontaneous drainage or only be localized swelling prior to the development of a discrete mass.

Laboratory Studies

Laboratory studies should, at a minimum, include cultures of the abscess. If there is suspicion for possible STD infection, cervical cultures for *N. gonorrhoeae* and *Chlamydia* should be sent.

Management

As for any abscess, incision and drainage with breaking of any loculations should be performed. Care must be taken not to incise the keratinized labial skin; rather, the incision should be made on the mucosal surface. It should be parallel to the posterior margin of the hymenal ring.[2] There is a high incidence of recurrent infection with this method, and future marsupialization may be required. Treatment with a Word balloon catheter is an alternative approach, which may eliminate the need for future marsupialization. Routine antibiotic therapy should not be needed if there is no associated cellulitis and adequate incision and drainage have been performed. If cultures return positive for *N. gonorrhoeae* or *Chlamydia*, appropriate treatment must be initiated. Initial follow-up can occur in the urgent care setting following incision and drainage, but all patients should be referred to their gynecologists for ongoing treatment.

If the patient presents prior to full abscess formation, a trial of antibiotic therapy may be indicated. Discharge instructions should include warm soaks, gynecologic follow-up, and an immediate recheck for worsening or new symptoms.

Pelvic Inflammatory Disease

 History

Patients presenting with PID typically complain of bilateral lower abdominal pain. It is important, however, to keep in mind that patients can also present with unilateral lower abdominal pain, back pain, or pain radiating to the right upper quadrant. Other symptoms that may be present include a history of irregular bleeding, nausea, vomiting, and urinary complaints. Of note, up to three-quarters of patients with PID will present just after menstruation or actually during their menses.[3]

 Physical Examination

On physical examination, it is important to document blood pressure, pulse rate, and temperature. Fever or mild tachycardia may be present, and when hypotension is present, more serious manifestations of PID must be considered. A detailed abdominal examination should be performed, which may reveal bilateral lower-quadrant tenderness, unilateral tenderness, right-upper-quadrant tenderness, or peritoneal signs (rebound and guarding), depending on the extent of the infection. On direct visualization, the pelvic examination may be positive for a mucopurulent discharge and an inflamed cervix; bimanual palpation may show evidence of adnexal tenderness, uterine tenderness, and cervical motion tenderness (the classic "chandelier sign"); if a tuboovarian abscess has developed, either adnexal fullness or an adnexal mass may be found. A rectovaginal examination may reveal tenderness of the posterior uterine wall or may identify an inflamed retrocecal appendix.

Laboratory

Laboratory evaluation should include a CBC with differential, a wet prep of vaginal secretions, cervical cultures (specifically for *N. gonorrhoeae* and *Chlamydia*), and uri-

TABLE 11-4

DIFFERENTIAL DIAGNOSIS OF PELVIC INFLAMMATORY DISEASE

Ectopic pregnancy	Endometriosis
Spontaneous abortion (threatened, septic)	Upper urinary tract infection
Ovarian cysts (ruptured)	Ovarian tumor
Ovarian cysts (intact)	Gastrointestinal disease (appendicitis,
Torsion	diverticulitis, gastroenteritis, etc.)

nalysis. A pregnancy test should be performed on all women of childbearing age who are sexually active and are capable of becoming pregnant. Those patients with a strong possibility of PID should also be evaluated for HIV disease, syphilis, and hepatitis B. Blood cultures should be drawn on all toxic patients.

Additional ancillary evaluation may include pelvic ultrasound looking for ovarian cysts, torsion, or tuboovarian abscesses; an ultrasound should be obtained whenever a mass is present in the face of possible PID or when clinical examination is limited secondary to marked tenderness.

Diagosing PID
The diagnosis of PID may be straightforward and clear-cut, depending on the patient's history and clinical examination. Unfortunately, however, PID will often present with a confusing clinical picture, making a definitive diagnosis difficult. Many of the findings of PID are part of a long differential (Table 11-4), adding to the difficulty of diagnosis. As a result, and in an attempt to decrease missed diagnoses, sequelae associated with PID (Table 11-5), and the transmission of STDs, the Centers for Disease Control and Prevention (CDC) have formulated criteria for diagnosing PID (Table 11-6). It is important, however, to realize that without confirmatory laboratory or laparoscopic evidence, these clinical recommendations can result in overdiagnosis of the disease.

 Management
Once a diagnosis of PID has been made, the first determination for treatment is the decision for inpatient versus outpatient treatment. Patients who have any of the following should be transferred, either for further diagnostic evaluation or, in consultation with an accepting gynecologist, for hospital admission:

- Confirmed pelvic abscess by ultrasound
- Suspected pelvic abscess based on clinical examination
- Pregnancy
- Adolescence
- Immunocompromised status

TABLE 11-5

SEQUELAE OF PELVIC INFLAMMATORY DISEASE

Ectopic pregnancy	Chronic pelvic pain
Infertility	Development of a tuboovarian abscess

TABLE 11-6

CRITERIA FOR THE DIAGNOSIS OF PELVIC INFLAMMATORY DISEASE

Minimal criteria (all three must be present in
the absence of an established cause
other than PID)
   Lower abdominal tenderness
   Adnexal tenderness
   Cervical motion tenderness

Additional criteria (improve specificity)
   Temperature >38°C (100.9°F)
   Abnormal cervical or vaginal discharge

Elevated erythrocyte sedimentation rate
Elevated C-reactive protein
Cervical culture positive for *N. gonorrheae*
   or *C. trachomatis*

Elaborate criteria
   Endometritis on endometrial biopsy
   Tuboovarian abscess on sonography or
     other radiologic test
   Demonstration of disease by laparoscopy

SOURCE: Pearlman and Tintinalli,[1] with permission.

- Toxic status (includes peritoneal signs, hypotension, high fever, recalcitrant vomiting or nausea)
- Outpatient treatment failure
- Unclear diagnosis or potential surgical diagnosis (presence of peritoneal signs)
- IUD[4]

Patients who are toxic should have an intravenous line placed for hydration and an initial dose of antibiotic therapy administered while awaiting emergency transport. The receiving hospital should be notified of all treatment provided in the urgent care center and the results of any tests that have been obtained. For patients with an unclear diagnosis who will require further diagnostic evaluation, transport arrangements will be determined in part by the clinical picture.

For patients not requiring inpatient treatment, one of the regimens in Table 11-7 can be used.

All patients treated on an outpatient basis must have arranged follow-up within 72 h. Discharge instructions must include signs and symptoms that would prompt immediate reevaluation.

TABLE 11-7

OUTPATIENT TREATMENT OF PELVIC INFLAMMATORY DISEASE[a]

Regimen A
   Cefoxitin 2 g IM plus 1 g probenecid
   concurrently PO
   OR
   Ceftriaxone 250 mg IM
   AND
   Doxycycline 100 mg PO b.i.d. for 14 days

Regimen B
Ofloxacin 400 mg PO b.i.d. for 14 days
AND EITHER
Clindamycin 450 mg PO q.i.d. for 14 days
OR
Metronidazole 500 mg PO b.i.d. for 14 days

[a]Follow up in 72 h.
SOURCE: Pearlman and Tintinalli,[1] with permission.

Errors to Avoid

- Failure to obtain a pregnancy test
- Failure to consider other diagnoses in a patient with a previous history of PID
- Failure to diagnose a tuboovarian abscess
- Failure to arrange follow-up (should be documented on patient's chart)
- Definitively stating that a patient has PID based solely on clinical criteria
- Failure to counsel against sexual intercourse (or to use condoms for any sexual activity) until negative laboratory results are documented or until completion of treatment and follow-up evaluation
- Failure to counsel (including chart documentation of this) on the importance of completing the full course of oral antibiotics unless directed otherwise

 Key Points of Documentation

- Temperature, blood pressure, and pulse
- A history of any underlying medical disorders
- The ability to take medication PO
- Results of pregnancy test (or why test was not required)
- Type of contraception used (specifically the presence of an IUD)
- Detailed abdominal and pelvic examination (including adequacy of examination, the presence or absence of cervical discharge, the specific location of any tenderness, the presence or absence of cervical motion tenderness, and the presence or absence of adnexal fullness or masses)
- Specific follow-up arrangements
- Review of discharge instructions with specific symptoms for reevaluation including:
    Failure to improve
    Any worsening or development of new symptoms
    Fever
    Vomiting and inability to take medications
    Persistent or severe pain

Vaginal Bleeding

Patients presenting to the urgent care setting with complaints of vaginal bleeding represent a wide spectrum of disease entities. The first step in evaluation is the assessment of hemodynamic stability. Any patient with evidence of hemodynamic compromise requires standard stabilization along with simultaneous assessment. Stabilization includes placement of two large-bore intravenous lines, continuous monitoring, and preparation for transport to an emergency setting capable of gynecologic evaluation.

- Any patient presenting with unstable vital signs, abdominal pain, and abnormal vaginal bleeding should be assumed to have a ruptured ectopic pregnancy until proven otherwise and should be treated accordingly.

Patients who are hemodynamically stable can be evaluated further in the urgent care setting. Evaluation can then include determination of the site and possible cause of bleeding, any urgent treatment required, and the development of a treatment plan for any further evaluation or treatment.

Differential Diagnosis

The differential diagnosis of vaginal bleeding can be divided into two major categories (Table 11-8):

- Vaginal bleeding associated with pregnancy
- Vaginal bleeding in the nonpregnant patient

Vaginal bleeding in the nonpregnant patient can further be categorized as anovulatory or ovulatory. In the urgent care setting, this distinction is not key, since definitive diagnosis is not required; what is required, however, is the diagnosis of conditions calling for acute management and follow-up, as indicated.

Evaluation

A full history and physical examination are the first steps in the evaluation of abnormal vaginal bleeding. A detailed history should be obtained, including the frequency, severity, and character of the bleeding as well as any associated symptoms. The physical examination should focus on determining the source of bleeding, if possible, including evaluation for nongynecologic sources of bleeding (i.e., gastrointestinal or urinary). Examination should document the presence or absence of any vaginal tears, cervicitis, or other localized findings. The general examination should look for evidence of systemic disease including thyroid disease, coagulopathy, or liver disease. Since the first step in the assessment of a patient with abnormal vaginal bleeding is determining whether or not the patient is pregnant (Fig. 11-2), a pregnancy test is indicated in all patients of childbearing age. Other laboratory studies, depending on the clinical presentation, include a CBC, thyroid function test (TFT), and coagulation studies.

 Management

See "Vaginal Bleeding in Pregnancy," below, for the management and treatment of the pregnant patient.

TABLE 11-8

CAUSES OF VAGINAL BLEEDING

VAGINAL BLEEDING IN THE PREGNANT PATIENT	VAGINAL BLEEDING IN THE NONPREGNANT PATIENT
Ectopic pregnancy	Menstruation
Spontaneous abortion	Dysfunctional uterine bleeding
Placenta previa	Bleeding related to contraception use
Abruptio placentae	Medical disorders
Bloody show	Gynecologic lesions/tumors
Local trauma	Trauma
	Infection

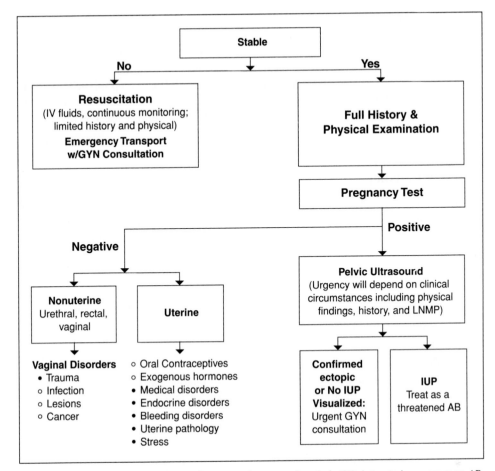

FIGURE 11-2   Vaginal bleeding. (LNMP, last normal menstrual period; IUP, intrauterine pregnancy; AB, abortion.)

For the stable nonpregnant patient who presents with vaginal bleeding, little acute intervention is generally required. In most patients, gynecologic follow-up is all that is necessary. For some patients, hormonal treatment may be beneficial, particularly for protracted or heavy bleeding. Hormone treatment, which may include the use of oral contraceptive pills, conjugated estrogen therapy, or progesterone therapy, should generally be initiated only in concert with the following physician.

THE PREGNANT PATIENT

Vaginal Bleeding

When one is evaluating a pregnant patient with vaginal bleeding in the urgent care setting, it is of prime importance to diagnose any life-threatening conditions or conditions requiring emergent intervention, the most likely being that of ectopic pregnancy. Other diagnoses that are likely to present in early pregnancy include spontaneous abortion (threatened, inevitable, or complete), implantation bleeding, cervicitis, and local trauma. Both cervicitis and local trauma should be evident on physical examination; in the urgent care setting, implantation bleeding is a diagnosis of exclusion and therefore should not be listed as a discharge diagnosis (implantation bleeding cannot be distinguished from a threatened abortion in this setting). Gestational trophoblastic disease, which occurs in 1 in 1700 pregnancies in North America,[4] should be considered in patients who present with vaginal bleeding, hyperemesis, and a uterine size that is greater than expected for gestational age.

Ectopic Pregnancy

Ectopic pregnancy is the number one cause of maternal death in the first trimester of pregnancy and must be ruled out in any patient presenting in early pregnancy with vaginal bleeding. (See Table 11-9 for risk factors for ectopic pregnancy.) Although ectopic pregnancies typically present between the sixth and eighth weeks of pregnancy, they can present as late as the twelfth or fourteenth week (most commonly when located in the fornix of the uterus, which allows for greater fetal growth before rupture).

- Ectopic pregnancies occur in up to 50 percent of patients who become pregnant after tubal ligation, particularly after laparoscopic tubal electrocautery.

Clinical Presentation

The diagnosis of ectopic pregnancy on history is unreliable, particularly in the ability to distinguish it from the diagnosis of a threatened abortion; a high index of suspicion, therefore, must be maintained in order not to miss this diagnosis. On history, patients may complain of vaginal bleeding, irregular menses, or spotting and abdominal pain. Some patients may report having had a syncopal episode. In patients in whom rupture has occurred, severe localized abdominal pain and peritoneal symptoms may be present, along with complaints of shoulder pain secondary to diaphragmatic irritation.

On physical examination, there may be peritoneal findings, hypotension, and shock if rupture has occurred. It should be noted that in these circumstances, a relative bradycardia might be present, even in the face of shock. For those patients who have not yet ruptured, physical findings can be variable. Vital signs may be normal or may show mild abnormalities. There may be tenderness on abdominal examination. Pelvic examination may be positive for bleeding from the cervical os or blood in the vaginal vault. The bimanual examination may show adnexal tenderness, adnexal fullness or a mass, or cervical motion tenderness. The uterus may or may not be enlarged.

TABLE 11-9

RISK FACTORS FOR ECTOPIC PREGNANCY

Previous history of pelvic inflammatory disease	Tubal ligation
Previous ectopic pregnancy	Tubal abnormalities
Fallopian tube surgery	Current IUD use

Management

Patients who are hemodynamically unstable or who show signs of rupture (even without significant hemodynamic changes) require immediate emergency transport to a facility with gynecologic surgical capabilities. Both the receiving facility and the consulting obstetrician must be notified of the patient's condition and physical findings. Fluid resuscitation with two large-bore intravenous lines should be started using normal saline or lactated Ringer's solution and the patient kept in the Trendelenburg position while awaiting transport.

For patients in whom the diagnosis is uncertain and those in whom the diagnosis cannot be *unequivocally* excluded, further diagnostic testing is indicated. Typically, a transabdominal or transvaginal ultrasound is the procedure of choice. In stable patients with minimal symptoms, particularly very early in pregnancy, these examinations can be ordered urgently from the urgent care setting. If there is any concern for potential deterioration, the patient should be sent to a hospital radiology facility with emergency department notification or sent for radiographic evaluation by way of the emergency department.

When ultrasound results show a normal intrauterine pregnancy with normal adnexa, the diagnosis of ectopic pregnancy can be eliminated and other causes should be sought for the patient's presenting complaints.

When an ectopic pregnancy is diagnosed, by visualization either of embryonic cardiac activity outside the uterus or of an empty uterus along with a pelvic mass or free pelvic fluid, emergent gynecologic referral is indicated. Treatment, depending on the stage of fetal development along with other factors, may be surgical or medical (in which case a baseline quantitative beta-HCG should be obtained). Patients should be referred directly to the treating physician and not discharged for follow-up at a later date.

Patients who pose more of a diagnostic dilemma include those in whom an equivocal ultrasound is found. Gynecologic consultation is key in these circumstances in order to appropriately arrange for further evaluation.

Spontaneous Abortion

Patients who present with vaginal bleeding prior to the 20th week of pregnancy are at risk for spontaneous abortion. In these patients, the major differential diagnosis to exclude, particularly in early pregnancy, is that of ectopic pregnancy. This differentiation can be difficult to make based on either the history or physical examination given that many of the presenting symptoms are the same. In these cases, ultrasonography may be key in patient evaluation. Differentiation between these two diagnoses is made easier if the patient has had a documented intrauterine pregnancy (IUP) by ultrasound, if the patient is further into the pregnancy than the point at which a viable ectopic pregnancy could present (generally over 10 weeks of pregnancy), or if there has been passage of fetal tissue.

- Twin pregnancies with an IUD and an ectopic site of implantation can occur.

Clinical Presentation

Patients with spontaneous abortions usually present with a history of vaginal bleeding. There may already be a confirmed diagnosis of pregnancy, or the patient may give a history of missed menses, spotting, or irregular bleeding. Other complaints may include abdominal pain and cramping or, depending on the stage of abortion, a history of passage of fetal tissue. On history, it is important to obtain information regarding the last menstrual period, including irregular menses, abnormal bleeding patterns, and the character of the last menses. On pelvic examination, the size of the uterus, along with any tenderness, adnexal fullness, or adnexal masses, should be noted. Additionally, the pelvic examination can help differentiate between a threatened, inevitable, incomplete, or complete abortion, depending on the appearance of the cervical os. In a *threatened abortion*, the os is closed and there has been no passage of fetal tissue. Typically, there is only mild bleeding and mild to moderate cramping. When the cervical os is open but there has been no passage of tissue, the diagnosis is that of an *inevitable abortion*. Symptoms associated with an inevitable abortion include moderate cramping and moderate, persistent bleeding. In contrast, an *incomplete abortion* is present when the cervical os is open and there has been incomplete passage of fetal tissue. Bleeding is usually more significant and persistent, as is the degree of cramping. With a *complete abortion*, there has been complete passage of the products of conception; little bleeding is generally noted, and typically there is resolution of cramping and abdominal discomfort.

 Management

Patients with a diagnosis of threatened abortion can generally be discharged home with arranged obstetric follow-up. Discharge instructions should include bed rest or low levels of activity, no tampon use, and no sexual intercourse. Patients should be told that unless there is a specific reason, such as an incompetent cervix, little can be done to actually prevent the progression of a miscarriage.

Patients who have an inevitable, incomplete, or complete abortion require further gynecologic consultation urgently in order to determine the next step in treatment. Patients with an incomplete abortion will need transport for dilatation and curettage.

- Tissue noted at the cervical os requires removal, but removal should not be done when there is an intact attachment to the endometrium, as severe bleeding can occur upon separation.
- Pregnant patients with vaginal bleeding who are Rh-negative and unsensitized require therapy with Rh immunoglobulin. It is extremely important, therefore, to inquire about the Rh status of all patients.

Vaginal Bleeding in the Second and Third Trimesters

Patients with vaginal bleeding in the second and third trimesters of pregnancy will need transfer to a facility capable of obstetric evaluation and treatment. These patients should all have an intravenous line started and should be positioned on their left side. In addition to notifying the receiving facility, the treating obstetrician should also be contacted. Fetal heart tones should be documented and monitored along with maternal vital signs. The differential diagnosis includes abruptio placentae, placenta previa, preterm labor, and onset of labor with a bloody show. Localized cervical or vaginal lesions may also be a source of vaginal bleeding.

Placenta Previa

Placenta previa occurs when the placenta implants over the cervical os. The chief symptom is that of painless, bright red bleeding. Speculum or bimanual examination should *never* be performed, as this may precipitate severe hemorrhaging.

Abruptio Placentae

Abruptio placentae occurs when there is premature separation of the placenta from the uterine wall. This may occur spontaneously or as a result of trauma. Symptoms include abdominal pain, back pain, uterine tenderness, and uterine irritability. Vaginal bleeding generally presents with dark red blood except in cases of a concealed abruptio, in which case vaginal bleeding may not be present. Depending on the severity of the bleed, hypotension and/or shock may be present.

Preeclampsia

Preeclampsia is defined as a triad of hypertension, generalized edema, and proteinuria in a pregnant patient. When seizures occur in addition to the symptoms of preeclampsia, the condition is known as *eclampsia* (which if untreated, is often fatal). Symptoms of preeclampsia may include generalized peripheral edema, headaches, visual changes, nausea, and vomiting. All pregnant patients that present to the urgent care setting should have their blood pressure documented; if an elevated blood pressure is noted, urine should be obtained and screened for evidence of proteinuria. Additionally, patients with symptoms of preeclampsia should also have blood drawn for a CBC, platelets, liver function tests (LFTs), blood urea nitrogen (BUN), and creatinine as well as urinalysis; arrangements for a 24-h urine for protein and creatinine may also be needed.

- Preeclampsia does not develop before the 20th week of pregnancy unless trophoblastic disease is present.

 Management

Gynecologic consultation is required on all patients with elevated blood pressure or any evidence of preeclampsia in order to determine inpatient versus outpatient management. Patients with a sustained blood pressure equal to or greater than 140/90, along with related symptoms, will generally require hospitalization.

In patients who present with elevated blood pressure and seizures (e.g., patients presenting with eclampsia), treatment should be initiated with magnesium intravenously at a rate of 4 to 6 g over 15 min followed by an infusion of 1 to 2 g/h. Treatment should be initiated while awaiting emergency transport to a facility capable of providing obstetric care.

Hyperemesis Gravidarum

Nausea and vomiting are common occurrences during early pregnancy. Hyperemesis gravidarum, however, is present when vomiting becomes intractable, with associated dehydration, weight loss, and ketonuria. Weight loss may be up to or greater than 5 percent of the total body weight. In general, hyperemesis gravidarum is limited to the first trimester of pregnancy.

- When hyperemesis gravidarum is associated with abdominal pain, other diagnoses should be considered and appropriately evaluated.

  Evaluation of patients with hyperemesis gravidarum must include evaluation for other causes of emesis, including pyelonephritis, gastroenteritis, biliary disease, and other gastrointestinal etiologies. The history and physical examination should be directed at excluding these other causes. Laboratory studies should include urinalysis to rule out infection and check for evidence of ketonuria, glucose, or bilirubinemia. Electrolytes should also be checked to evaluate for any abnormalities. Other laboratory procedures may include a CBC, LFTs, and an amylase, depending on the history and physical findings.

 Management

Treatment consists of intravenous hydration with a glucose-containing solution (i.e., D_5NSS or D_5 lactated Ringer's). For many patients, rehydration may be all that is required; for others, judicial use of antiemetics may be indicated. Use of antiemetics, as with most medications prescribed during pregnancy, is best discussed with patients following consultation with their obstetrician (Table 11-10).

TABLE 11-10

ANTIEMETICS

ANTIEMETIC	BRAND NAME	FDA CATEGORY	ORAL	RECTAL	INTRAVENOUS
Acute intervention for both N/V and HG					
Promethazine	Phenergan	C	25 mg q4h	25 mg q4h	25–50 mg IV push 50 mg in 500 mL 0.9% normal saline over 2 h
Prochlorperazine	Compazine		10 mg q6–8h	25 mg q12h	10 mg over 2 min Maximum of 40 mg q24h
Chlorpromazine	Thorazine	C	10–25 mg q4–6h	100 mg q6–8h	25 mg in 500 mL 0.9% normal saline at 250 mL/h
Maintenance therapy for N/V					
Doxylamine with pyridoxine	Unisom Vitamin B_6		25 mg every evening 25 mg q8h		
Diphenhydramine	Benadryl	B	25–50 mg q6h		
Cisapride	Propulsid	C	10 mg q6h		
Maintenance therapy for HG					
Metoclopramide	Reglan	B			10 mg over 1–2 min q4–6h or 1 mg/kg in 50 mL D_5 in 0.45% normal saline over 30 min
Trimethobenzamide	Tigan	C	250 mg q6–8h	200 mg q6–8h	Should not be given IV May be given 200 mg IM q6–8h

Key: N/V=nausea and vomiting of pregnancy; HG=hyperemesis gravidarum.
SOURCE: Pearlman and Tintinalli,[1] with permission.

TABLE 11-11

CRITERIA FOR DISCHARGE IN HYPEREMESIS GRAVIDARUM	
Able to take oral fluids	Resolution of ketonuria
Normal hydration status postrehydration	Normal electrolytes

Other measures that can help with nausea and vomiting include:

- Avoidance of strong odors
- Small, frequent meals
- Eating prior to rising from bed
- Avoidance of fat-containing foods
- Avoidance of sweet drinks

The criteria for discharge of patients with hyperemesis gravidarum are given in Table 11-11.

Urinary Tract Infections in Pregnancy

Patients with urinary tract infections (UTIs) in pregnancy are at increased risk for developing pyelonephritis and preterm labor; therefore, all pregnant patients with symptomatic UTIs require a urine culture and a full 7- to 10-day course of antibiotic treatment. Patients who are found, during evaluation, to have asymptomatic bacteriuria also require urine culture and, depending on the patient, treatment pending culture results. Given the increase risks associated with UTI in pregnancy, there should be a low threshold to check a urinalysis in pregnant patients presenting to the urgent care setting, even when symptoms may not be directly referable to the urinary tract.

- Pregnant patients with symptoms of pyelonephritis should be admitted for inpatient treatment.

BREAST DISEASE

Trauma, breast tenderness, a newly discovered mass, nipple discharge, or signs of infection are the most common complaints of women who present to an urgent care facility for evaluation and treatment of breast disease. The majority of these patients, with the exception of the patient with acute mastitis, will not require acute intervention. Nonetheless, a careful history and examination is warranted; when appropriate, diagnostic evaluation should be initiated. Referral for follow-up care is key. Whenever feasible, fears regarding carcinoma should be addressed and reassurance given if possible.

 History

On history, important information to obtain (particularly in women who present with tenderness or a mass) includes previous history of breast disease, any family history of breast disease, history of nipple discharge, trauma, and fever. In women of child-bearing age, the

TABLE 11-12

DRUGS THAT INCREASE PROLACTIN

Antidepressants	Haloperidol	Cocaine
Phenothiazines	Fluoxetine	Marijuana
α-Methyldopa	Reserpine	Opiates
ACE inhibitors	H_2 antagonists	

possibility of pregnancy should be assessed, as well as the timing of complaints in relation to the menstrual cycle. In patients who are nursing, information regarding the frequency and adequacy of nursing should be determined, as well as any difficulties with nursing, during delivery, or in the postpartum period. Patients with complaints of nipple discharge should be questioned specifically regarding the characterisics of the discharge, involvement of multiple ducts, the presence of blood, and whether an associated mass has been noted. In addition to the previous concerns, patients who present with galactorrhea should be evaluated for the possibility of increased prolactin production, including medication use (Table 11-12), hypothyroidism, and symptoms of a pituitary tumor.

 Physical Examination

Physical examination requires a patient and methodical approach; this is particularly true in patients who seek evaluation for a small, difficult-to-palpate, or poorly defined mass. Examination should begin with inspection, evaluating for skin changes, erythema, dimpling, and marked asymmetry. Palpation should include thorough palpation of the axilla, the supraclavicular space, the cervical lymph nodes, and the mamillary tail. The nipple should be checked for any discharge or other abnormalities. Examination should be performed in both the sitting and the supine position.

Mastitis

Infection of the breast occurs primarily in the first month of breast-feeding but rarely before the first postpartum week. Infection can be limited to a cellulitis or may develop into a breast abscess. The most frequent organism associated with mastitis is *Staphylococcus aureus*. Symptoms include breast pain, fever and chills, and malaise. Erythema or induration may be noted on physical examination. If an abscess is present, localized fluctuance may be noted. A CBC should be considered, depending on the clinical presentation, particularly for patients who present with fever or who are toxic-appearing.

 Management

Outpatient management of acute mastitis without abscess formation includes a 7- to 10-day course of oral antibiotics, continued breast-feeding or pumping, and gentle massage (Table 11-13).

TABLE 11-13

MASTITIS: OUTPATIENT MANAGEMENT

1. Oral antibiotics
   Cephalexin 500 mg PO qid
     OR
   Dicloxacillin 250 to 500 mg PO qid
     OR
   Erythromycin 500 mg PO qid (if penicillin allergic)
2. Continued nursing or mechanical pumping
3. Gentle massage
4. Pain medications (as indicated, which may require mechanical pumping and the discarding of breast milk)
5. Compresses (either warm compresses or ice packs)
6. Clinical follow-up in 48 h (sooner as indicated)

Patients with a suspected abscess will require further evaluation either by aspiration of the fluctuant area or via ultrasound. If an abscess is confirmed, surgical drainage is usually required. The exception to this is small subareolar abscesses at an early stage, in which a trial of antibiotic treatment can be tried.

Patients who are toxic on evaluation will require admission for parenteral antibiotics. These patients may present with an elevated temperature and elevated white blood cell count (WBC). Patients with underyling immunosuppresion should also be referred for inpatient management.

The indications for immediate surgical referral or hospitalization are given in Table 11-14.

 Errors to Avoid

- *Failure to consider the diagnosis of inflammatory carcinoma.* In nonlactating women who present with mastitis, or in women who do not respond appropriately to standard treatment, the diagnosis of inflammatory carcinoma should be considered and the appropriate referral for further evaluation made.

Breast Masses

Patients presenting with a complaint of a breast mass rarely require urgent treatment. Examination should verify the presence of a palpable mass as well as rule out a possible breast abscess. Such patients will generally require referral for further diagnostic evaluation (to rule out cancer) or for ongoing management, surveillance, and education

TABLE 11-14

MASTITIS: INDICATIONS FOR IMMEDIATE SURGICAL REFERRAL OR HOSPITALIZATION

Breast abscess
Toxic (fever, elevated WBC, tachycardia, ill appearance, signs of sepsis)
Immunocompromised status

(i.e., patients with fibrocystic breast disease). In patients in whom a discrete palpable mass is appreciated, a mammogram or ultrasound may be ordered to expedite follow-up care, but this should generally be ordered in concert with the following physician.

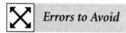

Errors to Avoid

- Failure to arrange follow-up in patients with a complaint of breast mass when no palpable mass is identified on examination.

Mastodynia

Evaluation of patients presenting with mastodynia (pain in the breast) should be limited to a search for any acute underlying cause requiring urgent treatment. Causes of mastodynia include hormonally induced pain associated with the menstrual cycle, infection, trauma, referred pain, cystic disease, or tumor. On physical examination, evidence of infection, mass, fibrocystic changes, or underlying chest wall tenderness should be sought. If no acute cause (particularly infection or trauma) can be determined, patients should be referred for ongoing management and further evaluation if indicated. Patients in whom a mass is palpated should be referred for further diagnostic evaluation. NSAIDs may be prescribed for acute discomfort. Patients who present with cyclic pain may benefit from caffeine avoidance and smoking cessation.

Nipple Abnormalities

Patients presenting with a complaint of nipple discharge or persistent nipple irritation require referral for specialty evaluation. Nipple irritation may be the result of friction or atopic dermatitis, but persistent nipple irritation, especially if associated with weeping lesions, may be a manifestation of Paget's disease and requires further evaluation, including possible mammography and cytologic testing. Similarly, women who present with a complaint of discharge, particularly bloody discharge, will need further evaluation and should be referred expediently. Examination of nonlactating women who present with galactorreha should include blood work for hypothyroidism and a detailed neurologic evaluation for evidence of a pituitary tumor. If neurologic symptoms are present, these patients should be sent for computed tomography scanning urgently. Other diagnostic tests can be initiated in consultation with the following physician.

REFERENCES

1. Pearlman MD, Tintinalli J: *Emergency Care of the Woman.* New York: McGraw-Hill; 1998:552, 602.
2. Roberts JR, Hedges JR: *Clinical Procedures in Emergency Medicine*, 2d ed. Philadelphia: Saunders; 1991:600.
3. Centers for Disease Control and Prevention: Sexually transmitted disease treatment guidelines. *MMWR* 42:RR-14, 1993.
4. Tintinalli J et al: *Emergency Medicine*, 5th ed. New York: McGraw-Hill; 2000:695,715.

BIBLIOGRAPHY

American College of Obstetricians and Gynecologists: *Emergency Contraception*. ACOG Practice Patterns, Number 3. Washington, DC: ACOG; December 1996.

American College of Obstetricians and Gynecologists: *Hypertension in Pregnancy*. ACOG Technical Bulletin 219. Washington, DC: ACOG; 1996.

Centers for Disease Control and Prevention: 1998 guidelines for treatment of sexually transmitted diseases. *MMWR* 47(RR-14):1–118.

Kahn J, Walker C, Washington AE, et al: Diagnosing pelvic inflammatory disease. *JAMA* 266:2594, 1991.

Ory SJ: New options for diagnosis and treatment of ectopic pregnancy. *JAMA* 267:534, 1992.

12

PEDIATRICS

Thom A. Mayer

INTRODUCTION

Although the definition of pediatric patients varies from institution to institution, this is generally considered to comprise patients less than or equal to 16 years of age, although adolescent pediatrics extends to patients 21 years of age. Regardless of the age group in question, children represent a large percentage—as many as one-third—of visits to urgent care centers (UCCs) and emergency departments (EDs). The majority of such patients have relatively straightforward, simple, circumscribed, and often self-limited diseases. However, patients with more severe clinical problems and clear-cut emergencies also present to such centers; therefore UCC physicians should be well trained in the diagnosis and treatment of such illnesses. This chapter addresses the care and treatment of such children and is intended as a quick and accurate reference for UCC physicians on the care of pediatric patients.

ACUTE OTITIS MEDIA

Acute otitis media (AOM) refers to acute inflammation of the middle ear and is one of the most common reasons for presentation of children to UCCs and EDs, accounting for nearly 4 million visits per year. AOM typically presents with ear pain, fever, irritability, and variable degrees of anorexia or vomiting. When the eardrum is perforated, there may be drainage from the ear. In infants and neonates, symptoms are typically less well defined and include inability to feed, fussiness, and irritability. AOM is distinguished from otitis media with effusion, which includes secretory, serous, mucoid, or nonsuppurative diseases presenting as asymptomatic collections of fluid in the middle ear cavity. It is usually quite easy to distinguish between these entities, as fever and ear pain are by far the most common presenting symptoms for patients with acute otitis media. Bullous otitis media is caused by *Mycoplasma* and presents distinctively on physical examination because of the characteristic bullae on the eardrum. AOM is almost a ubiquitous disease in children, with nearly three-quarters of children aged 3 or older having had at least one episode. Up to 40 percent of index cases of AOM resolve spontaneously with antibiotic therapy, but there is no reliable way to distinguish clinically which cases will do so.

Etiology

Although viral and bacterial agents can cause AOM, bacterial causes predominate; the most common agents are *Streptococcus pneumoniae, Haemophilus influenzae,* and *Moraxella catarrhalis*. The use of *H. influenzae* widespread type B (HIB) immunization has vastly reduced the incidence of this disease. However, in areas where there are large numbers of patients who have not received HIB immunization, *H. influenzae* can still be an important cause of AOM. *Mycoplasma* species are a less common cause of otitis media but present the classic bullous myringitis described above.

One of the most important evolving aspects of the diagnosis and treatment of AOM is the emergence of drug-resistant *Streptococcus pneumoniae* (DRSP). This organism is not only the most common cause of AOM (causing 40 to 50 percent of cases) but also the least likely to resolve without treatment. Rates of DRSP infection vary among geographic areas from 8 to 34 percent, but they appear to be increasing nationwide. For this reason, the DRSP Therapeutic Working Group made specific clinical recommendations regarding treatment in 1999.[1] Those treatment recommendations are reflected below, under "Management." The bacteria flora responsible for AOM in children less than 6 weeks of age are primarily group B streptococcus, gram-negative enteric bacilli, *Staphylococcus aureus*, and additional scattered strains of isolates.

Diagnosis

The diagnosis of AOM is made largely on clinical grounds, based upon a symptom complex of fever, irritability, and ear pain with or without discharge from the ear canal itself. In addition, up to 10 to 15 percent of children with AOM also present with nonspecific gastrointestinal disturbances, including vomiting and loose stools, although frank diarrhea is less common. While tympanocentesis can definitively confirm the diagnosis and the organism responsible, this technique is rarely utilized in present-day practice. The most important and confirmatory tool is the use of pneumatic otoscopy. The normal eardrum is usually clear and pearly gray in color, although it may become injected or slightly reddened with crying. Most importantly, the eardrum, or tympanic membrane (TM), in the normal child without AOM should be freely mobile in response to fluctuating pressure from the pneumatic otoscope. Although the majority of children with AOM also have reddened eardrums with abnormal landmarks, the best diagnostic tool in the ED and UCC setting is a confirmation of abnormal movement of the tympanic membrane in response to the pneumatic otoscope. AOM can usually be distinguished from serous otitis media (SOM) in that both have an abnormal response to pneumatic otoscopy, but the TM is usually retracted with SOM.

 Management

Most physicians treat AOM with oral antibiotics, the mainstay of effective treatment. However, because of the high rate of self-resolution of AOM that is due to *H. influenzae* and *M. catarrhalis*, some authorities have recommended withholding antibiotic treatment for 48 h, at which time a repeat pneumatic otoscopy and examination is performed. If symptoms continue and the TM is abnormal on pneumatic otoscopy, treatment can then be started. However, because of the inconvenience involved in such follow-up, most clinicians have found that treating initially with antibiotics in the face of appropriate clinical findings is the best course. In addition, patients and families generally tend to prefer antibiotic treatment at the initial visit.

The DRSP Therapeutic Working Group has made the following recommendations regarding treatment of AOM. Amoxicillin remains the best oral antimicrobial agent, since no oral antimicrobial agent currently available would be consistently expected to treat DRSP better than amoxicillin. However, because of the safety of dosing amoxicillin at higher than standard doses and evidence that higher doses achieve more effective concentrations in middle ear fluid, the group recommended an increase in dosage from the traditional 40 to 45 mg/kg/day to 80 to 90 mg/kg/day in three divided doses. Although no controlled, double-blind clinical trials have directly compared standard-dose versus high-dose amoxicillin and the U.S. Food and Drug Administration does not approve amoxicillin at these higher dosages, the Working Group felt strongly that amoxicillin at 80 to 90 mg/kg/day should be the first-line therapy for most patients. In patients above 2 years of age without complications or immune deficiency, a shorter course of 5 to 7 days of therapy is recommended. The traditional dose of amoxicillin (40 to 45 mg/kg/day) can still be considered for patients above age 2 who have not been treated with antimicrobials in the preceding 3 months and who do not attend a day care center. Alternatives to amoxicillin should be selected with two criteria: (1) effectiveness against *S. pneumoniae*, particularly DRSP, and (2) effectiveness against beta-lactamase-producing *H. influenzae* and *M. catarrhalis*. Agents meeting these criteria include amoxicillin/clavulanate (particularly at higher doses), cefuroxime axetil, and intramuscular ceftriaxone. If higher doses of amoxicillin/clavulanate are used, the newer formulation, which contains a decreased amount of clavulanate, should be utilized, since clavulanate at higher doses (greater than 10 mg/kg/day) leads to an increased incidence of diarrhea. Cefuroxime axetil (Ceftin) can be given in a dose of 30 mg/kg/day in twice-daily doses. One potential advantage of therapy with ceftriaxone (Rocephin) is that it can be given as a single injection, which eliminates concerns regarding compliance. A single injection of 50 mg/kg gives high concentrations in the middle ear fluid and has an outcome similar to that of oral antibiotics.

A number of additional agents can be utilized for AOM; their characteristics and dosing schedules are listed in Table 12-1. In the past, trimethropim/sulfamethoxazole and macrolide antibiotics were utilized for AOM, but antibiotic resistance patterns suggest that the agents previously described provide better coverage.[2] Of interest, reports of up to 10 percent prevalence of erythromycin resistance have been confirmed in a number of areas, and pneumococci that are resistant to erythromycin also appear to be resistant to newer macrolide antimicrobials such as clarithromycin and azithromycin. Fluoroquinolone agents have also been utilized for respiratory tract infections including otitis media but are not approved for routine use in children. If clinical improvement is not noted after 3 days of treatment with high-dose amoxicillin, amoxicillin/clavulanate, or cefuroxime, alternate therapy should be considered, including intramuscular ceftriaxone or clindamycin.

The diagnosis and treatment of children under 6 weeks of age deserves special comment. Children in this age group with documented AOM should all receive a full septic workup, including blood count, blood culture, urinalysis, urine culture, chest x-ray, and lumbar puncture. In the past, all such children were admitted for presumptive treatment of bacteremia and/or sepsis and in order to rule out meningitis. More recent literature suggests that there is still a need for a complete septic workup but that inpatient

TABLE 12-1

TREATMENT OF ACUTE OTITIS MEDIA: CDC WORKING GROUP RECOMMENDATIONS AND OTHER ANTIBIOTICS[a]

CDC Working Group

First-line treatment	Amoxicillin 80–90 mg/kg/day bid
Second-line treatment	Amoxicillin/clavulanate 80/90 mg/kg/day
	Cefuroxime 30 mg/kg/day bid
	Ceftriaxone 50 mg/kg IM
Refractory cases	Ceftriaxone 50 mg/kg/IM
	Clindamycin 10–20 mg/kg/day qid
Risk groups	Day care
	Prior antibiotics
	≤2 years
Other antibiotics	
Azithromycin (Zithromax)	10 mg/kg/day 1, 5 mg/kg/day 2–5 qd
Cefprozil (Cefzil)	30 mg/kg/day, bid
Cefuroxime (Ceftin)	30 mg/kg/day, bid
Cefpodoxime (Vantin)	10 mg/kg/day, bid or 100 mg bid for 5 days
Cefdinir (Omnicef)	14 mg/kg/day, qd
Trimethoprim/sulfamethoxazole	8 mg/kg/day, bid

[a]All medications by mouth except those noted IM (intramuscular).

versus outpatient therapy should be guided by the results of those tests. In the UCC setting, all those under 6 weeks of age with acute otitis media should be referred to the pediatrician for septic workup, with a decision regarding hospitalization made jointly between the UCC physician and the pediatrician.[3]

In addition to appropriate antibiotic therapy, patients or their parents should be instructed regarding appropriate fluid therapy, fever control, and pain management. In the majority of children with AOM, adequate hydration is difficult to maintain because of pain and fever. The importance of appropriate fluid management and fever control is critical. In addition, the majority of patients with AOM can receive adequate pain control if they are adequately hydrated and given acetaminophen (Tylenol) or ibuprofen for fever. In some cases, a limited prescription of acetaminophen with codeine may be necessary to moderate pain during the initial phases of treatment. All patients should be referred for follow-up care and reevaluation of the ear within 7 to 10 days of initial therapy. In addition, patients should be given specific instructions to follow up within 3 to 4 days if clinical improvement is not noted on antibiotic therapy.

 Errors to Avoid

- Failure to use pneumatic otoscopy
- Utilization of antimicrobials without consideration of DRSP

- Failure to refer for appropriate follow-up
- Failure to treat pain, fever, dehydration
- Failure to consider bacteremia/sepsis in children less than 6 weeks of age

 Key Points of Documentation

- Signs/symptoms in the physical examination should clearly delineate the clinical picture of AOM and exclude sepsis, meningitis, etc.
- Antibiotic therapy should be clearly delineated in the treatment plan and the instruction
- Referral for follow-up should be clear and within a certain time frame

CROUP (LARYNGOTRACHEAL BRONCHITIS)

Etiology

Croup is an extremely common illness affecting children from 6 months to 3 years of age; it is most commonly caused by the parainfluenza virus or respiratory syncytial virus (RSV).[4] It is the most common cause of stridor outside the neonatal age group and is classically seen between the months of November and March, although it can present at any time of the year. The viruses causing croup infect the vocal cords and mucosa of the subglottic area, causing edema and an increase in mucous secretions. Because of the relatively small size of the pediatric airway, the edema and increased secretions inhibit the flow of air through the vocal cords and subglottic area, with the severity of symptoms closely related to the degree of airway narrowing.[5]

Diagnosis

The majority of patients present with an upper respiratory prodrome of low-grade fever and rhinorrhea followed by a cough, which develops quickly into the severe, barking cough of classic croup. Such patients are usually fairly easy to diagnose; indeed, the classic barking cough often makes the diagnosis evident even before one enters the patient's room. Spasmodic croup is an entity that may be seen either independently or in conjunction with infectious croup and is caused by spasm of the larynx. In spasmodic croup, the onset of stridor is extremely sudden and fever may or may not be associated with the disease. Spasmodic croup most commonly responds very dramatically to exposure to humidity and/or the cool night air. In many cases, the child's symptoms may have resolved before presentation to the ED or UCC.

Except for patients with extreme airway narrowing, those with croup usually present without toxicity and with mild rhinorrhea and variable degrees of inspiratory stridor interrupted by the classic barking cough. Depending upon the degree of inflammation and mucous secretion, there may also be tachypnea, sternal or substernal retractions, and inspiratory stridor.

Management

All patients with croup should be placed in a comfortable environment; pulse oximetry should be utilized to measure oxygenation. Following initial pulse oximetry (to identify oxygenation at rest on room air), humidified oxygen should be administered as rapidly as possible and the croup score calculated (Table 12-2), since this provides a readily documented way of assessing the level of severity of the child's symptoms as well as progression with treatment.

The treatment of croup depends upon the severity of symptoms (Table 12-3). In children with mild croup (croup scores of 0 to 4 who have minimal respiratory distress at rest, are well hydrated, and tolerate humidified room air), continued hydration, provision of humidified air with a vaporizer, and reassurance may be all that is necessary. However, all such children should be observed for at least 30 to 60 min in the UCC to make sure that they do not deteriorate. The use of steroids has produced clearly documented improvement in those with moderate to severe early croup. Less clear but strongly suggested are

TABLE 12-2

MODIFIED WESTLEY CROUP SCORE[a]

CLINICAL INDICATION	SCORE POINTS	
Inspiratory stridor		
None	0	
At rest, with stethoscope	1	
At rest, no stethoscope required to hear	2	_____
Level of consciousness		
Normal	0	
Altered	5	_____
Air entry		
Normal	0	
Decreased	1	
Severely decreased	2	_____
Cyanosis		
None	0	
Agitated	4	
Resting	5	_____
Retractions		
None	0	
Mild	1	
Moderate	2	
Severe	3	
	Total =	_____

[a]NOTE: Multiple variations of this are used in the literature. When discussing scores, one must know which scale is being used. Score of 8 or greater indicates respiratory failure.
SOURCE: Adapted from Super DM, Cartelli NA, Brooks LJ, et al: A prospective randomized double-blind study to evaluate the effect of dexamethasone in acute laryngotracheitis. *J Pediatr* 115:323, 1989, with permission.

TABLE 12-3

TREATMENT OF CROUP

Mild croup (croup scores 0–4)	Humidified oxygen
	Pulse oximetry
	Hydration
	Reassurance
	Consider steroids[a]
	Observe 30–60 min
Moderate croup (croup scores 4–5)	Above plus
	Epinephrine therapy[b]
	Observe 1–2 h
	Steroids[a]
Severe croup (croup scores >5)	Above plus
	Continued epinephrine
	Steroids[a]
	Observe 2 h
	Consider need for hospitalization

[a]Steroid doses: Dexamethasone 0.6 mg/kg IM, prednisone/prednisolone 2 mg/kg/dose q8h × 3.
[b]Epinephrine doses: Racemic epinephrine 0.5 mL in 2.5 mL NS, L-epinephrine 3 mL of 1:1000 with 2.5 mL NS.

the benefits of steroids in mild croup. For patients who present within the first 3 to 4 days of illness, dexamethasone 0.6 mg/kg as a single intramuscular dose or prednisone 2 mg/kg per dose every 8 h for three doses is the recommended treatment.[6]

In children with moderate to severe croup (significant stridor at rest and croup scores greater than 4 or 5), the above measures should be utilized with the addition of treatment with epinephrine. In the past, racemic epinephrine, which comprises a nearly equimolar mixture of D and L isomers of epinephrine, was utilized under the assumption that it was more effective than L-epinephrine, the pure isomer used in classic Advanced Cardiac Life Support (ACLS) resuscitation.[7] However, more recent studies have shown that L-epinephrine is as effective as racemic epinephrine in the treatment of patients with croup.[8] Epinephrine can be given in the racemic mixture by giving 0.5 mL mixed with 2.5 mL of normal saline via nebulizer. If L-epinephrine is used, 3 mL of 1:1000 (3 mg) epinephrine may be drawn out of a multidose vial or out of ACLS injections and mixed with 2.5 mL of normal saline and administered to the child. The dose need not be adjusted for weight or age as the patient self-limits the dose by the tidal volume. In cases of severe croup, doses may be repeated continuously until clinical response occurs.

One of the enduring controversies regarding management of croup is the phenomenon of "rebound" and the necessity for hospitalizing children who have received epinephrine therapy. As the practice of pediatric emergency medicine has matured and careful studies have focused on this issue, it has become apparent that true rebound almost undoubtedly does not occur; rather, children with severe croup in whom epinephrine has been administered experience a decrease in edema, effectively increasing the airway diameter and thereby appreciably improving the clinical symptoms. In these severe cases, once the effects of the epinephrine have diminished, the edema increases, relatively speaking, and the airway narrows to a "critical mass," at which time the symptoms re-appear, sometimes dramatically. Thus, in children with mild to moderate croup, administration of epinephrine is safe and effective and no substantial rebound effects occur.

Patients with moderate to severe croup should be observed for a sufficient length of time to assure that subsequent diminution of the airway size will not result in recurrent symptoms. From a practical standpoint, the majority of symptoms in croup will recur within 2 h following administration of epinephrine nebulizer treatment. Thus, all children treated in UCCs should be observed for this period of time to determine their response both to the therapy itself and to the withdrawal of such therapy. If symptoms recur within this 2-h interval, it is likely that the child will need further therapy in either an ED or an inpatient setting. Children whose symptoms do not demonstrably recur within this 2-h window can safely be discharged with appropriate follow-up instructions regarding care. In all cases, the child's parents should be instructed to follow up with the pediatrician within 24 to 48 h to reassess progress. They should also be clearly instructed to return to the nearest ED if there are dramatic changes in symptoms.

Discharge

As indicated previously, after appropriate observation for 2 h, patients who have received epinephrine therapy can be discharged safely if there is no deterioration in the clinical findings. The parents of all children with croup should be given clear instructions to return the child immediately to the nearest ED if there is a dramatic change in airway symptoms. The family should also be given instructions for the outpatient use of humidified air, fluid therapy, and fever control. In general, parents should be given explicit discharge instructions to see the primary care physician within 24 to 48 h of the UCC visit. Careful instructions regarding the lack of indication for antibiotics should also be given.

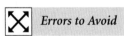

Errors to Avoid

- Failure to systematically access and document the patient's level of severity based on careful physical examination and/or croup score
- Failure to use steroids in appropriate cases
- Failure to use either racemic or L-epinephrine for fear of "rebound"
- Failure to observe patients for 2 h following epinephrine therapy

Key Points of Documentation

- Clinical progress following nebulization therapy, including physical examination and croup score
- Steroid dose and route of administration
- Follow-up instructions including what to do emergently if symptoms worsen
- A clear referral to a primary care physician in 24 to 48 h

Epiglottitis

Epiglottitis is a dramatic and life-threatening infection that can cause immediate airway obstruction and death. This rapidly progressing illness is usually seen in the preschool age group (between 2 and 5 years) and is almost universally caused by *H. influenzae* type B (80 to 90 percent of cases).[9] For that reason, the introduction of HIB immunization among children has all but eliminated cases due to this agent. However, other agents causing epiglottitis include *S. aureus, N. catarrhalis,* and the pneumococcus. In addition, this entity is still seen among isolated populations who have not received HIB vaccination (particularly immigrants), and the UCC physician should be capable of recognizing and treating it rapidly and effectively.

Diagnosis

Unlike croup, epiglottitis has no prodromal phase. The child usually presents as acutely ill with a body temperature between 102 and 104°F. Most children are toxic-appearing with significant stridor; many will have the classic "tripoding posture," sitting on the edge of the bed with the arms extended to the bed behind the patient and the neck and the mandible thrown forward to maximize airway patency. Patients typically refuse to lie down because dyspnea increases dramatically in the supine position. The voice may be muffled and secretions are difficult for the patient to handle. In most cases, a well-penetrated cross-table lateral film will show either a clear and nicely delineated epiglottis or the presence of the classic "thumb sign" reflecting a swollen epiglottis (Fig. 12-1).

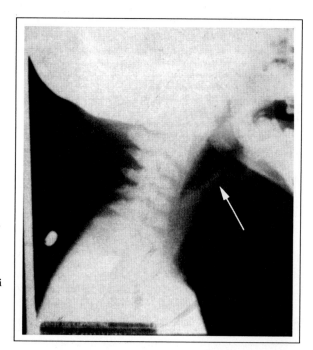

FIGURE 12-1   Lateral neck view of a child with epiglottitis. (From Tintinalli JE et al: *Emergency Medicine: A Comprehensive Study Guide,* 5th ed. New York: McGraw-Hill; 2000. With permission.)

Physical examination of the child should be undertaken with great care, since manipulation of the airway may cause laryngospasm, swelling of the epiglottis, and death.

 Management

When epiglottitis is confirmed or strongly suspected, an immediate call should be placed to the Emergency Medical Service (EMS) via 911 and the nearest ED alerted that a child with possible epiglottitis is en route, so that definitive airway management may be prospectively arranged. In patients with mild symptoms where there is some question regarding the diagnosis, cross-table lateral films of the neck can be undertaken to determine whether radiographic findings of epiglottitis are present.

All children suspected of having epiglottitis should have 100% oxygen administered either by mask or via "blow by" if the child cannot tolerate the mask. A pulse oximeter should be placed on all such children to measure their clinical course. In the event that airway compromise occurs (which may happen dramatically and suddenly), initial attempts at bag-valve-mask ventilation should be undertaken, since many children with respiratory compromise due to epiglottitis can be effectively ventilated (at least on a temporary basis) by this technique. The pulse oximeter should be followed closely during the course of therapy to determine success. In the vast majority of cases, bag-valve-mask ventilation will temporize until the child can be transferred to the ED for definitive airway management. If complete respiratory obstruction occurs and bag-valve-mask ventilation cannot provide adequate pulse oximetry readings, either endotracheal intubation or needle cricothyroidotomy should be undertaken to ventilate the child during transport.[10]

While epiglottitis is an increasingly rare disease, it is important that UCC physicians recognize the signs and symptoms and be able to diagnose and treat the illness in the most expeditious fashion possible. As mentioned previously, the disease tends to occur in areas where children have not been immunized with HIB vaccine, particularly among immigrant children who have not yet entered the school system (where such vaccinations are required to attend school).

BRONCHIOLITIS

Bronchiolitis is by far the most common respiratory tract infection in infants, affecting nearly one-half of children by the age of 1 year and virtually all children in one form or another by the age of 2. It typically begins in the late fall and early winter but can occur at any time of the year.

Etiology

The most common agent causing bronchiolitis (80 to 90 percent of cases) is RSV, although influenza virus, parainfluenza virus, and adenovirus can also cause the disease.[11] Regardless of the viral agent causing the symptoms, it is a highly infectious process and strict attention to hand washing and use of masks and gloves can help prevent transmission. Regardless of the viral agent causing the disease, the pathophysiology is similar: airway wall edema, inflammation, the production of cellular debris, and mucous occlusion of the airway impeding flow and increasing the work of breathing and airway resistance.

Diagnosis

Bronchiolitis is a clinical diagnosis based upon the symptom complex and presenting physical examination and supported, where appropriate, by radiographic studies. The infection typically begins with nasal discharge; it then progresses to cough and symptoms of airway obstruction with or without wheezing. Fever is typically present in the first few days of illness and may occasionally produce temperatures as high as 104°F. Patients usually present to the UCC or ED because of increasing respiratory symptoms, nasal congestion, and difficulty feeding. In any child with difficulty feeding as a presenting complaint, respiratory compromise should be considered, particularly in those within the bronchiolitis age group.

Physical findings almost universally include tachypnea, often with dramatically increased respiratory rates, with 50 to 60 breaths per minute not being uncommon. The majority of children also present with tachycardia, mild to moderate conjunctivitis, and additional respiratory symptoms depending upon the severity of the disease, which may include frank sternal and intercostal retractions, prolonged expiration, a hyperresonant chest on percussion, wheezes, and even hypoxemia if the disease is severe. All such children should receive pulse oximetry monitoring during the course of their visit. The combination of clinical findings, with particular emphasis on tachypnea and pulse oximetry readings, helps assure that the diagnosis is made appropriately.

Blood counts and serum chemistries are neither confirmatory nor particularly helpful in making the diagnosis of bronchiolitis and should be used only when other diagnoses are being considered or when dehydration is noted on clinical examination. Chest radiographs of children with bronchiolitis may reveal simple hyperinflation, with some peribronchial thickening due to the edema and mucous plugging. In some cases atelectasis may also be present, including segmental atelectasis. In the majority of cases, these patchy areas on the chest x-ray are usually due to atelectasis, but this always raises the question of whether a concomitant or secondary pneumonia has occurred as well.

Infant Apnea

The mechanisms causing RSV-induced apnea in young infants is not well understood but is probably related to hypoxemia and upper airway obstruction. Infants at highest risk for apnea are less than 6 weeks old; they have a history of prematurity, apnea of prematurity, or other related respiratory diseases in the neonatal period. There is also an association of the degree of oxygen desaturation with the potential for apnea.

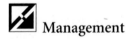 Management

A vast majority of patients with bronchiolitis can be treated on an outpatient basis in the UCC setting with appropriate follow-up with their private pediatrician or primary care physician. In the midst of RSV epidemics, there may be a large number of patients seeking care at both EDs and UCCs. The mainstay of treatment in bronchiolitis is supportive, comprising monitoring of oxygen saturation, appropriate oxygen therapy guided by the clinical findings and pulse oximetry readings, adequate fluid replacement, fever management, and, where appropriate, provision of bronchodilator therapy. Which children should receive bronchodilators and by what method remains an area where personal experience is as persuasive as the existing literature.

The first issue is who should receive bronchodilator therapy. In general, bronchodilator therapy is a safe and variably effective treatment for bronchiolitis, producing minimal side effects. Some authors recommend a "test treatment" to determine which patients respond to bronchodilators. In general, bronchodilator therapy can be safely used in any child who presents to the UCC or ED with respiratory obstruction and wheezing consistent with a diagnosis of bronchiolitis. The bronchodilator chosen may include epinephrine, racemic epinephrine, or albuterol; each has its proponents and detractors. Careful consideration of the literature indicates that this is largely an area of personal preference and experience and that all three agents can be utilized safely.[11] In patients with repeated episodes of wheezing or those presenting outside of RSV season and in whom there is a strong family history of asthma, many clinicians would choose albuterol, under the presumption that there is an asthmatic component to the presenting child's bronchospastic disease. Following bronchodilator therapy, children should be observed to determine their return to baseline, particularly in cases in which oxygen saturation is impaired as measured by pulse oximetry.

An additional issue is what steroids should be used in bronchiolitis. Steroids have been effective in croup (in which there is virally mediated airway edema) and in asthma (in which there is inflammatory disease with bronchospasm), so there is some logic to why they might potentially work in bronchiolitis, where both types of pathophysiology are involved. However, studies have been equivocal regarding this issue and the use of steroids in bronchiolitis is largely a matter of personal experience and conformity to existing practices within the pediatric and pediatric pulmonary community. Nevertheless, some general principles apply. First, children with severe bronchiolitis who are markedly symptomatic and have changes in oxygen saturation should probably receive steroids in the UCC or ED. Second, children with a strong family history of asthma or recurrent wheezing suggestive of asthma would probably benefit from steroid therapy as well. Third, in children with substantial underlying pulmonary disease such as bronchopulmonary dysplasia, steroids should be strongly considered and be given in the doses recommended for croup.

Children with refractory disease, those with persistent respiratory rates >60, those with substantial dehydration, and those with a history of bronchopulmonary dysplasia, congenital heart disease, immunocompromise, apnea, prematurity, or age <6 weeks should be hospitalized. At a minimum, the primary care pediatrician responsible for their care should be consulted prior to any disposition decisions.

Patients with mild disease who tolerate fluids well and whose symptoms have improved during their UCC visit may be discharged home with fever-control instructions, provision of humidified air, and bronchodilator therapy as indicated clinically. Albuterol in syrup form can be initiated for children who respond to this medication in the UCC setting. Cigarette smoking and the presence of other noxious stimuli should be avoided and the family should be instructed to return if symptoms worsen.

Asthma

Asthma is a chronic disease of the tracheobronchial tree, including elements of airway obstruction, hyperreactivity, and inflammation.[12] The pathophysiology is generally the same in adults and children, but there are some important anatomic differences in children that place them at higher risk of respiratory failure. These include the fact that their airway walls are thicker, resulting in greater narrowing of the airway with bronchoconstriction, increased compliance of the infant rib cage, and immaturity of the diaphragm—resulting in paradoxical respirations and inward displacement of the ribs during inspiration—and the fact that young lung tissue lacks the degree of elastic recoil present in adults. This last can result in atelectasis and the earlier development of ventilation/perfusion mismatch. The pathophysiology of asthma includes aspects of airway inflammation, airway trapping, and ventilation/perfusion mismatch (producing variable degrees of hypoxemia, carbon dioxide retention, and respiratory failure in the most extreme cases).

Diagnosis

A majority of children with asthma presenting to UCCs have had previous episodes of the disease, although first-time presentations are not uncommon. Risk factors associated with the development of asthma include low birth weight, family history of asthma and other atopic diseases, urban low-income households, and certain ethnic predispositions (children of Asian, Hispanic, and African-American descent). In most cases, airway obstruction and wheezing are predominant symptoms in the presentation of the asthmatic patient, although the typically broad spectrum of symptoms may be seen in both adults and children. Pulse oximetry readings should be undertaken (preferably prior to the administration of oxygen, although oxygen supplementation should never be delayed for children with significant respiratory distress). It is important to have a planned and careful approach to both the diagnosis and treatment of asthma, so that therapy can be initiated rapidly. Figure 12-2 shows the diagnostic and treatment algorithm used at our large pediatric ED, which has resulted in a clear and well-delineated approach to care in these patients. In addition to clinical examination and pulse oximetry, the use of peak flow meters to determine peak expiratory flow rates (PEFR) and forced expiratory volumes in 1 s (FEV_1) can be helpful in determining the severity of the attack. A major limitation in children is the ability to cooperate with such tests, which is severely limited in children below 4 to 5 years of age.

Management

The mainstay of treatment for the acute bronchospastic component of asthma is bronchodilator therapy geared toward the $beta_2$ receptor. The most commonly used bronchodilator is albuterol via nebulizer or metered-dose inhaler (MDI).[13] MDI therapy can be used in children over 6 years of age, although patient compliance is usually the rate-limiting factor in administering MDIs in the UCC setting. The safest and most reliable means of therapy is via nebulizer, which may be given sequentially or as a continuous 1-h nebulization treatment. In many cases, symptoms will resolve following albuterol

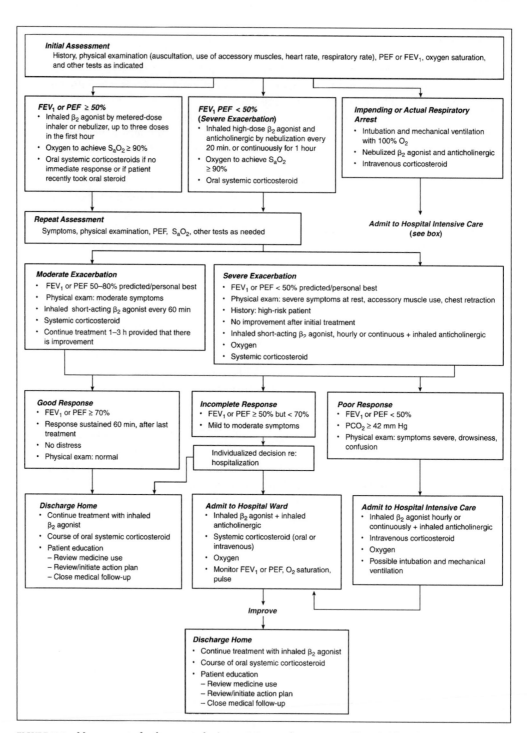

FIGURE 12-2 Management of asthma exacerbations: emergency department and hospital-based care. (From the National Institutes of Health, National Heart, Lung, and Blood Institute.)

therapy, after which the child should be observed for 30 min to 1 h for recurrence of symptoms. If symptoms do not recur, the child can be discharged on appropriate outpatient bronchodilator therapy, with adequate provision of hydration and steroids as indicated (see below). If the patient does not respond clinically or by pulse oximetry readings after the first hour of therapy, additional therapy should be considered both with beta agonists and with other agents. In most cases, if the child does not respond clinically to a substantial degree within the first 2 h of continuous nebulization therapy, ED referral and/or hospitalization should be considered and steroids should be administered as well.[14]

Corticosteroids have a well-known and important role in asthma, serving to inhibit the secretion of leukotrienes and prostaglandins. Early administration during the acute phase of the disease is recommended for all patients with substantial clinical findings as well as those in which the PEFR is less than 50 percent of predicted. In addition, many patients and/or families have a clear sense of whether the attack is severe enough to require steroid therapy. It is always good advice to adhere to the preferences of the patient/family in this regard, since most asthmatics know their disease and baseline status well, including when steroids are likely to be beneficial. In patients who cannot tolerate medication by mouth, intravenous methylprednisolone (Solu-Medrol) 2 mg/kg should be given. In milder cases and in those patients who can tolerate medication by mouth, prednisolone or prednisone can be given in a dose of 2 mg/kg. Prednisolone comes as Pediapred 5 mg/5 mL or as Prelone 15 mg/5 mL. If corticosteroid therapy is started in the UCC, it should be continued for a dose and duration that is coordinated with the pediatric pulmonologist or primary care physician who will be following the patient on an outpatient basis. In general, steroids are given for 7 to 10 days in a tapering dose.[15]

Additional mainstays of therapy include adequate hydration provided either by mouth or intravenously as clinically indicated. Subcutaneous epinephrine therapy has largely been abandoned except in those cases where patients are unresponsive to nebulized bronchodilator therapy or respiratory distress is so dramatic that inhalation is severely compromised. Other agents that can be used in the care of asthma include terbutaline, anticholinergic agents, magnesium sulfate, and other therapy.[16] However, in the UCC setting, such therapies are rarely needed and such patients should be referred to the ED if symptoms continue after adequate provision of oxygen, fluids, nebulized bronchodilators, and corticosteroids.

Discharge

A vast majority of pediatric patients presenting with asthma to the UCC can be discharged safely after the measures listed above. All such patients should be discharged with instructions to follow up immediately if symptoms worsen dramatically and to either call or visit their primary care physician on the following day regardless of symptoms.

Pneumonia

Both viral and bacterial pneumonia are common causes of illness in pediatric patients, although far less so than diseases such as AOM, pharyngitis, croup, and bronchiolitis. Pneumonia is defined clinically as the presence of pulmonary infiltrates on a chest radiograph due to infection; it is associated with clinical findings such as cough, fever, chest pain, and tachypnea.

Etiology

In the majority of pediatric pneumonias, a specific etiologic agent is not specifically identified.[17] Nonetheless, pathogens can usually be typified by the age of the patient, as indicated in Table 12-4. In the newborn age group (birth to 1 month), bacterial infec-

TABLE 12-4

COMMON CAUSES OF PNEUMONIA

AGE GROUP	PATHOGENS (IN ORDER OF DECREASING FREQUENCY)
0–1 month	Group B streptococcus *Escherichia coli* *Klebsiella* or Enterobacteriaceae *Listeria*

1–3 months	Pneumonitis syndrome (afebrile pneumonia)
	    Chlamydia trachomatis
	    RSV or other respiratory viruses
	    Bordetella pertussis
	    Ureaplasma urealyticum

1 month to 2 years	RSV or other respiratory viruses *Streptococcus pneumoniae* *Haemophilus influenzae* type B (HIB), non-type-B *H. influenzae* (NTHI), *C. trachomatis, Mycoplasma pneumoniae*
2–5 years	Respiratory viruses *S. pneumoniae* *Haemophilus influenzae* type B (HIB) or non-type-B *H. influenzae* (NTHI) *M. pneumoniae* *Chlamydia pneumoniae*
6–18 years	*M. pneumoniae* *S. pneumoniae* *C. pneumoniae* Non-type-B *H. influenzae* (NTHI) Adenovirus or respiratory virus

All ages	Severe pneumonia
	    S. pneumoniae
	    S. aureus
	    Group A streptococcus
	    Haemophilus influenzae type B (HIB)
	    M. pneumoniae
	    Adenovirus
	Immunocompromised (all of the above plus):
	    P. carinii
	    Cytomegalovirus
	    Fungi

SOURCE: From Tintinalli JE et al: *Emergency Medicine: A Comprehensive Study Guide,* 5th ed. New York: McGraw-Hill; 2000. With permission.

tions are actually more common than viral agents as the leading cause of pneumonia. In all other groups, viral agents are somewhat more common than bacterial. In the preschool age groups, viruses, *S. pneumoniae*, *H. influenzae*, and *Mycoplasma* are the most common, followed by *Chlamydia*. Once children reach school age, the most common bacterial cause is *Mycoplasma pneumoniae*, followed by *S. pneumoniae*. The widespread use of HIB vaccine decreases the incidence of pneumonia from *H. influenzae*.[18]

Diagnosis

The clinical findings in children with pneumonia vary widely depending upon age, the respiratory pathogen, severity of the disease, underlying illnesses, and other factors. However, by far the most common finding in pneumonia is tachypnea. Because respiratory rates are age-dependent, it is important to understand the upper limits of normal for such respiratory rates (Table 12-5). In general, pneumonia is highly unlikely to be present in children in the absence of tachypnea. Many children also present with fever, nonspecific respiratory findings, chest pain, and other symptoms. In children with lower lobe pneumonia, abdominal and gastrointestinal complaints including pain may be present. On physical examination, tachypnea should be noted, as well as the work of breathing. Auscultatory findings are notoriously inaccurate in children, particularly younger children. This is due to the vagaries of the transmission of sound in the pediatric chest, in which a clearly delineated pneumonia may be seen on chest radiograph and yet no findings from the stethoscope. When present, auscultatory findings can be helpful in focusing the diagnosis and may include rales, wheezing, or signs of decreased air entry, including egophony. Atypical pneumonia frequently has a more gradual onset of symptoms, including headache, nonproductive cough, low-grade fever, and headache. In neonates, symptoms are typically ill defined and may include difficult or poor feeding, lethargy, fever without a localizing source, apnea, and even vomiting and diarrhea. Neonates with pneumonia may also present with grunting, which is a physical finding produced by the forcing of air against a closed glottis, representing a physiologic attempt to keep the airway open. Grunting in an infant should be considered a sign of pneumonia until proven otherwise.

Chest radiography is the most pragmatic way to confirm a diagnosis of pneumonia in a child and should include both posteroanterior (PA) and lateral films. Some authorities have attempted to correlate specific radiologic findings with etiologic agents, but more carefully documented studies indicate that antibiotic therapy is better guided by the age of the patient, the symptom complex, and known bacteriologic resistance pat-

TABLE 12-5

STANDARDS FOR TACHYPNEA IN INFANTS AND CHILDREN

Age, Months	Upper Limit of Normal Respiratory Rate, Breaths per Minute
<2	55
2–12	45
>12	35

SOURCE: From Tintinalli JE et al: *Emergency Medicine: A Comprehensive Study Guide*, 5th ed. New York: McGraw-Hill; 2000. With permission.

terns within the community or region. Additional laboratory studies often undertaken in pneumonia include blood counts, bacterial or viral cultures of the sputum, bacterial antigen testing, and blood chemistries (where dehydration is suspected). Cold agglutinin tests can be helpful in patients where there is a high suspicion of *M. pneumoniae*.[19] If there is suspicion of infectious mononucleosis, antibody testing may be confirmatory.

 Management

Not surprisingly, the treatment of pneumonia in children depends upon the age. Almost without exception, children from birth to 3 months of age with documented pneumonia should be considered for hospitalization for antibiotics and supportive therapy.[20] Oxygen saturation should be determined in all patients, and documentation of their respiratory rate and difficulty in breathing should occur. Hydrational status should be assessed and treated as appropriate, with administration of fluids, since most such patients are clinically dehydrated to some degree. In children 3 months of age or older, decisions on inpatient versus outpatient therapy are guided by the patients' overall work of breathing, oxygen saturation status, preexisting medical problems (including immunocompromised states), and ability of the family to care for the child at home. A majority of children over 3 months of age with pneumonia can be treated effectively as outpatients with close follow-up. Table 12-6 suggests antibiotic therapy for children with pneumonia. In those aged 3 months to approximately 5 years of age, outpatient antibiotic choices include amoxicillin, erythromycin, cefuroxime, clarithromycin, and azithromycin. In children 6 to 18 years of age, these agents can also be utilized, with the understanding that amoxicillin or ampicillin may produce the classically dramatic rash if the patient has infectious mononucleosis. For patients who are unresponsive to these therapies, consideration should be given to mycoplasmal or chlamydial infections as the cause and

TABLE 12-6

ANTIBIOTICS FOR PNEUMONIA BY AGE

AGE GROUP	ANTIBIOTIC AND DOSE[a]
Neonates (≤30 days)	Ampicillin 100 mg/kg plus cefotaxime 100 mg/kg Or Gentamicin 7.5 mg/kg/day
Young infants (30–90 days)	Ampicillin plus cefotaxime (admitted patient) Erythromycin 40 mg/kg/day Azithromycin 10 mg/kg/day 1, 5 mg/kg days 2–5 Clarithromycin 15 mg/kg/day
Older children (≥90 days)	Amoxicillin 50–100 mg/kg/day Amoxicillin/clavulanate 50–100 mg/kg/day Cefuroxime 30 mg/kg/day Erythromycin 40 mg/kg/day Azithromycin 10 mg/kg/day 1, 5 mg/kg/days 2–5 Clarithromycin 15 mg/kg/day Cefixime 16 mg/kg, day 1, 8 mg/kg days 2–5

[a]All doses are intravenous.

antibiotic therapy appropriately altered. When amoxicillin or amoxicillin/clavulanate is selected, some authorities use the higher-dose regimen indicated previously in the discussion of AOM.

The use of quinolone antibiotics in pediatric patients deserves some mention. The quinolones in general and levofloxacin (Levaquin) in particular are highly effective antibiotics for pneumonia and other lower respiratory tract infections. However, they are not currently approved for use in pediatric patients (under the age of 16) owing to the potential side effects on musculoskeletal growth and function. However, it is quite likely that the indications for these antibiotics, and levofloxacin in particular, will be broadened to include treatment of at least a broader range of pediatric patients than is currently recommended.

Discharge

Patients with severe symptoms and those who are unresponsive to therapy should be considered for hospitalization. In addition, all children under the age of 3 months with documented pneumonia should be hospitalized, in coordination with their pediatrician. The parents of those patients who are discharged home should have clear instructions for fever control, hydration, and appropriate antibiotic therapy where indicated. A follow-up appointment should be made with their primary care physician within 1 to 2 days, with clear instructions to return either to the UCC or to the ED if symptoms worsen, depending upon severity. Antibiotic therapy should be continued for 10 days unless specifically approved regimens are undertaken for short-course therapy.

BACTEREMIA AND SEPSIS

UCC physicians often see children who have a fever (temperature $\geq$39.0°C/102.2°F) and no obvious source of infection. The risk of occult bacteremia in such children ranges from 3 to 5 percent; an additional 2 to 6 percent will develop serious septic complications such as meningitis.[21] What are the current thoughts on how best to identify and treat such patients?

Etiology

S. pneumoniae accounts for greater than 90 percent of patients with these bacteremias, particularly since the advent of HIB vaccination. As heptavalent conjugate pneumococcal vaccines are widely developed and utilized, the bacteriologic agents responsible for bacteremia will certainly change or be eliminated. However, at present the existing guidelines, developed conjointly between the American College of Emergency Physicians and the American Academy of Pediatrics, recognize *S. pneumoniae* as the most common agent and treatment recommendations are based thereon.[22]

Diagnosis

Occult bacteremia consists of fever without a recognized source of infection despite a detailed history, physical examination, and supporting laboratory studies, including, where appropriate, chest x-rays and urinalysis.[23] The concept of the consensus approach to such patients rests on the understanding that a small but discrete number of such patients will develop occult bacteremia, and an additional percentage will develop septic complications. With these assumptions, risk stratification attempts to determine which patients, if any, will benefit from antibiotic therapy and close clinical follow-up.[24]

 Management

The current diagnostic and treatment recommendations are summarized in Table 12-7. The existing recommendations define a fever at 39.0°C, although newly developed but as yet unpublished studies indicate that the cutoff point of fever will be 39.5°C.[25] Thus, patients with a fever of 39 to 39.5°C or higher are more at risk for the development of occult bacteremia. If white blood cell counts and absolute neutrophil counts are obtained in these patients, further risk stratification can be done to guide therapy. In the absence of specific clinical risk (defined below), those patients with a temperature ≥39°C to 39.5°C and either a white blood cell count of 15,000 or greater or an absolute neutrophil count of 10,000 or greater are at increased risk of occult bacteremia and subsequent septic complications. All such patients should be treated with ceftriaxone 50 mg/kg and have a follow-up evaluation in 2 to 3 days. Additional risk criteria include temperatures >40 to 41°C or a temperature >39°C and age between 6 and 24 months, presence of sickle cell disease, absence of HIB vaccination, toxic appearance, or lack of availability for follow-up. In any of these categories, patients should be treated with antibiotic therapy and followed closely. If patients do not have a temperature either >39°C under the old criteria or >39.5° under the new criteria, antibiotic therapy may not be indicated, particularly if HIB vaccination and, eventually, pneumococcal vaccination has occurred. The current recommendation for ceftriaxone is based on its increased effectiveness compared to amoxicillin or amoxicillin/clavulanate in reducing

TABLE 12-7

EMERGING CRITERIA FOR ANTIBIOTIC TREATMENT OF PEDIATRIC FEVER WITHOUT SOURCE

RISK CRITERIA	ADDITIONAL CLINICAL RISK
Temperature > 39°C[a]	Temperature > 41°C
or	Temperature > 39°C + age 6–24 months
Temperature > 39.5°C[b]	Sickle cell disease
and	Toxic appearance
WBC > 15,000	No HIB immunization
or	No follow-up
Absolute neutrophil count > 10,000	

RECOMMENDED ANTIBIOTIC THERAPY
Ceftriaxone 50 mg/kg IM

[a]Based on 1993 Practice Guidelines
[b]Based on 2000 Consensus Conference (as yet unpublished)
WBC = white blood cell count; HIB = hemophilus type B.

septic complications in children with occult bacteremia. It is important to note that this benefit appears to be limited to *H. influenzae* infection, so these recommendations may change over the course of time. However, because of the risk of early bacterial meningitis presenting as occult bacteremia and fever without source, the current recommendation remains the use of intramuscular ceftriaxone 50 mg/kg.

Discharge

Pediatric patients between the age of 3 and 36 months with fever without source can be safely discharged according to the criteria indicated above. Clearly, if the patient is toxic appearing, has signs of meningitis or other serious infection, or has other significant risk factors, referral, consultation, and hospital admission should be considered. In any case in which meningitis is suspected, a lumbar puncture should be performed, and this usually requires referral to the ED.

MENINGITIS

Meningitis in the pediatric patient can present either as a fulminant neurologic infection or as one that is far more subtle in nature. In most cases, meningitis occurs as a result of bacteremia seeding the meninges; therefore the pathogenic organisms responsible closely parallel those seen with bacteremia and sepsis. Unfortunately, meningitis is still an important cause of death and disability in children.[26]

Etiology

In the neonatal period, group B streptococcus and *Escherichia coli* and other gram negative enteric organisms predominate, although *Listeria monocytogenes* may also be seen in neonates and young children. Outside of the neonatal age group, *S. pneumoniae* and *Neisseria meningitides* are the most common pathogens, with DRSP strains increasing in frequency. For those children who have not received the HIB vaccine, *H. influenzae* can also be an important pathogen.[27]

Diagnosis

The findings in patients with meningitis vary from extremely subtle to quite obvious, with all possible protean manifestations in between. For this reason, the classic "high index of suspicion" must be maintained in all pediatric patients who present with fever associated with altered mental status or, particularly in neonates, altered levels of function, including irritability, lethargy, difficulty in feeding, vomiting, etc. All such patients should be assumed to have meningitis until proven otherwise. The definitive diagnosis of meningitis requires a lumbar puncture (LP), which is usually not performed in the urgent care setting, not because of the expertise of the physician but because of the lack of adequate capacity of the laboratory to provide the studies needed in a timely fashion. No laboratory study can substitute for the lumbar puncture in either making or excluding the diagnosis of meningitis. Even in cases where aseptic meningitis is strongly suspected, any evidence of meningeal inflammation on history or physical examination warrants a lumbar puncture because of the possibility of bacterial infection, which in the case of meningococcus can be quite fulminant in nature. If fever is not present or if there is some question as to other intracranial pathology and the patient is stable, computed tomography (CT) of the head may be performed prior to the LP. However, if meningitis is strongly suspected on clinical grounds, neither a CT nor an LP should delay prompt and aggressive administration of antibiotics.

 Management

Antibiotic treatment for patients with meningitis varies by age owing to the different organisms responsible. Table 12-8 summarizes appropriate antibiotics and doses for patients with meningitis. For neonates, ampicillin (100 mg/kg) plus a third-generation cephalosporin such as cefotaxime or ceftriaxone at a dose of 50 mg/kg should be given. It is necessary to cover with ampicillin in neonates and young infants, because of the incidence of *L. monocytogenes*.

Because *S. pneumoniae* is the most frequent cause of bacterial meningitis outside of the neonatal and young infant group and the increasing prevalence of DRSP, vancomycin should be added to the initial antibiotic regimen in young infants and older children with suspected or confirmed meningitis until culture and sensitivity results can be obtained. In infants aged 30 to 90 days, ampicillin 100 mg/kg (to cover *L. monocytogenes*) plus cefotaxime or ceftriaxone 100 mg/kg (to provide broad-spectrum coverage) *and* vancomycin 15 mg/kg (to cover the possibility of DRSP) should be utilized. In children older than 90 days, cefotaxime or ceftriaxone 100 mg/kg plus vancomycin 15 mg/kg should be utilized.[28]

Some controversy remains regarding the use of steroid therapy in pediatric patients with meningitis. Studies have been quite clear that steroids decrease the incidence of

TABLE 12-8

ANTIBIOTICS AND DOSAGES FOR PEDIATRIC MENINGITIS

Age Group	Antibiotic and Dose[a]
Neonates (≤30 days)	Ampicillin 100 mg/kg plus Cefotaxime 50 mg/kg or Ceftriaxone 50 mg/kg
Young infants (30–90 days)	Ampicillin 100 mg/kg plus Cefotaxime 50 mg/kg plus Vancomycin 15 mg/kg
Older children (≥90 days)	Cefotaxime or Ceftriaxone 100 mg/kg plus Vancomycin 15 mg/kg

[a]All doses are intravenous.

neurologic complications substantially in bacterial meningitis *due to HIB infection* but show no benefit in meningitis due to *S. pneumoniae* or *N. meningitides.* In addition, some studies indicated that steroids may actually worsen neurologic sequelae in patients with meningitis *not* caused by HIB. As the risk of HIB infection declines with immunization, the utility of steroids is likely to change. However, current recommendations are to *consider* steroid therapy in cases of suspected bacterial meningitis. When used, dexamethasone 0.15 mg/kg IV should be given before or immediately after administration of antibiotics. All patients suspected of having meningitis should be transported to the nearest ED as quickly as possible, with EMS transport utilized for all but the most stable patients. In all cases, telephone consultation with the ED should be obtained to make sure that the emergency physician is aware of the reason for referral and the necessity of obtaining a LP.

URINARY TRACT INFECTIONS

Urinary tract infections (UTIs) not only are among the most important causes of febrile illnesses in children but also pose vexing problems in diagnosis and treatment. UTIs occur in 4 to 7 percent of febrile infants, since studies indicate that of children with documented UTIs, nearly two-thirds were thought to have other sources for their fevers by the examining physician.[29] This is largely due to the fact that the presenting signs and symptoms of UTIs are often nonspecific, particularly in infants and younger children. For this reason, UTIs should always be considered when the source of fever in children is equivocal, particularly during the first 2 years of life.

Etiology and Epidemiology

Age and gender are important in the prevalence of pediatric UTIs. These infections occur three times more commonly in premature as opposed to full-term infants. Among infants, males and females have a comparable risk for UTI, although the risk of urinary infection is substantially higher in females beyond infancy because of the differences in the external female genitalia. In addition, the risk of UTI in uncircumcised males is much higher. Additional risk factors for UTI in children include the presence of immunologic or systemic disease and a number of anatomic urinary tract abnormalities, the most common of which is vesicoureteral reflux (VUR), which is present in 30 to 50 percent of children with UTIs but is extremely rare otherwise. In the neonatal period, UTIs presumably occur because of hematogenous spread, whereas infections after the neonatal period are largely ascending urinary tract infections following perineal colonization.[30]

Table 12-9 lists the most common organisms causing UTIs, among which *E. coli* accounts for the overwhelming majority (80 percent of cases) and is responsible for virtually all first infections. Other organisms include *Proteus mirabilis, Klebsiella pneumoniae, Pseudomonas, Enterobacter* species, *Streptococcus viridans,* and coagulase-negative staphylococci. It is important to note that adenovirus can also cause a specific form of acute cystitis that is more common in young male children, who present with fever, intense dysuria, and gross hematuria.

UTIs can be divided into two general categories: uncomplicated lower tract infections and more complicated upper tract infections. Upper tract infections are those in

TABLE 12-9

ORGANISMS RESPONSIBLE FOR URINARY TRACT INFECTIONS

Escherichia coli	Coagulase-positive *Staphylococcus*
Proteus mirabilis	*Neisseria gonorrhoeae*
Klebsiella pneumoniae	*Chlamydia trachomatis*
Pseudomonas aeruginosa	*Candida albicans*
Enterobacter species	Adenovirus
Streptococcus viridans	

which kidney parenchymal injury can be demonstrated, which has traditionally been referred to as pyelonephritis but is more commonly known now as upper tract infection. Lower tract UTIs include both cystitis and urethritis, but only the former is discussed here.

Diagnosis

UTIs in children are among the most underdiagnosed and mismanaged diseases owing largely to the lack of specificity of symptoms localized to the urinary tract. And yet it is extremely important to identify UTIs for several reasons. First, implementation of appropriate treatment at the earliest time is critical to the best possible outcome. Second, because of the frequency of anatomic urinary tract problems in children with UTI, appropriate follow-up studies must be arranged, as discussed below. Third, untreated or partially treated UTIs can result in renal scarring, producing significant morbidity including hypertension and the possible development of end-stage renal disease. The classic symptoms of dysuria, frequency, and urgency are clearly seen more commonly with lower tract or uncomplicated infections, but they are the exception, as opposed to the rule, particularly in younger children. Neonates with UTIs may present with poor feeding, irritability, and lethargy as well as jaundice. Older infants and young children often present not with urinary tract complaints but with gastrointestinal complaints such as nonspecific abdominal pain, vomiting, and poor feeding. In children outside of the neonatal age group, the most common symptoms of UTI include irritability (80 percent), poor feeding (65 percent), vomiting (40 percent), diarrhea (30 percent), and upper respiratory symptoms (15 percent). For all of these reasons, UTIs should be considered in the differential diagnosis of any child that has a fever without source or in those children who present with these symptoms even in the absence of documented fever.

Of particular concern is distinguishing between uncomplicated lower tract disease and complicated upper tract syndromes (pyelonephritis). At one end of the diagnostic spectrum are children who present with the more classic findings of fever, flank pain, and other systemic findings accompanied by dysuria, frequency, and urgency. Unfortunately, such clinical presentations are far less common in children, even when upper tract disease is present.

The "gold standard" for diagnosis of UTIs is a positive urine culture consisting of an uncontaminated urine specimen showing $>1 \times 10_5$ CFU/mL of a pathogenic organism. While urine cultures should certainly be obtained on infants and children in whom UTI is suspected, results of such tests are not available immediately to guide treatment decisions. Uncontaminated urine samples and the appropriate method of collecting them depend upon the child's ability to control voiding. In general, toilet-trained children (≤ 2 years of age) can, with appropriate supervision, produce voided midstream urine clean-catch samples. In young females, periurethral contamination can be avoided by having the female child sit facing the rear of the toilet, which maximizes labial retraction and exposure of the urethral meatus. In cooperative, toilet-trained males, clean-catch specimens are easier to obtain. In children from whom a clean-catch specimen cannot be obtained, either because of their young age or lack of cooperation, bagged urine specimens should be avoided, as contaminants are likely. Instead, a specimen for both urinalysis and culture should be obtained through direct bladder sampling, either by in-and-out catherization or by suprapubic aspiration. In the UCC, in-and-out catherization is far preferable in most cases unless the physician is comfortable with the technique of suprapubic aspiration. Both are safe and acceptable procedures for obtaining a specimen.

Because of the lack of availability of urine cultures to guide treatment decisions, indirect measures of UTI are utilized, including urinalysis, leukocyte esterase screening, and urinary nitrite screening. Leukocyte esterases are released into the urine after the breakdown of white blood cells, and provide presumptive evidence of urinary tract infection. Nitrates are converted to nitrites by gram negative urinary pathogens and provide indirect evidence of bacteriuria. The presence of pyuria (more than five white blood cells per high-power field) and bacteriuria on urine microanalysis are both time-honored methods of making a presumptive diagnosis of UTI, although the sensitivity of these tests is only about 65 percent. However, combining the standard urinalysis with urinary dip-stick screening increases the sensitivity in negative predictive values to the 95 percent range, making this combined approach a positive one for use in UCCs, particularly when coupled with obtaining an uncontaminated urine culture.

Management

Appropriate, aggressive treatment of UTIs clearly decreases the risk of renal damage and substantial morbidity in children. Figure 12-3 summarizes an approach to the care of such children with urinary tract disease, depending upon whether the patient has complicated upper tract disease or uncomplicated lower tract disease. For complicated upper tract disease in which there is presumed pyelonephritis, patients less than 3 months of age have traditionally been hospitalized and given parenteral antibiotics. However, more recent data suggest that children as young as 4 to 6 weeks of age with presumed upper tract disease can be managed on an outpatient basis using cefixime (16 mg/kg stat, followed by 8 mg/kg/day).[31] In the UCC setting, children under 3 months of age with evidence of UTI should have their care discussed with their treating pediatrician or primary care physician, as some controversy remains as to whether these children require hospitalization. If they are to be handled as outpatients, they need to be followed up closely and reexamined by the treating physician within 24 h of their initial care. Other children who should be considered for hospitalization include those who have a toxic, septic

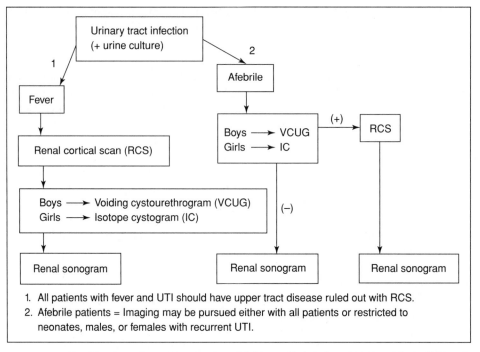

FIGURE 12-3   Algorithm for radiographic evaluation of children with their first UTI. (From Tintinalli JE et al: *Emergency Medicine: A Comprehensive Study Guide,* 5th ed. New York: McGraw-Hill, 2000. With permission.)

appearance, those with substantial dehydration who are unable to tolerate fluids by mouth, immunocompromised children, and those with known complicated urinary tract abnormalities, stents, or other urinary foreign bodies. All such cases should be discussed with the treating physician prior to referral. The majority of children with UTIs can be treated with an outpatient regimen consisting of appropriate hydration, fever control, and oral antibiotics. Table 12-10 lists the antibiotics most commonly used for UTIs. An understanding of the local antibiotic resistance patterns is, as always, important to guiding such therapy. In most regions of the country, increasing resistance to trimethroprim/sulfamethoxazole has led clinicians to use amoxicillin, amoxicillin/clavulanate, or cefixime as a first-line therapy for such children. The majority of first-time UTIs in children are due to *E. coli,* and each of these agents has good activity against this organism. The younger the child, the more likely it is that an undiagnosed upper tract, complicated infection may be present, which leads many people to use cefixime presumptively because of its demonstrated effectiveness in such cases.

A part of the treatment of such children is referral for appropriate radiographic evaluation with their first UTI. This should be carefully coordinated with the physician who will be following the patient, but an appropriate algorithmic approach is listed in Fig. 12-4, in which a combination of renal cortical scans, renal sonograms, and voiding cystourethrograms can identify those patients with anatomic abnormalities that require further follow-up.

TABLE 12-10

ORAL ANTIBIOTIC TREATMENT OF PEDIATRIC URINARY TRACT INFECTIONS
(5 TO 7-DAY COURSE)

Up to age 18
    Amoxicillin   40–50 mg/kg/day, tid
    Amoxicillin/clavulanate   50 mg/kg/day, tid
    Cefixime   16 mg/kg/day 1, 8 mg/kg/days 2–5
    Cephalexin[a]   25–50 mg/kg/day, qid
    Trimethoprim/sulfamethoxazole[a]   12 mg/kg/day TMP, 60 mg/kg/day SMZ[b]

Age 18 and above
    Agents listed above or
        Ciprofloxacin   250 mg bid
        Levofloxacin   250 mg bid
        Fosfomycin   3.0 grams × 1

[a]High resistance rates to these antibiotics in recurrent infections; local/regional resistance patterns should
guide therapy.
[b]TMP, trimethoprim; SMZ, sulfamethoxazole.

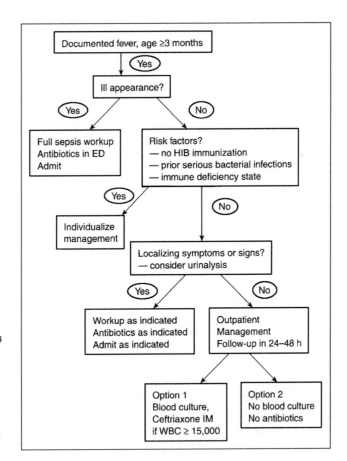

FIGURE 12-4 Management scheme for febrile infants aged 3 months or older. *Abbreviations:* ED, emergency department; HIB, *Haemophilus influenzae* type b. (From Tintinalli JE et al: *Emergency Medicine: A Comprehensive Study Guide,* 5th ed. New York: McGraw-Hill; 2000. With permission.)

Status epilepticus

Fortunately, children with status epilepticus (SE) rarely present to the UCC. However, because of the necessity for treating such children rapidly and effectively, a brief discussion of this entity in the pediatric age group is important and UCC physicians should know how to stabilize and initially treat such children prior to referral. SE is defined as a continuous seizure lasting longer than 30 min or the occurrence of two or more seizures without full recovery of consciousness during the seizure-free period.[32] By far the most common entity is a continuous seizure lasting longer than 30 min. Although any type of seizure can progress to SE, generalized tonic-clonic seizures are the most common.

The goals of therapy in such patients are threefold:

Rapid stabilization, including provision of airway and circulatory support
Expeditious termination of seizures
Clear delineation of the cause of seizures and treatment thereof

Rapid Stabilization

The initial management of seizures is to assure that cardiorespiratory stability is provided, including provision of an airway, securing of an intravenous line (where possible), and supporting the cardiovascular system to the extent necessary. A patent airway should be provided including adequate ventilation and oxygenation. In the vast majority of children, this will not require endotracheal intubation, although some children with severe and prolonged SE may require bag-valve-mask ventilation to support oxygenation. A pulse oximeter should be utilized to assess oxygen saturation and 100% oxygen should be administered to the patient. If an intravenous line can be placed, a blood glucose determination should be made and D_{50} 1 g/kg should be administered presumptively in the event the seizures are caused or exacerbated by hypoglycemia. Further details of supportive care should be according to ACLS and Pediatric Advanced Life Support (PALS) standards.

Expeditious Termination of Seizures

Profound and deleterious metabolic and hemodynamic changes occur during seizures, increasing morbidity as the length of SE continues. Thus, management of SE requires a prompt and aggressive approach to terminating it. Anticonvulsants such as phenytoin and phenobarbital, while excellent medications for ongoing seizure control, lack the ability to terminate the seizure as rapidly as is necessary in documented SE. For that reason, the initial drug therapy for SE is focused on various benzodiazepine agents, lorazepam (Ativan), diazepam (Valium), and midazolam. While diazepam is an effective agent used for SE since 1965, it is less commonly used in present-day practice than lorazepam for two reasons. While seizures can be effectively terminated within 15 to 20 min in up to 80 to 85 percent of patients with SE in whom diazepam is used, this agent redistributes to other parts of the body, decreasing its clinical effect over time. Second, diazepam suppresses respiratory effort and may cause respiratory arrest, particularly if used in high doses.[33]

TABLE 12-11

ANTISEIZURE MEDICATIONS FOR STATUS EPILEPTICUS

MEDICATION	DOSE
Lorazepam (Ativan)	0.1–0.5 mg/kg (maximum 4 mg) IV/IO
	0.1–0.4 mg/kg PR[a]
Diazepam (Valium)	0.3 mg/kg IV/IO
	0.5 mg/kg PR[a]

Key: IV, intravenous; IO, intraosseous; PR, per rectum.
[a]PR medications should be given with a well-lubricated insulin (3-mL) syringe, following which the buttocks should be taped and elevated with a folded rolled towel.

Lorazepam compares favorably to diazepam, although it is less lipid-soluble; therefore its onset of action is delayed for approximately 2 to 3 min. However, it causes far less respiratory depression than diazepam and its anticonvulsant effect is maintained for 6 to 12 h after administration. For this reason it has largely supplanted diazepam as the first-line agent for SE. In addition, it can be given by intraosseous or rectal routes. Table 12-11 summarizes the dosage and administration of these drugs.

Midazolam has been used to terminate SE in some cases; its duration of action is even shorter than that of diazepam and it is more of a respiratory depressant. For that reason, it is not commonly used as a first-line agent for SE.

The majority of patients presenting to urgent care centers with SE can have their seizures terminated with the use of the agents in support of therapy. Such patients should then be transported as quickly as possible to the nearest and most appropriate emergency department for further evaluation and antiseizure medications. Phenytoin, fosphenytoin, and phenobarbital are all effective agents; their administration should be coordinated with the treating physician or the emergency physician who will be responsible for the patient's care.

Delineation of the Cause of the Seizure

While the majority of patients presenting with SE do so following a known seizure disorder, SE can also follow meningitis, intracranial bleeds, intracranial tumors, and other acute and subacute causes. For this reason, patients should be referred for appropriate diagnostic workup, including, where indicated, further laboratory studies, CT or magnetic resonance imaging (MRI) of the head, and LP to rule out meningitis in appropriate cases. Patients who have suffered SE should be transferred by EMS and their care should be carefully coordinated with the EMS agency and the receiving physician.

DEHYDRATION

Dehydration is one of the most common problems facing ED and UCC physicians who treat pediatric patients, and it is usually due to acute gastroenteritis, which is discussed in more detail below. However, the following information is important in terms of understanding maintenance fluid requirements and rehydration of children in the UCC setting. While caloric expenditure and body fluid requirements can be estimated from body surface area, the most common means is through using body weight and percentage of dehydration. Clearly the easiest way to determine the percentage of dehydration is to compare normal body weight and current body weight. However, this information may not be obtainable in the UCC setting. Parents should be questioned regarding the child's most recent body weight, and, if the child has visited the pediatrician or primary care physician's office in the past 2 or 3 months, that body weight can also be determined by referring to him or her. A clinical estimate of dehydration can be determined by a careful physical examination, and weight loss is usually estimated as mild ($\leq$5 percent), moderate (6 to 10 percent), and severe (10 to 15 percent). Table 12-12 shows the best correlation of clinical findings with the degree of dehydration.

Normal maintenance fluid requirements can be summarized as follows:

- 0 to 10 kg: 100 mL/kg/24 h
- 10 to 20 kg: 50 mL/kg/24 h
- >20 kg: 20 mL/kg/24 h

By way of example, a 10-kg child requires 100 mL $\times$ 10 kg or a total of 1000 mL/24 h for maintenance fluid. An 18-kg baby requires 100 mL $\times$ 10 kg = 1000 mL + (50 mL $\times$ 8 kg) = 400 mL, for a total of 1400 mL/24 h. A 35-kg child requires 100 mL $\times$ 10 kg = 1000 mL + (50 mL $\times$ 10 kg) = 500 mL + (20 mL $\times$ 15 kg) = 300 mL for a total of 1800 mL/24 h.

Keep in mind that these are *maintenance* fluid requirements and that the percent of dehydration will need to be corrected for such children in addition to these maintenance requirements. The majority of children presenting with diarrhea present with isotonic dehydration, in which there are proportionally equal losses of sodium and water; therefore the serum sodium remains within normal limits. In diarrheal illness without vomiting as a primary symptom, isotonic dehydration is the most common form seen. When vomiting is a prominent symptom in the presentation of the illness, determination of serum electrolytes may be necessary, since prolonged vomiting can cause hypo-

TABLE 12-12

CLINICAL ESTIMATION OF DEHYDRATION

	MILD (<5%)	MODERATE (5–10%)	SEVERE (>15%)
Pulse	Normal	Slightly increased	Tachycardia
Mucous membranes	Normal	Drug	Extremely dry
Blood pressure	Normal	Normal	Orthostatic
Thirst	Slight	Moderate	Marked
Skin turgor	Normal to slight	Variable	Abnormal
Tears	Present	Decreased	Sunken eyes
Anterior fontanelle	Normal	Normal to sunken	Sunken
Capillary refill	Normal	Normal to slightly prolonged	Prolonged
Urine			
• Volume	Decreased	Oliguria	Oliguria/anuria
• Specific gravity	≤1.020	1.010–1.030	>1.035

chloremic, hypokalemic metabolic alkalosis, as is seen in children with pyloric stenosis (see below).

Following a careful physical examination to determine the cause of the dehydration and a correlation to determine the extent of dehydration, further evaluation and treatment must be planned. In cases of straightforward diarrhea without significant vomiting, serum electrolytes usually do not have to be measured and oral rehydration with solutions such as Pedialyte, Rehydralite, Resol, and Ricelyte is effective in rehydrating the child when given in small doses. Vomiting is clearly not a contraindication to administering oral rehydrating solutions, although the child may need to be given as little as 5 mL at a time every few minutes in order to avoid the vomiting reflex.

In children with moderate to severe dehydration, intravenous fluid replacement may be necessary to overcome the vomiting reflex and gastric atony. Children can initially be hydrated in the UCC or ED with an initial bolus of 10 to 20 mL/kg of normal saline or lactated Ringer's solution, followed by maintenance fluid therapy. After a period of 1 to 2 h, patients with moderate dehydration are usually able to tolerate fluids by mouth and may be discharged on oral rehydrating solutions with close follow-up. Children who fail this test (inability to tolerate fluids by mouth) and those with severe dehydration should be referred for hospitalization or treatment in a short-stay unit.

ACUTE GASTROENTERITIS

The term *gastroenteritis* is a bit of a misnomer in that true gastric involvement is uncommon. Most cases of noninflammatory infectious diarrhea are caused by viruses and, less frequently, parasites that localize to the proximal small bowel or by toxin-producing bacteria. The clinical syndrome produced in these cases is one of nausea and vomiting associated with profuse, watery diarrhea. While the term *gastroenteritis* is used, in fact the enteritis aspect is the true cause of the illness itself. *Diarrhea* is defined as an excessive loss of water in the stool compared to normal and is usually due to a variety of self-limited enteric infections caused by viruses or bacteria. The term *dysentery* is reserved for cases of inflammatory diarrhea. Children presenting with nausea, vomiting, and diarrhea constitute a large volume of patients seen in the UCC and ED setting and nearly every child has this illness at some point.

Various types of viruses, bacteria, or parasites can be isolated from 50 to 70 percent of children with diarrhea, with viral infection as the most common cause. Rotaviruses, the Norwalk virus, enteric adenoviruses, and astroviruses are the most commonly currently isolated viral pathogens, with rotavirus being a common agent which can be identified by enzyme immunoassay and latex agglutination tests. *E. coli* is by far the most common bacterial organism causing diarrhea in children, but other organisms—including *Campylobacter, Shigella, Salmonella,* and *Yersinia*—may also be found. *Giardia lamblia* is a common parasitic cause of diarrhea in infants and children.

The most important aspect of the management of children with acute gastroenteritis is an assessment of their hydrational status. As indicated previously, when possible, the current weight should be compared to a recent weight to assess the degree of dehydration (although this should always be coordinated with a careful physical examination) to determine whether the dehydration is mild, moderate, or severe. Dehydration should be treated appropriately with oral or intravenous fluids, depending on the severity of the disease. In most cases, it is not necessary to make a specific identification of the pathogen causing the diarrhea or gastroenteritis, although stool cultures and enzyme immunoassays can be helpful in outbreaks of diarrhea in day-care centers or other schools. In general, stool and viral cultures are reserved for these situations or those in which a child remains febrile, has more than 4 to 5 stools per day, or has bloody diarrhea, since there is a slightly higher incidence of identification of bacterial pathogens in this group. As stated above, dehydration caused by diarrhea is usually isotonic, although when vomiting is a prominent symptom, determination of serum electrolytes may be indicated to guide fluid therapy.

 Management

A majority of children with diarrhea and vomiting that present with dehydration can be managed with oral rehydrating solutions. Antiemetics can be used, but only very judiciously by the experience of the clinician and the amount of dehydration present in the child. Most children are able to tolerate oral fluids, even in very small doses, and for them antiemetics are not necessary. In cases of refractory vomiting, antiemetic therapy may be necessary both in the UCC and in the inpatient setting. In most cases, antiemetics are not necessary in children in the outpatient setting, but when utilized, they should be mild agents such as promethazine. Antimotility agents should also be avoided in general, particularly in cases that may be due to *E. coli*, since data suggest that the use of antibiotics, particularly trimethoprim/sulfamethoxazole, and antimotility agents promote the development of hemolytic-uremic syndrome after *E. coli* 0157:h7 infection.

A vast majority of the cases of infectious diarrhea are mild, resolve spontaneously, and do not require anything other than supportive treatment and correction of the dehydration. Antimicrobial therapy should be used only in patients with severe illness who present with fever and bloody stools, those in whom there are compromising medical conditions, or in young infants less than 6 months of age, where hospitalization is usually necessary to control dehydration, vomiting, and fever. As stated previously, there is an emerging sense that the combination of antibiotic therapy and antimotility agents can promote the development of hemolytic uremic syndrome. However, in patients where sepsis is a strong consideration or bacteria such as *Shigella* are likely to be the cause, antibiotics may have to be considered. One of the exceptions for treatment of diarrhea with antibiotics is in teenagers with travel-related diarrhea, where azithromycin has been shown to be effective without substantial side effects.

 Errors to Avoid

- Failure to document the degree of dehydration present
- Failure to treat mild degrees of dehydration
- Reliance on antibiotics, antiemetics, and antimotility drugs as opposed to supportive therapy
- Failure to provide close follow-up visits to determine the success of supportive therapy

Key Points of Documentation

- Degree of dehydration
- Response to oral hydration in the urgent care center
- Clear instructions to parents for follow-up
- Clear instructions on the use of oral rehydrating solutions and the lack of need for antiemetics, antimotility drugs, and antibiotics (except where indicated)

INTUSSUSCEPTION

Intussusception occurs when one portion of the bowel telescopes into the distal portion and becomes entrapped. If allowed to persist, venous congestion, edema, bloody diarrhea, and bowel necrosis can follow. Over 80 percent of intussusceptions are ileocolic, with the remaining 20 percent representing combinations of different anatomic patterns (which are more commonly associated with anatomic abnormalities, congenital abnormalities, or tumors). Seventy-five percent of children with intussusception are less than 2 years of age and 50 percent are less than 1 year. There is a male predominance by a 2:1 ratio and a strong seasonal prevalence for the summer months. Many patients who present with intussusception have had a viral illness within the 2 weeks prior to presentation with intussusception and 90 percent of patients show lymphoid hyperplasia.

The presenting symptoms of children with intussusception vary from the classic to the obscure. A majority of children with intussusception present with abdominal pain, and the classic story is that of a child with cramping abdominal pain of an intermittent nature who presents with the legs drawn up and crying inconsolably. While "currant jelly" stools are often described in intussusception, in fact only 50 percent of children have any blood present on rectal examination. At least 10 percent of children with intussusception present with less classic findings and may have a combination of milder abdominal pain, poor feeding, irritability, vomiting, and loose stools, which may be positive for blood.

Any child presenting within the first 2 years of life with either of these symptom patterns should be considered for the possibility of intussusception. Certainly those with the classic presentation should receive a thorough workup for intussusception. While plain films of the abdomen classically produce a pattern that shows a paucity of gas in the right lower quadrant, plain films of the abdomen are generally not recommended on such children. However, if the patient has had nonspecific symptoms and plain films have been obtained, this lack of gas in the right lower quadrant should alert the clinician to the possibility of intussusception. All children who are suspected of intussusception should be referred for abdominal ultrasonography, which confirms the diagnosis easily in the vast majority of cases. Once the diagnosis has been confirmed, the majority of children can have their intussusception reduced by air-contrast enema or by hydrostatic reduction enemas. In cases where the intussusception has been allowed to persist for long periods, perforation may result and abdominal surgery may be required. However, the vast majority of cases of intussusception present early and can be easily reduced via air contrast or hydrostatic enema. These children should thus be referred quickly to the nearest appropriate hospital capable of performing this procedure. Intravenous fluid therapy may be necessary if there is a long transport or if the child presents with substantial dehydration. The majority of cases, however, can be sent directly to the nearest ED for further evaluation and treatment.

Pyloric stenosis

Pyloric stenosis is an extremely common entity, occurring in 1 in 300 children. The classic description is the presentation of projectile vomiting in a firstborn male within the first 6 weeks of life. In fact, while there is a male predominance, pyloric stenosis can occur in females and also occurs well outside the classic 6-week period. A majority of children present with a fairly classic presentation of nausea and vomiting, with crying and inconsolability present as the child begins to develop dehydration. Up to 8 percent of children present with jaundice. Because the vomiting occurs above the level of the pylorus, children often present with hypokalemic, hypochloremic metabolic alkalosis due to the loss of the gastric secretions.

The pathognomonic finding in pyloric stenosis is a small "olive," which can be palpated just to the right side of the rectus abdominis sheath in the area of the pylorus. The olive represents hypertrophied pyloric tissue, which is more palpable because of the young age of the child and, in many cases, because of the dehydration present. While an olive can be palpated in 40 to 90 percent of children, it is difficult to detect it in a crying child unless the examiner is quite experienced.

In any child who presents within the first 6 to 12 weeks of life with substantial nausea and vomiting, whether projectile in nature or not, the possibility of pyloric stenosis should be considered. Such children should be referred for ultrasonography, in which the enlarged pyloric muscle can easily be visualized. Some centers still use upper gastrointestinal contrast series, but ultrasonography is by far the procedure of choice to make the diagnosis, as it is 97 percent sensitive and 100 percent specific. Children with substantial dehydration (>5 percent) with pyloric stenosis should have intravenous rehydration prior to surgery. The only effective treatment of pyloric stenosis is pyloromyotomy, but electrolyte imbalances should be corrected prior to surgery. Placement of a nasogastric tube prior to transport is usually not necessary, since the vomiting has emptied the stomach.

Pediatric dermatology

Rashes may be caused by a wide variety of viral, bacterial, immunologic, and idiopathic diseases and comprise a broad list of entities that account for a large number of visits to EDs and UCCs. This section is intended as a quick and easy reference to the initial presentation of these diseases and their most effective treatment. The disease entities are divided into the following categories in this discussion:

- Symptoms
- Etiology
- Rash
- Treatment

Bacterial Causes

Impetigo

Impetigo is a bacterial infection of the skin; it is most commonly confined to the epidermis. When the dermis is involved, the disease is known as ecthyma. Both diseases are caused predominately by phage group II staphylococci, although they may also be caused by group A streptococcus, including nephritogenic strains.

Symptoms The classic clinical appearance of skin lesions most commonly make for an easy visual diagnosis, with the patient presenting with a rapidly spreading vesicular and pustular rash, most commonly in children under the age of 6 years.

Etiology Phage group II staphylococci and group A streptococci.

Rash The rash is typically easy to diagnose and consists of erythematous macules and papules, which develop rapidly into vesicles and pustules. Classically, these rupture, producing a yellowish fluid. In many cases, the child presents with crusting lesions over the involved area, which often fosters spread by contact.

Management Since the diagnosis is largely made clinically, cultures are rarely necessary. Wound scrubbing and cleansing with a nonirritating soap should be undertaken and instructions should be given regarding the highly contagious nature of the disease both to the patient, through self-contamination, and to others. Topical antibiotics such as mupirocin or Neosporin ointment can be utilized, but most cases also require oral antibiotics such as dicloxacillin 50 mg/kg/day, cephalexin 50 mg/kg/day, or erythromycin or azithromycin 10 mg/kg on day 1, followed by 5 mg/kg per day on days 2 through 5.

Scarlet Fever

Symptoms Scarlet fever is an acute febrile illness that primarily affects young children and presents with an acute, often abrupt onset of fever, headache, vomiting, sore throat, and abdominal pain, followed by a distinct rash within 24 to 48 h. The patients typically present with pharyngitis and a bright red appearance of the tongue.

Etiology Group A beta-hemolytic streptococci, which produce an erythrogenic toxin.

Rash Beginning 24 to 48 h after the onset of the illness, a red punctate rash with the appearance of rough sandpaper appears on the axillae, groin, and neck and spreads rapidly to the trunk and extremities.

Management The diagnosis of scarlet fever is usually made on clinical grounds and cultures are unnecessary. Penicillin, ampicillin, or erythromycin may be used to treat the disease.

Viral

Roseola

Symptoms Roseola infantum (also known as exanthema subitum) is a common, self-limiting viral infection most commonly seen in infants. In children up to 3 years old, it presents with a high fever (up to 40.5°C) but with a paucity of additional findings, although mild cough, coryza, and difficulty in feeding may be present. The rash typically follows a febrile period by several days and lasts 1 to 3 days.

Etiology Human herpesvirus VI (most likely).

Rash The appearance of the rash usually coincides with the decline of the fever. It consists of discrete, light red or pale pink lesions usually 2 to 5 mm in size and macular or maculopapular eruptions. It fades with pressure and does not coalesce. The rash appears on the trunk initially and spreads outward.

Management There is no specific treatment for roseola other than antipyretic therapy during the febrile phase and reassurance to the parents.

Erythema Infectiosum ("Fifth Disease" or "Slapped-Cheek" Syndrome)

Symptoms Erythema infectiosum is also known as "fifth disease" or "slapped-cheek" syndrome (because of the child's typical rash). It is an acute febrile illness that occurs most commonly in the spring and may occur in epidemics, particularly among children between 2 and 15 years of age. In most cases, the appearance of the rash marks the onset of the disease and fever; prodromal symptoms are uncommon. Adolescents with the disease may also develop arthralgia or frank arthritis. In patients with chronic hemolytic anemias such as sickle cell disease, the etiologic agent may also cause aplastic crisis.

Etiology Parvovirus B 19.

Rash The classic form shows the classic slapped-cheek appearance, with diffuse erythema of the cheeks grouped in papules on an erythematous base. Pallor in the circumoral area is common and the eyelids and chin are usually not involved. After 24 to 48 h, after the appearance of the facial rash, a macular, erythematous, nonpruritic rash appears on the trunk and limbs.

Management There is no specific treatment for human parvovirus infection, although reassurance, fever control, and symptomatic therapy are helpful.

Measles

Symptoms Owing to the widespread use of immunizations, measles is a far less common disease than it was in the past. Nonetheless, with large numbers of immigrants and their children coming into the country, several thousand cases of measles are now seen each year, as verified by the Centers for Disease Control. Measles typically presents as a fever and malaise, with temperatures up to 40°C. Within 12 to 24 h, upper respiratory symptoms of cough, coryza, conjunctivitis, and spots on the buccal mucosa (Koplik's spots) appear. The rash itself erupts on the fourth or fifth day of the disease and is typically maculopapular in appearance, beginning on the face and neck and advancing down the trunk, followed by the extremities on about the third or fourth day of the illness, by which time the rash on the face is typically fading.

Etiology   Measles is a specific paramyxovirus that enters the body via the upper respiratory tact.

Management   In the past, physicians were familiar with the rash of the measles and its prodromal phase, which made the diagnosis quite easy. However, since it is now a far less common disease, the clinician must learn the disease pattern, which typically appears in unimmunized children, often recent immigrants to this country. If the disease is suspected, acute and convalescent measles titers can be drawn 1 to 2 weeks apart to verify the diagnosis. In most states, measles is a reportable disease, although treatment is most often supportive, as the disease runs a self-limited course except in the most severe cases. Rarely, measles may progress to a severe form of laryngotracheal bronchitis, lower respiratory tract infection, or central nervous system infection, all of which require hospitalization. For unimmunized contacts to index cases, immune serum globulin 0.25 to 0.5 mL/kg should be utilized.

Infectious Mononucleosis
Symptoms   Infectious mononucleosis (IM) is characterized by malaise, pharyngitis, fever, lymphadenopathy, and, in many cases, splenomegaly. It is an extremely common disease, since by late adolescence up to 90 percent of young people are seropositive for antibodies. The disease often begins insidiously with low-grade fever and malaise, progressing to sore throat, further respiratory symptoms, cough, and, in many cases, profound malaise. Lymphadenopathy is nearly uniformly present; it may be limited to the cervical region or may more commonly extend to the axillary and inguinal regions.

Etiology   The disease is caused by Epstein-Barr virus (EBV).

Rash   Only 5 to 10 percent of patients with IM present with a generalized, maculopapular, erythematous rash, often associated with petechiae on the soft palate. Interestingly enough, in patients with IM who receive ampicillin, the incidence of the rash and its severity increase dramatically. In fact, the rapid appearance of such a rash following administration of ampicillin in anyone should raise the possibility of IM.

Management   In general, hemoglobin, hematocrit, and white blood cell counts are not particularly helpful in either making or confirming the diagnosis, although there may be a high absolute lymphocyte count and many atypical mononuclear cells on the blood smear. The gold standard diagnosis of IM is the heterophil antibody test or related EBV-specific serology assay.

The vast majority of cases of IM are self-limited, although the course of the disease may be prolonged. The most important issues to be faced in the UCC setting are considerations of airway obstruction, since adenoidal and posterior pharyngeal hypertrophy are common, and there is the possibility of splenic rupture (careful studies indicate that this is rare). The patient should be assessed for splenomegaly and/or appropriate splenic imaging (usually by ultrasound) prior to allowing children with IM to return to physical activity and/or contact sports.

Varicella/Zoster

Symptoms   The virus causing varicella has two distinct clinical entities: varicella (chickenpox) and zoster (shingles). Varicella represents a primary infection with a virus, while zoster is a reactivation of latent virus, which presumably resides in susceptible nerve roots. Varicella is a frequent, nearly ubiquitous disease among children, although there are still many young adults who have not acquired the disease. Because the disease is much more severe in older children and adults, it is important to note if the child has ever been exposed to the disease in the past.

Children usually present with a mild prodrome, lasting 1 to 3 days, consisting primarily of fever and malaise. In the majority of cases, patients do not present until a frank rash has developed. While the disease is usually self-limited, a small but distinct group of children (particularly older children and young adults) may present with varicella pneumonia or encephalitis, which is a much more severe and less self-limited disease.

Varicella zoster usually appears quite abruptly and without a significant prodrome in the form of a painful vesicular rash.

Etiology   Varicella/zoster virus, which is a member of the herpesvirus family.

Rash   The rash of varicella initially appears as erythematous papules that rapidly evolve into vesicles and then pustules. A classic description is of multiple lesions and multiple states of healing, since macules, papules, vesicles, and crusted pustules may all be present on the patient simultaneously. The rash of zoster is also a vesicular, often confluent rash, which is typically quite painful in nature.

Management   The diagnosis of varicella and zoster is usually made on clinical grounds; the support of laboratory tests is not necessary unless signs and symptoms of more disseminated disease, such as pneumonitis or encephalitis, are present. While the majority of the patients can be treated symptomatically with warm baths (Aveeno bath) and appropriate cleansing to prevent superinfection, the rash is often profoundly pruritic and appropriate antihistamines may be needed to control the itching and help allow the patient to sleep. Temperature control should consist of appropriate hydration and acetaminophen, as aspirin and other nonsteroidal anti-inflammatory agents have been implicated in the subsequent development of Reye's syndrome.

Antiviral agents have been developed for use in patients with varicella zoster, but the recommendations for their use are fairly limited. Oral acyclovir is not recommended for routine use in the majority of children with varicella. Those in whom acyclovir should be considered are those with moderate to severe varicella (including pneumonitis and/or encephalitis), children older than 12 years of age, patients with chronic cutaneous or pulmonary disorders, patients on long-term salicylate therapy, and those who are receiving corticosteroids. In these patients, oral acyclovir in a dose of 80 mg/kg/day in four divided doses for 5 days should be considered. Patients with pneumonitis and encephalitis should be hospitalized and given intravenous acyclovir.

For unimmunized children exposed to varicella, the American Academy of Pediatrics recommends administration of a varicella vaccine to susceptible children within 72 h. In the event that exposure to varicella does not cause infection, this postexposure immunization should prevent the disease in the future. Varicella zoster immunoglobulin (VZIG) may be given to those at significant risk, including immunocompromised children who do not have a history of chickenpox and susceptible pregnant women, newborn infants whose mother had a history of chickenpox either within 5 days before delivery or within 48 h after delivery, or patients in whom the disease is expected to be both certain and/or severe. Herpes zoster infections are usually treated with oral acyclovir or other antiviral agents. The dose of oral acyclovir for zoster in immunocompetent hosts is 4000 mg/day in five divided doses for 5 to 7 days in patients greater than 12 years of age.

Diseases of Unclear Etiology

Kawasaki Disease (Mucocutaneous Lymph Node Syndrome)

Symptoms   Kawasaki disease or mucocutaneous lymph node syndrome (MLNS) is a febrile multisystem disease that is usually characterized by a rash and is of primary importance because of the risk of the development of coronary artery abnormalities following the disease. The illness is characterized by the onset of fever and other characteristic features including:

1. Conjunctivitis
2. Lymphadenopathy
3. Rash
4. Injection of the oral pharynx and lips with a "strawberry tongue"
5. Erythema and edema of the extremities

Diagnosis is made on a clinical basis in a patient with prolonged fever who has four of the five symptoms listed above.

Etiology   While the precise cause is not known, the characteristics of the disease strongly suggest an as yet unknown infectious agent.

Rash   The rash can take on many forms, including a generalized erythematous morbilliform rash, or even macular, papular, or scarlatin-form rashes. In some cases the rash may resemble erythema multiforme. In the second phase of the disease, desquamation of the fingers or toes is common.

Management   The primary risk of Kawasaki disease is the development of coronary artery abnormalities following the disease. While other complications—including urethritis, hepatic dysfunction, arthritis, aseptic meningitis, and gallbladder disease—have been described, the primary problems associated with the disease are due to the cardiac complications. When the diagnosis of Kawasaki disease or MLNS is made or strongly suspected, the patient should be treated with anti-inflammatory therapy (usually with salicylates), supportive care, and intravenous high-dose immunoglobulin therapy. For this reason, all children with suspected Kawasaki disease should have consultation with the appropriate physician and, in the majority of cases, admission to the hospital for consideration for immunoglobulin and supportive therapy.

Pityriasis Rosea

Symptoms   Pityriasis rosea (PR) is an extremely common dermatologic illness of unclear etiology that has occasional prodromal symptoms of headache, sore throat, fatigue, malaise, and arthralgia. The characteristic rash is usually diagnostic of the disease, as indicated below.

Etiology   The etiology is unknown but strongly suggests a viral pattern. The condition is more commonly seen in the spring and fall but rarely in the form of an epidemic. PR is not known to be contagious.

Rash   The classic rash of PR evolves over a period of at least 2 weeks and classically begins with a "herald patch," which is an erythematous lesion with a raised epidermal border in an oval shape. Such herald patches are often mistaken for tinea corporis, but patients often wait to be seen until they have developed the more classic rash of PR. This rash consists of salmon-colored maculopapillary lesions covered with dry epidermis, which frequently occur in lines parallel to skin tension, giving rise to the classic "Christmas tree" pattern seen on the chests or backs of patients with this illness. PR can often be mistaken for secondary syphilis, tinea corporis, and other viral exanthems. If tinea corporis is suspected, a potassium hydroxide preparation of the skin scrapings should distinguish between the two diseases.

Management   The most common therapy for PR is to assure that other diseases are not causing the rash and to provide supportive therapy. Patients who present with pruritus should be given appropriate antihistamines. Oatmeal baths and emollients can help with the dryness and irritation caused by the disease. The rash often responds to sunlight exposure, which shortens the duration of the disease, sometimes dramatically.

Eczema

Symptomatology

Eczema is an extremely common disease that can present in a wide variety of fashions. It is often called "the itch that rashes," since pruritus is a common and often dramatic finding. Patients often present because of the increasing rash, which is exacerbated by scratching.

Etiology   Eczema is an atopic disease.

Rash   The itching is classically more profound than the rash, which presents as a poorly demarcated scaling plaque that may include excoriations, weeping, or thickening from constant rubbing.

Management   Treatment of eczema requires a broad approach, including lubrication, elimination of pruritus, treatment of superinfections, judicious use of topical steroids, and appropriate patient education regarding the course of the disease and skin care. Lubricating agents should be liberally utilized, and should include creams such as Eucerin or other similar highly lubricating creams. In areas of severe irritation, petroleum jelly can also be utilized. Antihistamines should be used to control itching, and to assist with mild nighttime sedation to prevent scratching. Superinfections should be treated appropriately with antibacterial, antifungal, or antiviral agents. Superficial staphylococcal infections are common and may be treated with use of antibiotic ointment. For severe cases, topical steroids can be utilized twice a day, usually with triamcinolone 0.1% in an ointment base, which is more soothing and also adheres to the skin and is absorbed better. Patients should also be educated about the disease. Those whose disease is severe enough to have brought them to the UCC or ED should be referred to a dermatologist for follow-up care.

SCABIES

Symptoms   Scabies is quite possibly the "itchiest" disease on earth. It is also one of the most upsetting to patients because of its association with a specific mite. The majority of patients present with nearly excruciating pruritus, which also may be present in other members of the family.

Etiology   Scabies is an infestation of the skin by *Sarcoptes scabiei*. It is an extremely common disorder transmitted from human to human by close physical contact.

Rash   The rash most commonly occurs on the hands, feet, and flexor surfaces of the elbows and knees. The typical lesion is a burrow or fine erythematous linear or curved lesion with a central scale. The burrows are most easily seen when present in the web spaces of the digits, but burrows may often not be present.

Management   Diagnosis is usually made on a presumptive basis because of the association of intense pruritus with the classic rash. Topical agents effective against scabies are the treatments of choice and include permethrin 5% cream (Elimite) and lindane 1% lotion (Kwell). Both are effective and, while lindane is easier to apply, there have been reports of lindane resistance. For that reason, Elimite cream is more commonly used at the present time. Whichever preparation is selected, it should be applied from the neck down to the feet, with special attention to areas where the rash is present. All household members, sexual contacts, and others at high risk of acquiring the disease should be treated concurrently, even if they are not symptomatic. In addition, all clothing, towels, bed linens, etc., that have been used within the preceding 48 h should be bagged, washed, and dried on high heat to help eliminate the mite. Because of the intensity of the itching, triamcinolone cream 0.1% can be used to relieve it as well as appropriate antihistamines, including sedating antihistamines to help ensure sleep at night. All such patients should be referred for follow-up care or a revisit to make sure that the disease is fully treated.

REFERENCES

Acute Otitis Media

1. Dowell SF, Butler JC, Giebink GS, et al: Acute otitis media: management and surveillance in an era of pneumococcal resistance—a report from the Drug-Resistant *Streptococcus Pneumoniae* Therapeutic Working Group. *Pediatr Infect Dis J* 18:1–9, 1999.
2. Barnett ED, Klein JO: The problem of resistant bacteria for the management of acute otitis media. *Pediatr Clin North Am* 42:509–517, 1995.
3. Poole MD: Otitis media complication and treatment failures: implications of pneumococcal resistance: *Pediatr Infect Dis J* 14:s23–56, 1995.

Croup

4. Cordle R, Relich NC: Upper respiratory emergencies, in Tintinalli JE, Kelen GD, Stapczynski JS (eds): *Emergency Medicine: A Comprehensive Study Guide*. New York: McGraw-Hill; 2000.
5. Rothrock SG, Perkin R: Stridor: A review, update, and current management recommendations. *Pediatr Emerg Med Rep* 1:29–34, 1996.
6. Cressman WR, Myer NM: Diagnosis and management of croup and epiglottitis. *Pediatr Clin North Am* 41:265–269, 1994.
7. Prendergast M, Jones JS, Hartman D: Racemic epinephrine in the treatment of laryngotracheitis: can we identify children for outpatient therapy? *Am J Emerg Med* 12:613–617, 1994.
8. Waisman Y, Klein BL, Boenning DA, et al: Prospective randomized double-blind study comparing L-epinephrine and racemic epinephrine aerosols in the treatment of croup. *Pediatrics* 89:302–306, 1992.

Epiglottitis

9. Altieri MF, Mayer TA: Acute respiratory emergencies in children: croup, epiglottitis, bronchiolitis, pneumonia, in Schwartz GR, Hanke BK, Mayer TA (eds): *Principles and Practice of Emergency Medicine*, 4th ed. Baltimore: Williams & Wilkins; 1999.
10. Hickerson SL, Kirby RS, Wheeler JG, et al: Epiglottitis: a nine-year case review. *South Med J* 89:487–490, 1996.

Asthma and Bronchiolitis

11. Kou M, Mayer T: Pediatric asthma and bronchiolitis, in Tintinalli JE, Kelen GD, Stapczynski JS (eds): *Emergency Medicine: A Comprehensive Study Guide,* 5th ed. New York: McGraw-Hill, 2000.
12. National Institutes of Health: *Expert Panel Report II: Guidelines for the Diagnosis and Management of Asthma.* Publication #98-4051. Bethesda, MD: NIH; 1997.
13. Katz RW, Kelly HW, Crowley MR, et al: Safety of continuous nebulized albuterol for bronchospasm in infants and children. *Pediatrics* 92:666–670, 1993.
14. Reijnonen T, Korppi M, Pitkakangas S, et al: The clinical efficacy of nebulized racemic epinephrine and albuterol in acute bronchiolitis. *Arch Pediatr Adolesc Med* 149:686–692, 1995.
15. Tal A, Leby N, Bearman JE: Methylprednisolone therapy for acute asthma in infants and toddlers: a controlled clinical trial. *Pediatrics* 86:350–354, 1990.
16. Qureshi F: Management of children with acute asthma in the emergency department. *Pediatr Emerg Care* 15:206–214, 1999.

Pneumonia

17. Brown K, Terndrup TE: Viral and bacterial pneumonia in children, in Tintinalli JE, Kelen GD, Stapczynski JS (eds): *Emergency Medicine: A Comprehensive Study Guide,* 5th ed. New York: McGraw-Hill; 2000.
18. Davies HD, Matlow A, Petric M, et al: Prospective comparative study of viral, bacterial, and atypical organisms identified in pneumonia and bronchiolitis in hospitalized Canadian infants. *Pediatr Infect Dis J* 15:371–376, 1996.
19. Hammerschlag MR: Atypical pneumonia in children. *Adv Pediatr Infect Dis* 10:1–25, 1995.
20. Schidlow DV, Callahan CW: Pneumonia. *Pediatr Rev* 17:300–324, 1996.

Bacteremia and Sepsis

21. Kuppermann N: Occult bacteremia in young febrile children. *Pediatr Clin North Am* 46:1073–1109, 1999.
22. Baraff LJ, Bass JW, Fleisher GR, et al: Practice guideline for the management of infants and children 0–36 months of age with fever without source. *Ann Emerg Med* 22:1198–1210, 1993.
23. Bauchner H, Pelton SJ: Management of the young febrile child: a continuing controversy. *Pediatrics* 100:137–138, 1997.
24. McCarthy PL, Lembo RM, Baron MA, et al: Predictive value of abnormal physical examination findings in ill-appearing and well-appearing febrile children. *Pediatrics* 76:167–171, 1985.
25. Talan DA: New concepts of antimicrobial therapy for emergency department infections. *Ann Emerg Med* 34:503, 1999.

Meningitis

26. Schuchat A, Robinson K, Winger JD, et al: Bacterial meningitis in United States in 1995. *N Engl J Med* 337:970–976, 1997.
27. Talan DA, Gutterman JJ, Overturf GD, et al: Analysis of emergency department management of suspected bacterial meningitis. *Ann Emerg Med* 18:856–862, 1989.
28. Quagliarello VJ, Scheld WM: Treatment of bacterial meningitis. *N Engl J Med* 336:708–716, 1997.

Urinary Tract Infections

29. Shaw KN, Gorelick MH: Urinary tract infection in the pediatric patient. *Pediatr Clin North Am* 46:1111–1124, 1999.

30. Altieri MF, Camarca M, Mayer TA: Pediatric urinary tract infections, in Tintinalli JE, Kelen GD, Stapczynski JS (eds): *Emergency Medicine: A Comprehensive Study Guide*, 5th ed. New York: McGraw-Hill, 2000.

31. Altieri MF, Camarca MA, Bach GH: Pediatric urinary tract infections. *Pediatr Emerg Med Rep* 2:103–109, 1997.

Status Epilepticus

32. Haafiz A, Kissoon N: Status epilepticus: current concepts. *Pediatr Emerg Care* 15:119–129, 1999.

33. Treatment of convulsive status epilepticus. Recommendations of the Epilepsy Foundation of America's Working Group on Status Epilepticus. *JAMA* 270:854–859, 1993.

C H A P T E R

13
DERMATOLOGY

Tanise I. Edwards

Complaints referable to the skin are commonly seen in the urgent care setting and comprise a wide and varied differential. Fortunately, a small number of common conditions compose a vast majority of these complaints. This chapter covers some of the more common dermatologic diagnosis seen in the urgent care setting.°

OVERVIEW

In approaching the evaluation of patients with skin rashes, a detailed history is critical and may be the key to reaching a specific diagnosis. Important details to elicit on history include:

- Onset and duration of the rash
- Antecedent or concomitant illness
- Previous episodes of similar symptoms
- Home treatments or previously prescribed treatments and the response
- Any change in symptoms or distribution of rash since onset
- The presence of pruritus
- Any history of exposures: new medications, new foods, outdoor activities, new personal hygiene or laundry products, hobbies, occupational exposures, use of chemicals
- Associated symptoms: fever, cough, arthralgias, GI tract or urinary symptoms, etc.

Next, on physical examination, the location of the lesions, their pattern of distribution (see Table 13-1), and their characteristics may further narrow the differential and help formulate a working diagnosis. Specific areas to be examined include mucosal membranes; the scalp, hair, nails, palms, and soles; and covered body areas (perineum, etc.). Other aspects of the rash that should be noted on physical examination include:

- Symmetrical or asymmetrical distribution of the rash
- A distribution consistent with sun exposure

°Chapter 12, Pediatrics, covers many of the more commonly seen pediatric rashes, including impetigo, scarlet fever, roseola, rubella, measles, varicella (or chickenpox), erythema infectiosum (also known as fifth disease), and Kawasaki disease. These diagnoses, while occasionally seen in adults, are more specific to the pediatric population. Also covered in that chapter are pityriasis rosea, scabies, and eczema.

TABLE 13-1

DIFFERENTIAL DIAGNOSIS RELATIVE TO LESION DISTRIBUTION/PATTERN

DISTRIBUTION

Scalp	Trunk	Further subdivision of extremities:
Hair	Axilla	Upper vs. Lower
Face	Perineum	Proximal vs. Distal
Eyelids	Extremities	Wrists/Ankles
Mucosa (eyes, lips)	Nails	Hands/Feet
Mouth		

PATTERN

Sun-, clothing-, jewelry-, or agent-exposed	Hair-bearing	Apocrine
	Palmar plantar	Acneiform
Intertriginous	Pityriasis rosea	Acrodermatitis
Flexor/extensor		

SOURCE: Tintinalli J et al: *Emergency Medicine: A Comprehensive Study Guide*, 5th ed. New York: McGraw-Hill; 2000, with permission.

- Confluence of lesions
- Clustering
- Dermatomal patterns
- Lesion morphology (Table 13-2)
- Color
- Shape of the lesions
    Linear
    Annular (ring-like)
    Reticular (net-like or lacy)
    Serpiginous
    Bull's-eye or target-shaped

Laboratory Evaluation

Laboratory evaluations are usually not required for most dermatologic complaints seen in the urgent care setting. Laboratory tests should be considered when systemic symptoms are present in patients without a diagnosis, particularly in febrile or toxic-appearing patients. A complete blood count (CBC) with platelet count, erythrocyte sedimentation rate (ESR), prothrombin time and partial thromboplastin time (PT/PTT), urinalysis, and microbiology studies may sometimes be warranted. Patients with purpura or petechiae will generally require coagulation studies in addition to a platelet count. Depending on the morphology of the lesions and patient presentation, cultures, Wood's-light evaluation, and microscopic evaluation (with or without special preps such as Gram's stain, KOH, Tzank smear, etc.) may also be helpful in determining the diagnosis. Special laboratory tests [Lyme titers, rapid plasma reagent (RPR), etc.] are sometimes required, depending on the history and patient presentation.

TABLE 13-2

LESION MORPHOLOGY

DESCRIPTOR	MORPHOLOGY	DIFFERENTIAL CONSIDERATIONS
Macule	Flat, circumscribed discoloration 1 cm or less in diameter; color varies	—Drug eruption, nevus, tattoo, lice infestation, rheumatic fever, secondary syphilis, viral exanthem, erythema multiforme, meningococcemia, ecchymosis, tinea versicolor, cellulitis
Papule	Elevated, solid, palpable lesion less than 1 cm in diameter; color varies	—Acne, molluscum contagiosum, atopic dermatitis, urticaria, eczema, folliculitis, insect bites, poison ivy/oak/sumac, varicella, erythema multiforme, gonococcemia, vasculitis, basal cell carcinoma, melanoma, nevus, warts, skin tags
Plaque	Flat-topped elevation formed by confluence of papules greater than 0.5 cm in diameter	—Eczema, pityriasis rosea, tinea corporis, tinea versicolor, seborrheic dermatitis, urticaria, erythema multiforme, secondary syphilis, psoriasis
Nodule	Palpable solid lesion less than 1 cm in diameter	—Erythema nodosum, furuncle, lipoma, warts; basal cell, squamous cell, or metastatic carcinoma, melanoma
Wheal	Transient, edematous papule or plaque with peripheral edema	—Urticaria, angioedema, insect bites, erythema multiforme
Vesicle	Circumscribed, thin-walled, elevated blister less than 5 mm in diameter	—Herpes simplex, herpes zoster, varicella, impetigo, poison ivy/oak/sumac, scabies, burns, bullous pemphigoid, pemphigus vulgaris
Bulla	Circumscribed, thin-walled, elevated blister greater than 5 mm in diameter	—Bullous impetigo, poison ivy/oak/sumac, burns, toxic epidermal necrolysis, bullous pemphigoid, pemphigus vulgaris
Scales		—Pityriasis rosea, toxic infectious erythemas, secondary syphilis, tinea infections, tinea versicolor, dry skin, psoriasis
Crusts		—Eczema, tinea infections, impetigo, contact dermatitis, insect bites
Erosions	Ruptured vesicle/bulla with denuded epidermis	—Candidiasis, tinea infections, eczema, toxic epidermal necrolysis, erythema multiforme, brown recluse spider bite, bullous pemphigoid, pemphigus vulgaris
Ulcers	Epidermal/dermal tissue loss	—Apthous, chancroid, decubitus, friction, ischemia, primary syphilis, brown recluse spider bite, stasis ulcer, facitial, bullous pemphigoid, pemphigus vulgaris
Pustule	Vesicle containing purulent fluid	—Acne, rosacea, folliculitis, candidiasis
Petechiae	Nonblanching purple spots less than 2 mm in diameter	
Cyst	Sack containing liquid or semisolid material	
Abscess	Tender, erythematous, fluctuant nodule	
Tumor	Palpable solid lesion greater than 1 cm in diameter	

SOURCE: Tintinalli J et al: *Emergency Medicine: A Comprehensive Study Guide*, 5th ed. New York: McGraw-Hill; 2000, with permission.

Dermatologic Agents

The major dermatologic agents and indications for their use are shown in Tables 13-3 and 13-4.

TABLE 13-3

DERMATOLOGIC AGENTS AND INDICATIONS FOR THEIR USE

DERMATOLOGIC AGENTS	INDICATIONS FOR USE
Antihistamines • Diphenhydramine, hydroxyzine • (Second-generation): Loratadine, fexofenadine, cetirizine	Pruritus; allergic symptoms/reactions. (Can be administered orally, intravenously, or intramuscularly.)
H$_2$ blockers • Ranitidine, famotidine	May aid in allergic symptoms.

Topical antimicrobials
• Antibacterial:
  • Mupirocin
  • Neomycin
  • Bacitracin
  • Polymyxin B
• Antifungal:
  • Clotrimazole
  • Miconazole
  • Ketoconazole
  • Nystatin (for candidal infections)
  • Selenium sulfide
	Localized superficial bacterial or fungal infections.

Topical Corticosteroids (From lower to higher potency): • Hydrocortisone • Fluocinolone acetonide (Synalar) • Triamcinolone acetonide (Kenalog) • Fluocinomide (Lidex) • Fluocinolone (Synalar HP)	Allergic reactions/symptoms, inflammatory conditions (see Table 13-4). • *Do NOT use fluorinated steroids on the face, on infants, or on pregnant women.*
Systemic Steroids • Prednisone (oral), Prelone (oral), Solumedrol (IV or IM)	Allergic reactions/symptoms, severe inflammatory conditions (under certain circumstances). Must be aware of potential rebound effect seen in certain conditions.
Emollients • Eucerin Crème, Lac Hydrin	Dry skin.
Drying agents • Burow's solution, Aveeno, calamine lotion, zinc oxide	Weeping or oozing lesions; pruritus; can be used for its soothing effect.

TABLE 13-4

RECOMMENDATIONS OF CORTICOSTEROID POTENCY RELATIVE TO DERMATOLOGIC
DISEASE (GROUP I, HIGHEST POTENCY; GROUP VII, LOWEST POTENCY)

GROUPS I AND II	GROUPS III, IV, AND V	GROUPS VI AND VII
Psoriasis	Atopic dermatitis	Nonspecific dermatitis
Eczema, of hand	Stasis dermatitis	of face, eyelids,
(severe)	Seborrheic dermatitis	and perineum
Poison ivy (severe)	Tinea	
Atopic dermatitis	Scabies	
(severe)	Nonspecific dermatitis	
	of face (severe)	

SOURCE: Tintinalli J et al: *Emergency Medicine: A Comprehensive Study Guide*, 5th ed. New York: McGraw-Hill; 2000, with permission.

SPECIFIC DERMATOLOGIC DISORDERS AND DISEASES

Acne

Acne is a chronic inflammatory problem that is best treated by a dermatologist or primary care physician; treatment in the urgent care setting should be discouraged. Many regimens are available for the treatment of acne, and patients who present to the urgent care setting should be encouraged to follow up with their primary physician or a dermatologist. Patients with symptoms of acute infection should be treated as indicated.

Hidradenitis Suppurativa

Hidradenitis suppurativa is a disease of the apocrine sweat glands. It manifests primarily in the axillae, scalp, groin, breast, and anogenital region. Exacerbations begin with the development of inflammation, which may then progress to a cellulitis and abscess formation. *Staphylococcus* and *Streptococcus* are common pathogens found in the lesions, though groin lesions may also be positive for anaerobes and gram-negative organisms.

Characteristics: Hard, inflammatory, erythematous nodules or abscesses in the affected area, which are tender to palpation; nodules may drain spontaneously.
Associated Conditions: Obesity, poor hygiene, shaving.

 Management

Patients who have developed acute abscesses require incision, drainage, and surgical follow-up. Those patients who present with cellulitis or mild to moderate chronic disease but without abscess formation should be started on oral antibiotics. Appropriate choices include erythromycin, tetracycline, or minocycline. Antibiotic treatment may be needed for weeks. Patients should be referred for follow-up. Those who are toxic-appearing will require further evaluation and possible inpatient care.

Folliculitis

Folliculitis, an infection of the hair follicles, predominantly affects the face (particularly bearded areas), scalp, neck, legs, axillae, back, and buttocks.

Characteristics: Papules or pustules, which may rupture, causing superficial erosions and crusting; may develop into abscesses or furuncles; with acute infection, tender, erythematous nodules may be palpated on examination.

Associated Conditions: Diabetes, immunocompromised states. Seen more frequently in areas that are subject to shaving or other means of hair removal, such as waxing

If cultured, lesions may be positive for bacteria (*Staphylococcus, Pseudomonas,* gram-negative organisms), fungi, or viruses (herpesvirus). Cultures are not necessarily needed with straightforward, routine cases in healthy individuals; cultures should be sent if the lesions require incision and drainage or if the patient is immunosuppressed or has systemic symptoms.

 Management

Superficial folliculitis can be treated with warm soaks and topical antibiotics, such as mupirocin ointment, to the affected area twice a day. More severe forms should be treated with oral antibiotics (dicloxacillin, cephalexin, or erythromycin). If an abscess has formed, incision and drainage will be required.

Hot-Tub Folliculitis

Hot-tub folliculitis is caused by *Pseudomonas aeruginosa.* It is typically seen following the use of poorly maintained or communal hot tubs. Hot-tub folliculitis tends to resolve spontaneously but may be treated with ciprofloxacin 500 mg PO bid.

Apthous Ulcers

Apthous ulcers are painful, ulcerative lesions of the mucosal tissue.

Characteristics: Shallow, discrete ulcers with a sharp, erythematous edge that may be edematous. There may be a gray-white fibrinous coating centrally. Apthous ulcers can occur as single lesions or in multiples. Oral lesions are most frequently seen on the buccal or labial mucosa but may also occur on the floor of the mouth, the gums, or the tongue. Patients may report a history of antecedent tingling or burning prior to the appearance of the ulcers.

Associated Symptoms: Local mucosal trauma, stress; cervical adenopathy may be present.

 Management

Small ulcers tend to heal spontaneously. Symptomatic treatment includes topical Kenalog in orabase or diphenhydramine elixirs. Oral pain medications may also be used

as indicated. Patients should be encouraged to maintain good fluid intake in order to avoid dehydration.

Toxicodendron or *Rhus* Dermatitis (Poison Ivy/ Poison Oak/ Poison Sumac)

Toxicodendron dermatitis represents an acute contact dermatitis to the *Toxicodendron* plant species, which include poison ivy, poison oak, and poison sumac. It is contact with the milky sap found in these plants that causes the reaction, with symptoms appearing anywhere from 8 h to 10 days following exposure. (Typically, symptoms begin within 2 days of exposure.) Removal of the sap within 30 min of contact may help prevent a reaction.

> **Characteristics:** Lesions can range anywhere from mild erythema to erythematous papules to papulovesicular lesions to frank bullae. Intense pruritus is usually associated with the lesions; this itching may actually begin prior to the onset of a frank rash.

> **Distinguishing Feature**
>
> Papulovesicular lesions occurring in a linear configuration.

Toxicodendron dermatitis is a clinical diagnosis; laboratory studies are not necessary unless a secondary infection has developed and the patient appears toxic or has underlying disease.

 Management

Symptomatic treatment with topical agents such as calamine lotion is often all that is necessary. Cool compresses made from Aveeno baths or Burow's solution may also help provide relief from the itching, along with drying of any weeping lesions. Oral antihistamines may be needed if intense itching is present, particularly if there is evidence of excoriation. Patients with a history of severe reactions in the past, those who present with periorbital or genital lesions, and patients who have developed a severe dermatitis with a widespread distribution of bullae and vesicles will benefit from a course of systemic corticosteroids such as prednisone 40 to 60 mg/day (2 mg/kg/day in pediatric patients). Systemic corticosteroids require a 2- to 3-week course of treatment. Shorter courses may lead to a more severe rebound exacerbation.

Some patients develop a secondary id reaction or additional lesions over several days after onset of symptoms. This has led to the erroneous assumption that fluid contained in the vesicles is contagious. Note, however, that while the vesicle fluid is not contagious, the oils of the plant can remain on clothing or under unwashed nails for days to weeks, causing continued exposure or reexposure.

Contact Dermatitis

Contact dermatitis is an inflammatory disorder caused by irritants or antigens affecting the skin. Hands are the most commonly involved area of the body. Contact dermatitis can be an acute process or a chronic or recurrent illness. Pruritus is a common symptom and can be intense; pain can also develop as lesions ulcerate or skin fissuring occurs, or if the area becomes infected. Common causes of contact dermatitis include perfumed soaps, chemicals, foods, nickel (in jewelry), neomycin, rubber, and persistent exposure to moisture.

Characteristics: Lesions can vary in morphology from erythematous papules and plaques to nonumbilicated vesicles. These may begin to weep, leaking serum. At times, the rash can have a scaly, papulosquamous appearance. Fissuring can occur, as well as excoriation.

 Management

Contact dermatitis can be difficult to treat if the etiologic agent cannot be diagnosed or if contact with the irritant cannot be avoided. Topical steroids are used to treat mild to moderate cases of contact dermatitis, but severe cases may require systemic therapy over a 2-week period. Cool compresses with Burow's solution may provide some relief of the itching. Antihistamines should be prescribed as indicated by symptoms. Removal of the irritant is key to resolution.

Erythema Multiforme

Erythema multiforme (EM) is an inflammatory disease that develops secondary to infection, medication use (sulfonamides, barbiturates, penicillin, phenytoin), or malignancy.

Characteristics: The rash of EM is one of erythematous lesions in a symmetrical distribution; these are found primarily on the extensor surfaces, palms, and soles. The lesions may present as macules, papules, vesicles, or bullae. They may be painful or pruritic. If there is involvement of mucosal membranes, the disease is known as Steven-Johnson syndrome.

Distinguishing Feature

Classic "iris" or "target lesion": erythematous plaques with bright red borders and a dusky center.

 Management

Any inciting factors should be identified and removed. Symptomatic treatment with anti-inflammatories and analgesic may be all that is needed in mild cases. Compresses made with Burow's solution may provide some relief from the itching and pain. Systemic steroids are not recommended for minor cases of EM. Patients with a severe manifestation of EM will require transfer for inpatient care.

Tinea Versicolor

Tinea versicolor is a common superficial fungal infection seen more frequently in warmer temperatures and more humid conditions.

Characteristics: Lesions are typically hypo- or hyperpigmented macules with a scaly appearance; they are round to oval in shape. The lesions are usually multiple and are commonly scattered on the chest, back, abdomen, proximal extremities, and neck. Lesions can also involve the groin and scalp but are uncommon on the face. There may be an associated mild pruritus. Patients will often note that they are unable to tan on the involved skin.

Diagnosis

The diagnosis can often be made on the basis of clinical appearance. Scraping of the lesions and microscopic evaluation using KOH will demonstrate the presence of spores and short mycelia. Wood's-light evaluation may reveal fluorescence.

 Management

This condition can be treated with topical agents such as selenium sulfide (2.5%) lotion or shampoo; it should be applied to the affected area for at least 10 min a day (then showered off) for a period of 1 to 2 weeks. Alternatively, "azole" creams (ketoconazole, clotrimazole, miconazole) can be applied to the affected area once daily for 2 weeks. Oral treatment with ketoconazole can also be used but is not without risk and is better left to the dermatologist or primary care physician. Recurrences are not uncommon.

Molluscum Contagiosum

Molluscum contagiosum is a viral disease affecting the epidermis; it is caused by one of the poxviruses. These lesions are contagious via skin-to-skin contact.

Characteristics: Multiple papular, skin-colored lesions (mollusca) that are round, oval, or hemispheric in shape. Molluscum contagiosum may occur as a single lesion or as multiple lesions scattered over the body (most frequently on the face, trunk, and extremities). HIV-positive individuals may develop hundreds of mollusca. In adults, lesions may be found in areas of the groin and genitalia. They may be seen more frequently in wrestlers.

Distinguishing Feature

Pedunculated lesions with a white core and central umbilication.

 Management

Diagnosis can usually be made by clinical examination. In healthy individuals, the lesions are self-limited and resolve spontaneously (over months). In the urgent care setting, the goal of evaluation is diagnosis and education of the patient on the disease. More aggressive treatment includes curettage, cryosurgery, or electrodesiccation.

As molluscum contagiosum is spread via direct skin contact, patients should be cautioned to avoid skin-to-skin contact with others. The lesions can be spread by casual as well as sexual contact.

Tinea Corporis

Tinea corporis is a superficial fungal infection most commonly found on the trunk, arms, and legs. Transmission can occur via autoinoculation; through contact with infected persons, animals, or contaminated soil; or via contact with contaminated items such as shared towels.

Characteristics: The lesions of tinea corporis are typically sharply marginated plaques or papulosquamous lesions that may be singular or multiple. They are annular in shape, with central clearing and raised borders. They may be scaly or crusting and may develop small vesicles at their margins.

Diagnosis

Diagnosis can often be made clinically based on the appearance of the classic "ringworm" lesion; a scraping examined under the microscope using KOH will show budding yeast or hyphae. Wood's-light evaluation may show fluorescence of the lesions, though not all types (i.e., *Trichophyton*) will fluoresce.

 Management

Treatment is with topical antifungals such as clotrimazole, miconazole, or ketoconazole. Oral regimens are sometimes needed but are not without risks and may better be initiated by the primary care physician.

Lice

Lice appear as an infestation that can affect the head, body, or pubic area. Infestation of the hair and scalp is caused by *Pediculus capitis*; pubic infestation is caused by *Pthirus pubis*.

Head Lice

Infestation with *head lice* is spread by direct contact as well as by the sharing of combs, brushes, hats, and pillows.

Symptoms: Itching; scaling, crusting, and excoriated pustules, particularly on the occipital neck; posterior cervical adenopathy may be present. Nits, which are firmly adherent to hair shafts, and lice can be seen in the hair; live nits will fluoresce with Wood's-light examination.

Management Topical insecticides such as permethrin 1% cream rinse (Nix) or pyrethrins (Rid) can be used in the treatment of lice. Medication alone, however, will not "cure" the condition—*removal of the nits with fine-tooth comb is essential*. All household members should be checked and treated as indicated. It is imperative that household items be treated: clothing, bed linen, towels, etc., require washing in hot water and drying on hot cycles. Floors and furniture must be thoroughly vacuumed; combs and brushes must be soaked in hot water (over 20 to 30 min) or treated with insecticidal agents. Stuffed animals, pillows, etc., should be placed in a closed plastic bag for 21 days. Patients should be reevaluated in 7 to 10 days and will often require retreatment.

Pubic Lice

Infestation with *pubic lice* is spread through close physical contact, including shared beds and sexual contact.

Symptoms: Severe nocturnal pruritus; small erythematous papules may be noted in involved areas. Infestation can involve the eyelashes, axillae, and periumbilical areas. *Maculae ceruleae*, which are blue-hued macules, may be seen on the lower abdomen, buttocks, and proximal thighs. Embedded lice may be noted in the skin of the involved areas, or nits may be seen adherent to hair shafts. Eyelash involvement will show lice and nits adherent to the lashes.

Management As discussed above for head lice *except* for involvement of the eyelashes. Eyelashes should be treated with petroleum jelly or ophthalmic ointment twice daily for 10 days. All sexual contacts should be treated. Again, nit removal is key to treatment, as is decontamination of household items.

Lyme Disease

Lyme disease is a systemic infection spread through the bite of the *Ixodes* tick (deer tick). The offending organism is the spirochete *Borrelia burgdorferi*. Lyme disease, like syphilis, can be a great imitator, presenting in different stages and with different clinical manifestations. There may be a history of an antecedent tick bite, but the majority of patients diagnosed with Lyme disease recall no history of tick exposure. The majority of cases are seen in the spring and summer months, when outside activity is highest. Early, localized disease may present with symptoms of a viral febrile illness (headache, malaise, myalgias) and possibly the rash of erythema chronicum migrans (ECM). Later manifestations (weeks to months or years) include arthritis, neurologic complaints (cranial or peripheral neuropathies, aseptic meningitis), and carditis (including atrioventricular blocks).

Distinguishing Feature of Early Lyme Disease

Erythema chronicum migrans: an erythematous macular or papular lesion at the site of the bite which expands to leave a central clearing—the bull's-eye lesion; usually > 5 cm in diameter.

Characteristics: ECM can develop up to a month after tick exposure. While it is typically round or oval in shape, it can also be triangular. There may be a central punctate lesion at the site of the tick bite. ECM is typically neither painful nor pruritic. The edges may be raised.

Making the diagnosis of Lyme disease can be extremely difficult. At times, the diagnosis is clear-cut, i.e., a history of a tick bite from the deer tick, the classic nonspecific early symptoms including a low-grade fever, and the rash of ECM. What becomes more difficult is diagnosing those patients who present with nonspecific symptoms, no antecedent history of tick exposure, and no rash, or those patients who present in later stages of the disease and give no history of tick exposure. In the urgent care setting, maintaining a high index of suspicion for Lyme disease and referral for close follow-up is key. The approach to diagnosis will vary with patient presentation and the likelihood of a possible exposure. Serology testing includes enzyme-linked immunosorbent assay (ELISA), indirect fluorescent antibody (IFA), and Western blot tests; results may be negative depending on the timing in relation to the disease course. Consultation with an infectious disease specialist may be warranted for developing a treatment strategy including diagnostic testing and patient management.

 Management

Early Lyme disease can be treated with amoxicillin, doxycycline, cefuroxime axetil, erythromycin, azithromycin, or amoxicillin-clavulanate. Antibiotics should be administered for 10 to 30 days. Early disseminated disease without meningitis or high-degree heart block can also be treated with oral antibiotics, but this should be done only in consultation with the infectious disease specialist. Patients presenting with symptoms of meningitis, high-grade atrioventricular block, or radiculoneuritis require admission for intravenous antibiotic treatment.

Physical examination should include a search for the tick and its removal if found.

Shingles

Shingles are a reactivation of latent varicella zoster. Older patients and patients who are immunocompromised are most commonly affected, but the disease can occur in patients of all ages.

Characteristics: The rash of shingles is typically preceded by pain or paresthesias along the course of the affected dermatome. This prodrome of pain is followed by the development of the characteristic lesions seen in shingles. The rash initially begins with papular erythematous lesions that progress to form grouped vesicles and pustules and then crusting. The lesions develop along a unilateral dermatomal distribution and may cluster or coalesce. The thorax is the most commonly affected body site. If lesions are noted at the tip of the nose, the nasociliary branch of the trigeminal nerve is involved, indicating the potential for the development of ophthalmic zoster.

Distinguishing Feature

Dermatomal distribution of painful vesicular lesions on an erythematous base

---

 Management

Most cases of shingles can easily be diagnosed by physical examination once the lesions develop. The diagnosis is more difficult to make in the prodromal stage but should be

considered in any individual complaining of superficial burning pain in a dermatomal distribution. Antivirals such as acyclovir 800 mg PO every 5 h for 7 to 10 days have been noted to hasten healing and decrease the incidence of postherpetic pain if given within 48 h of the onset of the rash. Patients with ophthalmic involvement or lesions at the tip of the nose should receive slit-lamp evaluation with fluoroscein staining and ophthalmologic consultation. Ophthalmic zoster and patients who are immunocompromised should be admitted for intravenous acyclovir. Patients who are treated on an outpatient basis may require narcotic medication for pain control. Cool compresses with Burow's solution may provide some symptomatic relief.

Erysipelas

Erysipelas is a soft tissue infection caused by group A beta-hemolytic streptococci.

> **Characteristics:** Fiery red plaque with raised, sharply demarcated edges. The area is tender, with induration, and may appear hot to the touch. The rash is most commonly found on the lower extremities and face. Patients may complain of a prodrome of fever, chills, and malaise prior to the onset of the rash.

 Management

The diagnosis of erysipelas is generally made based on clinical history and examination. Adjunct labs, including a CBC, blood cultures, and antistreptolysin-O titers (ASO) may be warranted, depending on the patient's clinical appearance and underlying health. In nontoxic, healthy individuals, a trial of outpatient treatment is usually warranted. An initial dose of parenteral antibiotics can be instituted in the urgent care setting prior to discharge. Pencillin VK, dicloxacillin, or cephalixin are appropriate first choices for outpatient management. Erythromycin can be used in penicillin-allergic patients. Additionally, patients should be treated with antipyretics and analgesics as needed. Warm compresses should be applied to the affected area. Follow-up should be within 24 h or sooner for worsening. Patients who are toxic or with underlying disease may require inpatient treatment.

Disseminated Gonococcal Infection (DGI)

Disseminated gonococcal disease is a systemic infection caused by hematogenous spread of *Neisseria gonorrhoeae* from an untreated mucosal infection. Patients present with fever, chills, skin lesions, and symptoms of migratory polyarthralgias (asymmetrical), septic arthritis, and tenosynovitis.

> **Characteristics:** Lesions typically present as erythematous macules that progress to hemorrhagic, necrotic pustules over 1 to 2 days. Lesions can be seen near the small joints of the hands and feet, on the arms, and on the legs. The most commonly involved joints for septic arthritis are the knees, ankles, and wrists; involvement of the metacarpophalangeal and interphalangeal joints may also be seen. Gonococcal meningitis and endocarditis can occur.

> Diagnosis of DGI is primarily clinical, but cultures of mucosal sites (urethra, cervix, and at times the throat) are usually positive.

Management

Patients with DGI generally require inpatient treatment initially using an antigonococcal antibiotic regimen. Patients should be cultured and treated for *Chlamydia* as well.

Erythema Nodosum

Erythema nodosum is an inflammatory condition that occurs in the subcutaneous fat tissue. It is associated with infectious disorders (including beta-hemolytic strep and *Yersinia*), medications (including sulfonamides and oral contraceptives), and inflammatory diseases such as sarcoidosis, lymphoma, and ulcerative colitis.

> **Characteristics:** Lesions present as palpable nodules in the subcutaneous fat; they are associated with an erythematous appearance of the overlying skin. The nodules may be tender and indurated; distribution is usually bilateral and is seen more frequently on the extensor surfaces of the lower legs, the knees, and the arms. There may be associated fever, malaise, and arthralgia of the ankle joints.

 Management

The diagnosis of erythema nodosum can be made on the basis of the clinical picture, though cultures for underlying infection (strep, *Yersinia*, etc.) should be considered. A chest x-ray should be ordered to rule out evidence of sarcoid, tuberculosis, or hilar adenopathy. Any underlying disease processes should be treated and any potentially offending agents/drugs stopped. Spontaneous resolution generally occurs over the course of 6 to 8 weeks but may take months, depending on etiology. Treatment therefore is symptomatic and includes rest, elevation, compressive bandages, and anti-inflammatory agents. The use of systemic corticosteroids should be initiated only in consultation with and on the recommendation of the referring physician.

Moles in the Urgent Care Setting

At times, patients will present to the urgent care setting for the evaluation of a mole. This may be the presenting chief complaint or may come as a request in passing while being seen for another complaint. Given the potential for morbidity and mortality that can occur with improper diagnosis, extreme caution should be exercised in the evaluation of mole lesions without biopsy. When patients present for evaluation of moles, unless the lesion is a *classic* seborrheic keratosis or skin tag, they should be referred to a dermatologist for evaluation and biopsy as needed.

BIBLIOGRAPHY

Edwards L: *Dermatology in Emergency Care.* New York: Churchill Livingstone; 1997.
Fitzpatrick TB et al: *Color Atlas and Synopsis of Clinical Dermatology,* 3d ed. New York: McGraw-Hill; 2000.

Freedberg IM, Eisen AZ, Wolff K, et al (eds): *Fitzpatrick's Dermatology in General Medicine,* 5th ed. New York: McGraw-Hill; 1999.

Habif TP: *Clinical Dermatology*, 3d ed. St. Louis: Mosby; 1995.

Hurwitz A: Erythema multiforme: A review of its characteristics, diagnostic criteria and management. *Pediatr Rev* 11:217, 1990.

Knoop K, Stack LB, Storrow AB: *Atlas of Emergency Medicine*. New York: McGraw-Hill; 1997.

Resnick SD: Poison ivy and poison oak dermatitis. *Clin Dermatol* 4:208, 1986.

Tintinalli J et al: *Emergency Medicine: A Comprehensive Study Guide,* 5th ed. New York: McGraw-Hill; 2000.

14

GASTROENTEROLOGY

Z. Colette Edwards

The focus of the urgent care physician in evaluating patients with gastrointestinal (GI) disease or symptoms should be on the expeditious, high-quality, cost-effective diagnosis of the presenting complaints. Appropriate stabilization and emergency triage, or appropriate treatment and referral for subsequent care, as indicated, should follow this initial evaluation. Patients with GI complaints will generally fall into one of three classes, those in which:

1. Emergency treatment is needed
   - Unstable patients
   - Patients requiring hospital admission
   - Patients requiring specialty consultation on an emergent basis
2. Urgent care treatment is appropriate
3. Primary care physician referral for further evaluation and ongoing treatment is indicated

The first step in evaluating patients who present in the urgent care setting with gastrointestinal symptoms should be a detailed, GI-focused history, followed by a comprehensive GI-focused physical examination (Tables 14-1 and 14-2).

	TABLE 14-1

THE GI HISTORY—KEY POINTS OF DOCUMENTATION

Family History	Colon cancer, gallbladder disease, inflammatory bowel disease, liver disease
Social History	Tobacco, alcohol, and/or intravenous drug use/abuse, anal intercourse, travel
Past Medical History	Previous GI surgery, inflammatory bowel disease, cancer, menstrual cycle, lactose intolerance, esophageal varices, chronic liver disease
Diet	Fat, caffeine, and/or peppermint/spearmint intake, fiber intake, history of food intolerance
Symptoms	Abdominal pain, nausea and vomiting, change in bowel habits, weight loss/gain, acholic stool, heartburn, hematochezia/melena, coffee-ground emesis/hematemesis, fever, pruritus, easy bruising, dysphagia
Medications	NSAID/steroid use, recent antibiotic therapy, anticoagulants

TABLE 14-2

THE PHYSICAL EXAMINATION—KEY POINTS OF DOCUMENTATION

The abdominal exam	Pain on palpation of abdomen
The rectal exam	Organomegaly
The Presence *or* Absence of	Jaundice
Hypotension	Ascites
Orthostatic vital sign changes in blood pressure and heart rate	Palmar erythema
	Spider angiomata
Tachycardia	Purpura
Diaphoresis	Heme-positive stool

- One of the most helpful maneuvers the urgent care physician can make is to listen carefully to the patient, who will often provide the answers needed to make an accurate diagnosis. Failure to heed a patient's words may needlessly delay an evaluation or result in inappropriate treatment and/or unnecessary testing.

 Errors to Avoid

- Failure to consider a non-GI diagnosis in a patient with GI symptoms
- Reluctance to perform a rectal or anoscopic examination
- Reluctance to perform a pelvic examination
- Reluctance to obtain a sexual history
- Incomplete or abbreviated evaluation of "bounceback" patients
- Failure to obtain
  - Sexual history
  - Family history of GI disease
  - Travel history
  - History of tobacco, alcohol, and/or intravenous drug use
  - History of GI surgery

Common laboratory and x-ray studies that are helpful in the evaluation of patients presenting with GI symptoms or disease are given in Tables 14-3 and 14-4, respectively. Drugs commonly used in the treatment of GI disease are listed in Table 14-5.

TABLE 14-3

COMMON LABORATORY TESTS HELPFUL IN THE EVALUATION OF PATIENTS PRESENTING WITH GI SYMPTOMS OR DISEASE

CBC with differential and platelets	ESR
SMA-7	PT/PTT
LFTs-ALT/AST, bilirubin, total protein/ albumin, alkaline phosphatase, and LDH	Stool Gram stain (for detection of white blood cells)
Amylase and lipase	Tests for occult blood in stool

KEY: CBC, complete blood count; SMA-7, $Na^+/K^+/Cl^-/CO_2$/Glucose/BUN/Creatine; LFT, liver function test; ALT/AST, alanine aminotransferase/aspartate dehydrogenase; LDH, lactate dehydrogenase; ESR, erythrocyte sedimentation rate; PT, prothrombin time; PTT, partial thromboplastin time.

TABLE 14-4

COMMON X-RAY STUDIES IN THE EVALUATION OF PATIENTS PRESENTING WITH GI SYMPTOMS OR DISEASE

KUB and flat plate of the abdomen
Upright chest film (evaluates for free air under the diaphragm)

TABLE 14-5

DRUGS COMMONLY USED IN GASTROINTESTINAL DISEASE

DRUG TYPE	COMMONLY USED IN	USUAL DOSAGE (PO UNLESS OTHERWISE SPECIFIED)
H_2 *blockers*	*Acid-peptic disease*	
Zantac (ranitidine)		150 mg bid (acute); 150 mg qd (maintenance)
Pepcid (famotidine)		20 mg bid (acute); 20 mg qd (maintenance)
Tagamet (cimetidine)		300 mg qid or 400 mg bid or 800 mg qhs (acute); 400 mg qd (maintenance)
Axid (nizatidine)		150 mg bid (acute); 150 mg qd (maintenance)
Proton-pump inhibitors	*Acid-peptic disease; Zollinger-Ellison syndrome (ZES)*	
Prilosec (omeprazole)		20–40 mg qd; ≥ 60 mg qd in ZES
Prevacid (lansoprazole)		15–30 mg qd; ≥ 60 mg qd in ZES
Aciphex (rabeprazole)		20 mg qd; ≥ 60 mg qd in ZES
Protonix (pantoprazole)		40 mg qd; erosive esophagitis
Nexium (esomeprazole)		
Prokinetic/Promotility agents	*Acid-peptic disease; motility disorders; nausea and vomiting*	
Reglan (metoclopramide)		10 mg qid 30 min ac and qhs
Anti-inflammatory agents	*Inflammatory bowel disease*	
Azulfidine (sulfasalazine)		1 g qid (acute flare); 1 g bid (maintenance)
Pentasa (mesalamine)		1 g qid
Dipentum (olsalazine)		1 g bid
Asacol (mesalamine)		800 mg tid
Rowasa (mesalamine)		500 mg supp pr bid; 4 g suspension enema qhs
Remicade (infliximab)		5 mg/kg IV over at least 2 h; for fistulizing Crohn's, 5 mg/kg IV over at least 2 h at 0 weeks, 2 weeks, and 6 weeks
Immunosuppressive antimetabolites	*Inflammatory bowel disease*	
Imuran (azathioprine)		2.5 mg/kg/day
6-MP (mercaptopurine)		1.0–1.5 mg/kg/day

TABLE 14-5

(continued)

DRUGS COMMONLY USED IN GASTROINTESTINAL DISEASE

DRUG TYPE	COMMONLY USED IN	USUAL DOSAGE (PO UNLESS OTHERWISE SPECIFIED)
Anti–H. pylori *agent*	*Helicobacter pylori*	
Helidac (bismuth 262.4 mg tablets + tetracycline 500 mg capsules + metronidazole 250 mg tablets)		Four doses qd (at meals and bedtime); please note that 1 dose consists of 4 pills and each blister pack contains 4 doses
Tritec (ranitidine + bismuth)		400 mg bid
Prevpac (lansoprazole 30 mg + amoxicillin 500 mg + clarithromycin 500 mg)		daily administration pack
Hepatitis agents	*Hepatitis*	
Intron A (interferon alfa-2b)	Hepatitis B and hepatitis C	Hepatitis B: 5 million IU qd IM or SC or 10 million IU TIW Hepatitis C: 3 million IU TIW SC or IM
Rebetron (interferon alfa-2b + ribavirin)	Hepatitis C	Body weight ≤ 75 kg: 400 mg PO q am and 600 mg PO q pm + 3 million IU 3 times weekly SC Body weight > 75 kg: 600 mg PO q am + 600 mg PO q pm + 3 million IU 3 times weekly SC

TIW: Three times a week.

GASTROINTESTINAL EMERGENCIES

- GI bleeding
- GI tract perforation
- Biliary tract sepsis
- Foreign-body ingestion
- Food impaction

Gastrointestinal Bleeding

Clinical Presentation

GI bleeding can be characterized as life-threatening or non-life-threatening and can present either acutely or as a chronic condition. Acute bleeds may be ongoing, self-limited, or stuttering in nature. In contrast, a chronic bleed may be active or episodic. Patients complaining of GI bleeding may have multiple presentations depending on the site, severity, and duration of bleeding. In evaluating a patient with GI bleeding, it is important to assess him or her immediately for hemodynamic stability. Changes in orthostatic blood pressure and heart rate imply at least a 10 percent depletion in intravascular volume and the need for hospital transfer for further stabilization and evaluation. Depending on their underlying health status and the onset and duration of bleeding, patients exhibiting hemodynamic changes may also complain of diaphoresis, angina, presyncopal symptoms, or frank syncope.

- Patients with evidence of a microcytic anemia resulting from a GI bleed may present with complaints of chest pain, shortness of breath, fatigue, or weakness rather than a history of overt bleeding.

After the acute evaluation for hemodynamic stability, it is important to determine the patient's definition of bleeding, the duration and frequency of symptoms, the existence of risk factors for GI bleeding, and the presence of any associated symptoms.

- Risk factors for GI bleeding include the use of nonsteroidal anti-inflammatory drugs (NSAIDs), history of peptic ulcer disease, varices, a recent endoscopic procedure, vomiting, inflammatory bowel disease, a history of other GI pathology, and hemorrhoids.

Although there is no absolute correlation between the characteristics of blood in the GI tract and the site of bleeding, some signs may be useful to help determine the likely site of bleeding. For instance, upper-GI bleeding will often present as coffee-ground emesis, hematemesis, and/or melenic stool, though a very rapid upper-GI bleed can present as bright red blood per rectum (BRBPR). Lower-GI-tract bleeding, in contrast, will often manifest as maroon or burgundy-colored fecal material, clotted blood, or BRBPR. A detailed description of the stool's appearance (i.e., blood described as coating the outside of a normal stool versus bloody stools or frank melena) may also aid in identifying the exact site of bleeding.

- Of note, it requires at least 100 mL of blood to develop a melenic stool.

The differential diagnosis of GI bleeding is given in Table 14-6.

TABLE 14-6

DIFFERENTIAL DIAGNOSIS OF GASTROINTESTINAL BLEEDING

CAUSES OF GASTROINTESTINAL BLEEDING— UPPER GI TRACT	CAUSES OF GASTROINTESTINAL BLEEDING— LOWER GI TRACT
Acid-peptic disease—"itis," ulcer, reflux disease	Diverticular disease
Mallory-Weiss tear	Cancer
Varices	Benign neoplasm (e.g., polyp)
Medications—NSAIDs, anticoagulants	Hemorrhoids
Alcohol	Fissure
Cancer	Colitis—inflammatory bowel disease, ischemic, infectious, radiation
Arteriovenous malformation	Arteriovenous malformation
Dieulafoy's lesion	Meckel's diverticulum
Vascular-enteric fistula	Brisk upper-GI bleed
Trauma	Trauma
Oropharyngeal bleeding	

TABLE 14-7

PHYSICAL EXAMINATION FOR GI BLEED—KEY POINTS OF DOCUMENTATION

1. Vital signs with orthostatics
2. Findings on abdominal examination
3. Ear/nose/throat, cardiac, and genitourinary examinations as indicated
4. Rectal examination (including the presence of hemorrhoids, fissures, or masses)
5. Results of stool heme testing
6. Hematocrit

On physical examination, it is important, in addition to performing a thorough abdominal examination, to also perform cardiovascular, pulmonary, genitourinary, and basic ear/nose/throat examinations, which may help to identify non-GI pathology (Table 14-7). A digital rectal exam and anoscopy are also important tools for the detection and evaluation of rectal pathology such as hemorrhoids, fissures, or masses.

Laboratory and Ancillary Evaluations
A complete blood count (CBC) with differential and platelets should be obtained in virtually all patients complaining of GI bleeding. Liver function tests (LFTs), prothrombin time (PT), and partial thromboplastin time (PTT), while generally not available on a stat basis in the urgent care setting, may also be indicated depending on the clinical scenario. Blood chemistries are helpful for the evaluation of hydration, and an elevated blood urea nitrogen (BUN) can be seen in upper-GI bleeding. A fecal sample should be obtained and heme tested, since iron, bismuth, beets, certain food dyes, and charcoal can all blacken the stools. In contrast, red meat, raw vegetables, and fruit may produce false-positive results. Placement of a nasogastric tube should be done to help establish the site of bleeding and assess whether the bleeding is active at the time of presentation. Patients with complaints of cardiac symptoms, the elderly, and patients with a cardiac history require electrocardiographic (ECG) evaluation to help rule out evidence of cardiac compromise related to blood loss.

Treatment and Disposition (Tables 14-8 and 14-9)
Establishment of two large-bore intravenous lines (i.e., ≤18 Fr or large enough for blood transfusion) is mandatory for all patients presenting with acute, active, and large-

TABLE 14-8

MANAGEMENT OF ACUTE GI BLEED WITH HEMODYNAMIC INSTABILITY

1. Fluid resuscitation with crystalloid through two large-bore IV lines
2. Continuous cardiac monitoring
3. Frequent checking of vital signs
4. Oxygen supplementation with pulse oximetry monitoring
5. Mast trousers as indicated
6. Early notification of emergency medical services and emergency department for transport

volume bleeding or with hemodynamic instability. Fluid resuscitation should be started using crystalloid agents, with frequent monitoring of vital signs. Depending on the age of the patient, the symptoms, and the presence/absence of a cardiac history or underlying disease, oxygen supplementation may also be indicated, along with continuous cardiac monitoring. These patients should immediately be triaged to an emergency department for further stabilization, evaluation, and admission. The receiving facility should be notified as soon as possible of the transport and the hemodynamic condition of the patient. The threshold for transfer should be lower for patients with a history of esophageal varices or stuttering bleeding episodes for several days prior to presentation. Those with evidence of cardiopulmonary compromise or chronic liver disease also warrant transfer for ongoing care.

Patients with no evidence of significant blood loss or ongoing bleeding and who are stable can usually undergo evaluation as outpatients. Prior to discharge, however, arrangements should be made for prompt evaluation and follow-up by their primary care physician (PCP) or GI specialist. Potentially offending agents (e.g., NSAIDs) that may be causative or contributory should be discontinued, if possible, pending workup. Those in whom acid-peptic disease is suspected should be started on H_2-blocker or proton-pump inhibitor (PPI) therapy (see Table 14-3, "Drugs Commonly Used in Gastrointestinal Disease").

TABLE 14-9

GI BLEEDING—CRITERIA FOR DISCHARGE

1. No significant blood loss	4. No underlying medical problems or risk factors
2. No evidence of ongoing bleeding	
3. Hemodynamic stability	5. Arranged follow-up

 Key Points of Documentation in Discharge Instruction

- Advise not to use NSAIDs
- Make follow-up arrangements
- List criteria for reevaluation (recurrent bleeding, light-headedness, abdominal pain, new or worsening symptoms)

 Errors to Avoid

- Failure to recognize hemodynamic instability, leading to delay in transfer for definitive care.
- Failure to recognize hypovolemia with normal or elevated blood pressure.
- Failure to recognize high-risk patients with the potential for acute deterioration.
- Failure to recognize chronic GI bleeding presenting as anemia.
- Failure to identify vaginal bleeding as a presentation of GI bleeding.

- Failure to identify an ENT source as a cause of GI tract blood.
- Attributing a significant lower-GI bleed to hemorrhoids or fissures. *Major lower-GI bleeding is usually not due to these entities.*
- Assuming that a normal CBC rules out a significant or life-threatening GI bleed. *Patients with an acute GI bleed may have a normal CBC, depending on the timing of their presentation and the duration and rapidity of bleeding.*
- Failure to place a nasogastric tube secondary to the presumption that BRBPR excludes the diagnosis of an upper-GI bleed.
- Assuming that a clear nasogastric tube aspirate rules out an active or ongoing GI bleed.

GI Tract Perforation

Patients with perforation or impending rupture of the GI tract often present with complaints of severe abdominal pain, nausea, vomiting, fever, and change in bowel habits. Perforations can occur anywhere along the GI tract, from the esophagus to the rectum. The differential includes peptic ulcer disease, gallbladder disease, ingested foreign bodies, inflammatory bowel disease, appendicitis, and acute diverticulitis. On physical examination, patients may have evidence of hemodynamic compromise related to fluid shifts and sepsis. Important laboratory tests for the evaluation include CBC with differential and platelets, SMA-7, and an amylase. Abdominal films (flat and upright), along with an upright chest film, should be obtained to assess for free air, which may make the diagnosis of perforation.

- A posterior gastric perforation may erode into the pancreas and not produce evidence of free air on x-ray.

Any patient who presents with symptoms or signs suggesting perforation or an impending perforation should immediately be triaged and transferred for surgical consultation (Table 14-10). While awaiting transfer, two large-bore intravenous lines for fluid administration should be placed and broad-spectrum antibiotics started. The urgent care physician's responsibility in providing care to a patient having or suspected of having GI tract perforation is stabilization and prompt transfer to an acute care setting for surgical consultation. If at all possible, consultation should be arranged prior to transfer to help facilitate timely surgical management.

TABLE 14-10

SUSPECTED GI TRACT PERFORATION—ACUTE MANAGEMENT

1. Fluid resuscitation with crystalloid solution through large-bore IV lines
2. Frequent vital signs
3. Broad-spectrum antibiotic [e.g., cefotaxime, ampicillin sodium/sulbactam sodium (Unasyn), ceftriaxone, or ofloxacin]
4. Oxygen supplementation and cardiac monitoring as indicated by severity of patient's condition and underlying health status
5. Early surgical/emergency department notification for transport and definitive care

Biliary Tract Disease and Sepsis

- *Biliary colic* is abdominal pain secondary to passage of gallstones through the cystic or common bile duct.
- *Cholecystitis* is an inflammation of the gallbladder secondary to obstruction of the cystic duct. Cholecystitis can further be characterized as acute calculous cholecystitis (obstruction secondary to gallstones) or acalculous (obstruction with no stone formation). Acalculous cholecystitis occurs in approximately 5 to 10 percent of cases of acute cholecysitis.
- *Cholangitis* is inflammation and infection of the gallbladder and biliary tree secondary to obstruction of the common bile duct, which leads to increased intraluminal pressure and bacterial invasion usually involving gram-negative organisms, enterococci, or anaerobes.

Clinical Presentation

Patients with biliary tract disease usually present with complaints of right-upper-quadrant pain (which may radiate to the scapula), fever, nausea, and vomiting. They may also have or report a history of jaundice, acholic stool, dark urine, and change in bowel habits. Additionally they may give a history of previous attacks with similar symptoms or history of antecedent ingestion of fatty or fried food. A thorough history can help identify patients at higher risk for gallstone disease. Risk factors for (cholesterol) gallstones include family history of cholelithiasis, female sex, obesity, diabetes, hyperlipidemia, cystic fibrosis, ileal disease/bypass/resection, pregnancy, and use of exogenous estrogen. Acalculous cholecystitis is more commonly found in patients who are elderly or diabetic or who have chronic underlying disease. Patients at increased risk for developing cholangitis include the elderly and those with previous biliary tract disease.

On physical examination, patients will typically feel right-upper-quadrant pain on palpation. Murphy's sign (aborted inhalation on palpation of the right upper quadrant accompanied by increased pain) may be present or, less commonly, the gallbladder may be palpable. Fever is commonly noted in those patients with acute cholecystitis and cholangitis but not in those with uncomplicated biliary colic. Charcot's triad (pain, jaundice, and fever) may be noted in up to 70 percent of patients presenting with acute cholangitis.

The differential diagnosis of biliary tract disease is given in Table 14-11.

Laboratory

A CBC and LFTs should be obtained to evaluate common laboratory abnormalities seen in biliary tract disease, including leukocytosis (though the WBC may be low in over half

TABLE 14-11

DIFFERENTIAL DIAGNOSES

Acute pancreatitis	Acute hepatic disease
Peptic ulcer disease (especially with perforation)	Pneumonia (especially of the right lower lobe)
	Retrocecal appendix

the patients with cholangitis), hyperbilirubinemia, and increased AST/ALT (aspartate aminotransferase/alanine aminotransferase) and alkaline phosphatase. An amylase level should be obtained, as patients with acute pancreatitis, which is most often triggered by cholelithiasis, may have a similar presentation but without evidence of jaundice.

If abdominal x-rays are taken, they may show evidence of gallstones (only 20 percent are radiopaque) or, in patients with cholangitis, air in the biliary tree. Ultrasound, though not generally available in the urgent care facility, will allow not only visualization of gallstones within the gallbladder but also evaluation of the gallbladder wall, the liver, the pancreas, and the kidneys.

 Management and Disposition

Patients who present with simple biliary colic but no signs of sepsis or acute obstruction can usually be discharged. A follow-up appointment should be made with the primary care physician as well as arrangements for ultrasound evaluation to look for stones. The patient should be discharged on appropriate pain medication and advised to follow a low-fat diet. Criteria for discharge include resolution of pain, no associated peritoneal findings, no fever, and a normal CBC and LFTs.

- Meperidine, which does not affect the sphincter, is the pain medication of choice for biliary disease.

Patients with acute cholecystitis require hospital admission for surgical consultation and inpatient care including intravenous antibiotics and fluids. Patients with signs or symptoms of sepsis or acute obstruction, regardless of the specific diagnosis, will also require transfer to an acute care setting. It is important to recognize those patients with cholangitis secondary to impacted gallstones in the common bile duct, as these patients may decompensate to a life-threatening condition in less than an hour. Intravenous hydration should be started along with broad-spectrum antibiotic therapy, and arrangements for transfer to an acute care setting should be made immediately.

Foreign-Body Impaction (Esophageal) and Foreign-Body Ingestion

The esophagus is the most common site in the GI tract for a foreign-body impaction. General risk factors for foreign-body ingestion include denture use, alcoholic intoxication, dementia, and psychosis. People seeking secondary gains, such as members of the prison population, are also at increased risk for foreign-body impaction. In adults, food is the most common cause of esophageal foreign-body impaction. Patients with esophageal strictures related to acid-peptic disease or cancer are at greater risk for food impaction. Similarly, patients who have esophagitis or esophageal ulcers with accompanying edema can also develop significant enough narrowing to cause an impaction. The most common foods causing impaction include chicken, beef, and fish or chicken bones. In contrast to adults, coins are the most common culprits (80 percent) for esophageal foreign bodies seen in children. Other predisposing conditions that can lead to esophageal foreign-body impaction include esophageal rings (Schatzki's ring), webs, esophageal tumors, and Zenker's diverticulum.

TABLE 14-12

RADIOGRAPHIC DENSITY OF VARIOUS FOREIGN BODIES

FOREIGN BODY	DENSITY
Objects made of iron and steel	High
Chicken bones	> Body-tissue density
Aluminum (e.g., pull-top ring of soda can)	Low
Wood (< 24 h after ingestion)	Body-tissue density
Wood (≥ 24 h after ingestion)	Isodense with body tissue
Glass	High
Pennies	Low

Clinical Presentation

Patients with esophageal foreign bodies will usually present with a sensation of something being stuck in the throat and at times can point to the approximate location of the impaction. They will often complain of chest pain or, in the case of a tight or prolonged impaction, may report a problem in handling their own secretions. Other symptoms that may be present include odynophagia, choking or gagging, shortness of breath, wheezing, and coughing. Depending on the density of the foreign body ingested, radiographs of the chest or soft tissue of the neck may reveal the location of the impaction (Table 14-12).

Treatment

Patients who present with a food impaction will generally have to be referred to an emergency department for GI consultation and endoscopic removal (Table 14-13). Patients who exhibit any signs of respiratory distress require airway support. Supplemental oxygen should be administered, and care should be taken to prevent aspiration. The ABCs of life support (airway, breathing, and circulation) should be followed, including pulse oximetry monitoring, and emergency hospital transport should be arranged immediately. In stable patients without contraindications, an attempt can be made to relax the lower esophageal sphincter using sublingual nitroglycerin or nifedipine or intravenous glucagons (1 mg). This may allow spontaneous passage of a food bolus. An intravenous line should be started on all patients prior to administering medications. If there is no response to these maneuvers, the patient should be promptly transferred for endoscopic removal; the longer the food bolus is impacted, the more difficult removal becomes due to inflammation and edema at the site.

- Papain or other proteolytic enzymes should not be used in an attempt to dissolve impacted meat foreign bodies.

TABLE 14-13

ESOPHAGEAL FOREIGN BODIES—CRITERIA FOR HOSPITAL TRANSFER

1. Any respiratory compromise
2. Inability to handle secretions
3. Impaction without response to attempts to relax esophageal sphincter
4. Object with high potential for perforation or obstruction
5. Object containing toxic substances
6. Underlying GI disease (e.g., Crohn's)

In nonfood impaction, most foreign bodies pass through the GI tract within 7 to 10 days of ingestion without incident (Table 14-14). Small objects and objects that are rounded are more likely to pass through the GI tract without difficulty. One should be on the alert for objects with the potential to cause perforation (sharp or pointed objects) or obstruction (> 2 cm in width or diameter; > 5 cm in length), or those containing a toxic substance (e.g., a battery). Patients with such foreign bodies should be referred to the emergency department for emergent GI consultation and endoscopic removal. Patients with an underlying gastrointestinal condition such as Crohn's disease should also undergo GI consultation.

TABLE 14-14

ESOPHAGEAL FOREIGN BODIES—DISCHARGE INSTRUCTIONS FOR PATIENTS WHO DO NOT REQUIRE EMERGENCY TREATMENT

1. High-fiber diet
2. Avoidance of cathartics and enemas
3. Arranged follow-up

Esophageal Foreign Bodies

 Key Points of Documentation

- Stability of patient: document if patient is able to converse, to handle own secretions
- Respiratory status (is there any compromise present?)
- Description of object and relative risk factor for toxic effects, perforation, or obstruction
- Presence or absence of any underlying GI conditions
- Suspected location of object (should be distal to esophagus for safe discharge to home)
- Response, if any, to medications administered
- If discharged to home, strict criteria for reevaluation (especially signs of perforation/ obstruction)
- Arranged follow-up

NONEMERGENCIES

- Acid-peptic disease
- Pancreatitis
- Inflammatory bowel disease
- Diverticular disease
- Hepatitis
- Diarrhea

Though the diagnoses listed above are being discussed as nonemergencies, patients with these conditions *can* indeed present in a state that warrants emergency evaluation and treatment. *As always in medicine, each patient must be assessed as an individual, and the complete clinical picture must be taken into account in making a triage decision.*

Acid-Peptic Disease

Symptoms related to acid-peptic disease are among the most common GI complaints with which patients will present in the urgent care setting. Included in this category are peptic ulcer disease (PUD), gastroesophageal reflux disease (GERD), nonulcer dyspepsia, and the "itides"—esophagitis, gastritis, duodenitis. Some differentiation among these disease entities may potentially be made based on the location of the symptoms and the presence or absence of dietary and other contributory factors. Generally speaking, patients with acid-peptic disease will complain of discomfort in the chest, upper abdomen, or epigastrium. The pain may variably be described as burning or gnawing and is often related to food intake. Unless patients present with complications of their disease (e.g., stricture, gastric outlet obstruction, GI bleed, etc.), outpatient evaluation and treatment can be initiated in the urgent care setting. The patient can then follow up with the PCP or gastroenterologist for any further evaluation and ongoing care.

Gastroesophageal Reflux Disease (GERD)

Patients with GERD will usually complain of heartburn. Additional symptoms may include midepigastric discomfort, chest pain (especially if there is accompanying esophageal spasm), regurgitation, a brackish taste, cough, hoarseness, and early satiety. Symptoms are made worse with intake of alcohol, caffeine, peppermint or spearmint, tobacco, large meals, and fatty or fried foods. Symptoms are also exacerbated with weight gain and lying supine soon after eating. Some patients report an increase in symptoms with citrus foods, tomato products, spicy foods, and onions. While the physical examination, including abdominal and rectal examination, is generally unremarkable, evaluation of patients with GERD should include a search for any signs and symptoms suggestive of complications, including:

- Dysphagia, food impaction, or weight loss, which may be related to a peptic stricture
- Gastrointestinal bleeding (including melena and hematemesis), which may be related to esophagitis or esophageal ulceration
- Hoarseness, which may be related to inflammation or vocal cord nodules
- Episodes of coughing or choking or recurrent pneumonia, which may be related to aspiration

Examination should include a full pulmonary and cardiac examination, as well as indirect laryngoscopy as indicated. Additionally, if the history includes complaints of chest pain, *even with a diagnosed history of GERD*, a complete cardiac evaluation [including an electrocardiogram (ECG)] must be performed in order to look for possible cardiac disease.

Treatment of patients diagnosed with GERD includes use of antacids (Maalox, Mylanta, etc.), sucralfate, and prokinetic/promotility agents (see Table 14-3, "Drugs Commonly Used in Gastrointestinal Disease"). Patients should be advised to avoid the contributory factors previously listed, to eat 4 to 6 hours before lying down, and to lose weight if indicated.

Peptic Ulcer Disease (PUD), Nonulcer Dyspepsia, and the "Itides"

Patients with PUD generally complain of midepigastric discomfort or frank pain. These symptoms generally improve with oral intake in the case of a duodenal ulcer but worsen in the case of a gastric ulcer. Any use of NSAIDs, which may be etiologically contributory, particularly in the case of gastric ulcer disease, should be noted as well as symptoms suggestive of complications or cancer (e.g., weight loss, melena, nausea and vomiting, hematemesis). The history should also include information regarding any previous workup [e.g. upper GI (UGI), esophagogastroduodenoscopy (EGD), testing for *Helicobacter pylori*].

- Patients with gastritis or duodenitis will present with complaints similar to those seen in PUD, though the severity may be of a lesser degree.

Although abdominal discomfort on palpation may be present, the physical exam for PUD, gastritis, and duodenitis is often unremarkable. A rectal examination is mandatory to check for heme-positive stool. Any signs of blood loss (orthostatic changes, tachycardia, pale conjunctiva or nail beds, or heme-positive stools) warrants obtaining a CBC to rule out anemia or active bleeding.

- Without a GI workup, it is difficult to differentiate between patients with nonulcer dyspepsia and those with PUD. Symptoms are essentially indistinguishable and often respond to the same medical therapy.

Included in the differential of PUD are GERD, pancreatitis, acute myocardial infarction (MI), aortic dissection, biliary disease, and abdominal aortic aneurysm (AAA). Evaluation should include ruling out not only these potentially life-threatening diagnoses but also the presence of complications from ulcer disease, such as anemia, perforation, gastric outlet obstruction, or acute GI bleeding.

Treatment   PUD and the "itides" can be treated with antacids, H_2 blockers, or proton-pump inhibitors (PPIs) (Tables 14-3 and 14-15). With treatment, patients will usually experience relief of symptoms. While some patients will require a prokinetic agent to be added to their regimen, most will not require PPIs or prokinetic agents. The choice of medication will depend on the severity and duration of the symptoms as well as on other medica-

TABLE 14-15

GASTROESOPHAGEAL REFLUX DISEASE/PEPTIC ULCER DISEASE/"ITIDES"—
ACUTE MANAGEMENT

1. Obtain full set of vital signs, including orthostatics, as indicated
2. Evaluate for ischemic cardiac disease
3. Evaluate for acute complications (GI bleeding, perforation, gastric outlet obstruction, anemia)
4. Intravenous hydration as indicated
5. Antacids (Maalox, Mylanta, etc.)
6. H_2-blocker therapy (ranitidine/famotidine/cimetidine/nizatidine)
7. Consider proton-pump inhibitor therapy
8. Avoidance of NSAIDs, alcohol, caffeine, tobacco use

tions a patient may be taking that could cause adverse drug interactions. Patients should be instructed to avoid NSAIDs as well as alcohol and caffeine-containing products.

Patients with symptoms that suggest acid-peptic disease severe enough to prompt a visit to an urgent care center should have follow-up scheduled with their PCP so that any additional evaluation that may be indicated can be arranged. This follow-up is particularly important in the case of patients with symptoms of long duration, symptoms that are recurrent and/or persistent, symptoms refractory to previous therapy, and symptoms suggestive of complications or cancer. An *H. pylori* test may be ordered to help expedite further evaluation by the primary care physician.

Pancreatitis

Patients with pancreatitis may present with symptoms ranging from mild inflammation of the pancreas to life-threatening pancreatic hemorrhage and necrosis. Pancreatitis can be acute or chronic in nature. The most common causes in the United States are related to cholelithiasis and alcohol abuse. Table 14-16 outlines additional risk or causative factors that may predispose to the development of pancreatitis.

Clinical Presentation

Patients presenting with acute pancreatitis generally complain of mild to severe epigastric abdominal pain. The pain may radiate straight through to the back and may be noted to improve when the patient is upright and with leaning forward. Nausea and vomiting are common accompanying complaints. Additional symptoms that may be seen include fever, change in bowel habits, steatorrhea, and jaundice. On physical examination, patients typically have epigastric abdominal tenderness. There may be signs of abdominal distention or peritoneal irritation and, depending on the severity of the disease, tachycardia and hypotension. Physical examination should assess for any indication of cardiopulmonary compromise or evidence of fluid shifts related to sequestration requiring significant fluid replacement. Evidence of either would indicate the need for inpatient admission. The presence of Cullen's sign (a periumbilical bluish discoloration) or Turner's sign (bluish discoloration of the flanks) is indicative of hemorrhagic pancreatitis; these patients uniformly require hospitalization.

TABLE 14-16

CAUSES OF ACUTE PANCREATITIS

Cholelithiasis	Trauma
Alcohol abuse	Hypercalcemia
s/p ERCP	Renal disease—failure, transplantation
s/p Surgery	Infection—mumps, *Mycoplasma,*
Medications—thiazides, furosemide, steroids,	*Campylobacter,* Legionnaire's disease,
estrogen/oral contraceptives, tetracycline,	coxsackievirus
azathioprine, sulfonamides, valproic acid	Vasculitis
Hyperlipidemia	Cancer
Pregnancy	Scorpion bite
Abnormal pancreatic anatomy	

- Any intraabdominal process should be included in the differential of pancreatitis. PUD and biliary tract disease, however, are the entities that most closely mimic pancreatitis. Non-GI diagnoses in the differential should include left-lower-lobe pneumonia, MI, and ectopic pregnancy.

Laboratory

Laboratory studies that should be obtained in a patient presenting with symptoms of pancreatitis include an amylase, CBC with differential and platelets, an SMA-7, LFTs, calcium, and lipase. Lipase elevation will help distinguish between an increased amylase related to pancreatitis and those elevations related to other etiologies. Unfortunately, most of these studies are not readily available on a stat basis in the typical urgent care setting. This limitation of stat lab availability may in and of itself necessitate patient transfer to the emergency department for further evaluation and diagnosis. One should be aware, nonetheless, that the degree of amylase elevation does not necessarily correlate directly with the extent or severity of disease. For instance, in patients with renal disease, the amylase may be disproportionately elevated, and in patients with elevated triglycerides or "burned out" chronic pancreatic inflammatory disease, the level may be spuriously low.

An abdominal series may help in the evaluation of causes or complications of pancreatitis. Potential findings include the presence of (1) gallstones, which may be visualized in gallstone pancreatitis; (2) free air, as seen with a perforation; (3) pancreatic calcifications; and (4) a sentinel loop. On chest x-ray, there may be atelectasis or a left pleural effusion.

Treatment and Disposition

It is important to differentiate between those patients who can be treated on an outpatient basis with close follow-up and those who require hospital admission. Patients presenting with severe pain, inability to maintain hydration, any hemodynamic instability, or a poor prognosis based on the Ranson criteria (Table 14-17) should be admitted

TABLE 14-17

RANSON CRITERIA FOR ACUTE PANCREATITIS (NEGATIVE PROGNOSTIC FACTORS)

At Presentation	Within 48 h of Onset
Age > 55	Age > 55
WBC > 16,000	WBC > 15,000
Glucose > 200 (in nondiabetic)	Glucose > 180 (in nondiabetic)
LDH > 350	BUN > 16; increase in BUN > 5
AST > 250	Calcium < 8
	Drop in HCT > 10%
	Albumin < 3.2
	LDH > 600
	AST or ALT > 200
	Base deficit > 4
	PaO_2 < 60
	Fluid sequestration > 6 L

KEY: WBC, white blood cell count; LDH, lactate dehydrogenase; AST, aspartate aminotransferase; BUN, blood urea nitrogen; HCT, hematocrit; ALT, alamine aminotransferase.

TABLE 14-18

PANCREATITS—CRITERIA FOR DISCHARGE HOME/OUTPATIENT MANAGEMENT

Good prognosis based on Ranson criteria	Ability to maintain hydration
Stable patient	No significant underlying medical conditions
Controlled pain	

for inpatient care. Those patients with more severe disease or evidence of instability should have an intravenous line placed. Fluid replacement should be initiated while arranging for hospital transport. Oxygen supplementation, cardiac monitoring, and frequent checking of vital signs are also indicated. If pain control is required, meperidine, as the drug of choice, should be used judiciously.

Patients who are deemed stable for outpatient treatment and evaluation (Table 14-18) must be able to take clear liquids without a problem. Intravenous hydration prior to discharge may aid in the ability of a patient to be discharged home. Patients should be discharged on analgesics and should be instructed to follow a low-fat diet. A follow-up appointment should be arranged with a PCP *prior* to discharge. If gallstones are suspected, abdominal ultrasound should be arranged as well. Alcohol and NSAIDs should be avoided, and consideration should be given to a short course of H_2-blocker therapy.

 Errors to Avoid

- Relying on amylase values to make a diagnosis
- Underestimating the severity of the disease
- Inappropriate pain therapy

 Key Points of Documentation for Discharge

- Stable vital signs
- Abdominal examination without peritoneal signs
- Ability to tolerate fluids by mouth
- Appears nontoxic
- Arranged follow-up
- Instructed on:
  - Low-fat diet
  - Alcohol abstinence
  - Criteria for immediate reevaluation (worsening or persistent symptoms, inability to take fluids by mouth, increasing pain, fever, jaundice, new symptoms)

Inflammatory Bowel Disease (IBD)

- ***Ulcerative colitis***
- ***Crohn's disease***

Patients presenting with inflammatory bowel disease (IBD) have often been previously diagnosed and will usually complain of a flare of their typical symptoms, the constellation of which varies from patient to patient. Common complaints include diarrhea, abdominal pain with cramping, fever, weight loss, fatigue, dehydration, and, in patients with Crohn's disease, perirectal fistulous drainage. Patients with ulcerative colitis are more likely to complain of bloody diarrhea than those with Crohn's disease, but bleeding may be present in both disease entities. For both ulcerative colitis and Crohn's disease, patients can present with extraintestinal symptoms of their disease including uveitis, rashes, and arthritis.

On history, important points to obtain include duration and extent of disease, recent endoscopic findings, steroid/6-mercaptopurine (6-MP)/azathioprine use (which is an indication of more severe or refractory disease), fever, unusual bowel habits, and recent travel or antibiotic use that might be risk factors for diarrhea. The presence of nausea and vomiting, which may suggest possible bowel obstruction, should be noted.

- Many patients have diarrhea chronically even when "well"; therefore a change in bowel habits is more important than just a history of diarrhea.

It is particularly important in patients with known inflammatory bowel disease to obtain their input regarding their symptoms. These patients are usually able to gauge the severity of the presenting bout compared with previous episodes. If their clinical picture is atypical for them, it may suggest other potential etiologies or may increase the likelihood that hospitalization may be required.

On physical examination, a thorough evaluation of the abdomen should be performed as well as a general examination assessing for complications associated with inflammatory bowel disease (IBD), such as dehydration, bowel obstruction, bowel perforation, significant GI bleeding, toxic megacolon, and infection. A rectal exam is also a mandatory component of the evaluation of all patients with symptoms of IBD.

Laboratory Evaluation

Laboratory tests that should be obtained include a CBC with differential, platelets, an erythrocyte sedimentation rate (ESR), and an SMA-7 (looking for electrolyte imbalance). If the history or physical examination suggests the possibility of perforation or obstruction, abdominal films and an upright chest film should be obtained. Findings on abdominal films may include intramural gas (which develops secondary to air in the colon wall), free air, toxic megacolon (> 6 cm dilation of a portion of the colon), or air-fluid levels consistent with obstruction.

Treatment and Disposition (Table 14-19)

In general, patients who appear toxic or septic, have complaints of abdominal pain out of proportion to the physical examination, cannot be adequately rehydrated over the course of several hours, or about whom there is ambivalence regarding admission, should be hospitalized. There should also be a lower threshold for admission for patients who are on steroids. In patients who potentially can be discharged, it is important to assess whether liquids can be taken in sufficient amounts by mouth to maintain a hydrated state. Initiating therapy or revising a medical regimen should be done only after consultation with the patient's PCP or gastroenterologist. Among the medications used to treat IBD are anti-inflammatory agents (including steroids), immunosuppressants, antimetabolites, judicial use of antidiarrheal agents, and, as indicated, antibiotics. Prompt follow-up should be arranged with the PCP or gastroenterologist prior to discharge.

TABLE 14-19

CRITERIA FOR HOSPITAL ADMISSION

1. Persistent dehydration
2. High fever
3. Toxic-appearing
4. Symptoms consistent with surgical complications (perforation, impending perforation, toxic megacolon, obstruction, significant GI bleeding)
5. Abdominal pain in the face of steroid use

Diverticular Disease

Patients with diverticular disease usually present either with symptoms of diverticulitis or with a diverticular bleed. These two conditions rarely present concomitantly. Patients with diverticular disease tend to be older adults who have had similar bouts in the past.

Diverticulitis

Clinical Presentation Patients with diverticulitis will typically complain of abdominal pain (most often in the lower quadrants—left > right), change in bowel habits (diarrhea or constipation), and fever. They may present with nausea and vomiting, which suggests an ileus or obstruction, or may complain of tenesmus and/or urinary frequency. Physical examination is remarkable for abdominal pain on palpation, generally in the left lower quadrant, and a low-grade fever (though both findings may be affected by the severity of the illness). There may be voluntary guarding or rebound found on palpation of the abdomen; in some patients, an inflammatory mass may be palpated. Rectal examination may reveal left-sided tenderness.

- Older patients and patients who are immunosuppressed may not have typical findings on physical examination.

Laboratory
A CBC with differential and platelets should be obtained, which typically shows an increased white blood cell count (WBC) and left shift on differential. If dehydration is present, blood for an SMA-7 should be taken to rule out free air or findings consistent with obstruction.

Treatment and Disposition With a mild to moderate bout of diverticulitis without evidence of systemic toxicity, treatment as an outpatient with close follow-up may be appropriate. A 7- to 10-day course of antibiotic therapy should be initiated with broad-spectrum agents that will cover gram-negative bacteria and anaerobes (Table 14-20).

Patients should be instructed to maintain a low-fiber diet during the acute episode and to avoid nuts, seeds, and popcorn.

- Once the acute attack has resolved, patients should be instructed to switch to a high-fiber, low-fat regimen.

TABLE 14-20

ANTIBIOTIC REGIMENS FOR DIVERTICULITIS

1. Trimethoprim/sulfamethoxazole (Bactrim DS) bid + metronidazole 500 mg q6h
                                    OR
2. Cipro (ciprofloxacin) 500 mg bid + metronidazole 500 mg q6h
                                    OR
3. Amoxicillin/clavulanate (Augmentin) 875 mg bid

Those with evidence of toxicity/sepsis, peritonitis, or a suspected abscess or perforation should be promptly transferred for further evaluation (e.g., CT scan), intravenous antibiotics, and admission.

Diverticular Bleed

Patients with a diverticular bleed may or may not carry a diagnosis of previous diverticular disease. Typically, patients complain of a history of lower-GI bleed with passage of burgundy or maroon stools, passage of clots, or diarrhea with more blood than fecal material present. On physical examination, the patient may exhibit evidence of intravascular volume depletion (e.g., orthostatic changes and tachycardia), depending on the amount of bleeding. The abdominal examination may be entirely unremarkable, but rectal examination will most often be consistent with nonhemorrhoidal GI bleeding. Patients with suspected diverticular bleed should be treated promptly (see "Gastrointestinal Bleeding," above) and transferred to an emergency department for further evaluation (e.g., red cell scan if actively bleeding) and admission.

Hepatitis

Clinical Presentation

Patients with hepatitis often present with nonspecific symptoms such as malaise, fatigue, nausea, and anorexia. Additional complaints may include jaundice, right-upper-quadrant tenderness, acholic stool, dark urine, fever, itching, vomiting, and, in smokers, a loss of a taste for tobacco.

- In the urgent care setting, patients with hepatitis may present for other reasons, and it is only during the course of evaluation that signs of hepatitis such as jaundice or worsening LFTs may be noted.

On history, an attempt should be made to pinpoint potential risk factors that may give some indication of the type of hepatitis contracted. Potential risk factors include travel, intravenous drug use/abuse, blood transfusion, alcohol abuse, homosexual activity, day care or health care work, military service, needle-stick injury, hemodialysis, medication, and exposure to someone with known hepatitis. A medication history should be elicited, as many drugs have been implicated in the development of hepatitis (Table 14-21).

Common physical findings, depending on the etiology of the hepatitis and stage of the illness, include hepatomegaly, splenomegaly, jaundice, right-upper-quadrant tenderness, ascites, and palmar erythema.

TABLE 14-21

MEDICATIONS IMPLICATED AS CAUSES OF HEPATITIS

Acetaminophen	Erythromycin	Lovastatin
Allopurinol	Anabolic steroids	Chlorpromazine
Isoniazid	Phenytoin	Halothane
Nitrofurantoin	Tetracycline	Amiodarone
Birth control pills	NSAIDs	Cocaine
Quinidine	Alpha methyldopa	

Laboratory

Patients suspected of having hepatitis should have a urinalysis and blood drawn for a CBC with differential and platelets, PT/PTT, and LFTs (liver enzymes, alkaline phosphatase, direct and indirect bilirubin); blood should also be sent for hepatitis A, B, and C serologies (Table 14-22). In addition to the laboratory work, patients who present with

TABLE 14-22

LABORATORY EVALUATION—HEPATITIS

HEPATITIS A

	Hep A Antigen	IgM Hep A Antibody	Total Hep A Antibody
Acute			
Early	+++	+++	+++
Late	−	+	+++
Recovery	−	−	+++
Transmission	Enteric		
	Can be from blood or body fluids (rarely).		
Incubation	15 to 50 days		

HEPATITIS B

	Hep B s Antigen	Hep B s Antibody	Hep B c Antigen IgM	Hep B c Antigen IgG	Hep B e Antigen	Hep B e Antibody
Acute	+	−	+	−	±	±
Chronic	+	−	±	+	±	±
Chronic carrier	+	−	±	+	−	±
Transmission	Blood					
	Body fluids (semen, saliva, blood)					
	Enteric					
Incubation	45 to 160 days					

HEPATITIS C

	Hep C Antibody	RIBA	viral RNA
Acute	±	±	+
Chronic	+	+	+
Transmission	Blood		
	Sexual transmission is possible		
Incubation	15 to 160 days		

jaundice and abdominal pain should be sent for an urgent abdominal ultrasound to help rule out cholelithiasis or a mass.

Treatment and Disposition

In the triage decision making, the physician should assess for evidence of compromise of hepatic function, chronic liver disease, or hepatic decompensation (e.g., bleeding, elevated PT/PTT, ascites, change in mental status, intractable vomiting, history of new or recent easy bruising, and peripheral edema). Any of these symptoms indicates the need for hospital transfer for inpatient care. Additionally, patients who are pregnant or have underlying medical disorders, such as immunosuppressed states, should also be transferred for inpatient care.

When a patient is deemed stable for discharge and outpatient follow-up, he or she should be given advice to return for acute exacerbation or worsening of symptoms. Additionally, patients should be advised to avoid activity that would expose others (e.g., enteric and sexual precautions in the case of suspected viral hepatitis), to reduce their level of physical activity, and to avoid alcohol, acetaminophen, NSAIDs, and other hepatotoxic agents. The importance of follow-up evaluation, including laboratory tests, must be stressed.

Household Contacts

Household or other close contacts of patients with hepatitis A should be treated with immune serum globulin (0.02 mL/kg IM as soon as possible or within 2 weeks of exposure) and, in the case of hepatitis B, treated with immune serum globulin (0.06 mL/kg IM) followed by the hepatitis B vaccine series of injections.

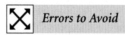 *Errors to Avoid*

- Failure to diagnose a treatable etiology for the hepatitis
- Failure to counsel appropriately regarding communicability
- Failure to counsel regarding prophylactic treatment for contacts
- Failure to avoid hepatotoxic medications or to adjust for altered hepatic metabolic clearance
- Assuming normal LFTs rule out severe hepatic disease and compromise of hepatic synthetic function

Diarrhea

Patients evaluated for complaints of diarrhea often present a challenge, given the vast number of potential causes of their symptoms. With regard to urgent care evaluation, however, the urgent care physician should focus on answering the following basic questions when making a triage decision:

- Is there evidence of dehydration?
- Is there evidence of systemic toxicity?
- Is there evidence of electrolyte imbalance?
- Is the patient able to maintain a hydrated state?

Etiology

Viruses such as rotavirus or the Norwalk virus are the most common cause of diarrhea, responsible for up to 60 to 70 percent of acute cases. The most common bacterial causes of diarrhea include *Shigella, Salmonella, Campylobacter, Escherichia coli,* and *Staphylococcus aureus. Giardia lamblia* and, at an increasing rate, particularly in the immunosuppressed, *Cryptosporidium* and *Listeria* are common parasites that may result in diarrheal illnesses. In patients with recent antibiotic use, *Clostridium difficile* should be considered as an important potential cause of diarrhea.

 History Taking

Important questions to ask in attempting to ascertain a potential etiology—and therefore an approach to treatment—include:

- Any history of foreign travel
- Medication use (laxatives, magnesium antacids, colchicine, misoprostol, theophylline, furosemide/thiazides, quinidine, digoxin)
- Recent antibiotic use
- History of inflammatory bowel disease
- Well-water use
- Camping with spring, lake, or river water ingestion
- Milk or gluten intolerance
- History of radiation therapy with the abdomen included in the ports
- Chemotherapy
- HIV/AIDS
- Raw food ingestion
- Shellfish ingestion
- History of bowel surgery
- History of diverticular disease
- History of weight loss
- History of pancreatitis
- Heavy caffeine intake
- Contacts with similar symptoms, particularly following fast food/restaurant meal
- History of thyroid disease

Note should be made of any accompanying symptoms such as fever, nausea and vomiting, abdominal pain, rash, hematochezia, melena, or weight loss. On physical examination, orthostatic vital signs should be obtained to assess for possible dehydration, and thorough abdominal and rectal examinations should be performed.

Diarrhea History

 Key Points of Documentation

- Hydration status/orthostatic vital signs
- Frequency/quantity of stools

- Quality of diarrhea (Often increased bowel movements or slightly softer stools are reported as frank diarrhea.)
- Presence or absence of abdominal pain or fever
- Presence or absence of blood in the stool

Depending on the patient's presentation, CBC with differential and platelets, SMA-7, and abdominal films should be obtained. If symptoms have been persistent, stool Gram stain should be performed looking for white cells, and stool culture should

TABLE 14-23

POSSIBLE ANTIBIOTIC TREATMENT REGIMENS IN DIARRHEA

ETIOLOGY	SPECIAL FEATURES	POSSIBLE TREATMENT REGIMENS (ORAL)
Viral	Associated N/V, low-grade fever, myalgias/malaise	Supportive
Salmonella	Fever; foul smelling stool; occasional blood; may have N/V; transmitted by eggs, poultry, water, and turtles	In severe cases, systemic disease, or immunocompromised host: Ciprofloxacin (Cipro) 500 mg bid for 3–7 days OR Norfloxacin (Norflox) 400 mg q12h for 3 to 7 days OR Trimethoprim/sulfamethoxazole (Bactrim DS) bid for 3 to 7 days
Shigella	May have N/V; fever (may be up to 104°F); blood in stools; may present in a child with a febrile seizure; transmitted via water, food, animals/humans	For severe cases, systemic disease, or immunocompromised host: as in Salmonella
Escherichia coli	N/V; transmitted via water and food; watery diarrhea; generally self-limited	Supportive For severe cases, systemic disease or immunocompromised host: as in Salmonella
Campylobacter	Similar to Shigella	Ciprofloxacin 500 mg bid for 5 days OR Norfloxacin 400 mg q12h for 5 days OR Erythromycin stearate 500 mg qid for 5 days OR Azithromycin 500 mg qd for 3 days
Giardia	Prolonged, chronic course; may have malabsorptive stools; may have previous history; transmitted via water (ask about well water); stools to be checked for parasites; may need multiple samples	Quinacrine hydrochloride: metronidazole (500 mg tid for 7 to 10 days), but not approved for this use
Cryptosporidium	Immunosuppressed patients at risk; transmitted via food and water; profuse and watery diarrhea; usually self-limited	In general, no effective therapy; paromomycin may be effective in immunocompromised patients

KEY: N/V, nausea and vomiting

be ordered. Patients with evidence of dehydration should receive intravenous fluids, and electrolyte imbalances should be corrected. Antibiotic therapy should be considered in patients with a suspected bacterial etiology (Table 14-23).

In patients found to be stable for discharge, work-up (if indicated) can be performed on an outpatient basis. Patients should be advised to avoid lactose-containing foods. Over-the-counter preparations such as Pepto-Bismol and Lomotil may be helpful in controlling symptoms, but antimotility drugs should be avoided if a bacterial or parasitic etiology is suspected. Patients should follow up with their primary care physician if symptoms persist for > 7 days, symptoms worsen, systemic toxicity develops, they are unable to maintain a hydrated state, diarrhea has been bloody, or stool studies are positive.

Hemorrhoids

Hemorrhoids often present with symptoms of bright red bleeding from the rectal area, with or without pain or itching. Patients will often give a history of previous episodes of hemorrhoidal disease or may report antecedent constipation with straining upon defecation. Bleeding from hemorrhoids is generally noted with defecation, but patients may also complain of blood soiling their underwear. Generally, the blood is described as coating the surface of the stool or noted as blood in the toilet or on tissue after wiping. Patients who complain of change in stool color or complain of blood mixed with the stool have a higher likelihood that another etiology is responsible for the bleeding. If the hemorrhoids have become thrombosed, the patient may complain of severe pain with defecation that slowly improves. Severe pain without evidence of thrombosis, however, should lead to further investigation into other causes of the patient's complaints.

 Physical Examination

Examination of the patient with hemorrhoids includes both direct visualization and digital examination. External hemorrhoids will be readily visible on direct visualization as dilated, engorged veins at the anal verge. Ideally, an anoscopic examination should be performed to evaluate for internal hemorrhoids, which cannot be palpated on digital examination unless they are thrombosed. If thrombosis has occurred, there will be a palpable cord at the site of thrombosis.

Treatment

Treatment of simple hemorrhoids consists of sitz baths. Patients should avoid any periods of prolonged sitting, including time spent on the commode. They should adhere to a high-fiber diet with adequate water intake (at least eight 8-oz glasses per day). Stool softeners may be beneficial, but any use of bulk laxatives *must* be accompanied by adequate water intake or constipation and frank impaction may ensue. Most thrombosed hemorrhoids resolve spontaneously; therefore treatment is initially the same as for non-thrombosed hemorrhoids, including sitz baths and bulk laxatives. In patients with severe pain, evacuation of the clot should be considered (Table 14-24).

TABLE 14-24

THROMBOSED HEMORRHOIDS—EXCISION AND EVACUATION

1. The area of evacuation should be prepped and anesthetized with a local anesthesic (lidocaine with epinephrine)
2. An elliptical incision should be made to expose the thrombosed vein
3. The clot should be excised with the overlying flap of skin tissue, and any retained clots should be evacuated
4. A pressure dressing or surgical foam dressing should then be applied
5. The patient should be instructed that the first sitz bath should not be taken until at least 6 h after the procedure
6. Any excessive bleeding, fever, or pain requires immediate reevaluation

 Errors to Avoid

- Attempted incision of a nonthrombosed hemorrhoid. *Incision of a nonthrombosed hemorrhoid is the same as incision of a vein, which can lead to the complication of severe and prolonged bleeding.*

Any hemorrhoids that are protruding should be manually reduced unless there is evidence of incarceration or strangulation, which would prompt immediate surgical referral. Surgical referral is also indicated for intractable pain, persistent bleeding, and/or severe pruritus.

- Narcotic pain medication will generally cause constipation and may actually delay resolution of symptoms.

Fissures

Fissures are linear tears at the anal canal. Patients with a fissure will typically give a history of severe pain on defecation which persists up to several hours after completion of the bowel movement. Bright red blood may be noted in the toilet water or upon wiping, and there may be an accompanying complaint of sphincter spasm. On physical examination, the fissure is readily noted by direct visualization and is usually located in the midline, most typically posteriorly. Fissures not located in the midline should lead to a high level of suspicion of other entities such as Crohn's disease, ulcerative colitis, or carcinoma. Treatment of anal fissures includes sitz baths, stool softeners, a high-fiber diet, and good anal hygiene. Use of local analgesics and hydrocortisone-containing products may also have a therapeutic role.

Bibliography

American Liver Foundation and American Digestive Disease Health Foundation: *Viral Hepatitis: An Epidemic in the Making? New Approaches to the Prevention, Diagnosis, and Treatment of Viral Hepatitis.* 1997:2–26.

Banks PA: Practice guidelines in acute pancreatitis. *Am J Gastroenterol* 92:377–386, 1997.

Colombel JF, Lemann M, Cassagnon M, et al: A controlled trial comparing ciprofloxacin with mesalazine for the treatment of active Crohn's disease. *Gastroenterology* 112:A951, 1997.

The diagnosis and management of chronic viral hepatitis: update 1998. *Clin Courier* September 1998, pp. 1–8.

EASL International Consensus Conference on Hepatitis C Panel: Consensus statement. *J Hepatol* 30:956–961, 1999.

Everson G, Lin T: Overview of viral hepatitis. *Gastroenterol Endosc News* September 1998, pp. 25–28.

Farrell RJ, Peppercorn MA: Diagnostic features of inflammatory bowel disease. *Gastroenterol Endosc News* 52(3):24–25, 2001.

Friel CM, Matthews JB: Diverticular disease of the colon. *Clin Perspect Gastroenterol* 3(4): 187–197, 2000.

Grendell JH: Acute pancreatitis: *Clin Perspect Gastroenterol* 3(6):327–333, 2000.

Gross JB: Clinician's guide to hepatitis C. *Mayo Clin Proc* 73:355–361; 1998.

Hoofnagle JH, DiBisceglie AM: The treatment of chronic viral hepatitis. *N Engl J Med* 336:347–356, 1997.

Jailwala J, Imperiale TF, Kroenke K: Pharmacologic treatment of irritable bowel syndrome: a systematic review of randomized, controlled trials. *Ann Intern Med* 133(2):136–147, 2000.

Ko CW, Lee SP: Gallbladder disease. *Clin Perspect Gastroenterol* 3(2):87–96, 2000.

Laine L, Schoenfeld P, Fennerty MB: Therapy for *Helicobacter pylori* in patients with non-ulcer dyspepsia. *Ann Intern Med* 134(5):361–369, 2001.

Lemon SM, Thomas DL: Vaccines to prevent viral hepatitis. *N Engl J Med* 336:196–204, 1997.

Leung J , Lee J: Nonvariceal upper gastrointestinal bleeding. *Gastroenterol Endosc Clin North Am* 7(4), 1997.

Liang TJ, Rehermann B, Seeff LB, Hoofnagle JH: Pathogenesis, natural history, treatment, and prevention of hepatitis C. *Ann Intern Med* 132(4):296–311, 2000.

McCallum RW: An update on gastrointestinal pharmacotherapy. *Pract Gastroenterol* 22(5):15–34, 1998.

McHutchison JG, Gordon SC, Schiff ER, et al: Interferon alfa-2b alone or in combination with ribavirin as initial treatment for chronic hepatitis C. *N Engl J Med* 339:1485–1492, 1998.

Maddrey WC: Update in hepatology. *Ann Intern Med* 134(3):216–223, 2001.

Martin P, Friedman LS: Viral hepatitis. *Gastroenterol Clin North Am* 23(3), 1994.

NIH Development Conference Panel Statement: Management of hepatitis C. *Hepatology* 26 (suppl 1):2S–10S, 1997.

Physicians Desk Reference, 55th ed. Montvale, NJ: Medical Economics Company, 2001.

Prantera C, Zannoni F, Scribano ML, et al: An antibiotic regimen for the treatment of active Crohn's disease: a randomized controlled clinical trial of metronidazole plus ciprofloxacin. *Am J Gastroenterol* 91:328–332, 1996.

Ranson JHC: Etiologic and prognostic factors in human acute pancreatitis: a review. *Am J Gastroenterol* 77:663, 1982.

Ranson JHC: Risk factors for acute pancreatitis. *Hosp Pract* 4:69, 1985.

Reichard O, Norkrans G, Fryden A, et al: Randomised, double-blind, placebo-controlled trial of interferon alfa-2b with or without ribavirin for chronic hepatitis C. *Lancet* 351:83–87, 1998.

Robinson M: Optimal healing and symptom relief for GERD. *Pract Gastroenterol* 24(10):14–27, 2000.

Sharara AI, Rockey DC: Medical progress: gastroesophageal variceal hemorrhage. *N Engl J Med* 345:669–681, 2001.

Shetty K, Younossi ZM: Diagnostic tests for viral hepatitis B and C. *Pract Gastroenterol* 22(5):39–47, 1998.

Shiffman ML, Hoffman CM, Thompson EB, et al: Relationship between biochemical, virological, and histological response during interferon treatment of chronic hepatitis C. *Hepatology* 26:780–785, 1997.

Sleisinger M, Fordtran JS (eds): *Gastrointestinal & Liver Disease*, 6th ed. Vols 1 and 2. Philadelphia: Saunders, 1998.

Update on liver & inflammatory bowel disease. *Can J Gastroenterol* 14(suppl C):1C–37C, 2000.

Viernes ME, Byrne TJ, McHutchison JG: Current therapy of chronic hepatitis C infection. *Pract Gastroenterol* 25(7):14–25, 2001.

Yamada T, Alpers DH, et al: *Textbook of Gastroenterology*, 3rd ed. Vols 1 and 2. Philadelphia: Saunders, 1999.

Zakim D, Boyer TD: *Hepatology: A Textbook of Liver Disease*, 3rd ed. Vols 1 and 2. Philadelphia: Saunders, 1996.

ORTHOPEDICS

J. Mark Evans

Orthopedic injuries are among the most frequent causes for emergency visits. This chapter offers an overview of the mechanisms, diagnosis, and emergency management of the most common injuries of the upper and lower extremities and the pelvic girdle. In each section, "red flag" injuries are also identified—i.e., those injuries that could cause long-term deleterious consequences if misdiagnosed or mistreated. Appropriate situations where an orthopedist should be more urgently involved in the care of the patient are also identified.

FRACTURE OVERVIEW

Fractures are conventionally described by several standard criteria, including (1) soft tissue disruption (open or closed injuries), (2) fracture pattern (transverse, oblique, spiral, and comminuted), (3) displacement (anterior, posterior, medial, or lateral), and (4) angulation (anterior, posterior, medial, or lateral). The displacement and angulation (Figs. 15-1 and 15-2) are described by the position of the distal fragment relative to the proximal fragment.

Pediatric fractures are also described using the Salter classification (Fig. 15-3), which describes various growth plate injuries. The classification is also prognostic for possible premature growth plate closure, with the higher-numbered injuries, types 4 and 5, posing a significantly higher risk of premature epiphyseal closure.

Incomplete fractures occur with plastic deformation or compression of one cortex of a long bone. The resulting fractures are torus and buckle fractures, respectively, as illustrated in Fig. 15-4.

GENERAL PRINCIPLES FOR THE EVALUATION OF FRACTURES

General principles for the evaluation of fractures include (1) examination, both anatomically and radiographically, of the extremity up to and including the joints above and below a fracture; (2) documentation of the vascular status distal to the fracture, includ-

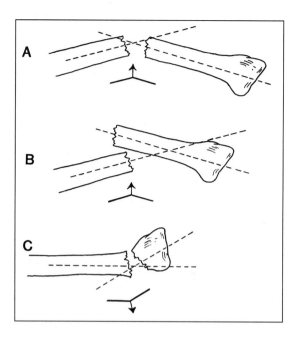

FIGURE 15-1   Fracture angulation. All figures depict 30-degree dorsal angulation. *A* and *B*. Direction is based on the apex of the angle indicated below the figures. *C*. Direction is based on that of the terminal fragment. (From Tintinalli J et al: *Emergency Medicine: A Comprehensive Study Guide,* 5th ed. New York: McGraw-Hill; 2000, with permission.)

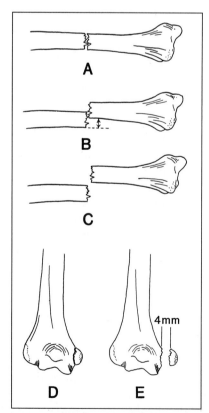

FIGURE 15-2   Fracture displacement and separation. *A*. No displacement, slight separation. *B*. Fifty percent dorsal displacement. *C*. Complete dorsal displacement. *D*. No displacement, no separation. *E*. A 4-mm separation. (From Tintinalli J et al: *Emergency Medicine: A Comprehensive Study Guide,* 5th ed. New York: McGraw-Hill; 2000, with permission.)

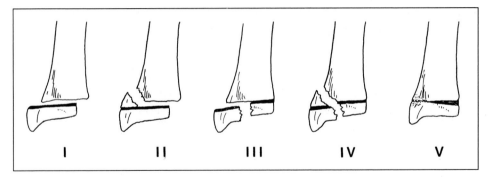

FIGURE 15-3   Salter-Harris classification. (From Tintinalli J et al: *Emergency Medicine: A Comprehensive Study Guide,* 5th ed. New York: McGraw-Hill; 2000, with permission.)

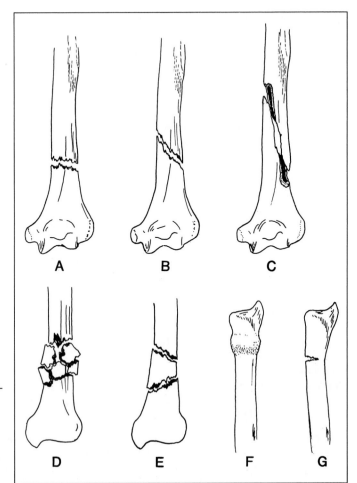

FIGURE 15-4   Fracture line orientation. *A.* Transverse. *B.* Oblique. *C.* Spiral. *D.* Comminuted. *E.* Segmental. *F.* Torus. *G.* Greenstick. (From Tintinalli J et al: *Emergency Medicine: A Comprehensive Study Guide,* 5th ed. New York: McGraw-Hill; 2000, with permission.)

ing pulses and capillary refill; and (3) evaluation of neurologic function, including sensation and motor strength distal to the fracture.

The universal principle in the emergent treatment of fractures is immobilization. The time-tested adage is to immobilize "one joint above, and one joint below" the fracture site. The goal is stable immobilization to prevent motion at the fracture site. This can be accomplished using aluminum splints, prefabricated splints, or custom-molded padded fiberglass splints. The splint should be secured without becoming tight enough to obstruct venous outflow or becoming a compression dressing, thereby avoiding the risk of creating a compartment syndrome.

GENERAL PRINCIPLES FOR THE EVALUATION OF DISLOCATIONS

General principles for the evaluation of dislocations include (1) evaluation of vascular status, including distal pulses and capillary refill both prior to and following reduction; (2) assessment of skin tenting prior to reduction and, if present, consideration of reduction even prior to x-ray evaluation; (3) documentation of x-rays following reduction, with attention to adequacy of the reduction and presence of fractures not noted prior to the reduction.

Table 15-1 lists the types of analgesics used for the reduction of fracture/dislocations.

SHOULDER INJURIES

In the urgent care setting, shoulder injuries typically present as (1) tendinitis/bursitis, (2) sprains or contusions, (3) dislocations, or (4) fractures.

Tendinitis/Bursitis

Bursitis in the shoulder, or subacromial bursitis, typically presents as an insidious onset of shoulder pain that is exacerbated with activity, particularly overhead activity.

TABLE 15-1

ANALGESICS UTILIZED FOR REDUCTION OF FRACTURES/DISLOCATIONS

MEDICATION	ROUTE OF ADMINISTRATION	DOSAGE
Morphine sulfate	IV	2–6 mg (adults)
Meperidine (Demerol)	IV/IM	25–50 mg (adults), 1 mg/kg (children)
Hydromorphone (Dilaudid)	IV/IM	1–2 mg (adults)

NOTE: These medications should be administered using standard conscious sedation protocols. Respiratory depression may occur, requiring airway and ventilatory support.

TABLE 15-2

NONSTEROIDAL ANTI-INFLAMMATORY DRUGS

MEDICATION	DOSAGE	FREQUENCY
Celecoxib (Celebrex)	100–200 mg	Daily
Diclofenac (Cataflam, Voltaren)	50–75 mg	tid–bid
	100 mg	Daily
Etodolac (Lodine)	300–400 mg	bid
	500 mg	Daily
Ibuprofen (Advil, Motrin)	200–800 mg	tid
Indomethacin (Indocin)	50–75 mg	tid–bid
Meloxicam (Mobic)	7.5–15 mg	Daily
Nabumetone (Relafen)	1000–1500 mg	Daily
Naprosyn sodium (Anaprox, Naprosyn)	375–500 mg	tid–bid
(Naprelan)	1000 mg	Daily
Piroxicam (Feldene)	20 mg	Daily
Rofecoxib (Vioxx)	25–50 mg	Daily

- The subacromial bursa is located between the acromion and the superior surface of the rotator cuff.

The typical patient with subacromial bursitis is under 25 years of age and has pain with resisted abduction at the shoulder and with full range of motion. The duration of symptoms may range from several days to several weeks. Treatment is directed toward cessation of aggravating activities and use of nonsteroidal anti-inflammatory drugs (NSAIDs) (Table 15-2). Initiation of range-of-motion and strengthening exercises should begin once symptoms improve. Patients with ongoing symptomatology should be reevaluated by their primary care physician or by an orthopedic surgeon within 2 weeks.

Patients with rotator cuff tendinitis often give a longer history of pain without a specific precipitating event. Patients often report worse pain at night or inability to sleep on the affected shoulder. Physical examination may demonstrate tenderness of the supraspinatus tendon insertion at the greater tuberosity and crepitus to range of motion, particularly rotation at the shoulder. There may be weakness to resisted abduction of the shoulder with the thumb pointed toward the floor (isolated testing for the supraspinatus tendon). Treatment consists of NSAIDs and range-of-motion exercises to prevent further fibrosis and scarring of the rotator cuff tendons. As with bursitis, follow-up should be with a primary care physician or orthopedic surgeon within 2 weeks.

Other possible causes of shoulder pain in the absence of an injury include glenohumeral arthritis, septic arthritis, and pulmonary lesions (Pancoast tumors). Radiographs are a useful differentiating tool. Arthrocentesis of the shoulder is diagnostic in septic arthritis of the glenohumeral joint. Patients with suspected septic arthritis should have emergent orthopedic evaluation. The risk of untreated or delayed treatment of septic arthritis is destruction of the articular cartilage and subsequent degenerative arthritis.

Sprains

This category includes the broad range of injuries from contusions to rotator cuff tears to biceps tendon ruptures. The physical examination is the primary means of differentiating between these entities.

Contusions

Contusion injuries occur as a result of a blunt injury, usually from a blow, running into a stationary object, or a deceleration injury such as a seat belt injury. Examination reveals tenderness along the deltoid muscle, pectoral muscles, or trapezial muscles. Depending on the time since injury and/or the severity of injury, there may be visible ecchymosis. Range of motion may show discomfort, but typically there is full range of motion to abduction, adduction, flexion, extension, and internal/external rotation. Motor strength, sensation, and distal pulses should be normal. X-rays of the injured area are normal. The treatment for this injury is supportive: sling immobilization, cold compresses, and NSAID therapy.

Rotator Cuff Tears

The rotator cuff is made up of four muscles, which provide the motor power for shoulder motion and strength as well as stabilization. The four muscles are the supraspinatus, subscapularis, teres minor, and infraspinatus. Mechanisms of injury include twisting/torque injuries, traction injuries such as catching oneself with an isolated extremity in a fall from a ladder, as well as loading injuries from falls onto an outstretched hand with a force applied to the shoulder through an extended elbow. The presenting complaint is usually pain and often an inability to raise the arm above shoulder level. Physical examination is significant for limited abduction and flexion of the affected extremity. The motor examination demonstrates weakness to resisted external rotation with the arm at the patient's side, weakness to resisted abduction at the shoulder, or inability to abduct the shoulder with only resultant shoulder shrug. The neurovascular examination is normal. There are no pathognomonic radiographic findings, but x-ray findings range from normal to rotator cuff calcifications to proximal migration of the humeral head. The last finding is caused by loss of the normal depression of the humeral head caused by the functioning supraspinatus tendon. Treatment for complete ruptures of the rotator cuff necessitates surgical repair or reattachment. Emergency treatment consists of sling immobilization, pain control, and referral for definitive treatment (Table 15-3).

Dislocations

There are four basic types or directions of shoulder dislocations: anterior, inferior, luxatio, and posterior. The immediate goal in all dislocations is to reduce the joint surfaces without doing further damage. In the evaluation of dislocations, biplanar x-rays are mandatory to document the type of dislocation as well as to rule out fractures of the humeral head, greater trochanter, or glenoid. In addition to a standard anteroposterior (AP) x-ray of the humeral head and proximal humerus, an additional view—consisting of a transthoracic view, trauma Y view, or preferably an axillary view—is necessary to ascertain the complete nature of the injury.

TABLE 15-3

STAGES OF IMPINGEMENT SYNDROME (NEER)

STAGE	ONSET	PATHOPHYSIOLOGY	OUTLOOK	TREATMENT
I	<25 years	Edema and inflammation	Reversible	NSAIDs, activity modification
II	25–40 years	Fibrosis and tendinitis	Pain with activity	PT, NSAIDs, possible surgery
III	>40 years	Rotator cuff tear	Disability	Surgical repair

KEY: NSAIDs, nonsteroidal anti-inflammatory drugs; PT, physical therapy.

Anterior Dislocations (see Fig. 15-6)
This subgroup of dislocations represents 60 percent of all shoulder dislocations. Mechanisms of injury include falls, longitudinal traction injuries, and twisting injuries. The physical examination is characteristic: the arm is held in a guarded or protected position, there is loss of the normal deltoid outline with a prominent acromion, and, in thin individuals, there is a palpable and visible prominence anteriorly at the deltopectoral interval. The presenting complaint is pain at the involved shoulder, exacerbated by any attempts at motion. A careful neurovascular examination is mandatory to rule out either a brachioplexus injury or injury to the axillary artery. The axillary nerve, in addition to supplying motor strength to the deltoid muscle, also provides sensation to a circular area immediately inferior to the acromion.

- In anterior shoulder dislocations, a neuropraxic injury or bruise to the axillary nerve is not uncommon, and should be ruled out.

Treatment of Anterior Dislocations   There are several described maneuvers for reduction of anterior shoulder dislocations (Fig. 15-5). In the traction-countertraction maneuver, longitudinal traction is applied through the hand/wrist, while an assistant applies countertraction using a sheet based at the junction of the axilla and the chest wall. The key to the reduction is adequate relaxation. This can be achieved via intravenous

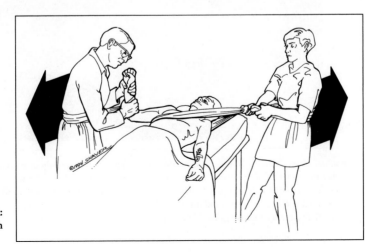

FIGURE 15-5   Shoulder dislocation reduction. (From Tintinalli J et al: *Emergency Medicine: A Comprehensive Study Guide,* 5th ed. New York: McGraw-Hill; 2000, with permission.)

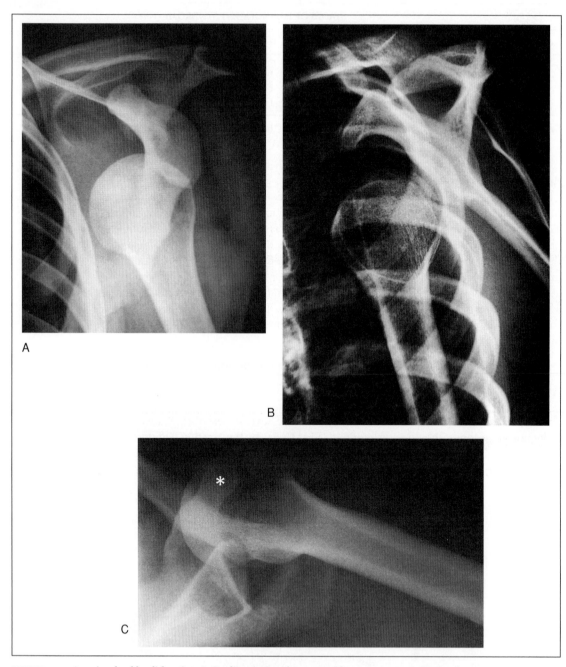

FIGURE 15-6   Anterior shoulder dislocation. *A.* On this AP view, the proximal humerus is greatly displaced from the glenoid fossa and lies in a subcoracoid position. The humerus is externally rotated and abducted. *B.* On the Y view, the humeral head is located anterior to the glenoid fossa, overlying the ribs. *C.* On the axillary view, the humeral head is displaced anterior to the glenoid fossa, overlying the coracoid process (*asterisk*). (From Schwartz DT, Reisdorff E: *Emergency Radiology.* New York: McGraw-Hill; 2000, with permission.)

sedation with appropriate monitoring and ventilatory support or, alternatively, using a shoulder injection of a combination of 1% plain lidocaine with 0.5% bupivicaine. Gradual traction is applied to overcome the muscles of the shoulder girdle. A successful reduction is usually appreciated both visually and palpably. There is usually immediate improvement in pain symptomatology following uncomplicated reductions. Scapular manipulation is an easy procedure that has been quite successful. With the patient in either a seated or prone position, gentle traction is maintained on the humerus while pressure is applied to the scapula anteriorly and laterally with the other hand, manipulating the humeral head over the glenoid rim. Following reduction, additional biplanar x-rays should be taken to document a successful reduction as well as to rule out an iatrogenic fracture. Postreduction immobilization consists of sling, sling-and-swathe, or shoulder velpeau immobilization and orthopedic follow- up. NSAIDs may be prescribed, and ice can be utilized to minimize swelling. Prognostically, the incidence of repeat dislocations is greatest in individuals who incur their first dislocation between the ages of 18 and 24. The incidence of repeat dislocations is lowest in patients above 35 years of age.

Luxatio Erecta /Inferior Dislocations

Luxatio erecta is a rare but unforgettable clinical presentation. The dislocation occurs as the result of a hyperabduction injury. The humeral head dislocates inferiorly, and the patient presents with the arm in an abducted position, a flexed elbow with the forearm resting on the top of the head, and severe pain symptoms (Fig. 15-7). Reduction is

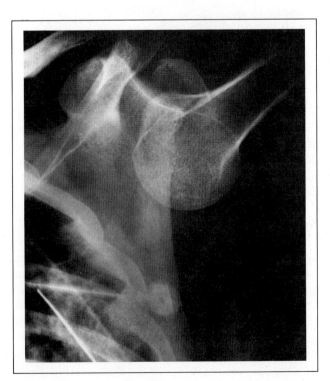

FIGURE 15-7   Luxatio erecta dislocation. (From Schwartz DT, Reisdorff E: *Emergency Radiology.* New York: McGraw-Hill; 2000, with permission.)

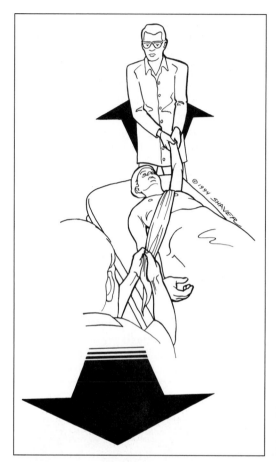

FIGURE 15-8   Reduction of luxatio erecta.
(From Tintinalli J et al: *Emergency Medicine:*
A Comprehensive Study Guide, 5th ed.
New York: McGraw-Hill; 2000, with permission.)

accomplished by the traction-countertraction method, with the countertraction provided by a sheet draped over the clavicle (Fig.15-8). Postreduction management consists
of immobilization of the shoulder. Associated injuries may include rotator cuff detachment, neuropraxic injury to the brachioplexus, and inferior capsular tears. These injuries
can be followed conservatively and should resolve with time. Patients should be referred
for orthopedic follow-up.

Posterior Dislocations

This is the most infrequently noted dislocation; however, it is the most frequent misdiagnosis or missed diagnosis of all the shoulder dislocations. Mechanisms of injury
include forward falls onto outstretched hands and seizures. The presenting complaint
is pain at the affected shoulder. The physical examination differs in that while the arm is
held in a protected position, it will be held in a position of internal rotation. There is significant pain with attempts at passive external rotation at the shoulder. The neurovascular examination should be checked closely, as noted in the previous sections, for
evidence of a brachioplexus injury. Radiographic changes are subtle, but with appropriate views, they are key to making the diagnosis (Fig. 15-9). AP x-rays show a "snow cone"

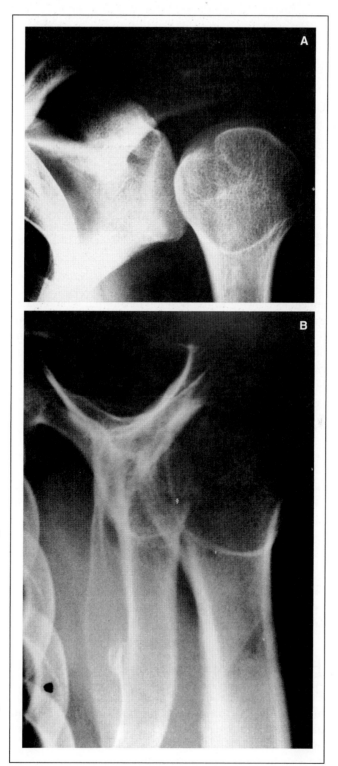

FIGURE 15-9 Posterior shoulder dislocation. *A.* On the AP view, the humeral head is displaced lateral to the rim of the glenoid fossa and there is diminished overlap between the humeral head and the glenoid fossa. The proximal humerus is fixed in internal rotation and looks like a "light bulb on a stick." *B.* On the Y view, the humerus is displaced posterior to the glenoid fossa (away from the ribs). (Copyright David Schwartz, M.D. From Schwartz DT, Reisdorff E: *Emergency Radiology.* New York: McGraw-Hill; 2000, with permission.)

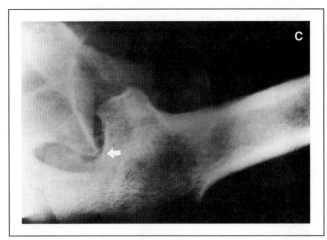

FIGURE 15-9   *(continued)*
C. The axillary view in another patient shows the humeral head displaced posterior to the glenoid fossa (opposite the coracoid process). This patient had prior posterior dislocations and has a large impaction fracture on the anterior surface of the humeral head. This is referred to as a "reverse Hill-Sachs" fracture (*arrow*). (Copyright David Schwartz, M.D. From Schwartz DT, Reisdorff E: *Emergency Radiology.* New York: McGraw-Hill; 2000, with permission.)

appearance owing to the position of internal rotation at the shoulder. An axillary view will show the definitive finding of posterior dislocation of the humeral head with respect to the glenoid. The technique for reduction is traction-countertraction with gentle external rotation. Postreduction management care is sling immobilization, with early gentle range-of-motion exercises and orthopedic follow-up.

 Key Points of Documentation

- Neurologic examination for possible axillary nerve neuropraxia
- Presence of peripheral pulses
- Absence of hematoma or pulsatile masses in the axilla
- Postreduction x-rays for adequacy of reduction and treatment of fractures

 Errors to Avoid

- Failure to look for other injuries distal to the shoulder
- Failure to confirm diagnosis and/or reduction with axillary or Y view x-ray

FRACTURES OF THE HUMERUS

Fractures of the humerus are divided into three categories: (1) fractures of the proximal humerus, (2) fractures of the humeral shaft, and (3) fractures of the distal humerus, including intraarticular fractures about the elbow. Fractures at the elbow are covered under "Elbow Injuries," below.

Proximal Humeral Fractures

These injuries are sustained in falls onto the outstretched hand, typically from a height. The presentation is one of acute onset of pain following a fall. Often, there will be an inability to move the extremity owing to the severity of the pain. Depending on the length of time between the injury and presentation, there may be early ecchymosis at the shoulder area. Neurovascular injury is possible but is less likely without concomitant dislocation of the humeral head.

 Errors to Avoid

- Failure to test and document sensation, capillary refill, and distal pulses.
- Failure to check lateral x-ray view (axillary, Y-view, or transthoracic lateral view) to rule out dislocation.

Definitive diagnosis of humeral fractures is based on radiographic evaluation. The proximal humerus has four segments, based on work done by Neer: (1) the head/neck, (2) the greater tuberosity, (3) the lesser tuberosity, and (4) the shaft. In order for these to be considered separate fragments, there must be either 1 cm of displacement or 45 degrees of angulation at the fracture site. Without one of these criteria, there may be a fracture but there are no separate fragments. Stated simply, a nondisplaced fracture of the humeral neck is considered a one-part fracture (Fig. 15-10). Displacement of the fractures occurs due to pull of the attached muscles, as follows:

- The subscapularis attaches to the lesser tuberosity.
- The supraspinatus, infraspinatus, and teres major all attach to the greater tuberosity.
- The pectoralis major attaches to the proximal humeral shaft.
- The deltoid attaches to the proximal third of the humerus.

Urgent care management of proximal humeral fractures *without* dislocation consists of sling immobilization. Two-part fractures with significant displacement or angulation, three-part fractures, and some four-part fractures require treatment with open reduction and internal fixation (ORIF). Four-part fractures and head-splitting fractures are usually treated with replacement of the proximal humerus with a prosthesis. Patients with proximal humeral fractures without displacement should be referred and evaluated by an orthopedist within 1 to 2 days so that definitive care can be initiated. Patients with two-, three-, or four-part fractures require emergent orthopedic evaluation for definitive management. More problematic, however, are patients who present acutely with a fracture of the proximal humerus and a dislocation of the humeral head. As compared to the standard shoulder dislocation, there is no connection between the shaft of the humerus and the dislocated humeral head. In this situation, longitudinal traction on the humerus via the hand or arm is not transmitted to the dislocated humeral head. In order for there to be a chance at closed reduction of the humeral head, there must be complete muscular relaxation, which is best achieved in the operating room. If a reduction cannot be obtained in a closed fashion, then ORIF or proximal humeral replacement is necessary, depending on the severity and type of the fracture.

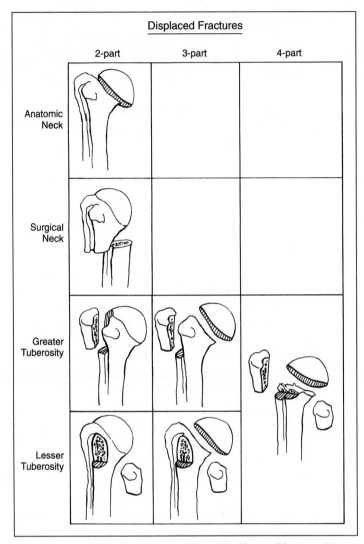

FIGURE 15-10 Neer classification system for proximal humeral fractures. (From Tintinalli J et al: *Emergency Medicine: A Comprehensive Study Guide,* 5th ed. New York: McGraw-Hill; 2000, with permission.)

Humeral Shaft Fractures

Fractures of the humeral shaft, unlike humeral head fractures, are categorized as open or closed and by the fracture configuration—transverse, oblique, or spiral. There are a variety of mechanisms that cause these injuries, including falls onto the extremity, motor vehicle accidents, and direct blows. These injuries can also be caused iatrogenically, by forceful manipulation of a stiff shoulder joint. The initial presentation of humeral shaft fractures is one of pain, with the arm held in a protected position. There may be visible angulation of the upper arm, possibly with tenting of the skin at the fracture site. Care should be taken during the exam, as well as during positioning for x-rays, to avoid converting a closed injury into an open one. Key descriptive points to note on the x-rays of the fracture include the longitudinal alignment or angulation (on both the AP and lateral views), the fracture pattern, the amount of displacement, and comminution if present. Patients with humeral shaft fractures should be carefully evaluated for possible median, ulnar, or radial nerve injury as well as a possible injury to the brachial artery or brachial vein. Oblique fractures of the distal third of the humerus (Holstein-Lewis fractures) should be evaluated carefully on physical examination for injury to the radial nerve. Radial nerve function should be evaluated both initially and following splint application to rule out dysfunction. This is easily identified by having the patient demonstrate dorsiflexion (extension) of the wrist and fingers, and by evaluating radial nerve sensory function at the dorsal first web space between the index finger and thumb.

Treatment

Initial treatment is directed toward immobilization of the fracture. The type of immobilization depends on the location of the fracture. The most versatile form of immobilization is the sugar-tong splint, which extends from the axilla, around the olecranon, and up the lateral aspect of the upper arm, ending in the region of the acromioclavicular (AC) joint or distal clavicle. This can be used for humeral shaft fractures as well as distal-third humeral fractures. Sugar-tong splinting should not be used for fractures of the proximal humerus, since the medial aspect of the splint would end at the fracture site, preventing adequate immobilization. The splint should be supported using a shoulder immobilizer, primarily for the sake of comfort. Range-of-motion exercises for the hand and fingers should be encouraged so as to limit finger swelling. Orthopedic follow-up should occur within 5 to 7 days.

Significantly displaced or angulated fractures as well as open fractures may require surgical treatment and should have emergent orthopedic evaluation.

 Key Points of Documentation

- Intact radial pulse
- Radial, median, and ulnar nerve function
- Fracture displacement, and/or skin tenting

CLAVICULAR FRACTURES

Clavicular fractures are divided into fractures of the distal third (including intraarticular fractures into the acromioclavicular joint), middle third, and proximal third. These occur 15, 80, and 5 percent of the time, respectively. The usual mechanism is either a direct blow or more typically compression (rolling onto the affected shoulder). Fractures of the middle third of the clavicle may occur medial to the coracoclavicular ligament and present with significant displacement of the medial end of the clavicle. Barring significant displacement of the fracture fragments, treatment for closed clavicular fractures is immobilization in a shoulder immobilizer or sling and swathe. These injuries typically heal in 3 to 4 weeks. The evaluation should be sure to assess for fractures of the first rib, which may be a harbinger of a more significant injury, including a pneumothorax or injury to the subclavian vessels or brachioplexus.

Errors to Avoid

- Failure to diagnose a fracture of the first rib

 Key Points of Documentation

- Skin tenting
- Neurovascular status
- First rib fractures

SCAPULAR FRACTURES

Fractures of the scapula can involve the body, spine, intraarticular glenoid, rim of the glenoid, neck of the glenoid, coracoid, and acromion. Fractures of the body of the scapula are rare injuries; they result from high-energy impact, typically motor vehicle accidents (MVAs), motorcycle collisions, or a direct blow. Associated injuries are common, and include injuries of the cervical spine, rib fractures, pneumothorax, and injuries to the great vessels. A full evaluation for associated injuries is mandatory. Additionally, a careful neurologic examination of both the upper and lower extremities should be performed, as well as assessment for peripheral pulses. Radiographs of the chest and shoulder should reveal the presence and extent of the scapular fracture. These films should also be used to evaluate for a pneumothorax, hemothorax, and widening of the mediastinum, which could be associated with injury to the great vessels. Intraarticular fractures can be further evaluated by computed tomography (CT). For isolated fractures of the scapular body, initial treatment is sling immobilization. Impacted or nondisplaced fractures of the glenoid neck can be treated with immobilization, followed by an aggressive range-of-motion exercise program to preclude loss of motion at the glenohumeral joint. Displaced glenoid fractures or unstable fractures of the glenoid neck require urgent orthopedic evaluation. These injuries may be treated with manipulative reduction and immobilization or may require operative reduction and stabilization.

 Errors to Avoid

- Failure to evaluate chest x-rays for pneumothorax or mediastinal widening
- Failure to evaluate for cervical spine injury

 Key Points of Documentation

- Chest x-ray
- Intact radial pulse
- Intact neurologic function

ACROMIOCLAVICULAR SEPARATION

Acromioclavicular (AC) separations are divided into six types, depending on the extent of injury to the AC ligament, injury to the coracoclavicular ligament, and displacement of the distal end of the clavicle (Fig. 15-11). Type 1 injuries represent a partial injury to the AC ligament alone. Physical examination reveals tenderness at the AC joint without

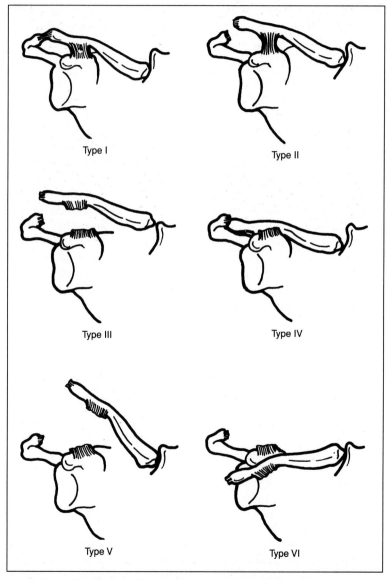

FIGURE 15-11   Classification of acromioclavicular dislocations. Types IV, V, and VI are usually associated with major traumatic injuries. Types I, II, and III are usually more localized injuries due to moderate degrees of trauma. (From Perry CR, Elstrom JA, Pankovich AM: *Handbook of Fractures.* New York: McGraw-Hill; 1995, with permission.)

significant elevation of the distal clavicle. Type 2 injuries involve a complete tear of the AC ligament without injury to the coracoclavicular ligament. Physical examination findings are the same as for type 1 but with slight prominence at the AC joint. Radiographic examination may show slight elevation of the distal clavicle but without significant widening at the coracoclavicular interval. Weight-bearing x-rays are negative, showing no increase in the coracoclavicular interval.

- *Weight-bearing x-rays should be taken with the weights suspended from the wrists and not held in the hands.* In the latter scenario, patients will often tense their shoulders, thus elevating the acromion and giving a false-negative x-ray.

Treatment of both types 1 and 2 is the same, consisting of sling immobilization.

Type 3 injuries involve complete tears of both the AC and coracoclavicular ligaments. Physical examination findings are similar to those for type 2 but with a more prominent bump visible at the distal clavicle. Weight-bearing x-rays are pathognomonic, with an increase in the coracoclavicular interval of 25 percent compared with the contralateral side. Current treatment recommendations for type 3 injuries are controversial; however, most orthopedic surgeons favor conservative treatment with sling immobilization. Studies have demonstrated that there is no statistical difference in outcome in patients treated with sling immobilization versus those treated with surgical reconstruction of the coracoclavicular ligament.

Types 4, 5, and 6 injuries involve complete tears of both the AC and coracoclavicular ligaments, with posterior, superior, or inferior displacement of the distal clavicle, respectively. All three injuries require urgent orthopedic evaluation and operative intervention, as there is either muscle or other soft tissue blocking reduction of the AC joint or significant displacement of the distal clavicle, leading to skin tenting. Although a careful neurologic examination should be performed in patients with these injuries, the incidence of brachial plexus injuries is low.

PROXIMAL BICEPS TENDON RUPTURE

Ruptures of the proximal end of the biceps usually occur at the long head of the biceps, which originates from the coracoid as part of the conjoined tendon. The short head of the biceps originates from the glenoid labrum and is rarely involved in tendon ruptures. The clinical presentation of a biceps tendon rupture is usually that of a middle-aged man who reports hearing a pop in the shoulder while lifting a heavy object. The physical examination may show early ecchymosis but typically is significant only for distal migration of the biceps musculature, with a "Popeye arm." The etiology of the proximal biceps rupture is usually related to intraarticular pathology within the shoulder joint, either from chronic impingement, intraarticular spurring, or rotator cuff tears. If the patient was asymptomatic prior to the rupture, treatment is supportive, with a brief period of immobilization followed by early range-of-motion exercises. A history of pain prior to the biceps rupture indicates the need for more aggressive treatment, with options including intraarticular steroid injection as well as possible arthroscopy with debridement, rotator cuff repair, and tenodesis of the distal end of the ruptured biceps tendon. Orthopedic evaluation should be arranged within 4 to 5 days.

ELBOW INJURIES

The elbow is a hinge joint with motion in the flexion-extension plane. The radial and ulnar collateral ligaments provide medial and lateral stability. Examination of the elbow should include inspection (looking for lacerations, swelling, erythema, bruising, or obvious deformity), palpation (evaluating for crepitus, areas of tenderness, increased warmth, or bony/soft tissue defects), and range-of-motion assessment, including a stability examination.

Epicondylitis

Medial and lateral epicondylitis represent two of the more common causes of atraumatic pain at the elbow. Both are forms of overuse injuries to the muscle/tendon origins at the elbow. Lateral epicondylitis, or tennis elbow, is inflammation of the common extensor origin at the lateral epicondyle of the elbow. The presenting complaint is pain at the lateral elbow exacerbated by lifting with the affected hand, particularly with the arm in pronation. The physical examination is notable for tenderness at the lateral epicondyle or just distal to the epicondyle, pain with resisted extension at the wrist, or more specifically pain with resisted extension of the middle finger. The differential diagnosis includes radial head fracture, lateral epicondylar fracture, and supinator syndrome (compressive neuropathy of the posterior interosseous nerve at the elbow). Radial head fractures and lateral epicondylar fractures can be differentiated by a history of trauma as well as on the radiographic examination. Supinator syndrome can be identified by tenderness over the supinator muscle and pain on resisted supination of the forearm. Treatment consists of NSAIDs, rest, ice, and—in more severe presentations—long arm splinting.

Medial epicondylitis, also known as golfer's elbow, is inflammation of the common flexor tendons at the medial epicondyle of the elbow. The presenting complaint is pain at the medial elbow, which is made worse with lifting or carrying. The physical examination demonstrates tenderness at the medial epicondyle or just distal to it and pain on resisted flexion at the wrist or fingers. The differential diagnosis includes medial epicondylar fractures, which are distinguished by a history of an injury, as well as x-ray findings. Initial treatment is identical to that for lateral epicondylitis.

Dislocations

Posterior dislocations comprise the majority of dislocations of the elbow, with the articular surface of the olecranon being displaced posterior to the distal humerus (Fig. 15-12). The primary mechanism is a fall onto an outstretched hand. The clinical presentation is a combination of pain, swelling, and inability to move the elbow. Physical examination reveals obvious deformity at the elbow. There will be prominence at the olecranon, often with an indentation just proximal to it. Associated injuries may include fractures of the medial or lateral epicondyles, coronoid fractures, or fractures of the radial head/neck. Neurovascular injury can also occur with ulnar neuropathy and brachial artery injury. Prereduction x-rays are important to ascertain the diagnosis and rule out any of these associated injuries. The reduction is accomplished using a combination of

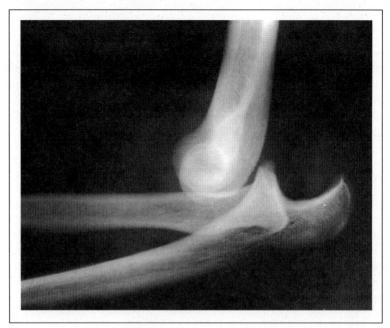

FIGURE 15-12   Posterior elbow dislocation. (From Schwartz DT, Reisdorff E: *Emergency Radiology.* New York: McGraw-Hill; 2000, with permission.)

adequate sedation/relaxation, distraction, and longitudinal traction. Longitudinal traction is applied through the wrist, with distraction applied by dorsally directed pressure on the proximal forearm to disengage the coronoid. Care must be taken to avoid anterior traction with the elbow flexed to a right angle so as to avoid increasing the risk of fracture of the coronoid. The morbidity associated with coronoid fractures includes converting a stable elbow joint into an unstable one and producing intraarticular bone fragments. A careful neurologic examination should be documented prior to attempting reduction. There have been reported cases of intraarticular entrapment of both the median and ulnar nerves following reduction. These conditions require operative exploration, with extrication of the nerve and any associated soft tissue. The neurologic examination should be repeated following the reduction to rule out nerve entrapment. The elbow should be taken through a passive range of motion to assess stability of the reduction as well as ligamentous stability of the elbow. Following reduction, the elbow should be immobilized in a posterior splint. A sling can be utilized for additional comfort.

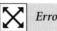 *Errors to Avoid*

- Failure to assess and document neurovascular status prior to reduction
- Failure to assess and document postreduction neurovascular status
- Failure to assess and document postreduction x-rays for fractures
- Failure to assess and document stable passive range of motion following reduction

Fractures

Elbow fractures can be divided into intraarticular and extraarticular fractures. Fractures in children can be more difficult to assess due to incomplete ossification about the elbow (Fig. 15-13). Supracondylar fractures of the humerus occur as the result of a fall onto the outstretched hand with the elbow extended. The fracture occurs through the olecranon fossa or at the flare of the distal humerus. The presenting complaint is pain, inability to move the elbow due to pain, and—in cases of displaced fractures—deformity of the elbow. The diagnosis is confirmed radiographically. In some cases, particularly in children, a clear fracture line is not apparent on the x-ray. However, in these cases, an elevated posterior and often anterior fat pad is visible on the lateral elbow, which, when combined with the history and tenderness on physical examination, should heighten the suspicion of a fracture of the supracondylar humerus (Fig. 15-14). Treatment for non-displaced fractures is with a posterior splint and sling immobilization, with orthopedic follow-up in 2 to 3 days. Displaced supracondylar fractures and intercondylar fractures need emergent orthopedic consultation for urgent operative treatment with reduction and stabilization.

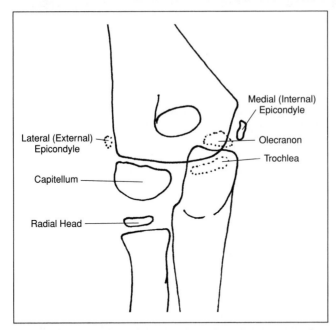

FIGURE 15-13   Secondary ossification centers of the elbow. Drawing of the elbow of a 6-year-old child showing age-appropriate ossification centers: capitellum, radial head, and medial epicondyle. Future ossification centers are indicated by the broken lines: trochlea, olecranon, and lateral epicondyle. The sequence of the ossification centers is given by the mnemonic CRITOE—capitellum, radial head, internal (medial) epicondyle, trochlea, olecranon, and external (lateral) epicondyle. (From Schwartz DT, Reisdorff E: *Emergency Radiology.* New York: McGraw-Hill; 2000, with permission.)

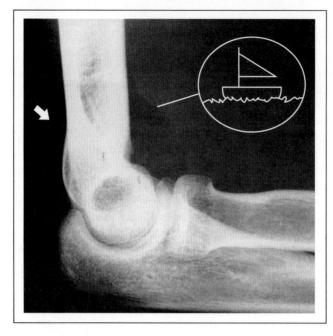

FIGURE 15-14 An anterior fat pad. (From Schwartz DT, Reisdorff E: *Emergency Radiology.* New York: McGraw-Hill; 2000, with permission.)

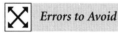 **Errors to Avoid**

- Failure to assess distal neurovascular status
- Splinting of the elbow in hyperflexion

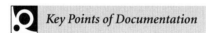 **Key Points of Documentation**

- Dimpling of the skin?
- Distal pulses intact?
- Distal neurologic status intact
- Displacement of the fracture

"Nursemaid's Elbow"

This is a common elbow injury seen in infants and toddlers, typically up to ages 3 or 4. The mechanism is one of a jerk on the hand of a child with the elbow in an extended and pronated position. Typically, this injury occurs in an attempt to prevent a child from falling. The child presents with refusal to utilize the injured arm, carrying the arm hanging by the side with the elbow in a flexed position. The pathology of the injury is one of subluxation of the annular ligament proximally into the radiocapitellar joint. The differential diagnosis includes fractures of the radial head/neck or lateral epicondyle, which can be ruled out by radiographic evaluation.

- Radiographs in cases of nursemaid's elbow should be negative.
- Positioning of the arm during x-ray will often reduce a nursemaid's elbow.

Reduction of a nursemaid's elbow is achieved via supination of the forearm, with hyperflexion of the elbow. Reduction is often accompanied by a palpable pop, though this does not occur in all situations. When the reduction is successful, the child will usually be moving the affected arm within several minutes. X-rays need not be repeated to assure reduction, as this can be evaluated clinically. Immobilization is unnecessary following successful reduction.

WRIST AND FOREARM INJURIES

The wrist and forearm are prone to multiple injuries, including fractures, dislocations, compartment syndrome, and tendinitis. The history is important in separating these entities, as is a careful physical examination. The examination should note visible abnormalities including skin disruption, soft tissue swelling, bruising, and obvious deformity. Palpable findings include tenderness, tendon or bony crepitus, subcutaneous emphysema, and increased soft tissue tension/pressure. Range of motion should be assessed at the forearm (rotation), wrist, and fingers. Sensibility at the forearm, hand, and fingers should be noted, as well as capillary refill at the fingers. The presence or absence of radial pulses should be documented where appropriate; additionally, in cases of inability to palpate a radial pulse or when there are injuries in the vicinity of either the radial or ulnar artery, Allen's testing should also be performed. Finally, the examination is completed with radiographic evaluation if indicated.

Fractures

Fractures at the wrist and forearm typically present following a fall onto the hand or arm or a direct blow. The presenting complaint is pain, exacerbated by attempts at motion. In more displaced fractures, there may be obvious deformity at the forearm or wrist. The definitive documentation is made with radiographic evaluation.

With *Monteggia fractures,* there are x-ray findings of a proximal fracture of the ulna, along with dislocation of the radial head. In light of this, evaluation of the elbow is key in all patients who present with a proximal ulnar fracture. In adults, this injury must be treated operatively with fixation of the ulna and reduction of the radial head. In children, this injury can often be treated by closed reduction of both the ulnar fracture and radial head dislocation. Orthopedic consultation should be obtained emergently to prevent converting a closed injury into an open one and to address the radial head dislocation. Initial treatment should be directed to pain control and temporary splint immobilization (Fig. 15-15).

Fractures of the radius and ulnar shaft, particularly when displaced, are immediately visible on examination. This injury in the adult requires operative stabilization with plate-and-screw fixation. In the child, this injury is usually amenable to closed reduction followed by casting or splinting. Orthopedic consultation should be obtained for reduction and ongoing care. Nondisplaced fractures of the radius and/or ulnar shaft can be treated emergently by sugar-tong splint immobilization with sling support of the extremity. Casting can be per-

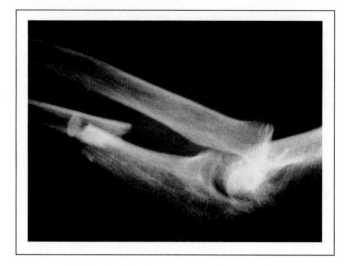

FIGURE 15-15　Monteggia fracture/dislocation, type I. There is a displaced fracture of the proximal ulnar shaft with anterior dislocation of the articulation between the radius and capitellum. (From Schwartz DT, Reisdorff E: *Emergency Radiology.* New York: McGraw-Hill; 2000, with permission.)

formed in 1 to 4 days, following elevation to decrease swelling. Long arm casts are continued for 6 weeks or until radiographic documentation of bony healing occurs.

Displaced fractures of the distal radius and ulna are treated by closed reduction and sugar-tong splint immobilization until definitive treatment by casting can be given. Subtypes of distal radial fractures include those with dorsal angulation and displacement (Colles' fractures) and volar angulation and displacement (Smith's fractures). Smith's fractures are further categorized into intraarticular fractures (Barton's fractures). While Colles' fractures can often be treated with closed reduction and immobilization, both Smith's and Barton's fractures are more unstable and frequently must be treated with ORIF. In nondisplaced fractures of the radius alone, splinting can be successfully achieved with a volar forearm splint.

- *A good rule of thumb for deciding between a sugar-tong and a short arm volar splint is the presence of pain with attempted active rotation of the forearm.* Pain with rotation implies increased instability; in these instances a sugar-tong splint will provide better immobilization and consequently better pain relief.

A variation of fracture of the distal radius is the *Galeazzi fracture.* In this injury, there is a fracture of the radius with concomitant dorsal subluxation/dislocation of the distal ulna at the distal radioulnar joint. This is often a subtle injury, but suspicion should be aroused by tenderness at the distal radioulnar joint on physical examination and either slight widening at the distal radioulnar joint on the AP x-ray or dorsal displacement of the head of the ulna on the lateral x-ray. This injury is treated by ORIF of the radial fracture with closed reduction of the distal ulna in injuries with a displaced radial fracture. In nondisplaced radial fractures, the arm should be immobilized in a sugar-tong splint with the forearm in supination, as this will reduce the distal radioulnar joint. Displaced fractures should have emergent orthopedic consultation for ORIF, while nondisplaced fractures should be referred for follow-up x-rays and cast immobilization in 2 to 3 days.

Key Points of Documentation

- Absence of skin disruption
- Intact distal pulses
- No tenderness at the distal radioulnar joint (to rule out a Galeazzi fracture)
- No tenderness or prominence at the radial head (to rule out a Monteggia fracture)
- No subluxation of the carpus (in Barton's fractures)

 Errors to Avoid

- Failure to include x-rays of the wrist and elbow with isolated radial or ulnar fractures (Monteggia or Galeazzi fractures)
- Failure to document active range of motion of the fingers (compartment syndrome)
- Failure to document intact skin (open fractures)

Wrist Dislocations

Along with open fractures and avascular limbs, joint dislocations are among the few orthopedic emergencies. Dislocations in the wrist typically involve lunate dislocations or transscaphoid perilunate fracture dislocations. The mechanism involves a fall onto the outstretched hand, resulting in hyperextension of the wrist. Physical examination demonstrates nonspecific findings of soft tissue swelling and decreased range of motion. The dislocated carpal bone(s) are not palpable discretely, although there may be a palpable fullness volarly just proximal to the wrist crease in instances of lunate dislocation. The hand should be examined carefully for evidence of a median neuropathy. In lunate dislocations, the median nerve is usually tented over the volarly displaced lunate. Patients may present with paresthesias or frank anesthesia in the median nerve distribution, affecting the thumb as well as the index and middle fingers and the radial aspect of the ring finger. AP x-rays reveal a triangular appearance to the lunate owing to its flexed position. Lateral x-rays are diagnostic and demonstrate the volar position of the lunate, with the "spilled teacup" sign. This injury requires surgery for open reduction of the dislocation and/or fracture and decompression of the median nerve where indicated. Emergent orthopedic consultation should be obtained. Other carpal bone dislocations may involve the scaphoid or triquetrium; however, these injuries are rare.

In instances of transscaphoid perilunate fracture dislocation, the lunate and proximal pole of the scaphoid remain reduced within the radiocarpal joint; however, the capitate, distal pole of the scaphoid and remainder of the carpus dislocate dorsally. Like lunate dislocations, transscaphoid perilunate dislocations are diagnosed definitively on radiographic examination. The AP x-ray reveals a fracture of the scaphoid, which is displaced. There is also overlap of the proximal capitate and distal lunate. The lateral x-ray demonstrates dislocation of the proximal capitate dorsal to the distal surface of the lunate. Emergent treatment is supportive, with splinting, elevation, analgesics, and cold compresses. Definitive treatment is urgent ORIF of the scaphoid, with reduction of the dislocation.

Carpal Fractures

Carpal bone fractures can involve—in decreasing order of frequency—the scaphoid, lunate, capitate, hamate, and trapezium. Seventy-five percent of carpal fractures involve the scaphoid bone, formerly known as the navicular or greater multangular bone. The inciting injury usually involves a fall onto a dorsiflexed hand or forced dorsiflexion. Patients often present some time after the actual injury, presuming that it represents only a sprain. The examination is significant for decreased range of motion, particularly to flexion. The pathognomonic finding is snuffbox tenderness on direct palpation. The diagnosis is confirmed radiographically, although a clear fracture line may not be visualized in acute fractures. The radiographs should be reviewed for displacement of the fracture site, with any displacement over 1 mm or distraction at the fracture representing a displaced fracture. The initial treatment consists of immobilization with a thumb spica splint. Definitive treatment of nondisplaced fractures consists of thumb spica cast immobilization for at least 6 weeks or until bony union is achieved. Displaced fractures will require ORIF followed by cast immobilization. Injuries involving snuffbox tenderness but no definitive fracture on radiographic examination should be treated as presumed scaphoid fractures, with thumb spica splint immobilization. Orthopedic referral should be within 5 to 7 days for cast immobilization.

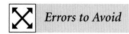 *Errors to Avoid*

- Failure to assess median nerve function (in lunate dislocations)
- Failure to evaluate lateral x-ray for lunate or perilunate dislocation
- Failure to immobilize an occult scaphoid fracture secondary to negative x-rays

Ligamentous Injuries

The most frequent ligamentous injury in the wrist involves the scapholunate interosseous ligament. As the name implies, this ligament connects the scaphoid and lunate bones. Injury to this intrinsic ligament occurs as the result of a fall onto the outstretched hand. The presenting complaint is typically one of pain and swelling at the dorsal surface of the wrist. Patients may describe a popping sound or feeling at the time of the injury. Physical examination may demonstrate soft tissue swelling at the dorsum of the wrist. Watson testing, or pressure over the scaphoid tubercle volarly while moving the wrist from radial to ulnar deviation, may cause a "clunk," which signifies reduction of a subluxed scaphoid within the scaphoid fossa of the radius. X-rays may reveal widening at the scapholunate interval on the AP view—also known as the Terry Thomas sign—with complete disruption of the scapholunate ligament. X-rays may also demonstrate shortening at the scaphoid on the AP view (the ring sign), due to flexion of the scaphoid with disruption of the ligament, as well as dorsal tilting of the lunate with flexion of the scaphoid on the lateral view (the DISI deformity—for dorsal intercalated segment instability) (Fig. 15-16). Urgent care treatment of this injury consists of thumb spica splint immobilization, elevation, and NSAIDs, with orthopedic referral within 2 to 3 days. For acute injuries, definitive treatment consists of closed reduction with pinning of the scapholunate interval or open reduction and repair of the torn ligament.

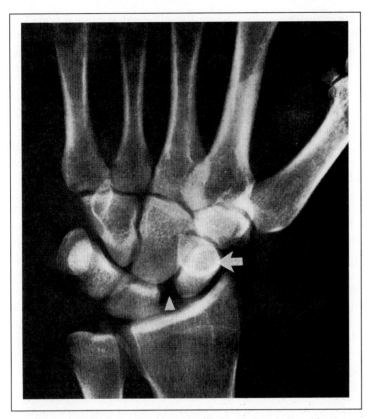

FIGURE 15-16   Scapholunate dissociation. Scapholunate dissociation with accompanying rotatory subluxation of the scaphoid. The scaphoid and lunate are separated by a gap of more than 3 mm (*arrowhead*) and the scaphoid appears to be shorter from rotation with a dense ring (cortical ring sign, *arrow*). (From Tintinalli J et al: *Emergency Medicine: A Comprehensive Study Guide,* 5th ed. New York: McGraw-Hill; 2000, with permission.)

Patients with a chronic scapholunate ligament injury may present complaining of increased pain following a relatively minor injury. In this instance, x-rays demonstrate the natural history of scapholunate ligament instability, with spurring at the radial styloid and varying degrees of degenerative arthritis at the wrist. Initial treatment for these injuries is the same as for acute injuries, with orthopedic referral in 5 to 7 days.

Hand injuries

The hand is involved in many acute presentations, including fractures, dislocations, tendon/nerve lacerations, clenched-fist injuries, and infections. The initial evaluation, following a careful history, is a thorough physical examination. This involves inspecting for lacerations, obvious tendon injuries, deformities consistent with fractures or dislocations, erythema, induration, or other evidence of infection as well as nonspecific soft tissue swelling. Palpation should reveal the presence of foreign bodies, any notable prominence consistent with dislocation, instability due to a fracture, or fluctuance. Range of motion should be assessed, assuring motion at each joint to rule out tendon injury. Neurovascular integrity can be verified by checking median, ulnar, and radial sensory nerve sensibility, capillary refill, and radial artery pulses.

Flexor Tendon Injuries

Lacerations are the predominant cause of flexor tendon injuries. Care should be taken to carefully evaluate the tendon function of any laceration over either the volar or dorsal surface of the hand, finger, or forearm. Failure to diagnose a tendon laceration or to appreciate the extent of a partial tendon laceration (which can convert to a complete disruption) can lead to severe consequences for both the patient and the physician. There is a normal flexion cascade in the hand. Laceration of both the sublimus and profundus tendons in the finger leads to loss of this cascade. These patients present with complete extension of the affected finger, with the normal flexion attitude at the adjacent digits. Examination is directed toward determining the number and extent of tendon injury. The sublimus tendon is responsible for flexion at the proximal interphalangeal (PIP) joint. Holding the adjacent digits in complete extension and having the patient flex the finger can test this. With an intact sublimis tendon, there is isolated flexion at the PIP joint. The profundus tendon is responsible for flexion at the distal interphalangeal (DIP) joint. Holding the PIP joint in extension and having the patient flex the finger tests integrity of this tendon. With an intact profundus tendon, this test results in flexion at the DIP joint.

- It is important to note that patients may have intact function even in the face of a near complete laceration of a tendon.

Open wounds should be examined carefully, inspecting for visible tendon or nerve injuries. Repair of flexor tendon lacerations, due to its complexity and the potential for injury to associated structures, should be undertaken only in the operating room. Acute treatment of these tendon injuries should include skin closure, splinting, elevation, and referral to a hand surgeon within 1 to 2 days.

Extensor Tendon Injuries

Extensor tendon injuries can occur in the forearm or over the carpus, metacarpals, or phalanges. These injuries result in inability to extend one or more digits. Physical examination should document the location and extent of the skin laceration, the patient's ability or inability to actively extend the digits, as well as impaired sensibility, which can occur with lacerations involving the dorsal sensory nerves of the radial or ulnar nerves. In cases where the patient complains of pain limiting active motion, integrity of the extensor tendons can be assessed via tenodesis. With flexion of the wrist, the extensor tendons are effectively tightened, resulting in extension of the fingers. Correspondingly, with extension of the wrist, there is flexion of the fingers. In cases of extensor tendon lacerations over the hand, resisted extension should be assessed. With lacerations at the level of the juncturae tendinum [i.e., on the dorsal hand, approximately one-third the distance from the metacarpal phalangeal (MP) joints proximally over the metacarpals], weak extension is possible using the adjacent extensor tendon through the juncturae tendinum. Extensor tendon lacerations in the hand distal to the juncturae tendinum can often be repaired in the urgent care setting by appropriately trained individuals. Lacerations proximal to the juncturae tendinum of the extensor tendons often retract proximally and are more difficult to repair outside the operating room.

 Errors to Avoid

- Repair of flexor tendon lacerations
- Failure to splint tendon lacerations
- Failure to diagnose tendon injury due to inadequate examination
- Assuming tendon is intact because ROM of the affected finger is intact

 Key Points of Documentation

- Location and depth of skin lacerations
- Intact radial and ulnar sensation
- Flexion or extension deficits to range of motion

Mallet Finger

Mallet injury or mallet finger occurs with a blunt blow to the tip of the finger. The pathophysiology represents detachment of the terminal extensor tendon from its attachment at the dorsal base of the distal tuft. This can occur as the result of a soft tissue avulsion of the extensor tendon from its bony attachment or as the result of a bony avulsion. X-rays, particularly the lateral view, assist in making this differentiation. Treatment in the preponderance of cases involves splinting the finger in full extension. This can be accomplished via a dorsal aluminum splint (the author's personal choice) or a volar aluminum splint. Splinting must continue uninterrupted—that is, without allowing flexion of the DIP joint—for a minimum of 6 to 8 weeks for soft tissue injuries and 3 to 4 weeks for bony injuries. Orthopedic follow-up should be within 7 to 10 days. Mallet fractures with involvement of greater than 30 percent of the articular surface may present with volar subluxation of the DIP joint. These are unstable injuries and should be splinted and referred emergently for orthopedic consultation for closed reduction and pinning (versus open reduction).

Boutonnière Injuries

Boutonnière injuries occur as the result of tip impaction, or jamming injuries to the fingers. These injuries occur during basketball, volleyball, or even baseball games. The pathophysiology involves avulsion of the central slip extensor tendon from its insertion at the dorsal base of the middle phalanx, at the PIP joint. The clinical presentation is one of swelling at the PIP joint, tenderness at the central slip insertion, and inability to extend the joint fully. Untreated, this injury may progress to a boutonnière deformity, with flexion at the PIP joint and DIP joint hyperextension. This results from lateral subluxation of the lateral bands of the extensor mechanism, with corresponding shortening of these tendons, producing the deformity. This condition can be difficult to differentiate from a simple PIP joint sprain. The treatment for a central slip avulsion consists of 6 weeks of extension splinting of the PIP joint, compared with only 1 week of splinting with a simple PIP joint sprain. If there is doubt, the finger should be splinted in extension and the patient referred for further evaluation and follow-up with a hand surgeon within 3 to 5 days.

Volar Plate Injuries

Volar plate injuries or avulsions occur as the result of hyperextension injuries to the PIP joint. This can occur with a fall onto the outstretched hand as well as with axial loading or impact injuries from ball sports. Presenting complaints include pain, swelling, and decreased motion at the PIP joint. Physical examination reveals soft tissue swelling at the PIP joint, with tenderness overlying the radial and/or ulnar collateral ligaments and particularly overlying the volar plate. Depending on the time of presentation, there can also be bruising over the volar PIP joint. There is typically good stability with stress testing of the collateral ligaments of the PIP joint. As opposed to the method of collateral ligament stress testing of the MP joint, stress testing of the collateral ligaments of the PIP joint is performed with the joint in extension. The volar plate is a thick ligamentous structure that extends from the neck of the proximal phalanx to the volar base of the middle phalanx. Avulsion of the volar plate can occur either as a tear at the insertion onto the base of the middle phalanx or with avulsion of a bony fragment. The latter situation results in a small bone fragment at the volar base of the middle phalanx which is visible on x-ray, particularly on the lateral view. There is usually no significant displacement of this fragment (Fig. 15-17). Although this injury is typically treated in the urgent care setting as a fracture, it is actually more of a ligamentous injury. Treatment consists of immobilization of the PIP joint with an aluminum splint, with the joint in extension. As compared with a typical fracture, this injury requires immobilization for only 1 week. Immobilization for longer periods can result in prolonged stiffness of the PIP joint. After 1 week, active mobilization of the finger is encouraged. Follow-up should be with a primary care physician or hand surgeon within 7 to 10 days.

Dislocations

Dislocations in the hand include such injuries as dorsal DIP dislocations, dorsal and volar PIP dislocations, MP dislocations, and carpometacarpal (CMC) dislocations.

DIP Dislocations

Dorsal DIP dislocations occur as the result of excessive loading, as in a jamming injury. Pain, deformity, and decreased motion are the typical examination findings. The diagnosis is confirmed radiographically. The x-ray should be carefully inspected both before and after reduction for evidence of fractures and also to ensure joint congruity. The key to successful reduction is adequate analgesia, which is usually obtained via a digital block. The reduction maneuver consists of longitudinal traction combined with slight hyperextension. The reduction of the joint is usually palpable. Stability is assessed postreduction by checking range of motion. DIP dislocations without fractures are stable following reduction and are treated by splint immobilization involving the DIP joint

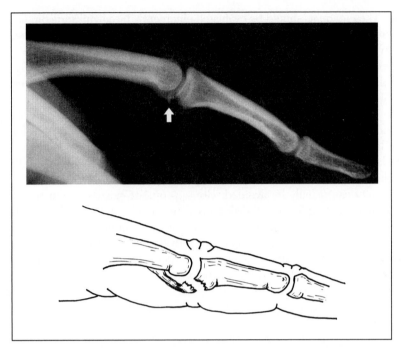

FIGURE 15-17   Volar plate avulsion. Hyperextension of the proximal interphalangeal joint tears the volar plate. A small avulsion fracture is often seen at the volar surface at the base of the middle phalanx. In some cases, a larger fracture is produced by a concomitant impaction and shearing. If a large portion of the articular surface is fractured, operative fixation with pins is necessary. (From Schwartz DT, Reisdorff E: *Emergency Radiology*. New York: McGraw-Hill; 2000, with permission.)

only. In general these injuries need immobilization for only 1 week, followed by range-of-motion exercises. Isolated DIP dislocations have a good prognosis for recovery of range of motion and function. Follow-up should be with the primary care physician or hand surgeon within 1 week.

PIP Dislocations

With axial loading of the finger, there is a continuum of injuries extending from simple sprains to volar plate avulsion to frank dislocation of the PIP joint. Dislocations can present in order of frequency as dorsal, radioulnar, and, more rarely, volar.

Dorsal dislocations represent the majority of dislocations in the hand. PIP dislocations also occur as the result of excessive loading. One of the key distinctions between dorsal and volar PIP dislocations is the associated injuries. Dorsal dislocations involve disruption of the volar plate, with a strain injury to the collateral ligaments. As with volar plate injuries, there can be a small bony avulsion fragment associated with this injury, at the site of the volar plate attachment. Closed reduction is accomplished via longitudinal traction, with slight hyperextension if necessary. As in DIP dislocations, stability is assessed following reduction by checking range of motion. Dorsal PIP joint dislocations with volar fractures involving more than 20 percent of the articular surface may not be stable in full extension. These patients should be evaluated emergently by a hand surgeon. Dorsal PIP dislocations without fractures are generally stable following reduction, and should be splinted in extension for 1 week to allow early healing of the volar plate injury.

Volar dislocations are the most rare of all the dislocations in the digits (Fig. 15-18). With a volar dislocation at the PIP joint, there is *always* disruption of the central slip tendon. Appreciation of this associated condition is mandatory to prevent the possible long-term sequela of this injury, which is a boutonière deformity. With a central slip tear, there is no tendon to extend the PIP joint, and a flexion contracture develops. With time, the lateral bands, which coalesce to form the terminal extensor tendons, begin to sublux volarly. Once these tendons pass volar to the plane of motion at the PIP joint, they produce flexion at the PIP joint and hyperextension at the DIP joint (Fig. 15-19). This deformity can usually be avoided with appropriate postreduction treatment. In contrast to the splinting for dorsal dislocations, which usually lasts only 1 week, immobilization for volar PIP dislocations should continue for a minimum of 6 weeks. The PIP joint must be splinted in full extension to return the central slip tendon to its proper position and then be maintained there until tendon-to-bone healing occurs. Given the time to healing as well as the possible sequelae, these injuries should be managed by a hand or orthopedic surgeon.

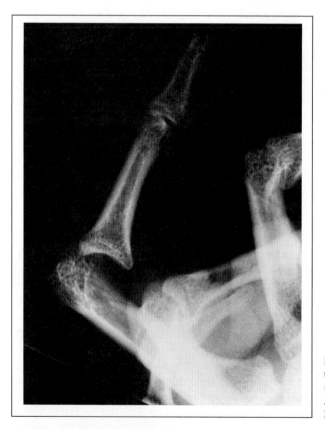

FIGURE 15-18　Volar dislocation of the proximal interphalangeal joint. (From Schwartz DT, Reisdorff E: *Emergency Radiology.* New York: McGraw-Hill; 2000, with permission.)

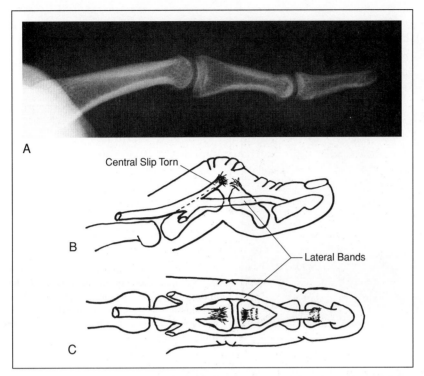

FIGURE 15-19   Boutonnière deformity. *A*. Slight flexion of the proximal interphalangeal (PIP) joint and extension of the distal interphalangeal (DIP) joint is seen. There is soft tissue swelling over the PIP joint. *B* and *C*. An extensor tendon injury at the PIP joint results in a boutonniere deformity. The central slip of the extensor tendon inserts on the base of the middle phalanx. It is torn by trauma to the dorsal surface of the PIP joint. The lateral bands of the extensor tendon then migrate volarly, causing flexion of the PIP joint and extension of the DIP joint. (From Schwartz DT, Reisdorff E: *Emergency Radiology.* New York: McGraw-Hill; 2000, with permission.)

Metacarpal Phalangeal Dislocations

MP dislocations occur infrequently. As with the two previous groups of dislocations in the digit, the mechanism is a loading injury. The characteristic physical examination includes hyperextension at the MP joint, a prominence in the palm caused by the metacarpal head, pain with attempted range of motion, and possibly dimpling in the palm. Adequate analgesia is mandatory for attempting closed reductions and can be accomplished by a wrist block. Unlike PIP and DIP dislocations, the reduction maneuver does not involve longitudinal traction.

- *Inadvertent longitudinal traction may convert a simple MP dislocation into a complex or irreducible dislocation.* This occurs by entrapping the volar plate between the base of the proximal phalanx and the dorsal metacarpal head.

Sensibility should be carefully assessed prior to attempting reduction, as one of the digital nerves is often tented over the prominent metacarpal head in the palm.

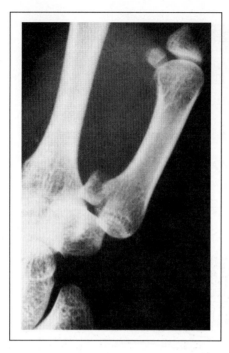

FIGURE 15-20 Bennett fracture. An intraarticular fracture at the base of the thumb metacarpal. The pull of the abductor pollicis tendon displaces the thumb's carpometacarpal joint. (From Schwartz DT, Reisdorff E: *Emergency Radiology.* New York: McGraw-Hill; 2000, with permission.)

Irreducible or complex MP dislocations must be reduced via an open reduction through either a dorsal or volar approach; appropriate hand surgical consultation should be obtained emergently. Following closed reduction, care consists of immobilization in a coaptation splint or spica cast for 3 weeks total.

Carpometacarpal Dislocations

Carpometacarpal (CMC) dislocations present in urgent care settings as either Bennett's fractures (fracture/subluxation of the thumb CMC joint), or reverse Bennett's fractures (fracture/subluxation of the fifth CMC joint) (Fig. 15-20). These injuries also present following falls onto the hand or thumb, with an axial loading injury. The presenting complaint is usually pain at the site of the injured joint. There may be moderate soft tissue swelling and the prominent metacarpal base may not be easily palpable. In these instances, careful evaluation of the x-ray is critical. Radiographic views should include an AP, a lateral, and—in the case of fifth metacarpal injuries—a 30-degree supinated view, which better documents subluxation at the fifth CMC joint. Although closed reduction can be obtained via longitudinal traction with volar pressure, this is an unstable injury. Consultation should be made with a hand surgeon for definitive treatment consisting of closed reduction with pinning of the CMC joint or, in difficult cases, open reduction.

Gamekeeper's Thumb

Gamekeeper's thumb, or, more modernly, skier's thumb, is disruption of the ulnar collateral ligament at the MCP joint of the thumb. This can occur as a tear in the ligament, usually from its distal attachment to the base of the proximal phalanx of the thumb, or as an avulsion of the ligament, again from its distal attachment along with a variable-sized bone fragment (Fig. 15-21). This distinction can be made with AP, lateral, and oblique radiographs. The injury typically occurs as the result of a forced radial deviation of the thumb. Historically, this occurred as a chronic injury with repetitive wringing of the necks of chickens. Presently, it occurs most commonly as the result of a fall onto the thumb, usually while skiing, but can also occur as the result of a fall from any cause with resultant stress on the ulnar collateral ligament. Examination is significant for soft tissue swelling and ecchymosis at the ulnar aspect of the thumb MP joint, with tenderness in this same distribution. The definitive test is stress testing of the ulnar collateral ligament. This is done with the thumb MP joint in flexion, so as to tighten the collateral ligaments. With the thumb in flexion at the MP joint, a radially directed stress is applied to the thumb. With complete disruption of the ligament, there is a giving way with stress testing with no firm endpoint. Complete disruption of the ligament usually requires surgical repair, but the acute injury can be treated with a thumb spica splint until orthopedic referral is obtained. Partial tears of the ligament have good stability to stress testing, and these injuries can be treated with immobilization in a thumb spica cast for 4 to 6 weeks or a thumb spica Velcro-type splint. Acute treatment of injuries to the ulnar collateral

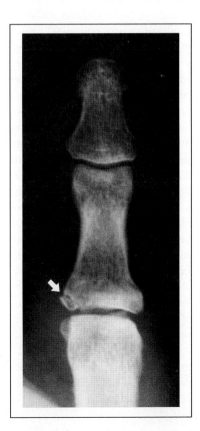

FIGURE 15-21   Gamekeeper's thumb. (From Schwartz DT, Reisdorff E: *Emergency Radiology.* New York: McGraw-Hill; 2000, with permission.)

ligament of the thumb consists of thumb spica splint immobilization, with follow-up with a hand surgeon within 2 to 4 days.

Carpal Tunnel Syndrome

Carpal tunnel syndrome represents an entrapment neuropathy of the upper extremity, presenting as pain and/or numbness/tingling of the hand in a median nerve distribution. This distribution classically involves the thumb, index, and middle fingers and the radial half of the ring finger. Carpal tunnel syndrome usually presents as a chronic condition or a phenomenon of gradual onset; however, it can, in certain situations, present acutely. Causes for acute presentation include acute distal radioulnar fractures, carpal dislocations, as well as falls onto an outstretched hand that produce an acute contusion to the median nerve.

Acute treatment consists of splinting with either a volar wrist splint or an ulnar gutter splint as well as rest, ice, elevation, and NSAIDs. Follow-up should be within 5 to 7 days.

Neurovascular Injuries

Neurovascular injuries can occur in the hand as a result of a laceration, fracture (usually open), or dislocation. Patients with crush injuries to the digits can present with absent sensation; these deficits usually represent neuropraxic injuries; as such, they can be expected to heal completely with time. There are three major nerves to the hand: the median, ulnar, and radial sensory nerves (Fig. 15-22).

At the level of the wrist, the median nerve is located volarly, at the center of the wrist. At this level, the median nerve is both a motor and sensory nerve. In the 85 percent of patients with a palmaris longus tendon, the median nerve lies immediately beneath this tendon. In lacerations where there is a visible laceration to the palmaris longus tendon, one should be particularly careful to assess for possible injury to the median nerve. A deficit can manifest itself by a sensory deficit or motor weakness of the abductor pollicis brevis or of the opponens pollicis. Median nerve motor deficit can be assessed by having the patient abduct the thumb against resistance. Weakness with this maneuver, particularly in the absence of pain, suggests a median nerve deficit.

The ulnar nerve at the level of the wrist is also both a motor and sensory nerve. The ulnar nerve is also located volarly, lying beneath the flexor carpi ulnaris tendon. The ulnar nerve is adjacent to the ulnar artery; therefore lacerations of the ulnar nerve are usually accompanied by moderate bleeding due to an associated laceration of the ulnar artery. In cases of suspected ulnar nerve injury, emergent hand surgery evaluation should be obtained, since operative treatment may be necessary. In addition to the sensory deficit involving the small finger and the ulnar aspect of the ring finger, there can be weakness of the intrinsic tendons to the fingers (manifest by weak abduction) and a weak pinch between the thumb and index fingers (Froment's sign).

The radial sensory nerve lies superficial to the radial styloid and supplies sensation to the dorsal and radial aspects of the hand. In contrast to the median and ulnar nerves, this nerve is a pure sensory nerve. Deficits can be manifest by numbness, dysesthesias, or hypoesthesias.

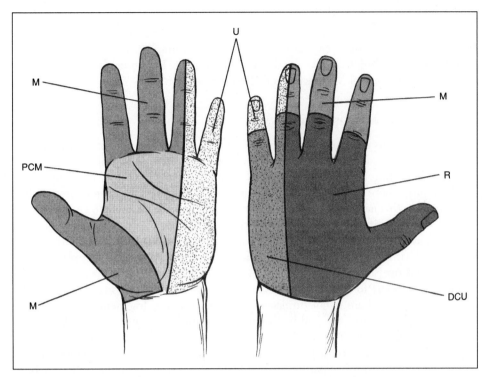

FIGURE 15-22   The cutaneous nerve supply in the hand. M, median; R, radial; U, ulnar; PCM, palmar branch of the median nerve; DCU, dorsal branch of the ulnar nerve. (From Tintinalli J et al: *Emergency Medicine: A Comprehensive Study Guide,* 5th ed. New York: McGraw-Hill; 2000, with permission.)

This group of injuries can be managed acutely with local wound care, including suturing and splinting of the extremity. They should be referred to a hand surgeon for definitive treatment within 1 to 2 days.

Fractures

Fractures in the hand can be subcategorized into open and closed injuries. The open injuries constitute orthopedic emergencies; therefore immediate consultation should be requested. Closed injuries, particularly when these fractures are nondisplaced or minimally displaced, can be treated with splinting and appropriate analgesics. Angulated or displaced fractures benefit from closed reduction and so usually require orthopedic consultation.

With hand fractures, there are typical displacement patterns caused by the pull of the intrinsic muscles. Metacarpal fractures usually present with volar angulation due to the forces of the intrinsic muscles. Fracture of the proximal phalanx presents with dorsal angulation due to the forces of the extensor mechanism. Fractures of the middle phalanx typically present with shortening due to the combined forces of the flexor and extensor tendons. Distal tuft fractures typically do not present with significant displacement due to the usual mechanism of injury, which is a crush injury. Fracture patterns have been discussed previously and include transverse, oblique, spiral, and comminuted fractures. Closed fractures can be treated with splint immobilization and referral to a hand surgeon within 2 to 5 days for definitive treatment. Fractures should be splinted with 70 to 80 degrees of MP flexion and IP joint extension.

Fingertip Injuries/Amputations

Partial amputations and fingertip injuries are among the more common injuries necessitating an urgent care center visit. These injuries occur as the result of closing a finger in a door or cutting the digit on a sharp surface. The resultant injury can range from a crush injury, where the distal tuft is fractured but there is no soft tissue laceration; to a crush injury with a nail-bed laceration causing a subungual hematoma; to an amputation of the distal end of the digit. Crush injuries that have corresponding nail-bed lacerations can be treated with removal of the nail plate and repair of the nail bed. This should be repaired with an absorbable suture, usually 5-0 or 6-0 Vicryl. The nail plate can be replaced back over the nail bed beneath the proximal fold, both to protect the nail bed and to give support to the distal tuft fracture. In nail-bed lacerations with subungual hematomas where there is not displacement of the fracture fragments, an alternative would be to decompress the nail bed by making a hole in the nail plate, either with a hollow-bore needle (an 18- or 20-gauge needle) or with a battery-powered electrocautery device. In cases of displaced fractures, the author prefers the method of nail-bed repair. In most cases, repair of the nail bed will result in reduction of the fracture. In a small percentage of cases, however, the fracture must be stabilized with a Kirschner wire, requiring consultation with a hand surgeon.

Partial amputations can be classified as transverse, oblique in the lateral plane, or oblique in the frontal plane. Treatment of these injuries varies by surgeon preference; therefore it is best to check with the hand surgeon providing follow-up *prior to* initiating treatment so as not to compromise his or her preferred method of treatment.

Digital Blocks

Digital blocks in the hand are useful for injuries to the dorsal and volar aspects of the fingers and thumb. In general, three agents are utilized for these blocks: lidocaine, mepivacaine, and bupivacaine. The agent administered depends on the desired duration of action. Lidocaine gives a 40- to 60-min block; mepivacaine a 4- to 5-h block; and bupivacaine an 8- to 10-h block. The advantage of lidocaine for digital blocks is its speed of onset, generally within 5 to 10 min. Bupivacaine, on the other hand, can take up to 30 min to take effect. Care should be taken to utilize only an agent *without epinephrine*. Use of epinephrine in the digits can result in ischemia or necrosis of the digit and therefore *should not be utilized!* Should hemostasis be desired, it should be achieved by direct pressure, use of a specially designed finger (Tourni-cot), ligation, or electrocautery.

Digital blocks in the border digits (index and small fingers) can be done as follows: Use a mixture of 5 mL of 1% lidocaine mixed with 5 mL of 0.5% bupivicaine. This mixture affords both speed of onset and useful duration of action. Inject 4 mL into the volar third of the web space using a 5/8-in. needle inserted to the hub. The injection should be made in the soft tissue volar to the level of the metacarpal heads. Following the injection of 4 mL, the web space should be noted to lose its concavity. The needle is then redirected to an area volar to the metacarpal head of the digit being blocked to anesthetize the proper digital nerve, which crosses over the metacarpal head. An additional 4 mL is injected at this site. Finally, the remaining 2 mL is injected into the subcutaneous tissue overlying the base of the proximal phalanx to anesthetize the skin over its dorsal aspect, extending to the dorsal PIP joint. Central digital blocks (the middle and ring fingers) are done in a similar fashion; however, two injections are required, one in each web space.

 Errors to Avoid

- Use of epinephrine
- Intravascular injections (always aspirate prior to injection)

 Key Points of Documentation

- A careful sensory examination should be performed and recorded prior to administering the digital block.

KNEE INJURIES

Evaluation and Management

Knee injuries can occur from a variety of mechanisms, including a fall from a height, impact or loading injuries from MVAs, twisting injuries from running sports, as well as blunt injuries from falls. The initial evaluation should be systematic, looking for lacerations, soft tissue swelling, obvious deformity, effusions, point tenderness, ligamentous laxity, reduced range of motion, crepitus, and compromised neurovascular status. Management is dependent on the specific diagnosis but generally consists of compression or immobilization, ice, elevation, rest, and crutch ambulation, or a cane to assist ambulation.

Fractures

Fractures about the knee can involve the patella, distal femur, or proximal tibia. Patellar fractures generally occur as the result of a low-injury fall onto the patella. Patients with displaced fractures are unable to ambulate because they cannot actively extend the leg. They may present with a palpable defect in the patella and inability to elevate the extended leg off the examining table. There is tenderness to palpation at the patella and a significant hemarthrosis at the knee. In the case of displaced fractures, the diagnosis is evident on examination, but the definitive diagnosis is made based on the AP and particularly the lateral radiograph. Fracture patterns include transverse, stellate or Y-shaped, and comminuted. The fractures can involve the midportion of the patella, the proximal third, and the distal third. The initial treatment consists of a compression dressing, knee immobilizer, and use of a crutch. These can be supplemented by a NSAID. Definitive treatment for displaced fractures is ORIF; however, this can be done electively, following orthopedic consultation, which should be obtained with 1 to 2 days. Nondisplaced fractures can be managed nonoperatively with immobilization only. Patients should be referred for orthopedic follow-up within 1 week of injury.

Distal femoral fractures can involve the supracondylar femur, or they can be intraarticular, involving the medial or lateral femoral condyles. These injuries occur as the result of a loading injury or a varus/valgus torqueing injury. Patients present with pain, inability to ambulate, and, in the event of displaced fractures, a varus or valgus deformity. The physical examination demonstrates tenderness to palpation and a hemarthrosis along with possible crepitus and ecchymosis. Radiographs will demonstrate the extent and configuration of the fracture. With displaced fractures, many orthopedists prefer urgent surgical treatment. This may necessitate transfer to a hospital setting following discussion with the treating orthopedist. Initial treatment is similar to patellar fractures, consisting of a compression dressing and a knee immobilizer. This will also provide better stability in the event of a hospital transfer. In condylar fractures, the displacement is caused by the attachment and pull of the collateral ligament. Definitive treatment consists of ORIF to restore joint congruity. Blood loss can occur in these fractures and intravenous fluid support may be required. A baseline hematocrit should be obtained.

Fractures of the proximal tibia can range from avulsion injuries, medial or lateral plateau fractures, and bicondylar fractures, to combined plateau fractures and ligamentous injuries. These fractures occur as the result of an axial loading injury, usually from a fall. They can also result from an axial load as the result of a MVA. Patients present with inability to ambulate, pain, swelling, and a hemarthrosis. Physical examination demonstrates tenderness, possible instability to collateral ligament stress testing, an effusion, and pain with attempted range-of-motion exercise. Radiographs will demonstrate the type of fracture and the extent of displacement or, more likely, depression of the fracture. Definitive treatment consists of ORIF, attempting to restore the articular congruity of the proximal tibial articular surfaces. Fractures with depression of the articular surface should have emergent orthopedic evaluation. Nondisplaced fractures should be evaluated within 1 to 2 days.

Dislocations

The most common dislocations in the knee are lateral dislocations of the patella and posterior dislocations of the knee. A posterior dislocation represents an orthopedic emergency due to the risk of an intimal injury to the popliteal vessels and possible arterial compromise as well as possible injury to the peroneal nerve. These injuries occur as the result of a posteriorly directed force to the proximal tibia, usually from an MVA or a direct blow in a football injury. Patients present with severe pain associated with the dislocation and/or obvious deformity of the knee.

Physical examination demonstrates a sag sign (due to disruption of the posterior cruciate ligament), possible hypoesthesia of the dorsal foot, inability to extend the ankle or toes, and diminished or absent dorsalis pedis and/or posterior tibial pulses. In severe cases, the foot may look dusky. Immediate treatment is reduction of the dislocation using intravenous sedation, longitudinal traction, and anteriorly directed pressure on the proximal calf. There is usually a palpable reduction with this maneuver. Even following reduction, the examination should be repeated to document a change in the findings noted above, particularly the distal pulses. The current recommendation is for an angiogram following reduction to assure integrity of the vascular supply to the leg as well as to rule out an intimal tear of the popliteal vessels. Other possible sequelae of posterior dislocation of the knee include compartment syndrome, fractures, patellar tendon ruptures, and collateral ligament ruptures. In the event of a vascular injury, emergent treatment is required to reestablish vascular supply to the leg. Additionally, stabilization in the form of ligament reconstruction or application of an external fixator is required to prevent redislocation. These patients should be transferred expeditiously to a hospital with facilities for vascular reconstruction and orthopedic stabilization. Reduction should take place prior to transfer.

 Key Points of Documentation

- Waiting for radiographic confirmation of an obvious dislocation with vascular compromise

 Errors to Avoid

- Palpable dorsalis pedis and posterior pulses both pre- and postreduction
- Active ankle dorsiflexion prereduction
- Intact sensibility at the dorsal and plantar foot
- Associated medial and/or lateral collateral ligament laxity postreduction
- Postreduction x-rays to rule out associated fractures

Ligamentous Injuries

There are four ligaments stabilizing the knee: the anterior cruciate ligament (ACL), the posterior cruciate ligament (PCL), the medial collateral ligament (MCL), and the lateral collateral ligament (LCL). The anterior cruciate ligament prevents anterior translation of the tibia on the distal femur. It is usually injured by a twisting movement, a blow to the lateral knee, or a sudden deceleration. Presenting patients report having heard or felt a pop in the knee. There is rapid onset of an effusion. On examination, the Lachman test is positive, as is the anterior drawer test. There may be associated injuries, including meniscal injuries and collateral ligament injuries. With football injuries resulting from a blow to the lateral knee, the evaluation may reveal the "terrible triad": an ACL injury, a MCL injury, and a medial meniscal tear. ACL tears are usually treated by reconstructive surgery; however, most orthopedists currently recommend regaining range of motion prior to reconstructive surgery. Acute care of these injuries consists of a compression dressing, knee immobilization, ice, crutch ambulation, and orthopedic referral.

Collateral ligament injuries result from a blow to the medial or lateral knee. They can also result from torqueing injuries to the knee, as in skiing injuries. The injury is usually accompanied by a popping sensation and onset of swelling overlying the injured ligament. Physical examination reveals tenderness over the injured ligament and, most important, laxity to stress testing of the affected ligament. Isolated collateral ligament injuries can usually be treated conservatively with immobilization, using a cylinder cast, a knee immobilizer, or a hinged knee brace. Immediate treatment consists of ice, elevation, a compression dressing, and knee immobilization. Orthopedic follow-up should be within 3 to 5 days.

Injuries of the PCL are relatively rare. They usually result from dashboard impacts or tackles with blows to the proximal tibia. The initial presentation is pain and swelling at the knee. Examination demonstrates an effusion, a posterior sag sign, and possibly a positive posterior drawer sign. Immediate treatment consists of compression and immobilization, with orthopedic referral for definitive treatment.

Meniscal Injuries

Meniscal injuries result from twisting movements to the knee. They may also be due to an impact or jarring. The presentation is pain, swelling, painful or limited range of motion, and difficulty ambulating. Patients can also present with locking of the knee, where they are unable to extend the knee. The examination reveals limited range of motion, an effusion, and joint-line tenderness overlying the injured meniscus. There may be a positive Apley compression test, with pain on compression and rotation of the tibia on the femur with the knee flexed 90 degrees. Meniscal tears usually require arthroscopic treatment; however, initial treatment is compression, knee immobilization, and orthopedic referral.

Tendon Injuries

Tendon injuries in the knee include both tendinitis and tendon rupture. Tendinitis results from overuse and presents with swelling and tenderness over the affected tendon. It can affect the patellar tendon, the pes anserine tendons (sartorius, gracilis, and semitendinosus), and the biceps femoris tendons. Treatment includes heat, rest, NSAIDs, and immobilization. These injuries are usually self-limited; however, patients with ongoing symptoms should be referred for orthopedic evaluation and treatment.

Tendon ruptures in the knee can involve the quadriceps, patellar, and plantaris tendons. These injuries usually result from sudden deceleration or jumping. With quadriceps and patellar tendon injuries, the patient is unable to ambulate. He or she usually reports having heard a popping sound in the knee. Physical examination reveals soft tissue swelling at the anterior aspect of the knee, and, with careful gentle palpation, one may be able to palpate a defect in the patellar or quadriceps tendon. The patient is unable to perform a straight leg raise owing to disruption of the extensor mechanism. In the case of a patellar tendon rupture, there may be proximal migration of the patella on examination and on x-rays. Definitive treatment requires surgical intervention; however, initial treatment calls for a compression dressing and splint immobilization. Orthopedic referral can be made for elective surgical treatment. In the case of plantaris tendon ruptures, the patient also reports having heard or felt a popping sensation. However, as opposed to the patient with extensor mechanism injuries, he or she is able to ambulate following the injury. Physical examination may reveal ecchymosis at the posteromedial aspect of the knee, with tenderness. There is good strength to resisted flexion and extension at the knee. There is usually no effusion. This injury responds well to a simple compression dressing and NSAIDs, with symptomatology resolving over a 1- to 2-week period.

Chondromalacia Patellae

Chondromalacia patellae is due to softening of the cartilage surface on the undersurface of the patella. While this is usually not an emergent condition, patients will occasionally aggravate it to the point of seeking acute treatment. There is usually a history of pain with negotiating stairs or with squatting. The typical presentation is one of pain localized to the patella, usually at the lateral margin. There is a positive patellar inhibition test, where active quadriceps contraction—with compression of the patellofemoral joint through pressure at the proximal patella—leads to pain and limitation of further testing. There can be crepitus to passive range of motion at the patella as well as with patellar inhibition testing. Depending on the severity of the presentation, the patient can present with an effusion; therefore there can be limited range of motion. Radiographs should show no acute abnormality. Emergent treatment includes rest and NSAIDs. Patients with ongoing symptoms can be referred to an orthopedic surgeon for continuing care, including supervision of a quadriceps-strengthening exercise program.

Osteochondritis Dissicans

Osteochondritis dissicans usually involves the medial femoral condyle of the knee. It can also be seen on the medial dome of the talus and the medial condyle of the humerus. The pathology is caused by loss of vascular supply to a portion of the subchondral bone. This loss of blood supply leads to loss of bony support to the articular cartilage and ultimately can cause fragmentation of the articular cartilage, with free fragments within the knee. The presentation is usually one of pain and an effusion and, in cases of a loose body, locking of the knee. Patients can also present complaining of the knee slipping or giving way due to temporary entrapment of the cartilage fragment between the articular surfaces. There are three stages of osteochondritis dessicans:

1. No radiographically visible lesion. These lesions can be visualized by magnetic resonance imaging (MRI) examination. The treatment is immobilization and/or activity modification.
2. The lesion is apparent on plain x-rays but is not displaced. This stage can also be treated by immobilization and/or activity modification.
3. The fragment is displaced and becomes a free fragment. This stage requires surgical intervention.

All three stages can be treated emergently by immobilization and the use of NSAIDs; orthopedic consultation should be obtained within 5 to 7 days.

Osgood-Schlatter Syndrome

Osgood-Schlatter syndrome is an apophysitis of the tibial tubercle. It is usually seen in adolescent and preadolescent children. There is a strong male predilection. Patients present complaining of knee pain, which is often bilateral. The pain is aggravated by running or jumping activities. Physical examination reveals prominence of the tibial tubercle, with moderate to severe tenderness. There is pain to resisted extension at the knee, but full extension is possible without resistance. Radiographs reveal widening of the epiphysis of the tibial tubercle. In the case of acute injuries or falls, there may be a fracture of the tubercle. Acute treatment consists of immobilization and avoidance of running and/or jumping activities. This condition may continue to flare periodically until the apophysis of the tibial tubercle fuses, usually at about age 15 in girls and age 17 in boys. Orthopedic follow-up may be required for patients with ongoing symptoms and should occur within 1 to 2 weeks.

INJURIES OF THE TIBIA AND/OR FIBULA

Proximal tibial fractures have been discussed above, with injuries of the knee. Fractures of the tibial shaft occur from a variety of direct blows and twisting movements. The initial presentation is one of pain, swelling, and—in most cases—inability to ambulate. Physical examination demonstrates soft tissue swelling, tenderness to palpation, possible angular deformity, and possible neurovascular compromise. The definitive diagnosis is made by x-ray evaluation.

 Key Points of Documentation

- Is there a skin laceration, making this an open fracture?
- Are the distal pulses intact?
- Is distal sensibility intact?

Nondisplaced fractures can ultimately be treated by cast immobilization following orthopedic referral. The initial treatment should consist of a compression dressing, long leg splint immobilization, non-weight-bearing ambulation with crutches, and ice. Displaced fractures of the tibia can pose skin problems if splinted in the displaced position. With skin tenting anteriorly over the fracture site, skin necrosis can develop. An emergent orthopedic consultation should be obtained in these instances for fracture reduction and stabilization. Definitive treatment of displaced fractures of the tibia/fibula includes the options of closed reduction and casting, intramedullary rod placement, and external fixator application. During the evaluation of these fractures at the urgent care center, careful assessment for compartment syndrome is in order (see below).

 Errors to Avoid

- Failure to document absence of compartment syndrome
- Splinting of the leg with anterior skin tenting

Compartment Syndrome

Compartment syndrome can occur at multiple sites, including the forearm, the hand, the lower leg, and the foot.

- The distinguishing characteristic of compartment syndrome is pain out of proportion to the findings on physical examination.

Patients complain of severe pain in the extremity, worse with movement. Complaints of numbness in the extremity come late and should not be depended upon for the diagnosis. Physical examination findings in the lower leg include increased tension in the anterior, lateral, or superficial posterior compartments; pain with passive extension of the great toe; and pain with active range of motion at the great toe. Late findings include diminished or absent pulses and decreased or absent sensibility in a superficial peroneal nerve distribution. The key to making the diagnosis in a timely fashion is to have a high index of suspicion (Table 15-4). The definitive diagnosis is made by compartment pressure monitoring. There are commercially available, portable wick catheter kits that can rapidly measure the pressure within the four compartments in the lower leg. If this device is unavailable at your urgent care center and you suspect that the patient has compartment syndrome, he or she should be transferred to the nearest hospital facility. The orthopedic consultant usually measures the compartment pressures if the diagnosis of

TABLE 15-4

COMPARTMENT SYNDROME IN THE LOWER LEG

COMPARTMENT	MUSCLES	NERVE	ARTERY	PROVOCATIVE EXAM
Anterior	Tibialis anterior, extensor digitorum longus, extensor hallucis longus	Deep peroneal nerve	Anterior tibial artery	Active dorsiflexion of the ankle and first toe Passive plantarflexion of the ankle and first toe Decreased sensation in dorsal first web space
Lateral	Peroneus longus, peroneus brevis	Superficial peroneal nerve	None	Active eversion of the foot Passive inversion of the foot
Superficial posterior	Gastrocnemius, soleus	Sural nerve	None	Active plantarflexion of the ankle Passive dorsiflexion of the ankle
Deep posterior	Tibialis posterior, flexor digitorum longus, flexor hallucis longus	Posterior tibial nerve	Posterior tibial artery	Active plantarflexion of the first toe Passive dorsiflexion of the first toe Decreased sensation in plantar foot

compartment syndrome is being considered. If these indicators are elevated, the patient will require emergent surgery for a fasciotomy to relieve the increased pressure prior to irreversible ischemia of the muscles within the compartment. Pressure measurements of greater than 30 mmHg are considered an indication for emergent fasciotomy.

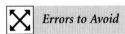 ***Errors to Avoid***

- Application of compression dressings in cases of suspected compartment syndrome
- Dependent positioning of the leg in suspected compartment syndrome

Peroneal Nerve Injuries

Peroneal nerve injuries result from blows to the region of the fibular neck, fractures of the proximal fibula, lacerations of the peroneal nerve, and compartment syndromes. Patients present complaining of numbness of the dorsal foot and inability to extend the ankle. Physical examination reveals tenderness at the fibular neck (in the case of fractures), inability to dorsiflex the foot, and absent sensibility at the first web space at the dorsum of the foot. With the exception of compartment syndrome and lacerations, the immediate treatment of this injury is posterior splinting in the neutral position, crutch ambulation, and orthopedic referral. Treatment of peroneal nerve palsies secondary to compartment syndrome is as outlined above. Lacerations involving the peroneal nerve should be treated by microvascular repair. The surgery can be performed electively, following skin closure, and posterior splinting in the urgent care center. Consultation with a hand surgeon or microvascular surgeon should be obtained to determine the timing of the nerve repair.

ANKLE INJURIES

The most commonly seen injuries to the ankle include sprains, fractures, dislocations, and Achilles' tendon ruptures.

Examination of the Ankle

Initial examination of the ankle should include an inspection looking for swelling, skin disruption, or obvious deformity. Palpation is performed for tenderness, defects associated with displaced fractures or tendon ruptures, or crepitus. Range of motion should be assessed at both the ankle and the subtalar joints. Pain with range of motion should be documented, as should crepitus with attempted range of motion. Neurovascular examination should assess for sensibility, intact dorsalis pedis and posterior tibial pulses, as well as strength to resisted inversion, eversion, dorsiflexion, and plantarflexion at the ankle. Examination of the ankle should include palpation at the base of the fifth metatarsal to rule out fracture at the base of the fifth metatarsal, which can occur along with twisting injuries. Palpation should also include the fibular head to rule out a fracture of the fibular neck with deltoid ligament disruption (Maisonneuve's injury).

- When a patient presents with an ankle injury, examination must always include palpation of the base of the fifth metatarsal and the fibular head in order to avoid missing associated injuries.

Sprains

There are five major ligaments stabilizing the ankle joint: the anterior and posterior talofibular ligaments, the calcaneofibular ligament, the anterior tibiofibular ligament, and the deltoid ligament. Ninety percent of ankle sprains are lateral sprains with injuries to the anterior talofibular and calcaneofibular ligaments. The majority of these injuries involve the anterior talofibular ligament. They are generally due to an inversion mechanism that occurs during running or, more rarely, with walking. The presentation is pain, swelling, and difficulty ambulating. Physical examination reveals soft tissue swelling and tenderness over the involved ligaments. There may be decreased range of motion at the ankle. Radiographs demonstrate soft tissue swelling but no bony injuries. Initial treatment consists of splinting—either in a posterior splint, sugar-tong splint, or air cast. Crutch ambulation is recommended for the first 2 to 4 days, as are NSAIDs and elevation. A referral to an orthopedic surgeon should be made for follow-up within 5 to 7 days.

Dislocations

Ankle dislocations occur as the result of twisting movements combined with axial loading. The predominant pattern is that of a posterior dislocation. The initial presentation is pain, swelling, deformity, and inability to ambulate. Physical examination reveals deformity, with prominence anteriorly at the distal tibia, tenderness at the anterior ankle, decreased range of motion at the ankle, as well as possible diminished sensibility and absent to decreased pulses. Radiographic examination reveals posterior dislocation of the talus on the distal tibia. There may be an associated fracture at the medial and/or lateral malleolus. Reduction of the dislocation is accomplished by anterior traction on the calcaneus performed with the ankle in slight plantarflexion. This is best performed with the patient under conscious sedation with intravenous agents for the sake of both pain control and muscle relaxation. Radiographs should be obtained following reduction to assure adequacy of the reduction and rule out new fractures or intraarticular fragments; neurovascular status should also be assessed and documented. Posterior splint or sugar-tong splint immobilization is utilized following reduction until orthopedic follow-up can occur, which should be within 2 to 3 days.

Fractures

Ankle fractures can be isolated lateral malleolar fractures, bimalleolar fractures involving both the medial and lateral malleoli, or trimalleolar fractures involving the medial malleoli, lateral malleoli, and posterior malleolus of the distal tibia. These injuries, which are due to inversion/eversion and twisting mechanisms, may be described according to the Lauge-Hansen and Weber classifications. The Lauge-Hansen system uses a combination of the position of the foot as well as the deforming vector. The Weber system classifies ankle fractures by the position of the fibular fracture. Weber A fractures have the fibular fracture at the level of the plafond of the distal tibia. Weber B fractures are at the level of the syndesmosis between the tibia and fibula. Weber C fractures have fibular fractures above the syndesmosis. These fractures require surgical reduction and stabilization (Fig. 15-23). If there is not significant displacement or skin tenting, these injuries can be treated emergently with splinting and orthopedic referral. If there is significant widening at the mortise of the ankle or if there is skin tenting at the medial aspect of the ankle, an emergent orthopedic referral should be obtained for reduction or reduction and stabilization.

 Key Points of Documentation

- Peripheral pulses intact pre- and postreduction in ankle fracture/dislocation
- Radiographic evidence of widening at the mortise

 Errors to Avoid

- Failure to obtain a full x-ray with isolated mortise widening of the tibia/fibula (Maisonneuve fracture)
- Failure to check postreduction x-ray for osteochondral fracture

Achilles' Tendon Ruptures

Achilles' tendon ruptures are the most frequent tendon ruptures in the lower extremity. The injury occurs with a sudden stress as the result of a forceful contracture of the Achilles' tendon with the ankle in a dorsiflexed position. There is an audible/palpable pop at the heel at the time of the injury. The patient is unable to walk on the ball of the foot following the rupture. Physical examination may reveal soft tissue swelling over the midportion of the Achilles' as well as a palpable defect in the substance of the tendon. Thompson's test, where the gastrocnemius muscle is squeezed with the lower leg in a horizontal position, fails to cause plantarflexion of the foot. With a palpable tendon defect, additional diagnostic tests are unnecessary. In cases where the tendon is not clearly ruptured, an MRI may be helpful in documenting the injury. Surgery to repair the tendon is the definitive treatment, so orthopedic referral is indicated. The acute treatment is posterior splinting of the ankle. The ankle should be splinted in plantarflexion. Non-weight-bearing ambulation is facilitated by crutch usage. NSAIDs, ice, and elevation are helpful in the acute management.

FOOT INJURIES

Evaluation of foot injuries should include examination to determine possible Lisfranc's fracture/dislocation, Chopart's injuries, calcaneal fractures, talar fractures, plantar fasciitis, stress fractures, as well as phalangeal fractures and dislocations. The examination should include assessment of soft tissue swelling, bony prominence, obvious deformity, skin disruption, tenderness, and neurovascular compromise. X-ray evaluation is impor-

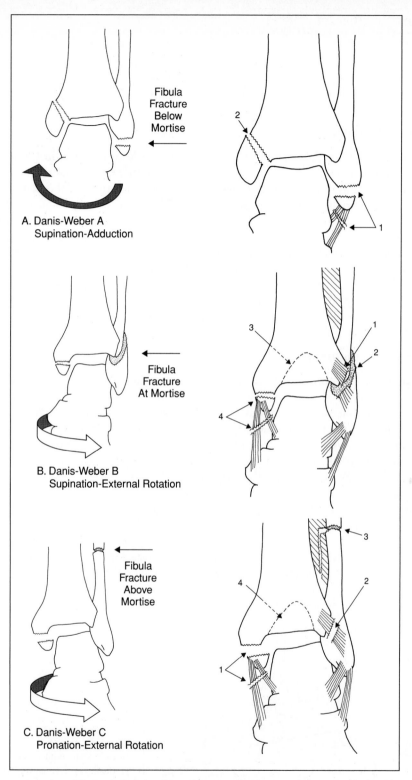

FIGURE 15-23 The Danis-Weber and Lauge-Hansen classification schemes of ankle injuries. (From Schwartz DT, Reisdorff E: *Emergency Radiology*. New York: McGraw-Hill; 2000, with permission.)

tant in determining the presence of fractures and dislocations. Range of motion should also be evaluated and documented.

Plantar Fasciitis

Plantar fasciitis is inflammation of the plantar fascial layer of tissue in the foot. The patient presents complaining of pain in the heel, particularly upon walking early in the morning. Physical examination may demonstrate tenderness at the plantar aspect of the foot at the distal portion of the calcaneus. There may be an antalgic gait favoring the affected heel. X-rays of the heel, in particular the lateral view, may demonstrate a spur at the distal plantar tip of the calcaneus. This is a traction spur, and the pain is not due to prominence at the site of the spur but rather to the inflammation and tension at the site of insertion of the plantar fascia. Initial treatment includes NSAIDs, rest, and Achilles' tendon stretching exercises. Patients with ongoing symptoms can be referred for orthopedic evaluation and treatment. Other treatment options include heel pads, orthotics, physical therapy, and possibly surgery for plantar fascial release.

Calcaneal Fractures

Calcaneal fractures occur as the result of falls from variable heights. With displaced fractures, there is a rapid onset of swelling. This may result in blistering, particularly if the foot is not placed in a compression dressing, splinted, and elevated. An orthopedic consultation should be requested urgently, since many orthopedists prefer to operate on calcaneal fractures acutely, prior to the onset of swelling. Radiographs, including axial and lateral views, should be obtained. The lateral view in particular should be evaluated to assess Bohler's angle. This is the angle formed by the intersection of a line connecting the superoposterior facet with the posterior calcaneal tuberosity with a line connecting the superoposterior facet with the anterior calcaneal process (Fig. 15-24). This angle should measure approximately 25 to 30 degrees. With calcaneal fractures, there is flattening of Bohler's angle due to axial loading of the talus into the calcaneus (Fig. 15-25). Acute treatment consists of compression dressing, posterior splint immobilization, elevation, and crutch ambulation, with no weight bearing on the affected extremity.

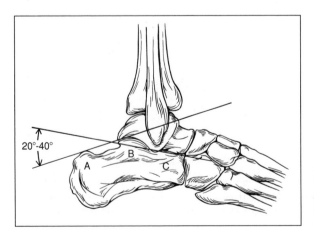

FIGURE 15-24 Bohler's angle. (From Tintinalli J et al: *Emergency Medicine: A Comprehensive Study Guide,* 5th ed. New York: McGraw-Hill; 2000, with permission.)

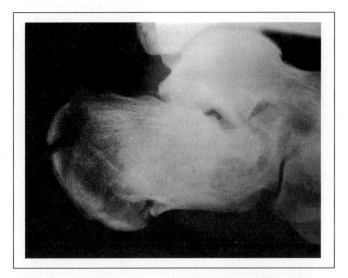

FIGURE 15-25   Calcaneal compression fracture. There is a comminuted compressed fracture of the calcaneal body and posterior tuberosity. Bohler's angle is flat (zero degrees). (From Schwartz DT, Reisdorff E: *Emergency Radiology.* New York: McGraw-Hill; 2000, with permission.)

Lisfranc's Fractures

Lisfranc's injuries consist of dislocations of the tarsometarsal joints of the forefoot, with a fracture of the base of the second metatarsal base. This occurs with excessive axial loading combined with a twisting mechanism. The initial presentation is one of swelling, pain, and inability to ambulate. The examination reveals soft tissue swelling at the midfoot, tenderness over Lisfranc's joint with a possible bony prominence at this location, and decreased range of motion at the ankle, forefoot, and toes. The first and second metatarsals should be moved in opposite dorsal and plantar directions checking for associated pain. X-rays are pathognomonic for this injury. On an oblique x-ray, the medial aspect of the second metatarsal should align with the medial second cuneiform. The medial aspect of the third metatarsal should align with the medial third cuneiform. Finally, the medial aspect of the fourth metatarsal should align with the medial cuboid. There are two types of Lisfranc's injuries, homolateral and divergent. In divergent dislocations, there is separation between the first and second metatarsals, with possible lateral dislocation of the third and fourth metatarsal bases with the second metarsal. There is no ligamentous attachment between the base of the first and second metatarsals. The ligamentous attachment is between the base of the second metatarsal and the lateral first cuneiform. A fracture at the base of the second metatarsal indicates disruption of this ligament. In homolateral injuries, the metatarsal bases all dislocate in the same direction, either medial or lateral (Fig. 15-26). Immediate orthopedic consultation should be obtained for these injuries. Definitive treatment consists of closed reduction and pinning of the tarsometatarsal joints, or open reduction and internal fixation of these joints with a screw.

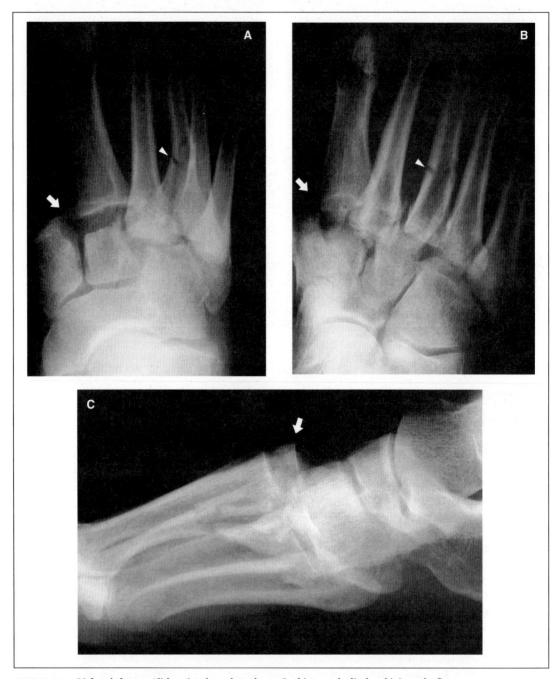

FIGURE 15-26 Lisfranc's fracture/dislocation, homolateral type. In this severely displaced injury, the first metatarsal is dislocated from the first cuneiform (*arrow*) (*A* and *B*). A fracture of the third metatarsal shaft is also present (*arrowhead*). (*C*) On the lateral view, the metatarsals are dorsally displaced relative to the midfoot. (From Schwartz DT, Reisdorff E: *Emergency Radiology.* New York: McGraw-Hill; 2000, with permission.)

Chopart's Joint

Chopart's joint comprises the calcaneocuboid and talonavicular joints. These injuries occur with a twisting mechanism. Patients present with pain, swelling, and inability to ambulate. As with Lisfranc's injuries, the x-rays confirm the diagnosis, demonstrating dislocation of the calcaneocuboid and/or the talonavicular joint, with possible avulsion fractures of the associated tarsal bones. Physical examination should inspect for ecchymosis, skin disruption, tenderness, and prominence at the midtarsal joints medially or laterally. Emergent orthopedic consultation should be requested, as surgical intervention will be required for reduction and stabilization.

 Errors to Avoid

- Failure to check alignment of second and fourth metatarsals in cases of fracture of the second-metatarsal base.
- Failure to assess for tenderness at Lisfranc's joint in cases of twisting foot injuries, resulting in inability to ambulate

Tarsal Fractures

Tarsal fractures can involve any of the hindfoot bones, including the calcaneus and talus; the first, second, or third cuneiforms; the cuboid; and the navicular. Fractures of the calcaneus have been discussed previously. The second most common tarsal fracture is the talus. These injuries occur with axial loading, as in falls or MVAs. The fractures can involve the body or the neck of the talus. The blood supply to the talus passes retrograde into the body of the talus through the neck. Fractures of the talar neck, and particularly fractures of the neck with dislocation of the body of the talus, can disrupt the blood supply to the talus, resulting in avascular necrosis (AVN). Physical examination should document tenderness medially at the midfoot over the talar neck, prominence medially or posteriorly indicating dislocation, decreased range of motion at the ankle, as well as neurovascular compromise. X-rays should be examined for fracture of the talar neck and dislocation of the body of the talus. Displaced talar neck fractures and particularly fracture/dislocations of the talus should receive emergent orthopedic consultation in order to reduce the fracture/dislocation as expeditiously as possible and not to jeopardize the talar blood supply. Nondisplaced talar fractures can be splinted in a posterior splint with a compression dressing and referred for orthopedic evaluation in 2 to 3 days.

Metatarsal Fractures

Metatarsal fractures occur due to direct blows or twisting of the foot. The fracture can involve the head, neck, shaft, and base of the metatarsal. X-rays can be utilized to assess the location, orientation, and displacement of the fracture. In minimally displaced or nondisplaced fractures, the patient can have the foot splinted in a posterior splint with subsequent orthopedic follow-up within 2 to 4 days.

A specific variant of the metatarsal fracture is fracture of the fifth metatarsal base. This injury occurs as the result of a twisting movement of the foot. The patient is unable to ambulate or finds ambulation to be painful following this injury. Physical examination may reveal ecchymosis, swelling, and tenderness at the fracture site. X-rays show one of two fracture patterns. One is a fracture at the proximal portion of the fifth metatarsal. The second is a fracture at the metaphyseal-diaphyseal junction of the fifth metatarsal, known as a Jones fracture (Fig. 15-27). This fracture has an increased risk of proceed-

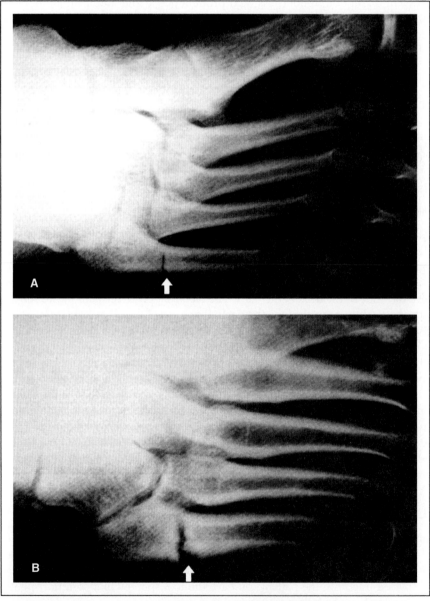

FIGURE 15-27   Jones fracture. *A.* Transverse fracture through the proximal shaft of the fifth metatarsal. *B.* This fracture is often complicated by nonunion. (From Schwartz DT, Reisdorff E: *Emergency Radiology.* New York: McGraw-Hill; 2000, with permission.)

ing to a nonunion, particularly if there is distraction at the fracture site. These fractures should also be treated by posterior immobilization acutely with subsequent orthopedic referral. In Jones fractures with more than 2 mm of distraction, more urgent referral should be obtained. This subset of fractures may have to be treated with ORIF.

Phalangeal Fractures

The majority of phalangeal fractures are nondisplaced, resulting from low-energy impact. The initial presentation is pain, swelling, and ecchymosis at the affected toe. The physical examination findings of tenderness to palpation are combined with x-rays to make a definitive diagnosis. Treatment of nondisplaced fractures is with buddy taping supplemented by a postoperative shoe. The fracture should be adequately healed within 2 to 3 weeks to allow discontinuation of immobilization. Patients with intraarticular fractures or ongoing symptoms should be referred for orthopedic evaluation.

BIBLIOGRAPHY

Green DP, Hotchkiss RN, Pederson WC (eds): *Green's Operative Hand Surgery,* 4th ed. New York: Churchill Livingstone; 1999.

Rockwood CA, Green DP, Bucholz RW, Heckman JD (eds): *Fractures in Adults,* 4th ed. Philadelphia: Lippincott-Raven; 1996.

Schwartz DT, Reisdorff E (eds): *Emergency Radiology.* New York: McGraw-Hill, 2000.

Tintinalli JE, Kelen GD, Stapczynski JS (eds): *Emergency Medicine: A Comprehensive Study Guide,* 5th ed. New York: McGraw-Hill; 2000.

NECK AND BACK

Daphne G. Golding

Cervical and/or lumbar pain is a common complaint in any busy clinical medical practice. It is prudent, therefore, for every physician involved in patient care to be skilled in the recognition and evaluation of conditions affecting the neck and back. Many medical conditions present with signs and symptoms originating in or referring to the cervical or lumbar spine (Table 16-1). This wide range of disorders should be kept in mind in evaluating patients complaining of neck or back pain. The patient's history and presentation will be useful in narrowing the focus.

Throughout this chapter, recommendations for the use of medications are made as part of the management of acute neck and back pain syndromes. As an overview, Table 16-2 lists commonly used anti-inflammatory medications, analgesics, and centrally acting medications that are frequently prescribed for the treatment of neck and back pain syndromes. The table is by no means complete but is meant only to serve as a guide. In prescribing medications, it is important to obtain a complete medical history including allergies and medical conditions such as ulcers or bleeding disorders that may prohibit the use of certain medications; it is also important to record the use of any current medications that could lead to adverse side effects or negative drug interactions.

TABLE 16-1

CONDITIONS AFFECTING THE NECK AND BACK

Rheumatologic	Infection
Inflammatory versus noninflammatory	Local versus systemic
arthropathies	Metabolic
Connective tissue disorders	Vascular
Tumors	Viscerogenic
Benign versus malignant	Musculoskeletal
Primary versus metastatic	Traumatic versus nontraumatic
Spinal versus nonspinal	

TABLE 16-2

EXAMPLES OF ORAL MEDICATIONS COMMONLY USED IN THE MANAGEMENT OF ACUTE NECK AND BACK PAIN[a]

DRUG	CLASS	ORAL DOSAGE	PROPERTIES/ INDICATIONS	COMMON SIDE EFFECTS
Acetaminophen		600 to 1000 mg qid	Analgesia for patients in mild to moderate pain	Hepatic toxicity with ingestion greater than 140 mg/kg.
Ibuprofen	NSAID	600 mg qid or 800 mg tid	Anti-inflammatory and analgesia for patients in mild to moderate pain	Gastrointestinal and renal. Use with caution in patients with impaired renal function.
Diclofenac	NSAID	50 or 75 mg bid	Anti-inflammatory and analgesia for patients in mild to moderate pain	Gastrointestinal and renal. Use with caution in patients with impaired renal function.
Hydrocodone	Opioid	2.5, 5.0, 7.5 mg qid	Analgesia for patients in moderate to severe pain Frequently used in combination with acetaminophen	Sedation, nausea, constipation. Physical dependence may occur after only 2 weeks of therapy.
Oxycodone	Opioid	2.5, 5.0, 7.5 mg qid	Analgesia for patients in moderate to severe pain Frequently used in combination with acetaminophen	Sedation, nausea, constipation. Physical dependence may occur after only 2 weeks of therapy.
Metaxalone	Centrally acting agent resulting in muscle relaxation	800 mg tid or qid	Use in patients with significant muscle pain and spasm	Nausea, vomiting, gastrointestinal upset, drowsiness. Use with caution in patients with hepatic dysfunction.
Carisoprodol	Centrally acting agent resulting in muscle relaxation	350 mg qid	Use in patients with significant muscle pain and spasm	Drowsiness, dizziness, nausea. Use with caution in patients with renal and hepatic dysfunction.
Diazepam	Benzodiazepine	2.5 or 5.0 mg bid or tid	Use in patients with severe muscle pain and spasm	Drowsiness, dizziness, fatigue, incoordination.

[a]This table represents suggestions of medications useful in the treatment of acute neck and back pain. The actions and side effects are not inclusive. Please refer to other sources for additional information.

Disorders of the Cervical Spine

Basic Functional Anatomy

A knowledge of basic clinical anatomy is necessary in order to understand the pathologic conditions of the cervical spine. The cervical spine is made up of seven cervical vertebrae, which are separated into upper (C1-2) and lower (C3-7) regions. The C1 (atlas) and C2 (axis) are unique in that the ring-like atlas has no vertebral body and articulates with the occipital condyles above and the axis below, while the axis has a vertebral body and spinous process as well as an odontoid process (also known as the dens) that articulates with the anterior arch of the atlas (Fig. 16-1). In contrast, the C3-7 vertebrae all have a vertebral body, spinous process, transverse processes, and facet articulations (Fig. 16-2). These vertebrae also have uncovertebral articulations (also called joints) that arise from their posterolateral margins and lie anterior to the exiting nerve roots. These articulations can degenerate, resulting in hypertrophy and osteophyte formation.

- The lower cervical spine accounts for most of the flexion, extension, and lateral bending of the neck. The greatest amount of flexion occurs at C4-5 and C5-6. Lateral bending occurs primarily at C3-4 and C4-5.

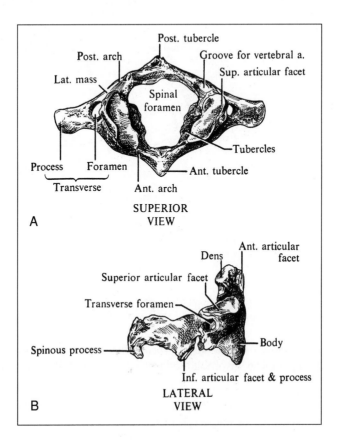

FIGURE 16-1 *A.* Atlas. *B.* Axis. (From Pansky B: *Review of Gross Anatomy*, 6th ed. New York: McGraw-Hill; 1996, with permission.)

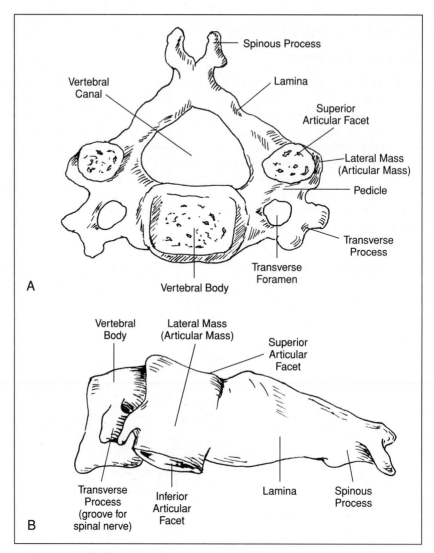

FIGURE 16-2   The lower cervical vertebra (C5). (From Schwartz DT, Reisdorff E: *Emergency Radiology.* New York: McGraw-Hill; 2000, with permission.)

The nerves of the cervical spine are formed by the union of the dorsal sensory roots and ventral motor roots after they exit from the spinal cord (Fig. 16-3). Each spinal nerve exits through the foramen formed by the uncovertebral joints anteriorly and the facet joints posteriorly. Because of these relationships, the nerves are subject to compression from pathology involving the facets, uncovertebral joints, and intervertebral disks.

- *Cervical nerves one through seven exit on top of their respective vertebrae; the eighth nerve exits between C7 and T1.* On x-ray evaluation, it is therefore critical to visualize the entire C7-T1 junction.

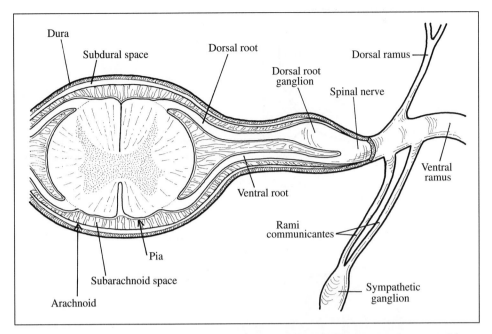

FIGURE 16-3 Spinal cord and meninges at thoracic level. (From Hollinshead W: *Functional Anatomy of the Limbs and Back*, 6th ed. Philadelphia: Sanders; 1991, with permission.)

In the cervical spine, *intervertebral disks* are located between the vertebrae from C2 through T1. Each intervertebral disk is made up of two parts, the outer annulus fibrosus and the central nucleus pulposus (Fig. 16-4). The annulus fibrosus is composed largely of fibrocartilage. The nucleus pulposus is a mass of gelatinous material containing a large amount of water, a small number of collagen fibers, and a few cartilage cells. Young disks are generally thick, malleable, and elastic. With advancing age, the water content of the nucleus pulposus diminishes and older disks become thin, rigid, and brittle.

- As a result of the changes that occur in disks with age, smaller forces are needed to injure "older" disks versus "younger" ones.

Numerous *ligaments* add stability to the cervical spine. In the upper cervical spine, the transverse, alar, and accessory atlantoaxial ligaments help maintain the integrity of the odontoid and C1 articulation (Fig. 16-5). The anterior longitudinal ligament passes the entire length of the spinal column just anterior to the vertebral bodies and disks. The posterior longitudinal ligament also passes the length of the spinal column, but it lies just posterior to the vertebral bodies and disks and reinforces the posterior annulus. Other ligaments include the supraspinous ligament, which connects the tips of the vertebral spines; the interspinous ligament, which runs between adjacent spines; and the ligamentum flavum, which connects adjacent laminae. The ligamentum nuchae, which is actually formed by the supraspinous and interspinous ligaments, extends from the spine of C7 to the external occipital protuberance (Fig. 16-6).

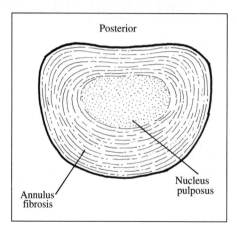

FIGURE 16-4 Structural components of the inter-vertebral disk, thoracic level. (From Bogduk N, Twomay LT: *Clinical Anatomy of the Lumbar Spine*. New York: Churchill Livingstone; 1988, with permission.)

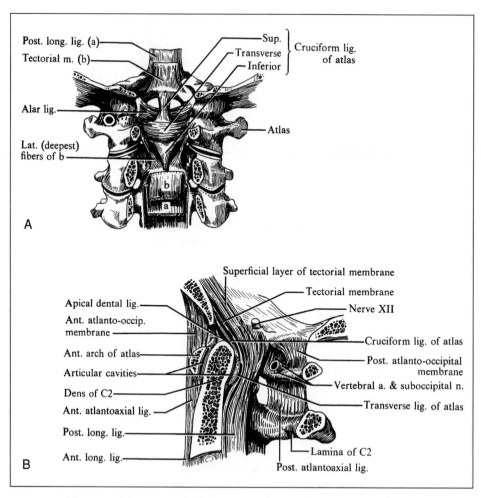

FIGURE 16-5 Ligaments of the upper cervical spine. *A.* Articulation. *B.* Median section. (From Pansky B: *Review of Gross Anatomy*, 6th ed. New York: McGraw-Hill; 1996, with permisssion.)

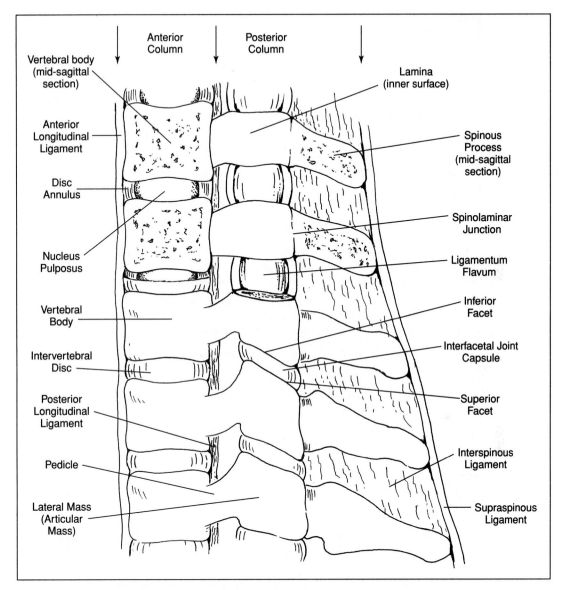

FIGURE 16-6 Anatomy of the cervical spine. (From Schwartz DT, Reisdorff E: *Emergency Radiology.* New York: McGraw-Hill; 2000, with permission.)

Pain Generators

Any innervated structure may be a source of pain. It should be noted, therefore, that in addition to nerve tissue, the vertebrae, the outer annular fibers of the intervertebral disks, the cervical muscles (or any other muscles that have attachments in the cervical region), and the ligaments may all contribute to pain syndromes in the cervical spine.

History

A detailed history is of paramount importance in evaluating the patient presenting with a complaint of neck pain. Often, following the history, a preliminary diagnosis may be formulated. This working diagnosis can then be confirmed or negated by subsequent physical examination and diagnostic studies.

 Errors to Avoid

- The most common error in obtaining a history is not asking.

  During the history, the following information should be obtained on all patients:

- The exact location (and radiation), onset, and duration of the pain
- The character and severity of the pain
- Any aggravating factors such as movement, specific activities, or positioning
- Specific positions, rest, or home remedies tried that alleviate the pain
- Associated symptoms such as headache, fever, malaise, constitutional symptoms, or pain in other regions that may suggest a systemic problem

When symptoms present as a result of trauma, details concerning the mechanism of injury are also important and can help direct the formulation of a differential diagnosis.

- Complaints of weakness and sensory abnormalities are suggestive of neurologic involvement.
- Complaints of bowel or bladder dysfunction are important and suggest myelopathy (i.e., actual spinal cord involvement).

 Physical Examination

- Patients who present with possible traumatic injury of the cervical spine should be examined in a neutral position; the neck should remain immobilized until fracture, dislocation, or instability has been ruled out.

For the patient who does not require immediate immobilization, a thorough examination of the neck begins with inspection. This should begin as the patient enters the examination room by observing his or her posture. The fluidity and coordination of movement should be noted, as any abnormal positioning of body parts may be secondary to pathology. Scarring, dermatologic processes, discoloration, swelling, and asymmetry are to be noted as well.

Palpation

The structures of the neck are best palpated with the patient relaxed in the supine position. Anteriorly, the hyoid bone (which lies opposite the C3 vertebral body), the thyroid cartilage (which marks the level of the C4-C5 vertebral bodies), and the first cricoid ring are all easily identified. These bony landmarks can be useful in locating the anterior soft tissue structures including the sternocleidomastoid muscles, the accessory muscles of the pharynx and larynx (often called the strap muscles), the anterior cervical lymph nodes, the thyroid gland, and the parotid glands. Any abnormalities in size, shape, or muscle tone as well as any swelling, tenderness, or nodules should be noted. Both the carotid pulses and the supraclavicular fossae should also be examined.

The posterior landmarks that are important to assess are the occiput, superior nuchal line, mastoid processes, spinous processes of the cervical vertebrae, and the region of the facet joints. It is important to note whether the normal lordosis of the cervical spine has been lost. The alignment of the spinous processes should be checked for, as well as any palpable tenderness. Of note, the soft tissue structures of the posterior neck are best examined with the patient seated. In this position, the trapezius and paraspinal muscles, the lymph nodes on the anterolateral aspect of the trapezius muscles, the greater occipital nerves, and the ligamentum nuchae can be examined.

Range of Motion

Both active and passive range of motion should be evaluated. The normal spine allows 45 degrees of flexion, extension, and lateral bending. Normal rotation is 60 degrees. During the clinical examination, range of motion can be estimated. This allows the physician to quickly assess whether neck motion is normal or significantly restricted. Neck flexion is usually normal if the patient can touch the chin to the chest with a closed mouth. Extension is normal if the face is almost horizontal as the patient goes into maximum neck extension. Lateral bending is normal if the ear can touch the shoulder with the shoulder in the neutral position. Rotation is considered normal if the chin can touch the shoulder.

Muscle weakness may limit active range of motion; it is important, therefore, to test passive range of motion in order to evaluate for limitation on a mechanical basis. Passive range of motion, however, should be tested only if cervical spine instability has been ruled out.

- Range of motion tends to diminish with aging.
- While it is important to test both active and passive range of motion, range of motion should be tested only in a stable cervical spine.

Neurologic Evaluation

The neurologic examination in the patient presenting with neck pain must include the neck and both the upper and lower extremities. Motor strength, sensation, and muscle stretch reflexes are significant components of the examination. Abnormalities may lead to a differential diagnosis that includes radiculopathy (pathology involving the nerve root), myelopathy (pathology involving the spinal cord itself), or other neuromuscular disorders. On motor examination, neck strength should be tested in flexion, extension, and rotation. The major muscle(s) responsible for moving the major joints of the upper and lower extremities should be evaluated for tone, bulk, and strength. Table 16-3 lists an established grading system for muscle strength. Table 16-4 lists the root level, peripheral nerve, and primary action for muscles of the upper extremity commonly evaluated in the patient with neck pain.

- The patient must be observed closely for asymmetry and signs of atrophy.

TABLE 16-3

COMMONLY USED GRADING SYSTEM FOR MUSCLE STRENGTH TESTING

NUMBER	WORD	DEFINITION OF MUSCLE STRENGTH
0	None	No movement
1	Trace	Movement with gravity eliminated but not through a full range of motion
2	Poor	Movement through a full range of motion with gravity eliminated
3	Fair	Movement through a full range of motion against gravity
4	Good	Movement through a full range of motion against gravity with slight (but not full) resistance
5	Normal	Movement through a full range of motion against gravity with normal resistance

- It is important to ensure that the prime movers of the joint are actually functioning and that secondary muscles are not performing the movement (i.e., substitution is not occurring).
- Note: Patients may seem weak because of pain rather than a true neuromuscular disorder.

The basic sensory evaluation includes light touch, pain (pinprick), vibration, and position sense. The light touch and pain portions of the sensory examination can best be achieved by initially testing an area of the body not expected to be involved in the

TABLE 16-4

NERVE ROOT LEVEL, PERIPHERAL NERVE, AND PRIMARY ACTION OF MUSCLES COMMONLY TESTED IN THE PATIENT WITH NECK PAIN

NERVE ROOT LEVEL	NERVE	MUSCLE	PRIMARY ACTION
C5,C6	Axillary	Deltoid	Abduction, flexion and internal rotation, extension and internal rotation of arm
C5, C6 (C5)[a]	Musculocutaneous	Biceps brachii	Flexion and supination of arm
C5, C6	Suprascapular	Supraspinatus	Abduction of arm
	Suprascapular	Infraspinatus	External rotation of arm
C6-C8 (C7)	Radial	Triceps	Extension of arm
C6, C7 (C6)	Radial	Extensor carpi radialis	Extension/abduction at wrist
C6, C7 (C6)	Median	Pronator teres	Pronation of forearm
C8, T1	Median	Abductor pollicis brevis	Abduction of thumb
C8, T1 (T1)	Ulnar	First dorsal interrossei	Abduction of index finger

[a]Parentheses denote a common segmental innervation. The actual composition of nerves may vary among individuals.

TABLE 16-5

COMMONLY USED GRADING SYSTEM FOR SENSORY TESTING

NUMBER	DESCRIPTION	NUMBER	DESCRIPTION
0	Absent	2	Normal
1	Impaired	NT	Not testable

pathology being evaluated (for example, the face); this allows the patient to understand normal sensation. Other areas can then be tested and compared to this "normal" area. Table 16-5 lists the commonly used grading system for the sensory examination involving touch and pain.

- It is important to always prompt the patient to be exact in describing the sensory change and the location of the change.

Based upon the patient's sensory evaluation, knowledge of peripheral nerve patterns (Fig. 16-7), and dermatomal distribution (see Fig. 16-8), some determination can usually be made as to whether there is peripheral nerve and/or nerve root involvement.

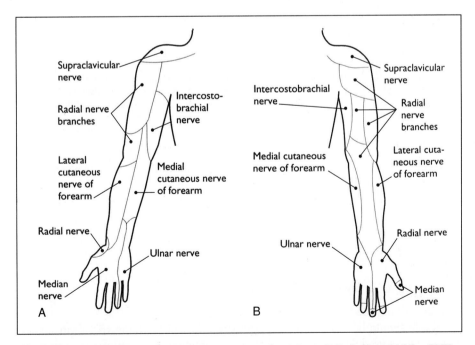

FIGURE 16-7　Peripheral nerve patterns of the upper extremity. *A.* Front. *B.* Back. (From McMinn RMH, Hutchings RT, Logan BM: *The Concise Handbook of Human Anatomy.* Stamford, CT: Appleton & Lange, 1998, with permission.)

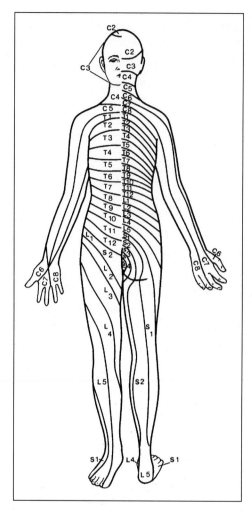

FIGURE 16-8   Dermatomes. (From Tintinalli J et al: *Emergency Medicine: A Comprehensive Study Guide,* 5th ed. New York: McGraw-Hill; 2000, with permission.)

- Of note, vibratory and position sense are both more likely to be involved early in radiculopathy. Unfortunately, in contrast to soft touch and pain, vibration is more difficult to localize to one dermatome.

 Errors to Avoid

- Interpreting "funny sensations" as sensory loss.

Reflex testing can be very helpful in localizing the area of pathology. Table 16-6 lists reflexes that should be tested in the upper extremities, while Table 16-7 represents the commonly used grading system for reflex documentation. Hyporeflexia is suggestive of a lower motor neuron process (one involving the root, brachial plexus, or peripheral

TABLE 16-6

COMMONLY TESTED MUSCLE STRETCH REFLEXES OF THE UPPER EXTREMITY

NERVE ROOT LEVEL	MUSCLE	SITE OF TAP
C5-C6	Biceps brachii	Antecubital
C5-C6	Brachioradialis	Radial wrist
C6-C8	Triceps	Distal arm
C7-C8	Ventral fingers	Finger flexors

nerve). Hyperreflexia and pathologic reflexes such as the Babinski and Oppenheim reflexes suggest an upper motor neuron process involving the brain, brainstem, or cervical spinal cord.

- A positive *Babinski* reflex is seen when, as a sharp instrument is run along the lateral foot, the great toe extends and the other toes flex and splay.
- A positive *Oppenheim* reflex is evoked by applying firm pressure along the tibial crest; the response is the same as for the Babinski reflex.

Hyporeflexia and hyperreflexia can be present together if the lesion involves both the central and peripheral nervous systems.

 Errors to Avoid

- *Use of improper equipment.* A heavy reflex hammer should be used to elicit a response properly.
- *Failure to recognize an inverted reflex.* An inverted reflex occurs when the antagonist of the muscle whose reflex is being tested actually responds. This may indicate root pathology.
- *Failure to note asymmetry.*
- *Assuming that all clonus represents pathology.* For some patients, a few beats of clonus can be normal.
- *Inappropriate interpretation of reflexes.* It is important to recognize that reflexes must be interpreted within the context of the complete neurologic evaluation.

Special Tests

Spurling's Test
The patient's head and neck are extended and laterally flexed while gentle but firm pressure is applied on the top of the head for up to 1 min. If pain, numbness, or tingling occurs into the ipsilateral shoulder and upper extremity in a dermatomal pattern, the test is considered positive. This is consistent with foraminal encroachment on an inflamed nerve root.

TABLE 16-7

COMMONLY USED REFLEX GRADING SYSTEM

NUMBER	DESCRIPTION
0	No reflex
Trace	Only a slight tendon movement regardless of method
1+	Requires facilitation to get the reflex
2+	Normal
3+	Brisk response, may carry over to other levels
4+	Brisk response with clonus

Adson's Maneuver

While the examiner is palpating the radial pulse, the arm is abducted, extended, and externally rotated. At the same time, the patient should take a deep breath and turn his or her head toward the symptomatic arm. This test is designed to determine compromise of the neurovascular bundle in thoracic outlet syndrome, a controversial condition that results in compression of the brachial plexus and/or subclavian vessels as they pass through the neck and superior thoracic outlet toward the axilla. If there is vascular compromise, the radial pulse will diminish. If there is neurologic compromise, the patient's neurologic symptoms will be reproduced. This test is sensitive but not very specific and has a high incidence of false-positives. If this condition is suspected, referral to a physiatrist, orthopedist, or neurologist is indicated for further evaluation.

Lhermitte's Sign

The examiner flexes the patient's head briskly. This test is positive if electric-like pain or shock sensations shoot down through the spine. A positive test suggests a spinal cord disorder or herniated cervical disks.

Distraction Test

With one hand under the patient's chin and the other on the occiput, the examiner slowly lifts the patient's head to decrease its weight on the neck. During the performance of this test, pain due to nerve root pathology secondary to narrowed neural foramina may be relieved.

Compression Test

Gentle pressure is applied to the top of the patient's head while he or she is in the seated position. An increase in neck pain or increased pain in the affected extremity is a positive test and may signify radiculopathy.

Diagnostic Studies

- In patients with a history of significant trauma or with neurologic complaints, the neck should remain immobilized in the neutral position inside a hard cervical orthosis with mandibular and occipital supports. Immobilization should be maintained until the spine can be "cleared." In some cases, the patient may need to remain immobilized and be transferred for further evaluation.

The radiologic evaluation is important in both traumatic and nontraumatic types of neck pain. Depending on the patient's presentation, history, and the extent and mechanism of trauma, a cross-table lateral x-ray should be obtained as the initial film for evaluation of cervical injury. It is of paramount importance that all seven cervical vertebrae and the full C7-T1 junction be visualized. If C7 cannot be completely visualized, the physician should gently pull the patient's shoulders down while the radiograph is being taken. If complete visualization is still difficult, the swimmer's view should be obtained. If full visualization still cannot be achieved, the patient should remain immobilized and should be transferred to an emergency department for further evaluation. In patients with a history of only minor trauma who have no neurologic complaints, an upright lateral may be ordered in place of a cross-table projection. Again, it is vital that all seven cervical vertebrae and the full C7-T1 junction be visualized.

Whether performed as a cross-table projection or in the upright position, a good quality lateral film will usually demonstrate most traumatic conditions of the lower cervical spine as well as injuries involving the anterior and posterior arches of C1, the odontoid process, and the anterior atlantal-dens segment. On this view, the bodies and spinous processes of C2-C7 can be fully visualized and the intervertebral disk spaces and prevertebral soft tissues evaluated. Additionally, the four contour lines of the normal cervical spine can be evaluated as well as the retropharyngeal and retrotracheal spaces (Fig. 16-9).

The lateral view alone, however, is inadequate to determine spinal stability and does not identify all cervical fractures. Other important projections to obtain in evaluating the cervical spine include the anteroposterior view, the open-mouth view, and bilateral oblique views. Flexion and extension radiographs may also be needed, particularly in those patients with severe pain in whom no bony injury or neurologic deficit has been identified. These films may reveal dynamic spinal instability secondary to severe ligamentous stretching or tearing.

To determine stability, the spine may be considered according to the three-column system. Column I includes the anterior longitudinal ligament and the anterior two-thirds of the vertebral body. Column II is composed of the posterior third of the vertebral body and the posterior longitudinal ligament. Column III is composed of the posterior elements including facet joints, the neural arch, and the spinous processes. On radiographic evaluation, any of the following findings represents instability:

1. Injury involving any two adjacent columns
2. Any angulation of two adjacent vertebrae that is greater than 11 degrees more than the angulation between each of those vertebrae and their adjacent vertebrae
3. Movement in the anterior, posterior, or lateral directions of one vertebra relative to an adjacent vertebra greater than 3.5 mm

• In patients with traumatic injury to the cervical spine, anterior soft tissue swelling seen on lateral films may be the only indication of an undetected fracture; in this situation, the neck should remain immobilized and the patient transferred for further evaluation including a CT scan of the suspicious area.

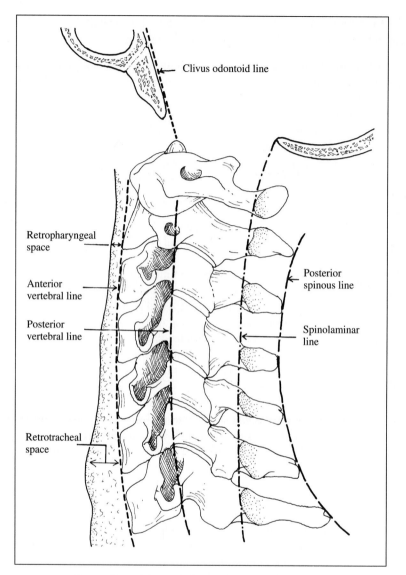

FIGURE 16-9 Contour lines of the cervical spine. (From Greenspan A, Montesano P: *Imaging the Spine in Clinical Practice.* London: Mosby Europe Limited; 1993, with permission.)

- For patients with nontraumatic causes of neck pain, radiographic evaluation should additionally include evaluation of disk height, calcific deposition within the disk space, degenerative changes, and evidence of lytic or blastic lesions.

Indications for Immediate Neurosurgical or Orthopedic Consultation

- Any new or worsening neurologic complaints including:
    Acute bowel or bladder dysfunction

Acute weakness or sensory loss in a myotomal or dermatomal distribution
- Dislocation, subluxation, or malalignment on x-ray
- Fractures on x-ray
- Ligamentous instability seen on flexion or extension radiographs
- An unclear or uncertain clinical or radiographic examination

 Errors to Avoid

- *Failure to visualize all seven cervical vertebrae and the superior margin of the first thoracic vertebrae.*
- *Failure to recognize ligamentous instability in the patient with severe pain and muscle spasm. Severe pain or muscle spasm may prevent full range of motion on flexion and extension films, thereby masking ligamentous instability.*
- *Failure to proceed with further testing in the patient with significant symptoms or examination findings and negative radiographs.*
- *Relying too heavily on radiographic findings. Findings alone do not assure a cause-and-effect relationship between the findings and the patient's complaints.*

 Key Points of Documentation

History	• Onset, location, radiation, duration of pain
	• Aggravating or remitting factors
	• Weakness, sensory loss, bowel or bladder dysfunction
	• Previous history of neck or back pain
	• Associated symptoms
Physical Examination	• Range of motion
	• Muscle weakness, sensory loss, abnormal muscle stretch reflexes
	• Painful musculature
Workup	• Presence or absence of radiologic findings

Nontraumatic neck pain

There are many medical and neurologic illnesses that may present with neck and upper extremity symptoms. These include processes that produce mass lesions, such as tumors or abscesses; general medical conditions such as rheumatoid arthritis; and neurologic disorders such as myasthenia gravis or multiple sclerosis. Many of these conditions have an insidious onset and are accompanied by symptoms in areas outside the cervical region including weight loss, fever, and/or intracranial symptomatology. The following discussion reviews only some of the more common causes of nontraumatic neck pain that may present for urgent care evaluation. The usual clinical presentation, diagnostic workup, and treatment are discussed. Note that when conservative treatment of acute neck pain is mentioned, this generally means rest, analgesia, and the use of passive modalities for additional pain relief. Table 16-2 lists commonly prescribed medications for the treatment of acute neck and back pain. When the acute pain subsides, a physical therapy program for neck stabilization can then be started. If appropriate, additional comments are made in reviewing the specific condition.

Cervical Spondylosis

This is one of the most common neck conditions affecting patients over the age of 50. As in osteoarthritis involving other joints in the body, there is a bony response to changes in the articular cartilage. Sclerosis and osteophyte formation occur. The uncovertebral joints and facet joints are the areas of the cervical spine most affected. Hypertrophy of the ligamentum flavum is a common pathologic finding. Dehydration of the intervertebral disk occurs. Tears in the annulus fibrosus can progress to disk herniation. The changes in the disk may further aggravate degenerative bony changes.

Clinical Presentation

The onset of symptoms is insidious. Neck pain and stiffness, particularly in the morning, that improves with movement is common. These complaints may be accompanied by radicular complaints if degenerative changes result in nerve root irritation. Examination findings are consistent with the physiologic changes that have occurred. Cervical range of motion is painful and decreased. Extension and lateral bending are affected early. With encroachment upon nerve roots, sensory loss, weakness, and diminished deep tendon reflexes may be seen in the appropriate dermatomes and myotomes. Tenderness in the paravertebral musculature is common.

Advanced cases of degeneration with or without posterior disk herniation can lead to severe neurologic deficit. This situation can produce spinal stenosis with actual spinal cord compression (i.e., cervical myelopathy); this is most likely to occur in patients with some degree of congenital spinal stenosis. These patients present with decreased range of motion, a positive Lhermitte's sign, and weakness that may involve all four extremities. Bowel, bladder, and sexual dysfunction may be present. Hyperreflexia may be seen in the lower extremities.

Diagnostic Studies

In the urgent care setting, plain radiographs are helpful to demonstrate degenerative changes. Magnetic resonance imaging (MRI) is useful for evaluating the disk integrity and computed tomography (CT) further demonstrates bony abnormalities.

Treatment

Most patients may be treated conservatively. A course of nonsteroidal anti-inflammatory drugs (NSAIDs) should be initiated and continued until symptoms have subsided. In severe acute cases, bed rest for not more than 2 to 3 days, temporary use of a cervical orthosis, and a course of steroids with a quick taper may be warranted. Physiatric or orthopedic referral is appropriate to direct further diagnostic workup and management. In patients with signs and symptoms of radiculopathy or those who have evidence of cervical myelopathy, additional treatment is needed and orthopedic or neurosurgical referral should be arrranged.

Rheumatoid Arthritis

- Approximately 50 percent of patients with rheumatoid arthritis have cervical involvement.

Rheumatoid arthritis is a progressive, chronic, proliferative inflammatory process affecting the synovium and resulting in the destruction of joints and ligaments. The process may occur alone or together with degenerative disease.

Clinical Presentation
As in degenerative disease, onset is insidious. The patient may complain of neck pain, often with symptoms consistent with radiculopathy, and may even give a history suggestive of myelopathy. Further questioning may reveal a history of fever, malaise, joint pain, and nonarticular findings consistent with this systemic disease.

Physical findings are similar to those seen secondary to degenerative disease. Tenderness in the paraspinal musculature as well as evidence of radiculopathy and myelopathy are not uncommon findings. Range of motion will generally be decreased and painful. Range of motion, however, should be tested with caution because instability, particularly in the proximal cervical spine, may be present.

Diagnostic Studies
If the patient has a known history of rheumatoid arthritis, laboratory studies may not be necessary. In patients without a known diagnosis of rheumatoid disease (which would be an unusual presentation), an erythrocyte sedimentation rate, rheumatoid factor, and joint fluid analysis may provide useful diagnostic information. On radiographic evaluation, lateral films of the cervical spine in neutral, flexion, and extension should be obtained (see Fig. 16-10 for possible findings seen in rheumatoid arthritis). Erosive changes may be seen in the odontoid process and apophyseal joints. Subluxation of the atlantoaxial joint is a common finding that may be accompanied by superior migration of the odontoid process. The intervertebral disks and adjacent vertebral bodies may be involved. Of note, three types of cervical instability may occur in patients with rheumatoid disease of the neck: atlantoaxial impaction, atlantoaxial subluxation, and subaxial subluxation. When present, subaxial subluxation most commonly occurs at C3-4.

Treatment
Treatment of the patient with a stable spine is conservative. NSAIDs may be given acutely; however, a referral to a rheumatologist for early aggressive treatment aimed at altering the disease's progression would afford the patient the best long-term outcome. Rest, gentle massage, heat, and judicious use of a soft cervical collar provide symptomatic relief. A carefully monitored isometric exercise within pain tolerance may help to strengthen and stabilize neck musculature and avoid further muscle weakening. Evidence of spinal instability and/or myelopathy warrants immediate orthopedic and/or neurosurgical referral.

Myofascial Pain Syndrome

Myofascial pain syndrome is a clinical syndrome that should be considered in patients presenting with neck pain that refers to the posterior shoulder girdle and/or upper

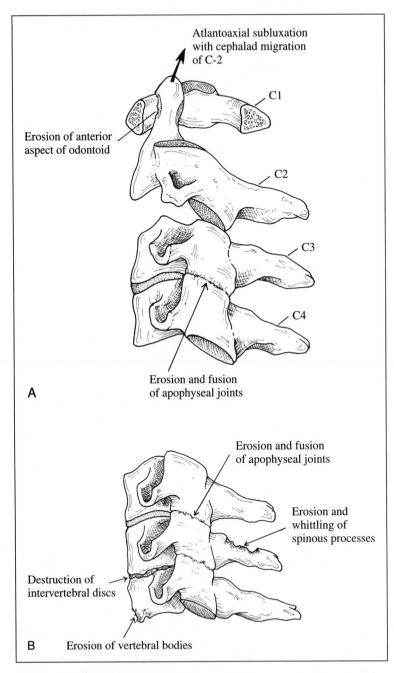

FIGURE 16-10   Morphologic features distinguishing the various arthritides as manifest in the spine. *A* and *B*. Rheumatoid arthritis. (From Greenspan A, Montesano P: *Imaging the Spine in Clinical Practice*. London: Mosby Europe Limited; 1993, with permission.)

TABLE 16-8

CLINICAL CRITERIA FOR THE DIAGNOSIS OF MYOFASCIAL PAIN SYNDROME CAUSED BY ACTIVE TRIGGER POINTS

To make the clinical diagnosis of myofascial pain syndrome, the findings should include five major criteria and at least one of three minor criteria. The five *major criteria* include the following:

1. Regional pain complaint.
2. Pain complaint or altered sensation in the expected distribution of referred pain from a myofascial trigger point.
3. Taut band palpable in an accessible muscle.
4. Exquisite spot tenderness at one point along the length of the taut band.
5. Some degree of restricted range of motion, when measurable.

The three *minor criteria* include the following:

1. Reproduction of clinical pain complaint, or altered sensation, by pressure on the tender spot.
2. Elicitation of a local twitch response by transverse snapping palpation at the tender spot or by needle insertion into the tender spot in the taut band.
3. Pain alleviated by elongating (stretching) the muscle or by injecting the tender spot (trigger point).

NOTE: Additional symptoms such as weather sensitivity, sleep disturbance, and depression are often present but are not diagnostic because they may be attributable to chronic severe pain perpetuated by multiple mechanical and/or systemic perpetuating factors.
SOURCE: Simons AG: Muscular pain syndromes, in Fricton JR, Awad EA (eds): *Advances in Pain Research and Therapy.* Vol 17: *Myofascial Pain and Fibromyalgia.* New York: Raven Press; 1990:18, with permission.

extremities. Typically, these patients complain of the slow onset of neck pain and stiffness radiating into the upper extremities, often accompanied by sleep disturbance and altered sensation. Dysesthesia, paresthesias, and weakness (secondary to pain) affecting the upper extremities may also be present, which may make this syndrome difficult to discern from radiculopathy; the presence of symptoms in a nondermatomal, nonmyotomal pattern will help in this regard. "Tender points" or "trigger points," which are firm, tender nodules that have a consistent pain referral pattern, must be found for this diagnosis. These areas are typically found within taut bands of muscle (i.e., a shortened group of muscle fibers) and can be best palpated by sliding the skin and subcutaneous tissues perpendicularly across the fibers of the muscle. Clinical criteria exist as guidelines to aid in the diagnosis (Table 16-8). All radiographic and laboratory studies are normal. This is a chronic condition that responds best to a chronic pain management program including medications, psychological support modalities, and a well-supervised exercise program.

TRAUMATIC NECK PAIN

Motor vehicle accidents account for the majority of presentations to the urgent care setting for the evaluation of traumatic neck pain. Other causes of traumatic neck pain include falls, participation in contact sports, and diving accidents. When a patient presents for evaluation, it is imperative that the physician maintain a high index of suspicion for fracture or dislocation. This suspicion may be increased or decreased based upon the patient's history. Details regarding the mechanism of injury—i.e., flexion, extension, compression, shearing, rotation, distraction—will assist in the investigation of the type of injury. Table 16-9 provides a classification of injuries to the cervical spine by mechanism of injury and stability.

TABLE 16-9

CLASSIFICATION OF INJURIES TO THE CERVICAL SPINE BY MECHANISM OF INJURY AND STABILITY

CONDITION	STABILITY
Flexion injuries	
Occipitocervical dislocations	Unstable
Subluxation	Stable
Dislocation in facet joints (locked facets)	
Unilateral	Stable
Bilateral	Unstable
Odontoid fractures	
Type I	Stable
Type II	Unstable
Type III	Stable
Wedge fracture	Stable
Clay-shoveler's fracture	Stable
"Teardrop" fracture	Unstable
Burst fracture	Stable or unstable
Extension injuries	
Occipitocervical dislocations	Unstable
Fracture of posterior arch of C1	Stable
Hangman's fracture	Unstable
"Extension teardrop" fracture	Stable
Hyperextension fracture–dislocation	Unstable
Compression injuries	
Jefferson fracture	Unstable
Burst fracture	Stable or unstable
Laminar fracture	Stable
Compression fracture	Stable
Shearing injuries	
Lateral vertebral compression	Stable
Lateral dislocation	Unstable
Transverse process fracture	Stable
Lateral mass fracture	Stable
Rotation injuries	
Fracture–dislocation	Unstable
Facet and pillar fractures	Stable or unstable
Transverse process fracture	Stable
Distraction injuries	
Hangman's fracture	Unstable
Occipitocervical dislocations	Unstable
Atlantoaxial subluxation	Stable or unstable

SOURCE: Greenspan A, Montesano P: *Imaging of the Spine in Clinical Practice.* London: Mosby Europe Limited; 1993, with permission.

In the evaluation of the patient presenting with a history of a traumatic neck injury, it is imperative that fractures, dislocations, spinal instability, and any neurologic deficits be recognized. During the initial evaluation, the cervical spine must first be secured in a neutral position with the use of a cervical collar and the patient assessed for life-threatening injuries. (See Chap. 19 for full assessment of the trauma patient.) During this initial assessment, any evidence of spinal instability or injury mandates full immobilization and immediate advanced life support transport to a facility capable of treating potential spinal cord injury. In patients without neurologic symptoms or initial evidence of spinal injury, cervical spine radiographs can be obtained, as discussed in the previous section on diagnostic studies (see also Appendix 2, "Radiographic Signs and Findings"). If any evidence of fracture, dislocation, or instability is identified, the spine must remain immobilized and the patient immediately referred for orthopedic or neurosurgical evaluation. If no abnormalities are identified or suspected, the examination can continue in the urgent care setting. At any time, however, if clinical evidence of spinal injury is noted, the patient should be immediately immobilized and transferred for neurosurgical evaluation.

Cervical Sprain and Strain

Injury to the cervical muscles is one of the most common etiologies of traumatic neck pain. Typically, this injury occurs following a motor vehicle accident in which an extension-flexion injury to the neck occurs as a result of a rear-end collision. This type of injury may also occur following other types of trauma, such as falls, participation in sports, or even housecleaning! While the primary injury is usually a sprain (injury to ligaments and/or tendons) or a strain (injury to muscle), nerve root injury from stretch or focal hemorrhages may also occur.

Clinical Presentation
In this type of injury, the patient typically presents with neck pain, often radiating into the shoulders and upper extremities. Headaches are a frequent associated complaint, and vague complaints such as light-headedness, nausea, paresthesias, and dysesthesias in a nonradicular pattern may occur. Symptoms usually appear within the first 24 to 48 h following the injury. In mild injuries, examination may reveal only painful restricted cervical range of motion and associated tenderness in the paraspinal musculature. Neurologic examination will be normal. In moderate to severe injuries, the patient may also complain of swallowing difficulties secondary to injury to the structures in the anterior neck. In these instances, cervical range of motion is significantly restricted and muscle swelling and tenderness are present. If injury to the zygoapophyseal joints has occurred, patients may complain of "spatial instability" and symptoms of disequilibrium and "veering" associated with changes in direction. In the patient who has suffered a stretch injury to the nerve root, true radicular signs may develop.

Diagnostic Studies
Plain radiographs should be obtained to rule out bony injury or ligamentous instability. Static as well as dynamic (flexion and extension) views are important in the patient with severe neck pain, even without positive neurologic findings. If any evidence of instability is seen, immediate referral for orthopedic evaluation is indicated.

Errors to Avoid

- *Failure to recognize ligamentous instability in the patient with severe pain and muscle spasm.* Severe pain or muscle spasm may prevent full range of motion on flexion and extension films, thereby masking ligamentous instability.

Treatment

Stable injuries are treated conservatively. Brief use of a soft cervical collar may provide comfort. The collar should be discontinued as soon as the symptoms subside; this is typically within 2 weeks. NSAIDs—and sometimes judicious use of narcotic analgesics—are helpful to control pain. While centrally active agents to decrease muscle tightness and pain are frequently used, it is not clear that this hastens recovery. Use of these and other sedating agents at night, however, may be useful in restoring a more normal sleep pattern and ultimately may have the indirect effect of lessening pain. In moderate to severe cases, bed rest for 2 to 3 days may be necessary. In the acute phase, the use of ice for 20 min every hour as needed may assist in pain relief as well as decreasing local swelling and inflammation of the soft tissues. A referral for physical therapy for additional modalities and mobilization can be effective. In an attempt to avoid chronic problems, follow-up with a physiatrist, orthopedist, or primary care physician familiar with the treatment of cervical sprain and strain is indicated to assure appropriate rehabilitation of these patients. The majority of patients improve within weeks to several months.

 Errors to Avoid

- *Failure to instruct patients using a soft collar not to use the collar while driving.* A soft collar will inhibit rotation, producing potentially unsafe driving conditions.
- *Failure to provide adequate acute pain relief and restore a normal sleep pattern.*

Acute Cervical Disk Disease

Cervical herniated nucleus pulposus (HNP) may occur acutely as a result of trauma and often accompanies the more chronic degenerative form of disk disease. HNPs may produce local nerve root irritation, resulting in radiculopathy.

Clinical Presentation

The patient with acute cervical HNP without radiculopathy will typically present with vague complaints of neck pain. Referred pain is usually in a nondermatomal pattern. In contrast, patients who have radiculopathy present with symptoms radiating into the upper extremity in a dermatomal pattern or into the shoulder. For both groups of patients, neck flexion and activities that increase pressure within the intervertebral disk—such as coughing, sneezing, and lifting—will tend to exacerbate the symptoms. Pain is aggravated by hyperextension and rotation of the neck to the involved side. The pain is relieved somewhat by bringing the patient's ipsilateral hand up behind the neck.

- *In the rare patient with a posterior herniation, cervical myelopathy may also develop.*

Examination of patients with cervical disk herniation is most significant for loss of range of motion. In these patients, axial compression may increase pain while distraction may lessen pain. Paraspinal muscle tenderness may also be present. Neurologic examination is normal unless radiculopathy is present. When neurologic symptoms are present, fasciculations, weakness, and loss of deep tendon reflexes may be noted. If cervical myelopathy develops, weakness and upper motor neuron signs can appear.

Diagnostic Testing

Although plain radiographs of the cervical spine are often normal, degenerative changes may be seen. Ultimately, an MRI is indicated to evaluate disk pathology, but this can be arranged by the following physician.

Treatment

Management is conservative. Significant radicular complaints may respond to a short trial of steroids with a quick taper. A cervical collar during the acute phase may provide symptomatic relief. When pain has subsided, a supervised therapy program is appropriate for neck stabilization.

In those patients in whom the history and physical findings suggest a posterior herniation, referral for neurosurgical evaluation is indicated.

Cervical Cord Syndromes

Several clinical syndromes are described in traumatic spinal cord injury involving the cervical spine. These syndromes include central cord syndrome, Brown-Séquard's syndrome, and anterior cord syndrome. The *central cord syndrome* is the most common and the one most likely to be encountered in the urgent care setting. It can be seen in elderly patients with degenerative spine disease who experience a hyperextension injury (frequently secondary to a fall). The cord is impinged upon by the ligamentum flavum posteriorly and by osteophytes anteriorly, resulting in injury to the central portion of the cervical spinal cord. The corticospinal tract is topographically organized, with the fibers for the upper extremities being more centrally located. Thus, this syndrome presents with upper extremity weakness greater than lower extremity weakness. Bowel and bladder dysfunction is varied. Patients presenting with a possible central cord syndrome should be immobilized and transferred for further diagnostic studies including an MRI, which will demonstrate the central cord lesion.

In *anterior cord syndrome*, trauma to the anterior spinal artery or direct trauma to the anterior aspect of the cord produces symptoms. These symptoms include variable weakness and loss of pain and temperature; proprioception (which is located in the posterior columns of the spinal cord) is spared. Flexion injury of the cervical spine or a retropulsed disk or bone fragments may produce this type of syndrome. Again, as with central cord syndrome, the patient should be immobilized and transferred for further diagnostic studies and continuing care.

Brown-Séquard's syndrome was initially described as injury secondary to hemisection of the spinal cord. It most commonly occurs from stabbing injuries with a knife or other sharp instrument. Patients who sustain this type of injury will present with ipsilateral motor weakness, ipsilateral loss of proprioception, and contralateral loss of pain and temperature. There is usually no fracture associated with this injury. It is unlikely that these patients would present in the urgent care setting. However, if this were to occur, transfer to an acute care setting that is prepared to care for patients with spinal injury is necessary.

LOW BACK PAIN

Anatomy

The lumbar spine consists of five vertebrae, each composed of a body, a spinous process, transverse processes, facet joints, laminae, and pedicles (Fig. 16-11). These vertebrae are the largest in the spinal column and carry most of the body weight borne by the spine. The intervertebral disks located in the lumbar spine are normally thicker anteriorly, which contributes to the normal lumbar lordosis.

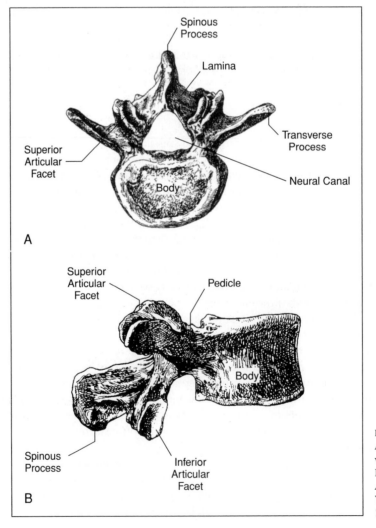

FIGURE 16-11
A typical lumbar vertebra. (From Pansky BL: *Review of Gross Anatomy,* 6th ed. New York: McGraw-Hill; 1996, with permission.)

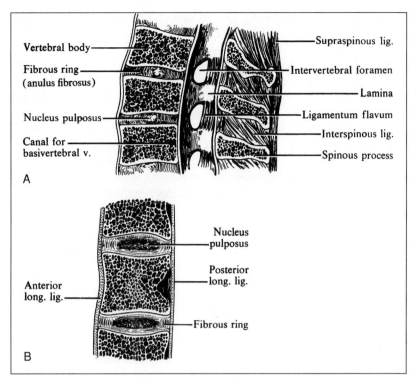

FIGURE 16-12   *A.* Median section—lumbar region. *B.* Sagittal seciton—lumbar region. (From Pansky B: *Review of Gross Anatomy*, 6th ed. New York: McGraw-Hill; 1996, with permission.)

- Some 75 percent of lumbar flexion and extension occurs in the lumbosacral junction, 20 percent at L4-5, and the remaining 5 percent at the other levels.

As in the case of the cervical spine, multiple ligaments add to the stability of the lumbar spine (Fig. 16-12). These ligaments include:

1. The supraspinous and interspinous ligaments. Together, they form the ligamentum nuchae in the cervical spine, but they are separate in the lumbar spine.
2. The ligamentum flavum, which connects the adjacent laminae and maintains the posterior facet joints.
3. The capsular ligaments of the facet joints. These allow for some movement at this level, which is necessary for normal range of motion.
4. The anterior longitudinal ligament and posterior longitudinal ligament, which run as continuous bands to the sacrum.

In addition to maintaining the axial stability of the vertebral column, these ligaments limit extension and flexion of the spine.

- In the lumbar spine, the posterior longitudinal ligament is wide over the intervertebral disks and narrow over the vertebral bodies. As it crosses the disk, its central portion is strong and its lateral portion weaker. Because of this (and the fact that the nucleus pulposus is eccentrically located more posteriorly), most disk herniations are posterolateral.

The vertebral column houses the neural elements. The spinal cord ends in the conus medullaris approximately at the level of L2. Below this is the cauda equina. The lumbar spinal nerve roots exit through the foramen formed by the vertebral pedicles superiorly and inferiorly, the facet joints posteriorly, and the bodies of the vertebrae and the intervertebral disk anteriorly. In the case of disk herniation, the nerve root is commonly compressed by the disk above the foramen. For example, the L4 root is compressed by the L3-4 disk, the L5 root by the L4-5 disk, and the S1 root by the L5-S1 disk. Severe central posterior disk herniations may result in cauda equina syndrome with lower extremity weakness as well as bowel and bladder dysfunction.

 History

A patient presenting with a complaint of low back pain may have pathology of either spinal or nonspinal origin. Essentially, the same processes that affect the cervical spine may also involve the lumbar spine (see Table 16-1). As in evaluating the patient with neck pain, an important first step in determining the etiology begins with a detailed history. The same types of questions asked for the evaluation of the patient with neck pain are appropriate in the evaluation of patients complaining of low back pain.

 Physical Examination

Examination of the low back begins with inspection, observing the fluidity of movement. The skin is inspected for any areas of discoloration or identifying markers that suggest underlying pathology, such as café au lait spots or skin tags (seen with neurofibromatosis) or lipomas (associated with spina bifida). On the lateral view, the examiner looks for the presence of the normal lordotic curve and evaluates the pelvis and paravertebral soft tissues. The pelvis should appear level and the paravertebral soft tissues symmetrical.

Palpation

Palpation of the lumbar spine is most easily achieved with the patient standing and the examiner sitting behind the patient. Posteriorly, the spinous processes and posterior aspect of the coccyx should be palpated. Other bony elements that should be examined include the posterosuperior iliac spines, iliac crests, greater trochanters, and ischial tuberosities.

- The only way to fully palpate the coccyx is by a rectal examination.

In addition to palpation of bony structures, there are several important soft tissue structures that should be evaluated posteriorly. In the midline, the area in which the supraspinous and interspinous ligaments lie should be examined. The thickness of the supraspinous ligaments is palpable over the vertebrae. While the interspinous ligaments lie between the spinous processes, and therefore cannot be directly palpated, tenderness in this region may be present if the ligaments have been ruptured. The paraspinal muscles must be examined for tenderness, evidence of muscle spasm, or atrophy. The sacral triangle, which is formed by the two posterosuperior iliac spines and the top of the gluteal cleft, is palpated. This is a common site of pain due to low back sprains or avulsion of a tendon from the posterosuperior iliac spines. Last, the sciatic nerve should be palpated where it lies halfway between the ischial tuberosity and the greater trochanter; irritation of the contributing nerve roots may result in tenderness of the peripheral nerve.

Anteriorly, though often with some difficulty, the L5-S1 articulation can be palpated. For this evaluation, the patient must lie supine with the knees bent to relax the abdominal musculature. The fingers are then placed just below the umbilicus and deep pressure is applied. Any tenderness should be noted. While the patient is still in the supine position, the anterior abdominal musculature should also be palpated. This is done with the patient lying supine, arms crossed over the chest, while a quarter sit-up is performed; any weakness or asymmetry is then noted.

Range of Motion

Both passive and active range of motion should be assessed. Normal motion in the lumbar spine includes 80 degrees of flexion, 20 to 30 degrees of extension, 35 degrees of lateral bending, and 45 degrees of rotation. Decreased or limited range of motion may be secondary to pain, muscle spasm, or structural pathology.

Neurologic Examination

The basic neurologic examination of patients with low back pain is the same as that performed for the evaluation of neck pain. As discussed above—under the neurologic evaluation of the cervical spine—motor strength, sensation, and reflex testing must each be examined. When muscle strength is being tested in the patient with low back pain, however, certain screening tests may be helpful. For example, in patients who can walk on their heels and toes, can deep knee bend or get out of a chair without using their arms, or can perform one sit-up, muscle strength is normal. If these maneuvers cannot be successfully performed, specific muscle strength tests must be done. Tables 16-10 and 16-11 list important major muscles to test and common reflexes that are useful in the neurologic evaluation. Figure 16-13 illustrates the peripheral nerve sensory distribution in the lower extremities and Fig. 16-7, as noted previously, illustrates dermatome patterns.

Special Tests

Valsalva Maneuver

Coughing, sneezing, laughing, and bearing down as if to move the bowels increase the intradiskal pressure and may reproduce back pain and/or pain radiating into the lower extremities. This is suggestive of disk pathology.

TABLE 16-10

NERVE ROOT LEVEL, PERIPHERAL NERVE, AND PRIMARY ACTION OF MUSCLES COMMONLY TESTED IN THE PATIENT WITH LOW BACK PAIN

Nerve Root Level	Peripheral Nerve	Muscle	Primary Action
L2-L4	Obturator nerve	Adductor longus and adductor brevis	Adduction and flexion at the hip
L2-L4	Femoral nerve	Iliopsoas	Flexion at the hip
L2-L4	Femoral nerve	Quadriceps femoris	Extension at the knee
L4-S2	Sciatic nerve	Hamstrings	Flexion of the leg at the knee
L4, L5	Deep peroneal nerve	Tibialis anterior	Dorsiflexion and inversion of the foot
L4-S1	Deep peroneal nerve	Extensor hallucis longus	Extension of the great toe and dorsiflexion of the foot
L4-S1	Superficial peroneal nerve	Peroneus longus and brevis	Eversion of the foot
L5, S1	Posterior tibial nerve	Tibialis posterior	Inversion of the foot
S1, S2	Tibial nerve	Gastrocsoleus	Plantar flexion of the foot

Pelvic Rock Test

In this evaluation, simultaneous pressure is placed on the iliac crests toward the midline; this may produce pain in the area of the sacroiliac joint, suggesting pathology in that joint.

Sciatic Stretch Tests

The following are several maneuvers that place tension or stress on the sciatic nerve. These tests are considered positive when they reproduce back pain that radiates down the leg of the involved extremity.

Lesegue. While lying supine, the patient's leg is raised with the knee fully extended. This test is considered positive if symptoms are reproduced when the leg is elevated to 60 degrees or less.

TABLE 16-11

COMMONLY TESTED MUSCLE STRETCH REFLEXES OF THE LOWER EXTREMITY

Nerve Root Level	Muscle	Site of Tap
L2-L4 (L4)[a]	Quadriceps	Patellar tendon
S1, S2 (S1)	Gastrocsoleus	Achilles tendon

[a]Parentheses denote common segmental innervations. Individuals may vary.

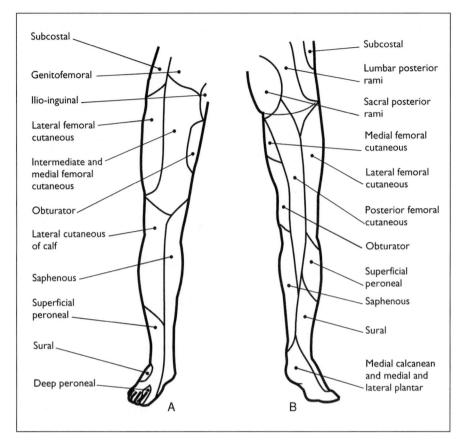

FIGURE 16-13   Peripheral nerve patterns of the lower extremity. *A.* Front. *B.* Back. (From McMinn RMH, Hutchings RT, Logan BM: *The Concise Handbook of Human Anatomy.* Stamford, CT: Appleton & Lange; 1998, with permission.)

Braggard. This test is the same as the Lesegue except that the foot is also dorsiflexed, further stretching the nerve.

Linder. In this test, the patient sitting with legs extended will have increased pain on flexion of the neck.

Bonnets. Pain is produced on adduction of the flexed hip.

Diagnostic Studies

The radiographic evaluation provides important information in the evaluation of low back pain. In situations involving trauma, this portion of the examination should be performed early, following assessment for life-threatening injuries and stabilization of the patient. The standard radiographic examination includes the anteroposterior (AP), lateral, and oblique views. These views will reveal the presence or absence of most major

TABLE 16-12

STANDARD AND SPECIAL RADIOGRAPHIC PROJECTIONS FOR EVALUATING INJURY
TO THE THORACIC AND LUMBAR SPINE

PROJECTION	DEMONSTRATION
Anteroposterior	Fractures of
	Vertebral bodies
	Vertebral end plates
	Pedicles
	Transverse processes
	Fractures–dislocations
	Abnormalities of intervertebral disk spaces
	Paraspinal bulge
	Inverted "Napoleon's hat" sign
Lateral	Fractures of
	Vertebral bodies
	Vertebral end plates
	Pedicles
	Spinous processes
	Chance fracture (seat-belt fractures)
	Abnormalities of
	Intervertebral foramina
	Intervertebral disk spaces
	Limbus vertebra
	Schmorl's node
	Spondylolisthesis
	Spinous-process sign
Oblique	Abnormalities of
	Articular facets
	Pars interarticularis
	Spondylolysis
	"Scotty dog" configuration

SOURCE: Greenspan A, Montesano P: *Imaging of the Spine in Clinical Practice.* London: Mosby Europe Limited; 1993, with permission.

spinal fractures or dislocations. The AP view demonstrates the vertebral bodies, transverse processes, and intervertebral disk spaces. The lateral view also visualizes the vertebral bodies as well as the superior and inferior end plates, spinous processes, and intervertebral disk spaces. The oblique view demonstrates the facet joints and lesions involving the pars interarticularis. Table 16-12 reviews standard and special radiographic projections for evaluating injury to the lumbar spine.

Plain radiographs are essential in the evaluation for spinal stability. AP and lateral films are standard. Bilateral oblique films may be particularly useful in evaluating the pars interarticularis. As in evaluation of the cervical spine, the three-column system is a useful approach (Fig. 16-14). If fractures involve only one column, the spine is considered stable. Two-column fractures may or may not be stable, depending upon the extent of injury. Three-column fractures are considered unstable.

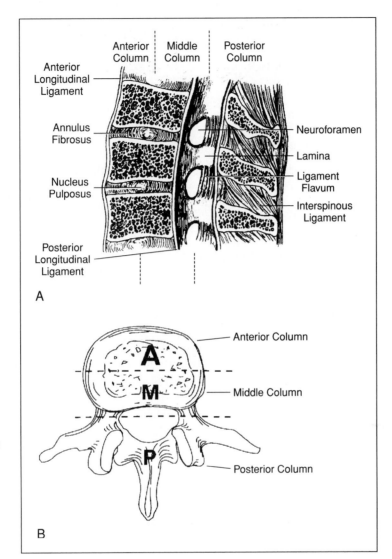

FIGURE 16-14 The three-column system of the lumbar spine. *A.* Sagittal section. *B.* Top view. (From Pansky BL: *Review of Gross Anatomy,* 6th ed. New York: McGraw-Hill; 1996, with permission.)

NONTRAUMATIC BACK PAIN

In evaluating nontraumatic back pain, an important distinction to make is whether the pain is of spinal or nonspinal origin. Problems within the abdominal cavity, pelvis, or retroperitoneal region may all present with back pain. The history and physical examination should help to distinguish back pain of nonspinal origin and help to direct the workup for these problems. Acute, life-threatening conditions such as a leaking abdominal aortic aneurysm must always be considered and ruled out in evaluating a patient with a complaint of low back pain.

Back Pain of Nonspinal Origin

- Pancreatitis
- Peptic ulcer disease
- Renal disease
- Neoplasm
- Aortic aneurysm
- Prostatitis
- Gynecologic processes

Back pain that occurs at rest, worsens during the night, awakens the patient from sleep, and is associated with fever and weight loss is ominous. These patients should be referred quickly for diagnostic evaluation to exclude major medical problems such as neoplasm or infection.

Degenerative Spinal Disease

Clinical Presentation

Degenerative spinal disease represents a process that occurs insidiously and typically becomes symptomatic as the patient ages. Classically, the patient with degenerative spinal disease presents with the complaint of morning stiffness and limitation of range of motion accompanied by pain. The physical examination is significant for decreased range of motion in the lumbar region. In the absence of neural involvement, the neurologic examination is normal. Hypertrophic changes, however, can compress nerve roots and cause radicular pain. Plain radiographs will demonstrate the hypertrophic changes in the bone.

- Symptoms of degenerative spinal disease may present at an earlier age in the patient who has previously sustained trauma.

Treatment

Conservative treatment includes analgesics as needed and physical therapy. Follow-up may be through the patient's primary care physician.

Facet Syndrome

Clinical Presentation

The articular facets are synovial joints that are subject to degenerative and inflammatory changes. The joint capsules are highly innervated; stretching of the capsule due to subluxation or joint fluid can produce pain. The degenerative process begins early; therefore patients presenting with complaints consistent with facet disease may be young to middle-aged. Typically, these patients present with sudden onset of localized back pain with a "catching" sensation in the lumbar spine. Pain may be referred to the buttock or thigh but rarely below the knee. Frequently patients experience morning stiffness or stiffness following prolonged inactivity. Recurrent episodes are common. On physical examination, range of motion, particularly in extension and rotation, is limited and painful. Paravertebral tenderness may be present. Neurologic examination is normal.

Diagnostic Studies

Plain oblique radiographs reveal evidence of facet hypertrophy and osteophyte formation. Very early in the process the radiographs are normal. CT scan, which rarely needs to be obtained on an urgent basis, will demonstrate greater detail of bony involvement and reveal the presence of foraminal stenosis.

Treatment

Conservative treatment consists of analgesics, NSAIDs, and local ice or heat. The patient should avoid hyperextension of the lumbar spine, and sleeping on the abdomen should be avoided. Follow-up should be arranged with a primary care physician, physiatrist, or orthopedic surgeon.

Frequently these patients, even if not treated, will improve within a few days. Manipulation, however, often gives dramatic relief. When the acute pain has subsided, a course of physical therapy directed toward strengthening the supportive musculature of the spine should begin. Patients who do not respond to this treatment may benefit from steroid injection in the facet joint under radiographic guidance. It is important to note that other degenerative spinal syndromes may occur concurrently.

Lumbar Degenerative Disk Disease

Clinical Presentation

Patients with lumbar disk disease will present with symptoms secondary to the degenerative changes that occur in the aging disk. As older disks become more dehydrated, loss of disk height and weakening and tears in the annulus fibrosus can develop. Subsequent degenerative changes in the surrounding bone result in restriction in range of motion and the development of muscle pain and spasm. Patients will often give a history of increased activity—particularly combined lumbar flexion and rotation, lifting, or trauma—that occurred prior to the onset of symptoms. On physical examination, there will be pain in the lower back on movement, decreased range of motion, and palpable muscle spasm in the paravertebral musculature.

Diagnostic Studies

Screening plain film radiographs that can be obtained in the urgent care setting will usually demonstrate loss of disk height. Hypertrophy of bone may be seen if degeneration has begun. An MRI, which is not typically needed on an emergent basis, will better evaluate actual changes within the disk.

Treatment

Conservative management is usually all that is required. Weight loss, analgesics, and physical therapy to include patient education in proper body mechanics and a back stabilization program will help to decrease the risk of chronic pain. Unfortunately, recurrence is common and these patients should be referred to an orthopedist, physiatrist, or their primary care physician for ongoing care.

Herniated Nucleus Pulposus

In the lumbar spine, disk herniations may occur secondary to trauma or as a result of degenerative disk disease. Posterolateral herniations may produce unilateral nerve root compression. In contrast, midline posterior herniations, if large, may produce bilateral nerve root compression or, if very large, cauda equina compromise with loss of bowel and bladder control.

Clinical Presentation

Patients with acute disk herniation are typically 30 to 50 years of age and present with localized low back pain or pain that radiates into the buttocks or thighs. Frequently there is a history of trauma, such as heavy lifting or a fall. Pain is increased by flexion, sitting, coughing, sneezing, or activity that increases the intradiskal pressure. The physical examination reveals decreased range of motion in the lumbar spine, particularly in flexion. Paravertebral tenderness secondary to muscle spasms may be present. If the disk is causing nerve root compression, weakness, sensory loss, and diminished muscle stretch reflexes specific to the involved nerve root(s) will be seen. Straight leg raising is limited in the affected limb, with radiculopathy.

Diagnostic Studies

Plain radiographs may demonstrate degenerative disk changes. The study of choice would be MRI to evaluate the integrity of the disk, but this rarely is needed on an emergent basis.

Treatment

In the absence of cauda equina syndrome or severe radiculopathy, initial treatment is conservative. Acutely, a period of relative bed rest not to exceed 2 to 3 days is appropriate. During this time, isometric exercises of the abdominal, hip, and leg muscles will prevent muscle deconditioning. The supine or side-lying position with the knees flexed is often the most comfortable. The sitting position should be limited acutely, since this increases the pressure within the intervertebral disk. Anti-inflammatory agents, analgesics, and judicious use of muscle relaxants will provide pain relief as well as decrease inflammation about the nerve root when present. A short course of steroids with a quick taper is indicated in the patient who presents with a significant radicular component. Following the acute phase, a physical therapy program is warranted for back stabilization. A cardiovascular conditioning program comprising activities such as walking or swimming will also help to prevent further injury. In uncomplicated cases, follow-up can be appropriately managed by the primary care physician or physiatrist. Any patient with evidence of significant neurologic findings, including profound weakness or loss of bowel or bladder function, requires immediate orthopedic or neurosurgical referral.

Spinal Stenosis

Spinal stenosis is a symptom complex that occurs secondary to a reduction in size of the central spinal canal, the nerve root canal, and/or the intervertebral foramen. It may be congenital, acquired, or both. Degenerative disk disease with narrowing of the intervertebral spaces, spur formation, ligamentous hypertrophy, facet hypertrophy, and subluxation all contribute to the decreased caliber. Because the acquired form is most common, it is seen more often in elderly patients with degenerative spinal disease.

Clinical Presentation

The pain noted in spinal stenosis often occurs in the buttocks or thighs and patients may or may not complain of any pain in the back. The hallmark of this syndrome is pain that occurs when walking or standing and that resolves when sitting down or flexing the waist; thus the term *pseudoclaudication* or *neurogenic claudication*, which has been used to describe the symptoms. These symptoms must be distinguished from claudication secondary to vascular disease (Table 16-13), in which the pain occurs with walking or exercising of the muscle and is relieved by rest.

- Symptoms of neurogenic claudication are diminished by flexing the spine because this alleviates neural compression.

The physical examination of patients with spinal stenosis will reveal lower extremity weakness and, in 40 to 50 percent, diminished deep tendon reflexes. Sciatic nerve stretch tests may be positive when involvement of the L5 or S1 nerve root occurs.

TABLE 16-13

DIFFERENTIATION OF VASCULAR AND NEUROGENIC CLAUDICATION

Factor	Neurogenic Claudication (Pseudoclaudication)	Vascular Claudication	Pitfalls and Remarks
Low back pain	Frequently present	Absent	Sometimes, coincidental degenerative joint disease can be present in patients with vascular claudication
Effect of standing	Provokes symptoms	Does not provoke symptoms	
Direction of radiation of pain in lower limbs	Usually downward	Usually upward	
Sensory symptoms	Present in 66% of patients	Absent	Some patients with vascular claudication can have distal sensory symptoms due to ischemic or diabetic neuropathy
Muscle weakness	Present in more than 40% of patients	Absent	
Reflex changes	Present in about 50% of patients	Absent	In older patients, especially if there is associated neuropathy, reflexes may be decreased or absent
Arterial pulses	Normal	Decreased or absent	In older patients, pulses may be reduced
Arterial bruits	Absent	Frequently present	
Effect of rest while standing	Does not relieve symptoms	Relieves symptoms	
Walking uphill	Symptoms produced later	Symptoms produced earlier	
Walking downhill	Symptoms produced earlier	Symptoms produced later	
Bicycling (stationary or regular)	Does not provoke symptoms	Provokes symptoms	

SOURCE: Sinaki M (ed): *Basic Clinical Rehabilitation Medicine,* 2d ed. St Louis: Mosby–Year Book; 1993, with permission of the Mayo Foundation.

Diagnostic Studies

Plain radiographs will reveal degenerative joint or disk disease with or without spondylolisthesis (see below). Electrodiagnostic evaluation and MRI or CT are useful in determining the extent of involvement.

Treatment

Conservative treatment includes analgesics and a physical therapy program directed at strengthening the abdominal muscles and lumbar flexors. Hyperextension of the spine should be avoided. Orthopedic referral is reasonable in these patients, who may wish to consider surgical options.

Spondylolysis and Spondylolisthesis

Spondylolysis is a defect in the pars interarticularis. It may be congenital, degenerative, traumatic, or secondary to stress fracture. The defect is more common at L5 to S1, then L4 to L5, followed by L3 to L4. Bilateral spondylolysis may result in spondylolisthesis, which is anterior slippage of a vertebral body on its adjacent inferior vertebral body. There are five types of spondylolisthesis (Table 16-14), and spondylolisthesis may be classified into four grades, depending upon the degree of relative displacement (Fig. 16-15).

Clinical Presentation

The presence of spondylolysis and spondylolisthesis in the patient who presents with back pain does not mean that a causal relationship is in effect. Not all patients with spondylolysis or spondylolisthesis are symptomatic. Patients under the age of 25, how-

TABLE 16-14

CLASSIFICATION OF SPONDYLOLISTHESIS

Type	Criteria
I	*Dysplastic:* The only truly congenital from of spondylolisthesis. The defect is a congenital dysplasia in the superior sacral facet or inferior L5 facet that allows L5 on S1 subluxation.
II	*Isthmic:* Defect (spondylosis) in pars interarticularis; the most common form of spondylolisthesis; typically involves L5 to S1. a. Lytic type, probably a fatigue fracture with hereditary predisposition. b. Elongated (attenuated) but intact pars, similar to type IIa, but the fatigue fractures have healed, resulting in elongated but intact pars. c. Acute fracture or pars due to trauma.
III	*Degenerative:* Secondary to degenerative changes at the disc and facet joints, most frequent at L4 to L5 followed by L3 to L4.
IV	*Traumatic:* Due to fracture of posterior elements other than pars (fractures of facet joints, lamina, pedicles).
V	*Pathological:* Due to pathological changes in posterior elements as a result of malignancy, primary bone disease, or infection.

SOURCE: Sinaki M (ed): *Basic Clinical Rehabilitation Medicine,* 2d ed. St Louis: Mosby–Year Book; 1993, with permission of the Mayo Foundation.

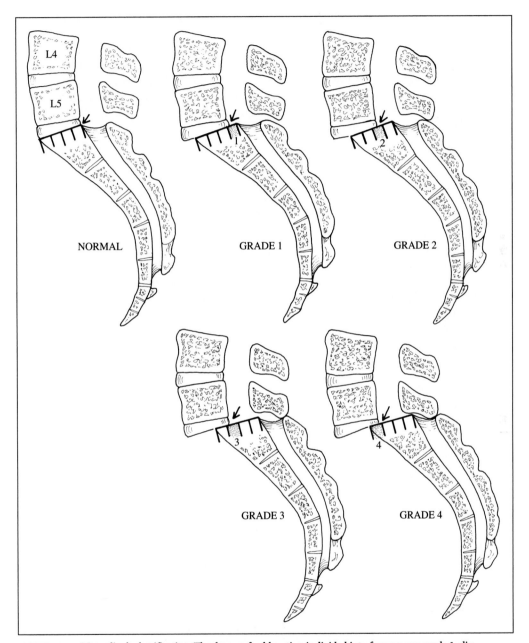

FIGURE 16-15   Meyerding's classification. The degree of subluxation is divided into four groups: grade 1, slipping on the vertebra less than one-fourth the distance of the lumbosacral angle; grade 2, less than half; grade 3, less than three-fourths; and grade 4, more than three-fourths. (From Mokri B, Sinaki M: Painful disorders of the spine and back pain syndromes, in Sinaki M (ed): *Basic Clinical Rehabilitation Medicine*, 2d. St. Louis: Mosby-Year Book; 1993: 489–502, with permission of the Mayo Foundation.)

ever, are more likely to have pain as a result of a pars defect, whereas this is an uncommon cause of back pain in the patient over the age of 40. On history, patients with symptoms referable to either of these entities will complain of back pain that is associated with activity and relieved by rest and that may radiate into the buttock and thigh. Radiculopathy may or may not be present. The physical examination reveals paravertebral muscle spasm with loss of the usual lumbar lordosis. Hamstring tightness is often noted. The neurologic examination is normal in cases where there is no nerve root irritation; if spondylolisthesis causes compression of nerve roots, radiculopathy will occur. In severe cases, when the spinal canal has become narrowed, neurogenic claudication may also be present.

Diagnostic Studies

Plain radiographs including AP, lateral, and oblique projections will reveal the defect. Occasionally, a bone scan may be necessary.

Treatment

Treatment is conservative for grades 1 and 2 spondylolisthesis. Analgesics, moist superficial heat, and massage provide pain relief. A therapeutic exercise program focusing on strengthening the abdominal musculature and stretching the hamstrings, hip flexors, and Achilles' tendons will help to relieve some of the stress on the lumbar spine. Patients with greater than grade 2 spondylolisthesis or who fail conservative treatment require orthopedic referral.

Osteoporosis

Osteoporosis develops as a result of a decrease in bone mass that occurs most frequently in the elderly. Fair-skinned postmenopausal women with a long history of decreased calcium intake are the most common patient population affected. Sedentary lifestyle, chronic steroid use, and smoking all increase a patient's risk for developing this condition. The process may also occur in males, but at a later age and with a slower rate of bone loss. In the axial spine, osteoporosis may lead to the development of wedge compression fractures.

Clinical Presentation

Patients with fractures secondary to osteoporosis may present in one of two ways. The first presentation occurs in patients who develop acute compression fractures as a result of a specific traumatic event. The trauma may be relatively minor; in severe cases of osteoporosis, even a sneeze or cough may result in a compression fracture. The second presentation occurs in patients who report continuous chronic back pain. In these patients, symptoms develop secondary to multiple ongoing microcompression fractures.

Physical examination typically reveals a stooped, kyphotic posture with localized, reproducible tenderness at the fracture site. The pain associated with these fractures can be severe, and radicular complaints may be present if collapse of the vertebra leads to nerve root impingement.

- Fractures caused by osteoporosis occur more commonly in the lower thoracic or upper lumbar vertebrae.

Diagnostic Studies

Plain AP and lateral radiographs will reveal a wedge-shaped compression fracture with injury confined to the anterior aspect of the vertebral body. Bone scan is particularly helpful in diagnosing the microcompression fractures that are not seen on plain radiographs. Bone density studies are helpful in identifying patients at risk for developing osteoporosis.

- Pathologic fractures are included in the differential of spinal compression fractures and should be considered in patients in whom the history, physical examination, or x-ray findings are suggestive of a metastatic or systemic bone lesion.

Treatment

Management includes analgesics, rest, and the use of a lumbosacral orthosis. In severe cases, hospitalization may be required. In cases with 50 percent or greater loss of vertebral height, orthopedic consultation should be arranged. Otherwise, follow-up with a primary care physician is appropriate. Calcium replacement will be necessary and, in the postmenopausal woman, the risks and benefits of estrogen replacement therapy and the use of biphosphonates should be addressed. When pain has improved, therapy for body mechanics, education to avoid flexion, and strengthening of the back extensors can be started.

Decompensation Syndrome/Mechanical Low Back Pain

Mechanical low back pain is one of the most common causes of back pain complaints. The syndrome is of insidious onset and no single cause can be identified.

Clinical Presentation

Patients with mechanical low back pain will often complain of pain that occurs with activity and is relieved by rest. The pain often varies in intensity and at times may radiate into the buttocks. These are often obese individuals, with weak abdominal and back musculature, leading a sedentary lifestyle. Physical examination will reveal pain on range of motion and difficulty or an inability to perform any of the following:

- One sit-up
- One hook-lying sit-up
- A prone leg lift for 10 s at 30 degrees
- One prone torso lift for 10 s
- One slow toe touch in the standing position

  These patients have a normal neurologic examination.

Diagnostic Studies

All diagnostic studies are normal, although this syndrome may be seen in combination with any other etiologies of low back pain.

Treatment

The majority of patients respond well to weight loss and exercise programs that strengthen the musculature of the abdomen, back, and lower extremity. NSAIDs may be used during acute exacerbations.

Arthropathies

In addition to osteoarthritis and rheumatoid arthritis, many inflammatory and non-inflammatory arthropathies have low back pain as a component of the disease. The pathophysiology and its effect on the spine will depend upon the exact etiology of the condition.

Common arthropathies include the following:

- Ankylosing spondylitis
- Diffuse idiopathic skeletal hyperostosis
- Reiter's syndrome
- Psoriatic arthritis
- Connective tissue arthropathy

Clinical Presentation

With arthopathies, the spine symptoms are usually insidious in onset. The patient may complain of morning stiffness or stiffness following periods of inactivity, pain, and limitation of movement. The patient's primary complaint, however, will frequently be that secondary to the primary disorder. Classic stigmata of the specific arthropathy will be seen in the extremities. In the absence of nerve root compromise, the neurologic examination is normal, but physical examination will confirm a limited range of motion in patients with arthropathies associated with inflammation. Findings on plain radiographs will depend upon the process involved.

Treatment

From the standpoint of back symptomatology, treatment is usually conservative. Disease-modifying agents, however, may be needed in cases of inflammatory conditions. These patients all require follow-up for ongoing evaluation, monitoring, and treatment.

TRAUMATIC BACK PAIN

Fractures and dislocation of the lumbar spine should always be considered in any patient who presents with back pain following a traumatic incident. This is especially true in the patient with additional complaints of numbness, paresthesias, weakness, or bowel and bladder dysfunction. The importance of diagnosing these injuries lies in the fact that the spinal column "houses" the neural elements. The spinal cord ends at the approximate level of L1 or L2. The cauda equina, composed of all lumbar and sacral nerve roots, ends in the sacrum. A spinal fracture or dislocation, therefore, has the potential to produce severe neurologic injury.

In those patients with symptoms of spinal injury, direct transfer to an emergency facility must be arranged immediately. It is imperative that the patient be evaluated and transported in such a way as to prevent further injury. In order to appropriately immobilize a patient with a lower spinal injury, he or she should be firmly secured to a fracture board that is as long as the patient and wide enough to accommodate the shoulders and pelvis. Life-threatening injuries and appropriate intervention needed to stabilize the patient should be addressed (see Chap. 19). Following these steps, a neurologic assessment must be made without moving the spine and the level of neurologic injury determined.

TABLE 16-15

BASIC TYPES OF SPINAL FRACTURES AND THE COLUMNS INVOLVED IN EACH

| | **COLUMN INVOLVEMENT** | | |
TYPE OF FRACTURE	**ANTERIOR**	**MIDDLE**	**POSTERIOR**
Compression	Compression	None	None or distraction (in severe fractures)
Burst	Compression	Compression	None or distraction
Seat-belt	None or compression	Distraction	Distraction
Fracture–dislocation	Compression and/or rotation, shear	Distraction and/or rotation, shear	Distraction and/or rotation, shear

SOURCE: From Greenspan A, Montesano P: *Imaging of the Spine in Clinical Practice.* London: Mosby Europe Limited; 1993, with permission.

In the ambulatory patient without neurologic symptoms or initial evidence of spinal injury on physical examination, films of the lumbar spine are an important aspect in the evaluation of injury and should be obtained as discussed above, in the discussion of diagnostic studies (see also Appendix 2, "Radiographic Signs and Findings"). The presence of a lumbar fracture and/or dislocation will often be seen on supine AP and lateral radiographs. These radiographs are crucial in determining the stability of the spine. See Table 16-15 for a list of the basic types of fractures and the columns involved in each fracture. The three-column system can then be used to determine stability. If any evidence of fracture, dislocation, or instability is identified or suspected, the spine must immediately be immobilized and the patient transported for orthopedic or neurosurgical evaluation. If these studies are negative and there is still suspicion of a possible fracture or dislocation, oblique films should be obtained.

- An immediate referral is necessary in patients with positive neurologic and/or radiologic findings. The patient is to remain immobilized until evaluated. Any patient with neurologic deficits requires neurosurgical referral. The patient with fracture or dislocation requires orthopedic referral. The patient with fracture or dislocation and neurologic deficits should have both neurosurgical and orthopedic referrals.
- If the index of suspicion for spinal injury or instability is high, even in the presence of a normal physical and radiographic examination, the patient should be transferred for further evaluation.

Lumbar Sprain and Strain

Clinical Presentation

Patients with lumbar sprain or strain will present with low back pain with or without a history of trauma. The precipitating event may be an acute injury or the condition may be related to a history of repetitive activity such as heavy lifting, frequent bending, or twisting. These patients will typically have acute onset of pain that may radiate into the buttocks or proximal lower extremity. Stiffness upon rising in the morning or following periods of inactivity is common. Examination may reveal painful limitation of lumbar movement, paravertebral muscle spasm, and tenderness on palpation. Loss of the usual lumbar lordosis secondary to muscle spasm is a frequent finding. The neurologic evaluation is normal.

Diagnostic Studies

Radiographs may reveal a straightening of the lumbar lordosis, but no abnormalities are seen in the bone.

Treatment

Treatment is conservative. Activity that causes pain should be avoided. Two to three days of bed rest may be indicated in patients with severe pain. Judicious use of a lumbosacral orthosis when out of bed may provide symptomatic relief. A back rehabilitation program should begin as soon as symptoms subside. Patients should be improved within a few weeks to several months, depending on the severity of the injury.

BIBLIOGRAPHY

American College of Rheumatology 1990 criteria for the classification of fibromyalgia: Report of the multicenter criteria committee. *Arthritis Rheum* 33:160–172, 1990.

Bogduk N: The anatomy and pathophysiology of whiplash. *Clin Biomech* 1:92–101,1986.

Bogduk N, Twomey LT: *Clinical Anatomy of the Lumbar Spine.* New York: Churchill Livingstone; 1988.

Cailliet R: *Neck and Arm Pain,* 3d ed. Philadelphia: Davis; 1991.

Cailliet R: *Soft Tissue Pain and Disability,* 2d ed. Philadelphia: Davis; 1988.

Cailliet R: *Low Back Pain Syndrome,* 4th ed. Philadelphia; Davis: 1988.

Crafts RC: *Textbook of Human Anatomy,* 2d ed. New York: Wiley; 1979:55.

Ellis H: *Clinical Anatomy: A Revision and Applied Anatomy for Clinical Students,* 6th ed. London: Blackwell; 1976:205.

Fast A: Low back disorders: Conservative management. *Arch Phys Med Rehabil* 69:880, 1988.

Frymoyer JW: Back pain and sciatica. *N Engl J Med* 318:291, 1988.

Greenspan A, Montesano P: *Imaging of the Spine in Clinical Practice.* London: Mosby Europe Limited; 1993.

Hollinshead W: *Functional Anatomy of the Limbs and Back,* 6th ed. Philadelphia: Saunders; 1991.

Kottke FJ, Mundale MO: Range of mobility of the cervical spine. *Arch Phys Med Rehabil* 40:379, 1959.

LaBan M: "Whiplash": its evaluation and treatment. *Phys Med Rehabil* 4:293–308, 1990.

Lagattuta FP, Falco FJE: Assessment and treatment of cervical spine disorders, in Braddom RL (ed): *Physical Medicine and Rehabilitation.* Philadelphia: Saunders; 1996:728–755.

Lind B, Schlbom H, Nordwall A, et al: Normal range of motion in the cervical spine. *Arch Phys Med Rehabil* 70:692–695, 1989.

Macnab I: Acceleration injuries of the cervical spine. *J Bone Joint Surg Am* 46:1797–1799, 1964.

Nachemson AL: The lumbar spine: an orthopedic challenge. *Spine* 1:59–71, 1976.

Roydhouse RH: Torquing of the neck and jaw due to belt restrain in whiplash-type accidents. *Lancet* 1:1341, 1985.

Saal JS, Saal JJ, Herzog R: The natural history of lumbar intervertebral disk extrusions treated nonoperatively. *Spine* 15:683–686, 1990.

Sinaki M (ed): *Basic Clinical Rehabilitation Medicine,* 2d ed. St. Louis: Mosby-Year Book, 1993:489–513.

Sinaki M, Mokri B: Low back pain and disorders of the lumbar spine, in Braddom RL (ed): *Physical Medicine and Rehabilitation.* Philadelphia: Saunders; 1996:813–850.

Simons AG: Muscular pain syndromes, in Fricton JR, Awad EA (eds): *Advances in Pain Research and Therapy.* Vol 17: *Myofascial Pain and Fibromyalgia.* New York: Raven Press; 1990:18.

CHAPTER

17

EVALUATION AND TREATMENT OF NONTRAUMATIC ABDOMINAL PAIN

Glenn G. Druckenbrod

Abdominal pain continues to present a diagnostic challenge for urgent care and emergency department physicians. Five to ten percent of the patients who present to the emergency department (ED) have abdominal pain. There are multiple etiologies of primary abdominal pain. Careful history and physical examination coupled with supplemental laboratory and x-ray data allow the physician to diagnose most causes of acute abdominal pain during the primary visit. It is important for the physician to understand the various presentations of acute abdominal pathology and to differentiate self-limited processes from progressive disease entities that require emergent medical or surgical intervention. The widespread use of abdominal imaging procedures, including standard computed tomography (CT), helical CT, ultrasound, and angiography, has made the rapid and accurate diagnosis of abdominal pain more accessible to treating physicians. One of the key issues in the urgent care center (UCC) is distinguishing patients who need to be referred for imaging from those who can be treated in the UCC. The American College of Emergency Physicians' clinical policy on nontraumatic abdominal pain is an extremely useful resource and is excerpted in Table 17-2 (see page 459).

CLINICAL EVALUATION

 History

The careful detailed history (Table 17-1) begins with the time of onset of pain, length of time the pain has been present, and rapidity of onset. Patients may often recall the exact time of onset, suggesting an acute process (i.e., kidney stone, dissecting aneurysm). Pain that persists throughout the night or awakens patients from sleep tends to be more serious. Pain that begins gradually and progressively worsens tends to be inflammatory (e.g., appendicitis). Pain that gradually improves without intervention tends to be of a more benign nature. A history of similar pain in the past with a known time course is also helpful (e.g., ruptured ovarian cyst). The next historical features are the location and character of pain. Quadrant-specific or localized pain is to be differentiated from diffuse pain. It is also important to note whether the pain is constant or intermittent, whether its intensity changes, its character (e.g., sharp versus dull, crampy, bloated or tearing) and whether the pain radiates to the groin, back, or shoulders. Pleuritic pain may suggest a diaphragmatic irritation or a nonabdominal cause of pain such as pneumonia. The severity of pain in older children and adults tends to conform to the severity of disease. It is important to realize, however, that catastrophic processes may present with relatively mild or generalized symptoms in the very young or the elderly, and a high index of suspicion is required in these patient populations.

Exacerbating and mitigating factors may be determined by asking whether the pain is worse with movement or cough. Peritoneal irritation is often made worse by anything that shakes the abdomen, such as a car ride. Other key points to be elicited on history include whether symptoms are made worse or improved by eating certain types of foods, and whether urination or defecation relieves the symptoms. Finally, the patient should be asked about any medications used (i.e., antacids, antispasmodics, etc.) and their effectiveness.

Associated symptoms—such as fever, nausea, vomiting, anorexia, constipation, or diarrhea—should be inquired about, as well as sore throat, cough, chest pain, back pain, urinary symptoms, vaginal bleeding, weakness or dizziness, and rashes. Syncope and abdominal pain very often point to a vascular or ischemic etiology.

The complete past medical history is of vital importance, including the gastrointestinal history for inflammatory disease, peptic ulcer disease, pancreatitis, hepatobiliary disease, or diverticulosis. The presence of systemic diseases such as diabetes, hypertension, or renal disease must be determined as well as, in female patients, a full gynecologic history. Recent trauma should be ruled out. A complete social history with a detailed questioning of alcohol use should also be taken.

TABLE 17-1

DIFFERENTIAL DIAGNOSIS OF ACUTE ABDOMINAL PAIN ACCORDING TO LOCATIONS

Diffuse	Right upper quadrant
Peritonitis	Acute biliary cholecystitis and biliary colic
Acute pancreatitis	Acute hepatitis
Sickle cell crisis	Hepatic abscess
Early appendicitis	Hepatomegaly due to congestive failure
Mesenteric thrombosis	Perforated duodenal ulcer
Gastroenteritis	Acute pancreatitis (bilateral pain)
Dissecting or rupturing	Retrocecal appendicitis
aneurysm	Herpes zoster
Intestinal obstruction	Myocardial ischemia
Diabetes mellitus	Right-lower-lobe pneumonia

TABLE 17-1
(continued)

DIFFERENTIAL DIAGNOSIS OF ACUTE ABDOMINAL PAIN ACCORDING TO LOCATIONS

Right lower quadrant
Appendicitis
Regional enteritis
Meckel's diverticulitis
Cecal diverticulitis
Leaking aneursym
Abdominal wall hematoma
Ruptured ectopic pregnancy
Twisted ovarian cyst
Pelvic inflammatory disease
Mittelschmerz
Endometriosis
Ureteral calculi
Seminal vesiculitis
Psoas abscess
Mesenteric adenitis
Incarcerated or strangulated groin hernia

Left upper quadrant
Gastritis

Acute pancreatitis
Splenic enlargement, rupture, infarction,
aneurysm
Myocardial ischemia
Left-lower-lobe pneumonia

Left lower quadrant
Sigmoid diverticulitis
Leaking aneurysm
Ruptured ectopic pregnancy
Mittelschmerz
Twisted ovarian cyst
Pelvic inflammtory disease
Endometriosis
Ureteral calculi
Seminal vesiculitis
Psoas abscess
Incarcerated or strangulated
groin hernia
Regional enteritis

 ## Physical Examination

A thorough and repeated physical examination is the cornerstone of care in patients with acute abdominal pain. While some physicians focus primarily on the abdomen, a complete head-to-toe evaluation must be done, beginning with an evaluation of the vital signs, including orthostatic changes if indicated. The patient's general appearance should be noted (e.g., whether sitting quietly or writhing in the bed). A complete head, neck, cardiac, lung, and back examination is to be performed, along with a thorough vascular examination. This establishes rapport and puts the patient at ease prior to the abdominal examination. The examiner's hands and stethoscope should be warm and the patient's knees bent to relax the abdominal musculature. The abdomen can then be inspected for distention and any evidence of previous surgery.

On auscultation, high-pitched bowel sounds may indicate an obstruction of the small bowel. Caution is in order, however, because the absence or presence of bowel sounds is nonspecific and may be misleading. Auscultation for the presence of a midline or renal bruit should also be done. Palpation is the most important part of the examination. The patient is asked to indicate the area that hurts most and the examiner begins at the area most distant from this. In examining children, the examiner may ask the child to place one of his or her hands on top of the examining hand; this helps to make the child feel in control of the examination, reduces tickling, and results in a more cooperative child and a more thorough physical examination. Palpation is done gently at first, noting the location and severity of tenderness. The presence or absence of rebound tenderness, both local and referred, is noted next. Organomegaly, masses, or a midline pulsatile mass is to be noted. The complete abdominal examination includes the groin to rule out a hernia. All patients should have a rectal examination to check for masses, tenderness, or blood in the stool. All males should have a testicular examination to rule out testicular torsion or a testicular mass. All females with abdominal pain should have a pelvic examination. The abdominal examination may then be completed by performing the iliopsoas test (i.e., flexing the thigh of the supine patient against resistance) and the obturator test (i.e., flexing the right thigh of the supine patient to 90 degrees and internally/externally rotating the hip).

Diagnostic Studies

In addition to a thorough history and physical, the clinician will often require the use of laboratory, radiography, and sonography to confirm suspected diagnoses (Table 17-2). Many patients with abdominal pain will require intravenous access for hydration and medication. Adequate hydration and control of pain and emesis not only provides excellent clinical care but the patient's response can also help to distinguish benign, self-limited pain from more acute etiologies. However, response alone does not exclude more serious diagnoses if suggested by appropriate history and physical examination findings on the initial clinical evaluation. A complete blood count helps differentiate infectious from noninfectious causes of abdominal pain, although many patients with surgical conditions (e.g., appendicitis) may have a normal white blood cell count initially. A complete blood count is also useful in diagnosing anemia and thrombocytopenia. The urinalysis is required to exclude urinary tract disease or diabetes. All women of childbearing age (i.e., approximate 12 to 50 years of age) should have a pregnancy test as part of their evaluation. Liver function tests may suggest gallbladder or hepatic dysfunction but are frequently normal. A lipase or amylase (or both) should be ordered if pancreatitis or a stone in the common bile duct is suspected. In patients with nonspecific abdominal pain, an electrocardiogram (ECG) should be performed, especially if there is no abdominal tenderness. Acute coronary syndrome may present atypically (e.g., with nausea, atypical chest discomfort, shortness of breath) in women, diabetic patients, and stroke victims.

Plain radiographs of the abdomen are helpful in identifying small bowel obstruction or free intraperitoneal air. Almost without exception, plain abdominal radiographs in the UCC setting should include a flat abdominal film, an upright abdominal film, and an upright well-penetrated chest radiograph. Free abdominal air from a perforated intra-abdominal viscus is best seen on a chest radiograph, while mechanical small bowel obstruction is best seen on the upright abdominal film. However, significant abdominal pathology may be present with normal plain radiographs. Ultrasonography is an excellent modality to elucidate gallbladder disease, abdominal aneurysm, ovarian cyst, ectopic pregnancy, or testicular torsion. Computed tomography (CT) scanning has developed a significant role in the evaluation of abdominal pain. As the CT scan has become more readily available, the evaluation of undifferentiated abdominal pain with CT has become more commonplace. CT is excellent for aneurysm, dissection, tumor, kidney stone, or appendicitis. Similarly, the HIDA scan remains an excellent modality for evaluating biliary obstruction. Of note, none of the tests indicated here has 100 percent diagnostic accuracy, and a negative test coupled with strong clinical suspicion demands close and repeated follow-up. Such entities as suspected appendicitis, ischemic bowel, and so on require surgical consultation even in the face of normal diagnostic testing. In the UCC setting, whether radiographic evaluation occurs urgently or in follow-up will depend on the working diagnosis and patient presentation.

TABLE 17-2

IMAGING MODALITIES AND LABORATORY TESTS OFTEN USED IN THE EVALUATION OF PATIENTS WITH SUSPECTED MAJOR ABDOMINAL CONDITIONS LISTED IN APPROXIMATE ORDER OF UTILITY FOR EACH CONDITION

PRESUMPTIVE DIAGNOSIS	TESTING	COMMENTS
Appendicitis	CT[a]	CT scanning has emerged as the imaging modality of choice in most patients with suspected appendicitis in whom an imaging study is indicated. Sensitivity approaching 100% and specificity of 95% to 98% are reported from one university group. Similar results have been reported in a community hospital setting.
		Liberal use of CT scanning has decreased negative appendectomy rates and may decrease the cost of hospital resources in patients with suspected appendicitis.
	Unenhanced CT	Sensitivity/specificity of 90% and 97%, respectively, have been obtained with helical CT technique without contrast.
	Ultrasound	Best reported sensitivity of 93% and specificity of 91%. This modality is generally preferred in children and pregnant patients but is also the test most subject to operator variation.
	Tc-99m WBC scan	Radiolabeled WBC scans are very effective in some hands with a sensitivity of 98% and specificity of 95%.
	Tc-99m immune globulin scan	Sensitivity of 91% reported. Inherent delays with this type of imaging, technical preparation, and large number of nonspecific findings make radiolabeled studies less useful in most institutions.
	Abdominal plain films	Abdominal plain films are not beneficial.
	WBC Count CRP	An elevated WBC count or CRP level is not sensitive for appendicitis; both tests demonstrate rather poor specificity.
Abdominal aortic aneurysm	CT Ultrasound	CT and ultrasound approach 100% sensitivity in detecting the presence of an aneurysm. In stable patients, a leaking aneurysm is best visualized by CT, and obtaining this study did not adversely affect outcome. Unstable patients with AAA have an increased mortality and morbidity if surgical evaluation is delayed for formal imaging studies. A bedside ultrasound scan during resuscitation in unstable patients may help to confirm or refute the diagnosis.
	MRI	Very accurate in delineating AAA anatomy but logistical concerns preclude its use in the emergency patient.
	Angiography	Less sensitive than CT or ultrasound scan in detecting AAA and neither practical nor appropriate in the emergent patient.

TABLE 17-2

(continued)

IMAGING MODALITIES AND LABORATORY TESTS OFTEN USED IN THE EVALUATION OF
PATIENTS WITH SUSPECTED MAJOR ABDOMINAL CONDITIONS LISTED IN APPROXIMATE
ORDER OF UTILITY FOR EACH CONDITION

PRESUMPTIVE DIAGNOSIS	TESTING	COMMENTS
Biliary tract disease	Ultrasound	Ultrasound scanning remains the preferred test for delineating biliary tract anatomy. Sensitivity for detecting cholelithiasis is approximately 91% and specificity 98%. Ultrasound scanning has practical advantages in imaging in that it is quick, inexpensive, and generally easier to obtain and should be considered the test of first choice.
	Radionuclide scanning	Radionuclide scan depicts function best—sensitivity 97% and specificity 90% for acute cholecystitis.
	CT/MRI	CT and MRI are superior to ultrasound scans for detecting common duct pathology and choledocholithiasis.
	LFT	Elevated LFTs are only approximately 50% specific for cholecystitis and relatively insensitive.
	WBC count	Up to 40% of patients with acute cholecystitis will not have an elevated WBC count.
Bowel obstruction	Abdominal plain films	Plain film sensitivity for diagnosing SBO is as high as 70% with a specificity of approximately 80%. Test of first choice.
	CT	CT is 94% to 100% sensitive and 83% to 96% specific in diagnosing SBO and can delineate the etiology of obstruction in up to 90% of patients. CT is also accurate in differentiating SBO from ileus.
	Ultrasound	The sensitivity and specificity of ultrasound scanning approximates 88% and 96%, respectively, in diagnosing bowel obstruction.
Diverticulitis	CT	CT demonstrates diverticulitis with sensitivities and specificities approaching 100%.
	Ultrasound	Graded compression ultrasound scanning has a sensitivity of 84% to 98% and a specificity of 93% to 97%.
	Barium contrast enema	Sensitivity of 80%, specificity of 100% has been reported.
Ectopic pregnancy	Ultrasound—endovaginal	The accuracy of ultrasound scanning is dependent on the operator and the gestational period as evidenced by the quantitative β-hCG value. The primary utility of ultrasound is detecting an IUP, thereby essentially excluding an ectopic pregnancy. A gestational sac can be seen at a β-hCG level of 1,000 to 2,000 mIU/mL (1 to 2 IRP). With a β-hCG <1,000 mIU/mL, there is only a 17% sensitivity in making the diagnosis of IUP or ectopic pregnancy.
	Ultrasound—transabdominal	Transabdominal ultrasound scanning may occasionally locate an ectopic pregnancy missed by an endovaginal examination.

TABLE 17-2

IMAGING MODALITIES AND LABORATORY TESTS OFTEN USED IN THE EVALUATION
OF PATIENTS WITH SUSPECTED MAJOR ABDOMINAL CONDITIONS LISTED IN
APPROXIMATE ORDER OF UTILITY FOR EACH CONDITION

(continued)

PRESUMPTIVE DIAGNOSIS	TESTING	COMMENTS
Mesenteric infarction/ischemia	Angiography	Angiography has 88% sensitivity for mesenteric infarction (92% arterial, 50% venous).
	CT	Sensitivity to 82%, specificity to 93%. CT more accurate for venous obstruction than angiography.
	Ultrasound	28% sensitive for infarction, although color Doppler can be helpful in differentiating ischemic bowel wall from inflammatory bowel wall.
	Abdominal plain films	Plain radiographs are typically normal in early disease, but can show pneumatosis intestinalis, portal vein gas, or thumb-printing in more advanced disease.
	Serum phosphate	Sensitivities quite variable: 26% to 85%, specificity as high as 85%.
Ovarian torsion	Color flow Doppler ultrasound	Color flow Doppler ultrasound was 100% sensitive in a small series for depicting ovarian torsion.
Pancreatitis	Amylase	Sensitivity approximately 80%, 90% specific. Using a cutoff of 3 times the traditional top normal value of amylase increases specificity to 100%, although a corresponding drop in sensitivity to 72%.
	Lipase	Sensitivity 97% to 100%, specificity 83% to 98%.
	CT/MRI/ultrasound	All depict pancreatic and peripancreatic fluid collections well. CT demonstrates pancreatic necrosis reasonably well and can aid in establishing prognosis.
Urinary stone disease	Unenhanced CT	Unenhanced helical CT depicts urinary stone disease with sensitivity of 97% to 98%, specificity of 96% to 100%.
	IVP	Sensitivity of 85% to 90%, specificity of 95% to 100%.
	Ultrasound plus KUB	Best reported sensitivity of 93%, with 100% specificity.
	KUB alone	Sensitivities approximate 60%, specificity 77%.
Testicular torsion	Color flow Doppler ultrasound	Sensitivities and specificities approach 100% in some reported series.
	Radionuclide scanning	Reported sensitivities of 85% to 98%, specificity to 100%. If acute torsion is suspected, urologic consultation should not be delayed for imaging studies.

TABLE 17-2
(continued)

IMAGING MODALITIES AND LABORATORY TESTS OFTEN USED IN THE EVALUATION OF PATIENTS WITH SUSPECTED MAJOR ABDOMINAL CONDITIONS LISTED IN APPROXIMATE ORDER OF UTILITY FOR EACH CONDITION

PRESUMPTIVE DIAGNOSIS	TESTING	COMMENTS
Urinary tract infection	Urine WBC	>10 WBC/hpf sensitivity 82% and specificity 80% for positive culture (>50,000 CFU/mL).
	Leukocyte esterase	Sensitivity 72% to 89%; specificity 68% to 92%.
	Nitrite	Sensitivity 40% to 75%, specificity 93% to 98%.
Salpingitis/PID	WBC	An elevated WBC count is generally not a sensitive indicator of PID (66% sensitive).
	ESR	60% to 81% sensitive, 53% to 57% specific.
	CRP	50% to 74% sensitive, 59% to 80% specific.
	Ultrasound	85% sensitive, 100% specific in a small series, but 63% sensitivity reported in a study primarily of adolescents.

KEY: CT, computed tomography; Tc-99m, technetium 99m; CRP, C-reactive protein; AAA, abdominal aortic aneurysm; MRI, magnetic resonance imaging; LFT, liver function test; SBO, small bowel obstruction; β-hCG, β-human chorionic gonadotropin; IUP, intrauterine pregnancy; IRP, International Reference Preparation; IVP, intravenous pyelogram; KUB, kidneys, ureter, and bladder; hpf, high power field; CFU, colony-forming unit; PID, pelvic inflammatory disease; ESR, erythrocyte sedimentation rate.

[a]There are differences in contrast administration protocols among the studies, making direct comparison or reports problematic.

SOURCE: Clinical Policy—Critical Issues for the Initial Evaluation and Management of Patient Presenting with a Chief Complaint of Non-Traumatic Acute Abdominal Pain. American College of Emergency Medicine Clinical Policies Committee. *Ann Emerg Med* 36(4):415–416, 2000.

Treatment

Nausea, vomiting, and abdominal cramping are all often improved with hydration alone. Antacids are helpful for gastritis or peptic ulcer disease, but the response should not be used as evidence of presumptive diagnosis. Antispasmodics may be helpful in certain cases (e.g., gastroenteritis, irritable bowel syndrome). Narcotic analgesia may be used for patient comfort after the initial evaluation and should not significantly change the examination. It is well to remember that all disease states from colonic spasm to aortic dissection respond to narcotic analgesia but that such a response does not indicate a more benign outcome. Abdominal pain is a spectrum of disease that develops over time; therefore a thorough evaluation requires repeated examinations. Approximately 40 percent of abdominal pain is nonspecific on initial evaluation. Consequently, an accurate diagnosis may not be made on the first clinical evaluation. Repeated examinations in the UCC and close follow-up with a referring physician are mandatory in all patients discharged without a definitive diagnosis. *Serial examinations are of key importance for any patient with abdominal pain.*

EVALUATION AND MANAGEMENT OF SELECTED ABDOMINAL DISORDERS

Table 17-3 provides a summary of this subject.

TABLE 17-3

EVALUATION, TREATMENT, AND DISPOSITION OF SELECTED ABDOMINAL DISORDERS

DISORDER	HISTORY	PHYSICAL EXAMINATION	DIAGNOSTIC EVALUATION (SEE TABLE 17-1)	DISPOSITION
Acute gastroenteritis	Colicky abdominal pain associated with nausea, vomiting, and diarrhea.	Dehydration, diffuse mild abdominal tenderness without rebound, present bowel sounds.	Consider CBC, stool guaiac, electrolytes, BUN, creatinine, and glucose. Also consider abdominal radiographs to exclude obstruction.	Most patients can be discharged with timely follow-up and complete discharge instructions.
Acute gastritis, peptic ulcer disease	Epigastric pain worse following meals. May be associated with NSAID use.	Epigastric tenderness, possible occult fecal blood.	Consider CBC, stool occult blood test, and ECG.	Admit with acute GI bleed or uncontrolled pain or emesis.
Acute cholelithiasis/ cholecystitis	RUQ pain worsened by fatty food. Associated fever, chills in cholecystitis. Pain is often episodic.	RUQ tenderness, and possibly rebound in cholecystitis. Positive Murphy's sign (i.e., inspiratory arrest). Possible jaundice.	CBC, liver enzymes, amylase, lipase, ultrasound or HIDA scan.	Admit patients with cholecystitis. Admit patients with cholelithiasis for intractable pain or emesis.
Appendicitis	Classically general abdominal discomfort followed by nausea, then RLQ pain and fever. Anorexia is common. Atypical presentations are frequent.	RLQ tenderness, guarding, and possibly rebound. Fever.	Consider abdominal CT in adults, especially females, and ultrasound in children.	If the diagnosis of appendicitis is considered, refer to a surgeon or emergency department for definitive evaluation and management.
Small bowel obstruction	Colicky, diffuse abdominal pain. Diminished or absent bowel movements and flatus. History of prior abdominal surgery.	Distended abdomen with either diminished or high-pitched bowel sounds. Look for abdominal scars.	Multiple differential air fluid levels on upright abdominal x-rays.	Refer for admission and surgical management.

TABLE 17-3

EVALUATION, TREATMENT, AND DISPOSITION OF SELECTED ABDOMINAL DISORDERS

(continued)

DISORDER	HISTORY	PHYSICAL EXAMINATION	DIAGNOSTIC EVALUATION (SEE TABLE 17-1)	DISPOSITION
Ruptured viscus	Prior symptoms suggesting peptic ulcer disease. History of NSAID use. Improvement in pain, followed by gradual worsening suggests peritonitis. Symptoms may be nonspecific in the elderly.	Diffuse tenderness with rebound. Diminished bowel sounds (late finding). Distended abdomen.	Free air seen on upright chest radiograph.	Refer emergently for surgical management.
Pancreatitis	Epigastric pain often penetrating, nausea, vomiting, history of alcohol use common.	Epigastric tenderness with guarding, dehydration.	Amylase, lipase, and consider liver enzymes, CBC, electrolytes, calcium.	Consider admission for severe pain, vomiting, fever, significant dehydration.
Ruptured abdominal aortic aneurysm	History of vascular disease, frequently among males. Sudden worsening of abdominal or back pain. Syncope.	Pulsatile mass, hypotension, generalized abdominal tenderness, diminished lower extremity pulses, bilateral leg weakness.	Do not allow diagnostic evaluation to delay treatment of unstable patients. CBC and either ultrasound or abdominal CT.	Immediate referral for operative management.
Ureteral calculi	Sudden onset of severe, often unilateral flank pain that may radiate to the groin. History of ureteral calculi. Male sex.	CVA tenderness. Soft abdomen.	Urinalysis, although hematuria may be absent in complete ureteral obstruction. Consider CBC, electrolytes, BUN, creatinine, spiral CT, and KUB.	Admit for severe pain, fever, intractable vomiting, complete ureteral obstruction.

TABLE 17-3

EVALUATION, TREATMENT, AND DISPOSITION OF SELECTED ABDOMINAL DISORDERS

DISORDER	HISTORY	PHYSICAL EXAMINATION	DIAGNOSTIC EVALUATION (SEE TABLE 17-1)	DISPOSITION
Ectopic pregnancy	Abnormal or absent menses, pelvic pain, vaginal bleeding, history of ectopic, history of PID, infertility.	Vaginal bleeding, unilateral adnexal tenderness, fullness, pelvic mass.	Quantitative serum hCG, pelvic ultrasound, CBC, type and Rh.	Referral to ED or OB/GYN for definitive management. Only attempt outpatient management following consultation with an OB/GYN physician.
Ovarian cyst	Sudden onset pelvic pain, typically at midcycle, with gradual improvement. Vaginal spotting.	Hypotension and shock may occur following rupture of hemorrhagic cyst. Unilateral adnexal tenderness. Ovarian fullness on bimanual examination.	CBC, hCG, pelvic ultrasound if diagnosis is in question.	Stable patients are referred for timely reevaluation by an OB/GYN physician. Admit for intractable pain, significant anemia, or signs of ongoing blood loss.
Diverticulitis	Fever, lower abdominal pain (typically left lower quadrant) that is progressively worse.	Tenderness, guarding, and possibly rebound in the left lower quadrant.	CBC and abdominal radiographs. Consider abdominal CT to exclude diverticular abscess.	Mild cases with known disease may be discharged on oral antimicrobials. Admit for intractable pain, fever, vomiting, signs of peritonitis, extremes of age, and intraabdominal abscess as diagnosed by CT.

KEY: NSAID, nonsteroidal anti-inflammatory drug; RUQ, right upper quadrant; RLQ, right lower quadrant; CBC, complete blood count; BUN, blood urea nitrogen; ECG, electrocardiogram; HIDA, dimethyl iminodialetic acid; CT, computed tomography; GI, gastrointestinal; CVA, cerebral vascular accident; PID, pelvic inflammatory disease; KUB, kidneys, ureters, bladder; hCG, human chorionic gonadotropin.

TABLE 17-4

DISPOSITION OF URGENT CARE PATIENTS WITH ACUTE ABDOMINAL PAIN

Treat and discharge
   Acute gastroenteritis
   Gastritis
   Pelvic inflammatory disease
   Acute cholelithiasis without signs of
      infection, vomiting, or intractable
      pain

Refer for further imaging and treatment
   Cholecystitis
   Appendicitis

Diverticulitis
Ovarian cyst

Send by EMS for definitive evaluation and
   management
   Suspected abdominal aortic aneurysm
   Ruptured abdominal viscus
   Ectopic pregnancy
   Bowel obstruction
   Gastrointestinal bleeding
   Ischemic bowel

DISPOSITION

Any episode of hypotension associated with abdominal pain requires aggressive evaluation for a vascular cause and admission to the hospital.

For patients with suspected surgical conditions such as appendicitis or cholecystitis, a rapid surgical consultation should be obtained with a view to possible admission. Under certain circumstances, urgent surgical consultation in the surgeon's office may also be appropriate. However, all patients with significant abdominal pain that is undiagnosed should be admitted for further evaluation and serial examinations. Once the decision to admit is made (see Table 17-4), further considerations include the level of transportation utilized [e.g., private vehicle, basic emergency medical services (EMS) unit, or advanced life support (ALS) paramedic ambulance unit] and whether the patient should be transferred to the ED or can safely be transported for direct admission.

Patients with improving symptoms or stable diagnoses may be safely discharged from the UCC with clear instructions on when to return for reevaluation (Table 17-5)

TABLE 17-5

SAMPLE DISCHARGE INSTRUCTIONS FOR PATIENTS WITH ABDOMINAL PAIN

1. Immediate repeat evaluation:

   ◆ New symptoms

   ◆ Worsening or change in symptoms

   ◆ Light-headedness or syncope (fainting)

   ◆ Persistent pain or abdominal distention

   ◆ Persistent vomiting or vomiting of blood or coffee-ground material

   ◆ Dehydration

   ◆ Fever or shaking chills

   ◆ Blood in urine or feces

   ◆ Development of shoulder pain

   ◆ Yellow coloring to skin or eyes

2. Avoid pain medication stronger than Tylenol.

3. Avoid aspirin, as it will prolong bleeding time.

4. Follow up with primary care physician in 24 to 48 h for recheck.

and when to schedule definitive follow-up. When possible, contact the referring physician to ensure timely follow-up and reevaluation. Explaining the uncertain nature of abdominal pain to your patient is good medical practice and also may be good medical legal protection.

"GOLDEN RULES"

1. Abdominal pain progresses over time. Repeated examination while in the UCC and close follow-up after discharge are essential.
2. Patients at the extremes of age may often not localize symptoms, and nonspecific complaints may often be signs of significant intraabdominal pathology. *An unimpressive examination or normal blood work does not preclude a serious diagnosis in these age groups.*
3. Hypotension or syncope related to abdominal pain demands a significant evaluation for underlying vascular or cardiac etiology.
4. Diagnostic tests are not 100 percent sensitive or specific and do not replace a good history and physical and sound medical judgment.
5. Missed abdominal pathology is a significant cause of medical malpractice litigation. Thorough evaluation and careful explanation to the patient coupled with close follow-up and repeated examinations minimize this risk.

REFERENCES

American College of Emergency Medicine: Clinical policy for the initial approach to patients presenting with a chief complaint of nontraumatic acute abdominal pain. *Ann Emerg Med* 23:906–922, 1994.

Barkin RM, Hayden S, Schaider JJ, Wolfe R: *The Five Minute Emergency Medicine Consult.* Philadelphia: Lippincott Williams & Wilkins; 1999.

Lukens TW, Emerman C, Effron D: The natural history and clinical findings of undifferentiated abdominal pain. *Ann Emerg Med* 22:690, 1993.

Silen W: *Cope's Early Diagnosis of the Acute Abdomen,* 18th ed. New York: Oxford University Press; 1991.

NEUROLOGY

Gary D. Johnson

Many physicians feel uncomfortable with the neurologic examination because they perceive it to be both time-consuming and complicated. In general, physicians are not taught to perform a focused examination tailored to the problem at hand. Such an examination requires consideration of the key elements that must be evaluated before actually examining the patient. Patient history provides a basis for hypotheses of localization and probable etiologies that can be tested through a focused neurologic examination. In other words, if physical signs support the hypothetical localization and etiology, then the probability increases that the hypothesis is correct. It must be kept in mind that the neurologic examination will assess normal as well as abnormal areas of the nervous system. Many symptoms may *sound* neurologic but are actually related to other systems. In this setting, demonstrating that pertinent areas of the nervous system are normal will be helpful in excluding neurologic dysfunction. As a review, the folllowing is a description of the components of the full examination. In each subsequent section a suggested focused examination is described.

MENTAL STATUS

The mental status examination is certainly the most challenging aspect of the neurologic examination. In detail, an hour or more may be spent testing various aspects of mentation. The examiner should remember, however, that this approach would not be practical in the urgent care setting and that a full mental status examination is not required to make some assessments regarding cortical function. Key elements of the mental status examination that should be assessed and documented include *alertness* and *attention*, *orientation*, *language*, and *memory*.

Alertness

A description of the state of wakefulness defines *alertness*. Somnolence or lethargy is the inability to remain awake. A stuporous patient is unable to be awakened by stimuli other than pain. *Coma* roughly refers to an inability to awaken with any stimulus. *Attention* is noted in the ability to follow conversation or a coherent stream of thought. An attentive patient follows commands quickly and does not lose track of conversation. Counting backward from 20 or repeating the months of the year backward tests concentration. Inattentive patients may pause or stop midtask. If this occurs, the patient should be asked if he or she recalls the task requested. Obviously, a patient who is not attentive will not be able to perform other, more complex mental tasks.

 Errors to Avoid

- Charting documentation using the term *lethargy* without a detailed description of what the patient or examiner actually means by the term. Many patients use the term *lethargy* or *lethargic* to describe tiredness, fatigue, or increased sleeping, not true lethargy (i.e., the inability to remain awake).
- Assuming that abnormal mental status is related to malingering, hysteria, drugs, or psychiatric symptoms. An abnormal mental status should always be assessed fully to rule out organic causes.

Orientation

Orientation should be assessed for recognition of person, place, time, and situation. Of note, patients who are disoriented may first lose sense of their situation or problem, followed by time, then place, and then person.

- An inability to know one's name, with recognition of the presenting problem, is usually psychiatric in origin. Patients who are in a confusional state, such as those with metabolic encephalopathy, are frequently inattentive as well as disoriented.

Language

Language testing assesses the function of the dominant hemisphere. In practice, this generally means left hemispheric function. Many aspects of language function are observed during normal conversational speech. The essential components are fluency, comprehension, naming, and repetition. Fluency is the ability to connect words in a sentence with a normal flow of speech. Nonfluent speech is halting or effortful. Testing of the patient's ability to follow multistep commands assesses comprehension. Observations of this ability can be made throughout the rest of the examination. If there is impairment of comprehension with normal attention, there may be impaired auditory comprehension. The naming of various common objects tests naming. Asking the patient to repeat a sentence assesses repetition.

- Language dysfunction can be further localized in the left hemisphere by considering that anterior lesions produce more fluency problems, whereas posterior lesions produce more difficulty with comprehension.

Memory

Memory is classified as immediate, short-term, and long-term. Each aspect is tested in patients with possible memory disturbance. Immediate memory is tested by immediate recall of selected words or phrases. Patients with difficulty in immediately recalling three words frequently have a disturbance of attention. Short-term memory is tested by the recall after 3 to 5 min. Long-term memory is tested by recall of prior historical or life events. Behavior and the patient's emotional state should also be taken into account in assessing memory. For instance, depression can present as a memory disturbance.

- Right hemispheric lesions produce inattention, confusion, and left spatial neglect.

CRANIAL NERVES

Examination of the cranial nerves serves to evaluate the status of brainstem function. This examination can easily be performed in a matter of a few minutes.

Cranial Nerve II

The fundi are examined for optic nerve swelling, hypertensive or diabetic vascular changes, and hemorrhages. The visual fields are examined by having the patient look straight ahead into the examiner's eyes as as he or she faces the patient; the patient is asked to count fingers in four quadrants; each eye is tested separately and the performance on one side is compared with that on the other. To complete evaluation of cranial nerve II, visual acuity in each eye is checked with a near card.

Cranial Nerves III, IV, and VI

Pupillary responses to light should be checked in a darkened room, looking for asymmetry in size, shape, and reaction. Extraocular movements in all directions of gaze are checked, observing for nystagmus and limitations of eye movement. If limitation of movement is observed in a particular direction, the patient is asked whether he or she notes diplopia.

- The pupils are examined in a darkened room (this will bring out any asymmetry or abnormal reactivity).
- Nystagmus at the extremes of gaze is not as important as unilateral nystagmus or nystagmus near the primary position of gaze.
- Ptosis associated with an ipsilateral small pupil suggests *Horner's syndrome*, while ptosis with an ipsilaterally large pupil could be a *third nerve palsy.*

Cranial Nerve V

Facial sensation is checked to pin or temperature in the three divisions (ophthalmic, maxillary, and mandibular) of the trigeminal nerve. (Note: the territory of the facial nerve does not include the ear or the angle of the jaw.) Any asymmetry is noted.

Cranial Nerve VII

The examiner looks for facial asymmetry at rest. A decreased nasolabial fold or widened palpebral fissure suggests mild facial weakness. Symmetry of smile and brow elevation should be noted.

Cranial Nerve VIII

Hearing to finger rub is tested. Weber and Rinne testing should be performed when hearing loss is suspected in order to classify the probable mechanism. With a conductive hearing loss (bone > air conduction), the Weber test lateralizes to the poor ear; with sensorineural hearing loss (air > bone conduction), the Weber test lateralizes to the better ear.

Cranial Nerves IX and X

The examiner looks for symmetrical elevation of the soft palate, *not* uvular deviation. The gag reflex is checked on each side.

Cranial Nerve XI

The bulk and strength of the sternocleidomastoid are checked on each side, as well as the strength of shoulder elevation.

Cranial Nerve XII

With the patient's tongue outstretched, the examiner checks for deviation, which would suggest weakness on the side of the deviation.

MOTOR EXAMINATION

Motor function is initially assessed by simple inspection, noting any preferential movements of one side of the body or apparent stiffness of an extremity. Muscle bulk, tone, and strength are checked. In the setting of suspected peripheral nerve disorders, isolated muscle groups should be tested to confrontation. Agonist and antagonist muscle groups around the large joints should be tested for evaluation of central processes. Muscle strength is graded in a 0-to-5 grading system. Notations of plus (+) and minus (−) may be used to further define degrees of strength (Table 18-1).

TABLE 18-1

GRADING SYSTEM OF MUSCLE STRENGTH

---

0 = No movement
1 = Trace movement
2 = Unable to resist gravity
3 = Able to resist gravity but not able to move against resistance
4 = Able to move against resistance but with less than normal strength
5 = Normal muscle strength

- Screening tests for more subtle hemiparesis include checking for a *pronator drift* by asking the patient, with eyes closed, to hold both arms outstretched at shoulder level in the supinated position. Pronation of the arm with a downward drift may be indicative of a mild hemiparesis.

CEREBELLAR FUNCTION

Coordination can be checked with finger-to-nose testing, rapid alternating movements, and heel-to-shin testing. The performance of one side is compared with that of the other, checking for appropriate speed of movement and accuracy and looking for any evidence of tremor or ataxia.

- Motor and sensory dysfunction can affect coordination and therefore affect the results of coordination testing.

REFLEXES

Reflexes should be compared side to side, observing for any asymmetry or difference between the upper and lower extremities. Reflexes should be checked at the biceps, triceps, radial, quadriceps, and Achilles' (ankle) tendons. The reflex response, like muscle strength, is graded on a system of 0 to 5+ (Table 18-2).

SENSORY EXAMINATION

Although the sensory examination is difficult in that it is entirely subjective, it can be used in the context of the presenting complaint, history, and prior examination to help refine hypotheses regarding anatomic localization. The primary modalities of the examination—pinprick and temperature, light touch, position sense, and vibratory sense—should therefore be examined in an effort to determine if there is a pattern consistent with the theorized localization.

While the sensory examination is being performed, the patient should have his or her eyes closed and the stimulus moved from the abnormal area to normal areas. This examination method is better able to map out the true area of sensory disturbance than a method utilizing random testing.

- The patient should be asked to point out the area that he or she feels is abnormal; this should serve as a starting point and guide to the examination.

TABLE 18-2

GRADING SYSTEM OF THE REFLEX RESPONSE

0 = No reflex response	3+ = Brisk reflex response
1+ = Reflex present, but diminished	4+ = Presence of unsustained clonus
2+ = Normal reflex response	5+ = Presence of sustained clonus

GAIT

Although gait analysis is frequently reserved for the end of the examination, it is a particularly good initial screen for neurologic signs and symptoms like hemiparesis, ataxia, bradykinesia, and sensory loss. In addition to the casual observation of gait, heel walking and toe walking are helpful in assessing distal leg strength and coordination or balance. *Romberg testing* is also helpful in gait evaluation as a screening test for proprioceptive or vestibular problems. When swaying is noted while the patient's eyes are open, the problem is vestibular or cerebellar in nature. Repeat testing with the patient's eyes closed is then not necessary.

- A truly positive Romberg test (i.e., swaying noted with feet together, arms at the sides, and eyes closed) that is not duplicated when the eyes are open suggests significant loss of position sense in the legs.

DOCUMENTATION OF THE NEUROLOGIC EXAMINATION

Precise and accurate documentation of the neurologic examination is crucial prior to transferring care of patients and for follow-up or serial evaluations. All observations should be recorded as they were observed. Whenever possible, the patient's own description of symptoms should be used. Vague terms like "neuralgia" are best avoided; specific descriptions such as "shooting," "electric-like," "sharp," and so on are more helpful. Unless all parties exactly understand the terms used to describe the particular sign or symptom, misunderstandings can occur.

 Errors to Avoid

- Performing an examination blindly. *It is important to decide ahead of time, based on presenting symptoms and history, what may be expected on examination.*
- Failure to perform an accurate examination.
- Assuming a "grossly nonfocal" examination without appropriate evaluation.
- Inappropriate interpretation of findings. (*Example: A Babinski without weakness, hyperreflexia, or increased tone is worthless.*)
- Assuming that an inability to obtain reflexes is due to anything other than frank pathology until proven otherwise.
- Failure to account for the effects of alcohol or other medications. *Alcohol will cause bilateral end-gaze nystagmus, limb and gait ataxia, and sedation. Stimulants cause tremor, pupillary dilatation, and occasionally hyperreflexia.*

BELL'S PALSY

Bell's palsy, or idiopathic peripheral facial weakness, is a fairly common disorder. The history and physical findings are usually quite characteristic and the disease process is generally benign and not associated with significant morbidity. Nonetheless, to some degree, Bell's palsy is a diagnosis of exclusion, since multiple disease processes—including Lyme disease, cerebellopontine angle tumors, otitis media, parotid tumors, Ramsay Hunt syndrome, and trauma may produce similar facial paresis or paralysis. For the patient, the immediate concern is usually whether the facial weakness is related to a stroke.

Evaluation

Patients presenting with symptoms consistent with Bell's palsy have a history ranging from acute to subacute (over a couple of days) onset of unilateral facial weakness. There may be a history of an antecedent viral infection, and frequently patients will describe an aching pain behind or around the ipsilateral ear that began prior to onset of actual weakness. On physical examination, weakness or paralysis of forehead elevation will be seen. There may also be an inability to perform eye and mouth closure on the affected side. In some patients, a Bell's phenomenon may be noted, in which efforts to close the eyelid on the affected side cause a rolling upward of the eye.

- Peripheral facial weakness is always on the side with decreased furrows on the forehead and decreased ability to close the eye. Patients may report that the other side is affected, but this is related to a sensation of pulling of the unopposed normal muscles on that side.

Ipsilateral hyperacusis, excessive tearing, and alteration in taste may also occur, since these functions are also innervated by the facial nerve (cranial nerve VII). A complete cranial examination should be performed, since the fifth and sixth nerves are adjacent to the seventh nerve in the brainstem. Of particular interest are facial sensation and the extraocular movements, both of which should be normal.

- Involvement of the upper part of the face, however, is the key sign to suggest a *peripheral* cause of the facial paralysis.

A complete ear/nose/throat (ENT) examination should be performed. The physician should check for signs of otitis media and mastoiditis as well as for the presence of vesicles in the ear, which would suggest a diagnosis of herpes. The testing of reflexes and motor responses should be performed with attention to the arm and leg on the affected side. Any apparent extremity weakness or hyperreflexia on the same side as the facial paresis suggests the possibility of a cerebral lesion instead of Bell's palsy. Similarly, any apparent weakness or hyperreflexia on the contralateral side suggests the possibility of a brainstem lesion.

 Management (Table 18-3)

In most cases, recognition of the disorder and exclusion of other abnormalities that might suggest a structural lesion is all that is required. Up to 90 percent of patients have significant if not complete improvement in the facial weakness over the course of approximately 3 to 8 weeks. The prognosis for complete and rapid recovery is greatest in those patients with incomplete or partial weakness; patients with complete paralysis are much less likely to have complete improvement. In patients with a history of a tick

TABLE 18-3

MANAGEMENT OF BELL'S PALSY

Neurologic referral and neuroimaging for any associated abnormalities
Prednisone 60 mg/day for 5 days, with rapid taper
Eyedrops and taping of eyelid to prevent corneal drying
Primary care follow-up within 1 week

bite or who have been in areas endemic for Lyme disease, Lyme titers should be checked. Treatment should be considered for high clinical suspicion or in the patient presenting with erythema migrans.

Patients with other abnormalities in addition to the unilateral facial weakness should be sent for neuroimaging, preferably magnetic resonance imaging (MRI), and referred for full neurologic evaluation.

Treatment options include a short course of steroids, particularly for those patients with periauricular pain or who present with complete paralysis. Prednisone 60 mg/day for 5 days can be given, followed by a rapid taper over a week or so. Lubricating eye drops or ointment should also be prescribed for patients who are unable to keep their eye closed.

 Errors to Avoid

- Failure to instruct patient on taping the involved eye to keep it closed during sleep, if indicated, in order to prevent drying or damage of the cornea from an inability to keep the eye closed

Bell's Palsy—

 Key Points of Documentation

- Involvement of upper face/forehead on physical examination. (The upper face is spared in central disease processes involving the brain and brainstem.)
- Patient's ability to keep eye closed

Dizziness

Patients and physicians frequently use the term *dizziness* to describe any sensation from light-headedness to true vertigo. Much of the difficulty in evaluation stems from a failure to correctly categorize the type of dizziness described by the patient. As always, the history is very important in determining the category of dizziness and therefore the subsequent examination, evaluation, and management. Once the symptoms are categorized into vertigo, disequilibrium, or light-headedness, the evaluation can be tailored to that particular type of dizziness.

Definitions

- *Vertigo* is an illusion of motion that is frequently but not exclusively rotational in nature. Occasionally, patients with vertigo may describe a sensation of being pulled or tilted to one side or the other. Vertigo is most often associated with vestibular dysfunction.
- *Disequilibrium* is an imbalance or unsteadiness primarily occurring while walking or standing. Difficulties with proprioceptive, motor, cerebellar, or visual functioning, alone or in combination, are frequent causes of disequilibrium.
- *Light-headedness* is predominantly a presyncopal sensation commonly described as "wooziness." Patients will frequently note the sensation of light-headedness in association with rapid positional changes, such as arising from a recumbent or seated position to standing. In general, a decrease in cerebral perfusion is the cause of light-headedness.

 History

On history, patients should be asked to describe the dizziness, without prompting, in an effort to truly assess what type of dizziness they are experiencing. Many patients, because of the anxiety associated with the symptoms, will readily conclude that the physician knows more about their problem than they do and will not volunteer descriptive information unless they are urged to do so. Questions should be asked using an open-ended format, thus avoiding "yes-no" responses. This approach will help to elicit a description that conforms to the above categories without bias. Of particular concern in the history are any features that suggest a central cause of the symptoms or an emergent etiology.

Dizziness—

 Key Points of Documentation to Elicit on History

1. Description of symptoms
2. Precipitating factors
3. Onset/duration of symptoms (acute vs. gradual; recurrent)
4. Time course of symptoms
5. Relationship to positional changes
6. Associated symptoms
   - Nausea
   - Vomiting
   - Headache
   - Neurologic symptoms
   - Chest pain

- Palpitations
- Fever
- Medications
- Hearing loss
7. Past medical history
8. Residual effects

 ## Physical Examination

In acute vertigo, most neurological disorders are peripheral in nature—i.e., outside the central nervous system. The examination, therefore, is focused on demonstrating the signs suggestive of this peripheral localization while ruling out involvement of the central nervous system or other disorders. This approach helps to confirm the diagnosis and rule out more emergent conditions. The examiner should note all vital signs and perform a brief general physical examination before proceeding to a detailed neurologic examination. The external auditory canal should be examined for the presence of infection or vesicles consistent with herpes zoster. The mental state should be evaluated and should be normal unless a central nervous system (CNS) lesion, infection, metabolic derangement, or drug intoxication is responsible. A detailed cranial nerve examination is mandatory.

- Any focal asymmetry of the cranial nerve examination in combination with vertigo should be considered evidence of CNS involvement.

Since the vestibulo-ocular system is frequently impaired in peripheral and central causes of vertigo, careful assessment of eye movements should be performed. Nystagmus in the primary position of gaze should be checked, as well as a full range of horizontal and vertical eye movements. Nystagmus in extreme gaze is not as diagnostic as nystagmus just off the primary position of gaze. Therefore, it is especially important to test for nystagmus with the hand held a couple of feet away to prevent convergence and to hold end positions of gaze for a couple of seconds.

- *Peripheral lesions* tend to produce nystagmus that is delayed with a latency of a few seconds, fatigues after repetitive maneuvers, is unidirectional, is inhibited by fixation, and is frequently associated with profound vertigo.
- Asymmetrical rotational nystagmus is most suggestive of a peripheral cause for vertigo.
- *Central lesions* tend to produce nystagmus that starts abruptly, does not fatigue, and is not usually associated with profound vertigo. Any vertical nystagmus should be considered secondary to a central cause.

Table 18-4 outlines several clinical findings of central versus peripheral vertigo.

Next, hearing should be evaluated for unilateral hearing loss or tinnitus, which is suggestive of eighth-nerve or brainstem dysfunction. Arm and leg movements should be observed, screening for motor dysfunction. Special attention to gait analysis and sensory examination of the legs, particularly proprioception, is very important. Coordination is tested to exclude limb ataxia suggestive of brainstem or cerebellar dysfunction. Any abnormalities observed require further evaluation with appropriate examination of the affected system.

TABLE 18-4

CENTRAL VERSUS PERIPHERAL VERTIGO

CLINICAL SIGNS	PERIPHERAL VERTIGO	CENTRAL VERTIGO
Latency period before onset of positional nystagmus	2–20 s	None
Duration of nystagmus	< 30 s	> 30 s
Fatigability of nystagmus	Fatigues with repetition	No fatigability
Direction of nystagmus	Unidirectional	Multidirectional in a given head position
Intensity of vertigo	Severe	May be mild or none
Response to head movement	Single position/movement elicits vertigo	Multiple positions elicit vertigo

Provocative maneuvers like *Barany's maneuver*, particularly in patients with positional vertigo, can be tested to help differentiate peripheral versus central lesions. Barany's maneuver is performed by moving the patient from a sitting position to a supine position with the head lying off the end of the bed and supported by the examiner's hands. The head should be extended 30 to 45 degrees from the horizontal plane. The patient is observed for the development of nystagmus and vertigo. If nystagmus is elicited, the latency, duration, direction, and fatigability of the nystagmus should be noted. The maneuver is repeated with the head extended and turned to the right and then repeated with the head turned to the left.

In patients with light-headedness, orthostatics should be checked, along with a full cardiac evaluation. Occasionally, the response to hyperventilation should be evaluated as well. Any precipitation of symptoms should be noted. Screening examination of cranial nerves, including pupils, extraocular muscles, and facial symmetry should be performed. Gait evaluation can be used to screen for motor asymmetry, while reflex and sensory examinations should be directed at evaluating possible neuropathies.

Dizziness

 Key Points of Documentation on Physical Examination

Complete ENT examination

1. Eye movements and visual fields
2. Nystagmus (rotational, vertical, horizontal, latency, fatigability, and duration)
3. Barany-Nylan test results
4. Cerebellar findings (ataxia, coordination, past pointing)
5. Gait abnormalities
6. Orthostatic vital signs
7. Cardiac examination, especially for rate, rhythm, and murmurs
8. Meningeal signs

Clinical Presentations

PERIPHERAL VERTIGO

Peripheral vertigo is commonly seen in the urgent care setting related to acute vestibu-lopathies, including vestibular neuronitis, benign positional vertigo, acute labyrinthitis, and Ménière's disease. Other causes may include trauma, ototoxic drugs, and acoustic neuromas.

Acute Vestibular Neuronitis In acute vestibular neuronitis, the symptoms are usu-ally sudden, severe, and acute in onset. Frequently, there are profound associated auto-nomic symptoms, with sweating, nausea, and vomiting. Precipitation of the symptoms by head movement is common, and there may be continued nystagmus toward the affected side. The symptoms may occur in episodes that become less frequent, less severe, and shorter in duration over a course of days to a couple of weeks. There is no specific eti-ology, though viral involvement of the vestibular system is likely, particularly as this condition may occur in epidemics.

Benign Positional Vertigo Benign positional vertigo (BPV) is seen with some fre-quency in the urgent care setting and tends to affect older patients. Symptoms are acute and often occur in the morning upon arising. Patients describe rolling over in bed or bend-ing the head back and noting the symptoms. The symptoms experienced with BPV tend to be similar to those seen in acute vestibular neuronitis, but the head movements that pro-duce vertigo in BPV are much more specific and better defined by the patient. BPV may occur spontaneously or after head trauma. The cause is postulated to be secondary to debris accumulating in the posterior semicircular canal. These particles stimulate hair cells and cause a sensation of movement.

Acute Labyrinthitis In acute labyrinthitis, cochlear and vestibular involvement occurs, usually secondary to bacterial infections, viruses such as mumps or measles, or in the con-text of meningitis. Along with profound vertigo, there may be associated fever, ear pain, and hearing loss. Acute labyrinthitis is a relative emergency requiring appropriate anti-biotic administration.

Ménière's Disease Ménière's disease is discussed frequently but is much less common than the above entities. The major clinical features of Ménière's are profound attacks of spontaneous vertigo associated with a feeling of fullness or pressure in the ear, tinnitus, and a fluctuating hearing loss. This last can be demonstrated on audiograms and pro-gresses over time. Ménière's is generally seen in patients over 50 years of age.

DISEQUILIBRIUM

Disequilibrium seen acutely is frequently related to new medications or to toxicity from the use of chronic medications. Patients with peripheral neuropathy, decreased vision, and presbyacusis often describe a sense of disequilibrium on a chronic basis. It should be noted that patients with multisensory deficits might present acutely with disequilibrium in the setting of a rather small brainstem, cerebellar, or cerebral stroke.

CEREBELLAR HEMORRHAGE

Of ominous concern is disequilibrium related to acute cerebellar dysfunction due to a cerebellar stroke or hemorrhage. Cerebellar hemorrhages or posterior fossa masses should be considered whenever acute disequilibrium is associated with headache, nausea (often with intractable vomiting), and neck pain. The concern for cerebellar hemorrhage should be particularly heightened when ataxia is associated with a headache, hypertension, or a coagulopathy. Although the physical examination may have no detectable focal signs and the patient may be quite alert early on, there is the potential for rapid deterioration to occur. *Cerebellar hemorrhage is a true neurologic emergency.*

LIGHT-HEADEDNESS

Light-headedness is most often associated with hemodynamic or cardiovascular disorders. A common presentation of light-headedness is the development of symptoms precipitated by standing that improve upon lying down. Frequently, acute events such as dehydration or a change in antihypertensive medication will precipitate light-headedness. Patients with a predisposition, particularly patients with diabetic neuropathy and autonomic involvement, are at increased risk. Alternatively, an acute episode of light-headedness is occasionally seen in patients with a cardiac dysrhythmia. Other etiologies of light-headedness include postprandial hypotension, vasovagal episodes, and a vasodepressor phenomenon. Ill-defined light-headedness may also be seen in the context of hyperventilation and anxiety disorder with panic attacks. In contrast to true vertigo or disequilibrium, positional changes of the head do not usually precipitate the symptoms.

 Management of the Patient with Dizziness

Emergency Transfers

If the history or examination suggests the possibility of a central process, the patient should be transferred for emergent CT scanning to exclude cerebellar hemorrhage, stroke, or brainstem lesion. An intravenous line should be placed and the patient should be monitored continuously while awaiting transport by emergency medical services (EMS). Oxygen therapy should be started as indicated by the patient's condition and underlying health status. The receiving facility should be notified regarding the patient's arrival, history, physical findings, and condition. In patients with a suspected cerebellar hemorrhage in whom rapid deterioration could occur, preparations should be made for possible emergency airway management.

Other conditions that will require transfer for emergent treatment include bacterial labyrinthitis, cardiac disease, and cardiac dysrhythmias. Patients with intractable symptoms who are unable to care for themselves or who have intractable vomiting will also need transfer for inpatient management.

- Many patients are evaluated for carotid disease because of complaints of dizziness; however, carotid stenosis in general—as compared with vertebrobasilar disease in particular—does not produce true vertigo.

TABLE 18-5

VESTIBULAR SUPPRESSANTS

NAME	DOSAGE	ROUTE OF ADMINISTRATION	SEDATING EFFECTS
Meclizine (Antivert)	12.5–25 mg q 8 h	PO	Somewhat sedating
Diphenhydramine (Benadryl)	25–50 mg q 6 h	PO; may be given IV or IM in the urgent care center	Very sedating
Diazepam (Valium)	20–50 mg q 8 h	PO; initial dose may be given IV in the urgent care center	Very sedating
Dimenhydrinate (Dramamine)	25–50 mg q 6 h	PO	Somewhat sedating
Promethazine (Phenergan)	12.5 or 50 mg q 6 h	PO; initial dose may be given IV, IM, or PR in the urgent care center	Very sedating

Outpatient Treatment

Patients with vertigo who do not require emergency transfer should be evaluated for evidence of dehydration occurring secondary to emesis or poor fluid intake. Intravenous rehydration for those patients may be needed. Blood work, including SMA-7 and a complete blood count (CBC), should be checked to exclude infection or electrolyte abnormalities.

Vestibular suppressants may be helpful for symptoms but will not improve the rate of recovery and should only be used acutely. Caution should be used in prescribing these to elderly patients, as they do not tolerate them well and, as a result, may return with an apparent increase in dizziness often related to the medications (Table 18-5).

 Management

Tables 18-6 and 18-7 describe management of the patient with dizziness.

Discharge Instructions

It is important to have the patient follow up with an internist or a neurologist, particularly if the symptoms are frequent and recurrent. Patients should be reassured that most cases of acute peripheral vertigo are self-limited and will improve on their own. If

TABLE 18-6

DIZZINESS—CRITERIA FOR TRANSFER

Inability to exclude cerebellar hemorrhage, stroke, or brainstem lesion
Suspected bacterial labyrinthitis or meningitis
Suspected cardiac disease or dysrhythmia
Intractable vomiting with an inability to care for self

TABLE 18-7

MANAGEMENT OF DIZZINESS

Transfer Patients

1. Intravenous infusion of D_5W at keep vein open (KVO)
2. Continuous cardiac and neurologic monitoring
3. Oxygen therapy as needed
4. Notification of receiving facility

Outpatients

1. Rehydration if there is clinical evidence of dehydration
2. Blood work for complete blood count and electrolytes *as indicated*
3. Vestibular suppressants/antiemetics *as indicated*
4. Primary care physician follow-up

vestibular suppressants are used, the patient must be warned against driving and advised to abstain from all activities that require mental alertness and dexterity.

For patients with symptoms of light-headedness and disequilibrium, further evaluation to determine the underlying etiology of their symptoms is required. Vestibular suppressants are not helpful in treating these patients.

 Errors to Avoid

- Failure to diagnose cerebellar hemorrhage or other central lesion
- Failure to caution patient against driving until symptoms have completely resolved
- Failure to caution patient against quick head movements or activities that precipitate symptoms
- Failure to advise patient against driving and activities requiring mental alertness/ dexterity while they are taking vestibular suppressants

GUILLAIN-BARRÉ SYNDROME

Guillain-Barré syndrome (GBS) is the most common acute paralytic syndrome diagnosed in the United States. It is not a disease but a syndrome caused by multiple etiologies. GBS should strongly be considered in the differential diagnosis of any patient presenting with acute generalized weakness. The generalized weakness seen in GBS is produced by acute demyelination of the peripheral nerves. In many cases the demyelination is autoimmune in nature, occurring after a flu-like illness, vaccinations, surgery, or drug use. It may also be idiopathic in nature. It is important to consider that many patients with GBS are not initially recognized as having the disorder because of vague symptomatology. Patients may complain of a feeling of "heaviness" or clumsiness. Early on, the examination may be relatively unremarkable. A clinical point in GBS is that the weakness is often noted more in the proximal muscles; this presentation is unusual for most neuropathies. Sensory loss is primarily seen distally but is not usually noticed as much as the weakness. Though areflexia is a hallmark of the disorder, initially the reflexes may appear normal or decreased and then develop gradual weakening over time. GBS may be rapidly progressive, with generalized weakness leading to respiratory muscle involvement. Autonomic dysfunction also occurs with cardiac arrhythmia, hypotension or hypertension, and difficulties with temperature regulation. The respiratory and autonomic involvement causes the majority of the morbidity and mortality associated with the disorder.

Due to the sequelae of GBS, any patient with acute to subacute onset of generalized symptoms or signs of proximal greater than distal weakness—especially if associated with decreased reflexes—should be considered to have GBS until proven otherwise.

The differential diagnosis of Guillain-Barré syndrome is given in Table 18-8.

 # Evaluation/Management

Vital signs should be documented as well as the respiratory status for signs of tachypnea or dyspnea. The neurologic examination should focus on motor, sensory, and reflex function. The common pattern is of proximal greater than distal weakness, with diffusely decreased or absent reflexes. The legs are usually more severely affected than the arms. Reflexes may initially be normal or decreased, but they become gradually weaker further into the course of the disease. Although facial weakness is sometimes seen, other cranial nerves are not usually affected.

The evaluation and management of patients suspected of having GBS is dependent on the rapidity of progression of the weakness and the degree of weakness or other complications. *Any patient that is suspected of having GBS should be transported to an acute care facility for further evaluation and observation.* If there is weakness that is impairing the ability to walk, the patient will likely require admission to an intensive care unit (ICU) for inpatient electrodiagnosis—electromyography/nerve conduction studies (EMG/NCS)—respiratory monitoring, and possible plasmapheresis. Plasmapheresis has been demonstrated to shorten the course of patients with GBS who have gait difficulties if they are treated within 2 weeks of the onset of illness.

Guillain-Barré Syndrome—

 ### Key Points of Documentation

1. Presence or absence of recent illness or antecedent event such as recent immunization or surgery
2. Reflex, motor, and cranial nerve examinations
3. Respiratory status

TABLE 18-8

DIFFERENTIAL DIAGNOSIS OF GUILLAIN-BARRÉ SYNDROME

Botulism	Myasthenia gravis
Polymyositis	Heavy metal poisoning
Tick paralysis	Acute alcoholic myopathy
Organophosphate poisoning	

Errors to Avoid

- Assuming that the patient is malingering or has a psychiatric disorder
- Failure to recognize the rapidly progressive nature of GBS
- Failure to examine for ticks in order to rule out tick paralysis
- Misdiagnosing GBS as disk disease
- Failure to intubate for any signs of respiratory fatigue prior to transport (*respiratory failure can occur rapidly with GBS*)
- Failure to recognize autonomic dysfunction in GBS

TEMPORAL ARTERITIS

Temporal arteritis is a systemic inflammatory disorder that affects medium to large arteries, particularly in the cranial circulation. It afflicts predominately older patients, usually older than 60 years of age. The main symptoms that generally lead to evaluation are headache and visual loss. Unilateral tenderness of the temporal arteries and pain with chewing may be noted, and patients may complain of pain with brushing their hair. Other primary complaints are systemic, such as low-grade fever, weight loss, malaise, or vague, nonspecific complaints. If visual loss is present in an elderly patient, temporal arteritis should be considered, particularly if there are other systemic symptoms. Loss of vision in an elderly patient who is suspected of having temporal arteritis is a medical emergency. This relates to the fact that in many cases, the vision loss may become permanent if it is not treated. Additionally, treatment with corticosteroids is quite effective at preventing complications of temporal arteritis, including blindness and stroke.

Evaluation

Palpation of the temporal arteries should be performed, which may reveal exquisite tenderness, pulselessness, and/or induration. The eyes should be examined for any retinal ischemic changes as well as for documentation of visual acuity. In addition to the neurologic evaluation, which should be normal, a general medical examination should also be performed in order to address other disorders that may produce similar systemic symptoms. An erythrocyte sedimentation rate (ESR) should be obtained. This will usually be elevated between 60 and 100 mm/h.

Management (Table 18-9)

When the ESR is elevated, prednisone, 60 to 80 mg/day should be initiated and the patient sent for urgent biopsy of the temporal artery. Although there are occasional false-negatives, a biopsy generally confirms the diagnosis. The biopsy can be performed by an ophthalmologist in an outpatient setting with local anesthesia. Corticosteroids should not be forgone because of concern regarding their effect on the biopsy, particularly in patients with a suggestive history and visual loss.

TABLE 18-9

MANAGEMENT OF TEMPORAL ARTERITIS

1. Prednisone, 60 to 80 mg per day
2. Ophthalmologist consultation for futher direction of care
3. Primary care physician/rheumatologist follow-up

In patients with headache or other constitutional symptoms but no other findings suggestive of temporal arteritis, an ESR should be obtained and the patients followed up by their primary care physicians within the next couple of days.

Temporal Arteritis—

 Key Points of Documentation

1. Visual acuity
2. Findings on palpation of the temporal artery, including the character and quality of the pulse
3. Funduscopic examination
4. Intraocular pressures, as indicated, to rule out acute glaucoma
5. Results of stat ESR
6. Findings on palpation of all large arteries (including character and quality of pulse and presence of bruits)

 Errors to Avoid

• Failure to recognize a presentation of *acute glaucoma* with headache and visual changes
• Failure to treat a patient suspected of having temporal arteritis with a presentation of visual loss

NERVE ENTRAPMENT SYNDROMES

Nerve entrapment syndromes comprise a group of disorders that present with symptoms localized to a specific nerve. The symptoms that develop occur secondary to the compression of the involved nerve.

Carpal Tunnel Syndrome

Carpal tunnel syndrome (CTS) is a common cause of pain and paresthesias of the hands. It is produced by compression of the median nerve in the carpal ligament in the wrist. The paresthesias frequently occur at night, with patients describing a burning or tingling feeling in one or both hands that occasionally awakens them from sleep. The symptoms may radiate into the forearm or rarely into the shoulder. Change in hand position or activities such as reading a book or driving may precipitate the symptoms. The symptoms may be intermittent or constant. Although CTS is more common among those who work with their hands, it is also frequently seen in pregnancy (particularly in the sixth and seventh months), diabetes, and hypothyroidism. Most patients describe symptoms that have been present for some time, though fairly acute cases do occur. Although weakness of the hand is a common complaint, true weakness is seen only in severe cases. The differential diagnosis includes a C6 radiculopathy, proximal median nerve compression, arthritis, or tendinitis.

Evaluation

The strength of the hand muscles innervated by the ulnar and median nerves should be tested. Tinel's sign and Phalen's sign should also be tested, as they are common positive findings in patients with CTS.

- *Tinel's sign:* paresthesias in the median nerve distribution that are noted when tapping the volar surface of the wrist.
- *Phalen's sign:* paresthesias reproduced by hyperflexing the wrist for 1 min

Strength of the proximal arm muscles and reflexes should also be tested to rule out abnormalities that suggest a C6 radiculopathy. Evaluation of passive range of motion of the digits and wrist should be performed to exclude arthritis or tendinitis as a component of the symptoms. Additionally, atrophy of the thenar eminence should be sought, since this finding suggests axonal damage to the median nerve.

- Combined weakness in the ulnar and median hand muscles suggests a C8 radiculopathy or a lesion of the lower brachial plexus

On the sensory examination, although patients may describe subjective abnormalities of the median side of the palm, testing will show no true sensory loss. This finding occurs because the palmar cutaneous branch of the median nerve arises proximal to the carpal tunnel in the wrist.

 Management

In patients with symptoms that are predominantly nocturnal, splinting of the wrists in the neutral position may relieve the symptoms. The patient can then follow up with his or her physician, orthopedist, or hand specialist. In patients with arthritis, nonsteroidal anti-inflammatory drugs (NSAIDs), if not contraindicated, may help to reduce acute inflammation. If there is weakness or atrophy of the thenar muscles, an aggressive approach should be taken and the patient should be referred to an orthopedist or hand surgeon for further evaluation.

If the clinical picture is not clear, electrodiagnosis with EMG/NCS may be helpful in excluding other diagnoses in the differential. It should be kept in mind, however, that patients can have symptoms of CTS without EMG/NCS abnormalities, particularly if the examination is performed in the first couple of weeks after the start of symptoms.

Ulnar Palsy

In an ulnar nerve palsy, the ulnar nerve is frequently compromised either by compression of the nerve at the elbow or, less commonly, by compression of the nerve at the wrist. The cause may be related to anatomic factors such as (1) a shallow ulnar groove at the elbow, (2) fibrous bands causing compression related to repetitive flexion and extension of the elbow, (3) a traumatic contusion of the nerve at the elbow or the wrist, or (4) a prolonged compression due to improper surgical positioning under anesthesia.

Patients will describe a feeling of tingling in the ulnar part of the hand that does not usually extend above the wrist. The intrinsic hand muscles may be involved, with weakness and atrophy of the hand. The differential diagnosis includes C8-T1 radiculopathy and thoracic outlet syndrome.

- Diabetes and other causes of neuropathy may predispose individuals to developing ulnar palsy.

Evaluation

A complete motor and sensory examination of the upper extremities should be performed. For a pure ulnar nerve palsy, abnormalities should be found only in the distribution of the ulnar nerve. Palsy caused by nerve compression at the wrist may present with weakness of the first dorsal interosseous (FDI) and abductor digiti quinti (ADQ). Palsy caused by compression at the elbow, however, will also include weakness of the distal flexor of the fifth digit. Electrodiagnosis may be helpful in localizing the symptoms.

- Weakness of the hand, predominantly involving the abductor pollicis brevis (APB) and with sensory abnormalities in the ulnar part of the hand, suggests thoracic outlet syndrome.
- The presence of Horner's syndrome ipsilateral to the ulnar distribution symptoms suggests a lesion of the lower brachial plexus.

 Management

When the only findings are pain and sensory changes without weakness, management is conservative, with padding of the elbow or splinting. If weakness ensues, referral to a hand specialist is indicated.

Radial Nerve Compression

Radial nerve compression commonly presents with acute wrist drop. It frequently occurs in the setting of intoxication or occasionally after improper surgical positioning under anesthesia. The symptoms seen are caused by prolonged compression of the radial nerve in the spiral groove of the forearm. This compression produces a deficit that, in almost all cases, is reversible. The symptoms are predominantly motor, with wrist drop developing secondary to weakness of the extensor muscles of the fingers and wrist. There may also be sensory abnormalities in the webspace between the first and second digits on the dorsum of the hand, with sensory changes extending into the wrist.

Evaluation

The neurologic examination should focus on a detailed motor and sensory evaluation of the upper extremities. The examination should show motor abnormalities only in the radial nerve distribution distal to the triceps. Lack of involvement of the triceps differentiates the radial palsy at the spiral groove from a C7 radiculopathy.

 Management

For most patients, splinting with a "cock-up" wrist splint and physical therapy are helpful in preventing complications such as contractures. NSAIDs should be prescribed for those patients without known contraindications. Improvement generally occurs over days to weeks. If there is profound weakness or if the patient presents with weakness that has lasted longer than 2 months, a referral to a neurologist is appropriate.

Meralgia Paresthetica

Meralgia paresthetica is a syndrome of numbness and occasionally burning discomfort in the anterolateral thigh. It is produced by entrapment or compression of the lateral femoral cutaneous nerve at the level of the inguinal ligament. The symptoms may be worse when the patient is lying down and better when sitting. This condition is frequently related to an increase in abdominal girth, as in ascites or pregnancy, or it may be related to compression by tight-fitting garments. Rarely, the disorder can be seen related to an intrapelvic mass.

Evaluation

On examination, sensory abnormalities restricted to the anterolateral thigh consistent with the distribution of the lateral femoral cutaneous nerve will be noted. There should be no associated motor abnormalities. A thorough abdominopelvic examination should be documented and is indicated to exclude an obvious mass.

 Management

Management is entirely conservative and supportive. This condition may resolve on its own or continue to produce annoying symptoms without disability. For patients with pain, a referral to the primary care physician is appropriate.

SEIZURES

Seizures are episodes of abnormal electrical discharges by the brain. They can occur in normal people under provoked situations such as head trauma, metabolic derangement, withdrawal syndromes, or drug use. Some individuals have a genetically determined or acquired tendency toward recurrent seizures. The condition of repeated or recurrent seizures without apparent provocation is epilepsy. Seizures may be focal, affecting one specific area of brain, or generalized. Focal seizures are frequently related to structural abnormalities, whereas generalized seizures are often related to a genetic predisposition. The diagnosis of seizures in the urgent care setting is primarily clinical, suggested by history and supported by investigation. The determination of the etiology of an initial event is sometimes difficult and should be left to the neurologist. Frequently, seizures are a symptom of another disorder such as a tumor, CNS infection, stroke, electrolyte abnormality, alterations in glucose levels, trauma, or drugs. The goals for the urgent care setting are to describe the spell, determine whether there are any clear precipitating factors, ensure the safety of the patient, and provide appropriate triage for subsequent management.

The differential diagnosis of seizures is given in Table 18-10.

Clinical Presentation

There are a number of historical features that are suggestive of a seizure. An abrupt onset, with the duration of seizure activity and resolution all occurring within a couple of minutes, is commonly seen. Seizures are usually quite similar in characteristics to each other or to those experienced in the past. Incontinence is seen frequently, as is tongue biting (particularly the sides of the tongue). The patient should be questioned as to whether a strange feeling (aura) preceded the seizure. Vague abdominal discomfort is a common aura. Uncommonly, olfactory hallucinations may also be observed as auras. Memory loss for the seizure is common; therefore both the patient and observers should also be questioned regarding the seizure.

- Observers frequently overestimate the duration of the seizure, and postictal drowsiness may confuse the question of the exact duration of seizure activity.

The patient or observers should be asked whether there was focality during the seizure—i.e., movement or lack thereof of one limb. Of course, a prior history of seizures and history of medication use is important. Other important factors to note from history include recent fever, infection, change in medications, alcohol ingestion or withdrawal, head trauma, and any past medical history.

Types of Seizures

Generalized seizures are secondary to nearly simultaneous activation of both cerebral hemispheres. The most common generalized seizure is the *grand mal seizure (GMS)*. Consciousness is usually lost early on. Frequently there is clonic jerking of the extremities, tonic posturing, or myoclonic jerking. The duration is usually 60 to 90 s. A brief

TABLE 18-10

DIFFERENTIAL DIAGNOSIS OF SEIZURES

Syncope	Hyperventilation
Migraine	Panic attacks
Transient ischemic attack	Psychogenic seizure-like activity
Narcolepsy	

period of apnea may be associated with cyanosis. There is gradual slowing of the clonic movements and then deep, labored breathing. A gradual return of consciousness follows.

Absence or *petit mal seizures* are also generalized seizures but with quite different manifestations. Staring or blinking without response to voice is common. The absence spells are very brief, lasting seconds at a time. There is abrupt onset and resolution, with resumption of the previous activity. There is no postictal state. Petit mal seizures occur mainly in children, usually resolving in adulthood, when other types of seizures may replace them. Note that the term *petit mal seizures* refers to a specific clinical-ECG syndrome and should not be used to describe small, partial, or limited seizures.

Focal or partial seizures are secondary to activation of a single area of brain. Frequently, focal seizures are related to a structural lesion. There is no alteration of consciousness. Clonic or tonic movements of an extremity are caused by seizure discharges in the contralateral motor cortex. Similarly, sensory symptoms (dysesthesias, burning, tingling) of an extremity are caused by seizure discharges in the contralateral sensory cortex. The duration is usually a matter of minutes. Occasionally, focal seizures can spread to involve the entire brain, in which case a focal seizure may secondarily become generalized.

Partial complex seizures are focal seizures that involve areas of the brain controlling attention, memory, and behavior. They are frequently of temporal lobe origin. The limbic system is often involved, producing hallucinations, automatic behavior, affective disturbances, and amnesia for the events. By definition, consciousness is impaired in partial complex seizures.

Status epilepticus is a neurologic emergency. It is defined as continuous seizure activity lasting 30 min or more or two or more seizures without full recovery of consciousness between attacks. This clinical situation must be quickly recognized and immediately triaged to the acute medical setting.

Seizures—

 Key Points of Documentation to Elicit on History and Physical Examination

1. Previous seizure history
2. Description of type of seizure
3. Duration of seizure activity
4. Duration of postictal state
5. Any history of antecedent trauma
6. Any history of trauma sustained during seizure activity
7. Medication history (anticonvulsants, other prescribed medications, street drugs, change in medication, alcohol use)
8. Complete set of vital signs
9. Complete neurologic examination

Evaluation

The general physical examination should be directed toward the assessment of injuries such as fractures, dislocations, head trauma, and tongue lacerations.

- After a true seizure, lacerations of the tongue are more often seen laterally than at the tip.

Seizure patients should be assessed for evidence of infection—i.e., fever, meningismus, otitis, pneumonia, or urinary tract infection—as well as signs of alcoholism. On neurologic evaluation, the patient's attention and concentration should be tested and documented and then serially followed. Progressive obtundation instead of gradual clearing after a seizure is an ominous sign suggestive of ongoing seizures; encephalopathy related to drugs, alcohol, or metabolic derangement; or an intracranial lesion. The remainder of the neurologic examination should be directed at identifying focal signs if present, particularly in partial seizures. Any observed asymmetries in the cranial nerves or in the motor, reflex, or sensory examination may be suggestive of a focal lesion and therefore mandate urgent imaging with CT scan or MRI.

 Management

There are few circumstances in which management of seizures is appropriate in the urgent care setting. A full examination and evaluation for underlying causes such as infection, intoxication, or trauma can generally be safely performed in the urgent care setting in a patient with known epilepsy who is taking anticonvulsants and who presents after an uncomplicated seizure and has a normal return of consciousness. Anticonvulsant levels and electrolytes, including glucose, calcium, phosphorus, and magnesium, should be determined. If no abnormalities are found during evaluation, the patient can be discharged. Close follow-up should be arranged with the patient's primary care physician. In general, the determination and manipulation of anticonvulsants should be deferred to the patient's neurologist. Frequent seizures require a more urgent follow-up, either with the patient's physician or with a neurologist.

New-onset seizures, prolonged seizures, or seizures complicated by focal signs or lack of return to baseline require the patient to be urgently triaged to an acute care facility for further evaluation and management, including CT scanning. The major nonneurologic issues of concern related to seizures are aspiration, injury, and metabolic derangement (particularly lactic acidosis, hypoxia, and hypotension). Indications for admission include a prolonged seizure or postictal state, repetitive seizure activity, seizures in the setting of a complicated medical condition, or seizures complicated by aspiration. The management of an ongoing seizure is primarily supportive, and preparations for transport should include the anticipation of possible recurrent seizure activity. It is important to keep a calm demeanor and to speak in a calm voice. The patient and observers should be re-assured that most seizures are self-limited. Aspiration and physical injury may be prevented by maintaining the patient in the lateral decubitus position with suction and oxygen readily available. Padded bed rails should be up and care taken not to restrain the patient. Only axillary temperatures should be taken, since no objects other than an oral airway should be put into the patient's mouth. Intravenous access with normal saline (preferably not in an antecubital vein) should be established; in patients with a history of coronary artery disease, oxygen should be administered by face mask or nasal cannula. Blood to determine a CBC, glucose level, magnesium, calcium, alcohol, toxicology screen, and anticonvulsant levels should be drawn. Glucose followed by thiamine should be given, especially if alcohol withdrawal is suspected.

Status Epilepticus

In general, seizures last no more than 3 min continuously; therefore if there is no return to consciousness between seizures or seizures are continuous for longer than 3 min, status epilepticus should be considered. As previously mentioned, status epilepticus is a neurologic emergency requiring emergent advanced life support (ALS) transport to an acute care facility with available neurologic consultation.

 Management of Seizures

The acute management of seizures is given in Table 18-11.

Alcohol Withdrawal Seizures

Alcohol withdrawal seizures do not necessarily require treatment with anticonvulsants. These seizures usually occur within 48 h of cessation of drinking.

- Although alcohol withdrawal seizures are seen mainly in alcoholics, there are some patients who have a predisposition for seizures in whom seizures may be provoked by alcohol cessation.

  If a patient with alcohol withdrawal seizures has a normal physical examination, the seizure was generalized, and there no evidence of trauma or an underlying medical condition, he or she can generally be referred for the treatment of the alcoholism. Thiamine, glucose, correction of electrolytes, and occasionally benzodiazepines are indicated in preparation for a referral to detoxification when appropriate. Any findings of focality, repetitive seizures, trauma, or underlying conditions require further evaluation.

TABLE 18-11

ACUTE MANAGEMENT OF SEIZURES

1. ABCs of ACLS to include:
   - Airway maintenance (use oral or nasal airway as needed)
   - Supplemental oxygen
   - Intravenous access with normal saline (do not use antecubital veins)
   - C-spine precautions as indicated
2. Cardiac and pulse oximetry monitoring
3. Protection from aspiration (suction should be ready and available)
4. Protection from injury (use of padded side rails)
5. Diazepam 5 to 10 mg IV over 2 to 3 min slow push for status epilepticus; lorazepam may be given 2 to 4 mg IV (or IM if no IV access)
   - Can repeat diazepam q 5 min up to 20 mg
   - Be prepared to support breathing
6. Finger-stick glucose and administer intravenous glucose as indicated for hypoglycemia
7. Immediate notification of EMS for ALS transport to an acute care facility

KEY: ABCs-airway, breathing, circulation; ACLS, acute cardiac life support; C-spine, cervical spine; EMS, emergency medical services; ALS, advanced life support.

HEADACHE

Headache is another common complaint seen in the urgent care setting. In most cases, headache is related to a primary headache disorder such as migraine, tension, or cluster headache. Secondary or symptomatic headache disorders are related to systemic diseases or to intracranial or extracranial disorders. The history is the most important part of the evaluation of headache, since overt signs or abnormalities do not always accompany many conditions causing headache. A history of one type of headache also does not exclude the presence of another type. For example, a patient with a history of migraine who has a new headache associated with visual symptoms could also have an occipital arteriovenous malformation. The goal of the history and examination is to determine whether there is evidence to support or refute a secondary cause for headache. There are several historical features that suggest an ominous cause for headache, such as new headaches in a patient with a history of cancer or AIDS, new headache in an elderly patient, or the sudden onset of a severe "thunderclap" headache. Progressive or continuous headaches may be seen with CNS tumors, hydrocephalus, or inflammatory conditions. Acute headache—especially with fever, neck pain, alteration in consciousness, or in relation to physical exertion—is suggestive of meningitis or subarachnoid hemorrhage. In order to characterize the headache, it is important to inquire about the onset, duration, location, and quality of pain, precipitating factors (food, menstruation, exercise), family history, prodromes, and prior headaches.

The differential diagnosis of headache is given in Table 18-12.

Headache—

 Key Points of Documentation to Elicit on History

1. Onset of headache (*sudden versus gradual*)
2. Duration
3. Quality/character of pain (*throbbing or pulsating, sharp, thunderclap, worst headache of patient's life*)
4. Location (*unilateral, localized-occipital, temporal, periorbital, frontal, diffuse*)

TABLE 18-12

DIFFERENTIAL DIAGNOSIS OF HEADACHE

Migraine headache	Glaucoma
Tumor	Tension headache
Hypertension	Cluster headache
Aneurysm	Subarachnoid hemorrhage
Hematoma (subdural/epidural)	Meningitis
Sinusitis	Abscess
Temporal arteritis	Metabolic (fever, hypoglycemia, etc.)

5. Prodromes (*flashes of light, visual changes, etc.*)
6. Headache history (*previous workup, medications, response to medications*)
7. Precipitating factors (*fasting state, activity, time of day, relation to menstrual cycle, food products*)
8. Associated symptoms (*nausea, photophobia, fever, neurologic findings, underlying illness*)
9. Comparison to previous headaches

Clinical Presentation

Migraine is diagnosed by establishing a history of episodic, primarily unilateral throbbing or pulsating headache associated with nausea, vomiting, or anorexia. It is important to note that many patients, because of a lack of diagnosis, do not have a prior history of migrainous episodes. For a true diagnosis of migraine, the headaches should occur at least five times in the patient's life with no other identifiable cause. The intensity of a migraine is moderate to severe, with a gradual onset that at times may build rapidly. Photophobia and sonophobia may also be present. In classic migraine, the headache may be preceded by a visual aura with features of bright, shimmery, zigzag lines or flashing lights. A key point in the course of migraine is a waxing and waning of intensity over a couple of hours to up to a day. Migraine headaches frequently improve with sleep and are worsened with physical activity. Tiredness, hunger, menstruation, stress, and certain foods are triggers for migraine (Table 18-13). A regular sleep schedule on weekdays and weekends, regular meals without skipping, as well as avoidance of highs and lows in stress and workload may all help to decrease the frequency of migraines. Occasionally, migraine may be associated with focal sensory complaints that gradually spread over 30 min or so. As a rule, it must not be assumed that focal neurologic symptoms are related to migraine unless there is a well-established prior history of the same deficit and that the symptoms resolve within 24 h.

Tension headache is generally mild to moderate in intensity. The headache is characterized as a squeezing, aching, or pressure-like sensation that does not vary much in intensity. Tension headache or muscle contraction headache is frequently holocephalic or bitemporal in nature. There is no change in intensity with physical activity. There is little or no photophobia or nausea. The headache may last for hours or days at a time.

TABLE 18-13

COMMON FOOD TRIGGERS FOR MIGRAINE HEADACHES	
Wine	Dairy products such as yogurt and sour cream
Beer	Aspartame
Liquor	Pickled foods
Bananas	Nuts, including peanuts
Chocolate	Hot dogs and processed sandwich meats
Chips	Citrus fruits
Raisins	

Occasionally, tension or muscle contraction headache is seen in combination with a tendency for migraine.

Cluster headache is classically described as occurring in recurrent episodes year after year, with the cluster period lasting for several weeks at a time. These peri-orbital headaches are brief but quite severe in intensity. The headache may last for 30 min to approximately 1.5 h, but it may occur repeatedly throughout the day. The onset may be acute and is particularly likely to occur during the middle of the night. The pain is unilateral; ipsi-lateral miosis, lacrimation, and nasal congestion are commonly seen. Cluster headache is seen predominantly in middle-aged men. Migraine, on the other hand, occurs predominantly in women. Alcohol frequently precipitates cluster headache. This type of headache is not associated with focal neurologic complaints or alteration in consciousness.

Subarachnoid hemorrhage (SAH) is a neurologic emergency and should be considered as a diagnostic possibility in a situation of acute headache of abrupt onset, with or without associated alteration in consciousness (which, if it occurs, may be brief). The pain of SAH is often characterized as the worst headache of the patient's life and may be described as a "thunderclap" headache that is either poorly localized or felt in the back of the head. Vigorous physical activity or the Valsalva maneuver commonly precipitates a SAH. Nausea, vomiting, and photophobia can occur and therefore may lead to an inadvertent diagnosis of migraine; it is imperative to remember, therefore, that migraine is a diagnosis of exclusion. Neck stiffness or nuchal rigidity is commonly found in SAH, though several hours may elapse before they become prominent. Localized neurologic findings aside from alterations in consciousness are rare. Rapid evaluation of these patients is very important, because the longer the SAH is present and surgically untreated, the more likely it is for complications such as hydrocephalus and vasospasm to occur.

Meningitis produces headache that builds gradually. The headache may be associated with fever, neck stiffness, and a change in mental status. The quality and characteristics of the pain are variable. There may be evidence of infection of the teeth, sinuses, ears, or a systemic infection. Other notable symptoms may include rash (meningococcemia) or focal neurologic findings. Kernig's and Brudzinski's signs should be checked for and documented.

Evaluation

A brief general medical examination as well as a complete set of vital signs is indicated in all patients with new or acute headache. Emphasis should be placed on signs suggestive of systemic illness or infection. The mental status examination should focus on the level of consciousness and quality of speech. Any abnormality in consciousness should be assumed to be related to the etiology of the headache and not, for example, to pain medications. Similarly, speech difficulties may indicate left hemispheric dysfunction. Examination of the cranial nerves should be complete and comprehensive. The fundi should be checked for papilledema, subhyaloid hemorrhages, or arteriovenous nicking, and the pupils should be screened for inequality (anisocoria), reactivity, and associated ptosis. The extraocular movements (EOMs) must be assessed and the patients questioned as to whether they experience diplopia. Visual fields and acuity are tested in patients with visual complaints. Any facial asymmetry should be noted. The motor, sen-

TABLE 18-14

INDICATIONS FOR URGENT COMPUTED TOMOGRAPHY

Any focality or abnormality on neurologic examination
Alteration of mental status
Change in headache characteristics (especially if progressive)
Headache in a patient with a history of a systemic disorder associated with intracranial lesions
Any signs of increased intracranial pressure
A history of the worst headache of the patient's life (followed by LP, if the CT is normal)
Trauma
Recurrent AM headaches
Headaches of uncertain etiology

KEY: CT, computed tomography; LP, lumbar puncture.

sory, and coordination examinations are guided by the patient's complaints. Any focality should be assumed to be related to an intracranial lesion, indicating urgent imaging to exclude hemorrhage or a mass.

Patients with any of these types of presentation, even with a prior history of migraine, should have a CT scan (Table 18-14). If the patient is stable and the history does not suggest an acute, ominous, or immediately progressive etiology, the patient may be sent directly for an urgent CT scan from the urgent care center. Specific arrangements must be made with both the patient *and* the radiology department for follow-up instructions. If *any* concern exists that the patient is not stable for an outpatient CT scan or that he or she could experience any deterioration during the evaluation, the patient should be sent for CT scan via the emergency department.

 Key Points of Documentation on Physical Examination

1. Complete vital signs, including temperature
2. Complete neurologic examination
3. Presence or absence of nuchal rigidity or Kernig's and Brudzinski's signs
4. Funduscopic examination, including presence or absence of papilledema
5. Presence or absence of a rash
6. Mental status
7. Temporal artery palpation
8. Intraocular pressures if indicated by age and presentation
9. Presence or absence of signs of infection (pneumonia, otitis media, etc.)

 Management

Patients with acute headache are frequently quite distraught and anxious. Evaluation and management in a quiet, darkened setting, if possible, is helpful. The patient's movement should be minimized, since it can worsen migraine as well as SAH.

Any patient with a history suggestive of a possible SAH or meningitis requires immediate triage to a hospital setting for further emergent evaluation. An intravenous line should be established prior to transport. For a possible SAH, the patient should be positioned with the head of the bed at a 30-degree elevation. Frequent monitoring of the neurologic status and vital signs is essential, and severe elevation of blood pressure should be treated, though ideally in a controlled hospital setting. Rapid changes in consciousness can occur with subarachnoid hemorrhages, as can respiratory failure. Respiratory support with intubation may be required, including hyperventilation for any evidence of increased intracranial pressure.

If meningitis is a consideration, empiric intravenous antibiotics (such as ceftriaxone 2 g) should be started while awaiting transport. Early administration of antibiotics is key, given that an important prognostic factor for patients with meningitis is the time between onset of illness and institution of antibiotic therapy.

- Precautions against *N. menigitidis* should be instituted as indicated and patient follow-up should occur in order to assess the need for prophylactic therapy to be provided to urgent care staff.

Table 18-15 outlines the criteria and management of patients requiring emergency transfer.

For patients presenting with headaches of a more benign nature, treatment can be initiated in the urgent care setting. Hydration and antiemetics are indicated in those with nausea and/or vomiting. Table 18-16 lists medications useful in the treatment of headaches. Abortive medications such as sumatriptan and ergotamine are indicated only in patients with a clearly established history and presentation consistent with

TABLE 18-15

HEADACHE

CRITERIA FOR EMERGENCY TRANSFER

1. Unstable patient
2. Any focality on neurologic examination including mental status alterations
3. Signs or concern for possible meningitis
4. Signs or concern for possible subarachnoid hemorrhage
5. Signs or concern for possible hematoma
6. Need for lumbar puncture
7. Intractable headache

MANAGEMENT OF THE TRANSFER PATIENT

1. ABCs of life support, including standby preparation for intubation
2. Intravenous administration of D_5W at keep vein open (KVO)
3. If SAH is suspected: keep head of bed at a 30-degree elevation
4. If meningitis is suspected: institute antibiotic therapy empirically as time permits
5. Arrange immediate EMS transport with notification of the receiving facility

KEY: ABCs-airway, breathing, circulation; SAH, subarachnoid hemorrhage.

TABLE 18-16

MEDICATIONS USED IN THE TREATMENT OF HEADACHES

Sumatriptan: 6 mg subcutaneous injection
25- and 50-mg tablets, orally
20-mg nasal spray

Ketorolac: 30 to 60 mg IM (initial dose)

Dihydroergotamine 45: 1-mg subcutaneous or intramuscular injection
(may take up to 3 h to work)
4-mg nasal spray (migranal)

Meperidine: 75 to 100 mg with hydroxyzine 25 to 50 mg, as tolerated

Prochlorperazine: 10 mg intravenously

Chlorpromazine: 10 to 12.5 mg q 15 min up to three doses

migraine. These medications should not be given in pregnancy or to patients with coronary artery disease (CAD), peptic ulcer disease, severe hypertension, peripheral vascular disease, or renal or hepatic dysfunction. Abortive medications must be used with extreme caution in patients with risk factors for CAD but who lack a documented history. See Table 18-17 for other contraindications in the treatment of migraine headache.

If the patient's history and evaluation do not suggest a particular headache type or there are contraindications to abortive medications, the use of analgesics such as ketorolac, chlorpromazine, or narcotics is indicated, depending on the intensity of the headache. Tension headache is managed with reassurance and simple analgesics.

For cluster headaches, abortive treatment, as with migraines, is indicated. Oxygen at 7 to 10 L/min by face mask, however, is quite helpful in patients who catch their cluster headaches at the onset. Intranasal lidocaine (1 mL of 4% lidocaine) administered to the ipsilateral nostril can also be tried.

Early follow-up by the primary care physician should be encouraged in all patients with headache. The fact that symptomatic treatment in the urgent setting does not substitute for long-term management by their primary care physician or headache specialist must be emphasized. The physician following the patient is in the best position to decide whether prophylactic treatment is indicated. Patients should be informed that the treatment of migraine/tension/cluster headaches requires an approach that addresses the likelihood of recurrence; otherwise they will find themselves having to make repeated visits to the urgent care setting.

TABLE 18-17

IMPORTANT CONTRAINDICATIONS IN THE TREATMENT OF MIGRAINE HEADACHES[a]

Dihydroergotamine and other vasoconstrictive medications should not be used within 24 h of each other
Meperidine must not be given to patients taking monoamine oxidase inhibitors

[a]See text for contraindications for sumatriptan.

General Discharge Instructions for Headache Patients

Recheck immediately for the following:

1. Worsening/new signs or symptoms
2. Change from typical headache pattern
3. Development of neck pain or stiffness
4. Fever
5. Weakness or numbness
6. Change in behavior
7. Intractable vomiting with dehydration

 Errors to Avoid

- Failure to diagnose an SAH sentinel headache
- Failure to diagnose meningitis
- Performing an inadequate history
- Performing an inadequate neurologic examination
- Failure to diagnose temporal arteritis as the etiology of a headache
- Failure to diagnose glaucoma, which may present with headache and vomiting
- Failure to diagnose sinusitis

STROKE/TRANSIENT ISCHEMIC ATTACK

Cerebral stroke is secondary to either ischemia or hemorrhage that causes an acute neurologic deficit corresponding to dysfunction in a particular vascular territory. If the degree of injury is profound enough, a permanent or persistent loss of function will result. Although there is no clear treatment for stroke, there are interventions that can be directed at limiting the deficit or preventing other episodes. Some of these therapies are particularly important to initiate at the onset or earliest point in the course of the stroke. In this regard, prompt recognition, evaluation, and triage of these patients to the appropriate medical setting is important. The term *TIA*, transient ischemic attack, refers to an acute, transient loss of neurologic function with subsequent improvement and resolution. TIAs usually last for minutes to hours, though by definition the deficits may be manifest for up to 24 h. The use of the term *TIA* is entirely clinical in that there are patients who appear to have had a TIA but who, on CT scanning or MRI, are found to have actually suffered a stroke. Once again, the recognition of this clinical situation is important in that there are therapies that may decrease the likelihood of future stroke (which likelihood is increased in patients with a recent history of TIA).

Clinical Presentation

The vascular territory involved as well as the pathologic process (ischemic versus embolic versus hemorrhagic) defines most stroke or TIAs. Risk factors for stroke include hypertension, coronary artery disease, atrial fibrillation, diabetes, and smoking. The occlusion of the *middle cerebral artery* (MCA) causes weakness and/or numbness of the contralateral face, arm, and leg, and is commonly associated with contralateral hemianopsia and hemisensory deficits. If the left MCA is affected, language deficits are observed as well. For example, a patient with acute weakness of the right face, arm, and leg with associated speech disturbance probably has a deficit corresponding to the distribution of the left middle cerebral artery. The *posterior cerebral artery* supplies the occipital lobe; its occlusion causes contralateral hemianopsia with occasional hemisensory deficits. Occlusion of the *anterior cerebral artery* causes contralateral lower extremity weakness that is greater than upper extremity weakness. There may also be a related gait abnormality and sensory changes. Insufficiency of the *vertebrobasilar artery* is associated with any combination of diplopia, vertigo, incoordination, facial numbness or weakness, dysarthria, or crossed signs (i.e., cranial nerve abnormalities on one side and hemiparesis or hemisensory deficits on the other). The patient may also give a history of syncope or sudden drop attacks. One of the more recognizable TIA syndromes is *amaurosis fugax,* or transient monocular blindness caused by retinal ischemia. Patients report an acute decrease in vision in one eye that occasionally is described as similar to a "shade being pulled down." Patients may describe blurring of vision or frank visual loss. Patients can only truly observe this after covering each eye separately and noticing the visual change in one eye only (otherwise it is possible that the visual symptom was present in both eyes and therefore is of cerebral localization). In most cases the cause is atherosclerotic plaque in the ipsilateral internal carotid artery leading to stenosis, occlusion, or embolism.

Ischemic strokes are usually large vessel occlusions, but they can also be produced by small vessel occlusion, as seen in lacunar strokes. *Lacunar strokes* present in syndromes such as pure motor hemiparesis, pure sensory stroke, and ataxic hemiparesis. Because lacunar strokes affect deep penetrating small arteries, there are no cognitive or mental status abnormalities associated with them. *Embolic stroke*, in particular cardioembolic stroke, is frequently seen in the context of atrial fibrillation, valvular disease, recent myocardial infarction, or cancer. *Hemorrhagic stroke* is related either to acute hemorrhage into the brain or to ischemic stroke that secondarily becomes hemorrhagic. Primary hemorrhages of the brain occur commonly in patients with a prior history of hypertension; their location is frequently in the basal ganglion, putamen, or cerebellum. Spontaneous hemorrhages or ischemic stroke with secondary hemorrhages are seen frequently in patients on anticoagulants.

 Evaluation/Management

In most situations, patients with acute symptoms suggestive of stroke will present to an emergency department; however, some patients do seek evaluation in the urgent care setting. Symptoms suggestive of an acute or evolving stroke or symptoms of a deficit that persists require emergent transfer to an acute care setting for further evaluation. Thrombolysis with tissue plasminogen activator (t-PA) is currently used by some hospitals in patients with disabling nonhemorrhagic stroke the onset of which was within 3 h of administration of the drug. Anticoagulants are also commonly used in nonhemorrhagic stroke, particularly in the setting of a possible cardioembolic stroke. Considering that these patients need CT scanning in addition to a rapid assessment, any patient who is felt to have an acute stroke should be emergently sent to a hospital setting. Vital signs,

TABLE 18-18

MANAGEMENT OF ACUTE STROKE OR TRANSIENT ISCHEMIC ATTACK

ABCs of life support (be prepared to intubate as needed)
Establishment of intravenous line with D_5W
Continuous cardiac monitoring
Pulse oximetry monitoring with supplemental oxygen administration
Sequential neurologic evaluation
Hospital notification with transport by emergency medical services

KEY: ABCs-airway, breathing, circulation.

a general examination with emphasis on the cardiovascular system, as well as a brief neurologic examination to define the presenting pattern and level of involvement should be performed. This evaluation, however, should not significantly delay transfer to the acute care setting. While awaiting EMS transport, an intravenous line should be established along with continuous cardiac monitoring and supplemental oxygen as indicated. The patient should be checked for any evidence of trauma, particularly head trauma, and evaluated for any evidence of a bleeding disorder.

Table 18-18 describes the management of acute stroke and TIA.

Patients who suffer either a minor, nondisabling stroke or TIA and whose symptoms began within 2 to 3 days of their evaluation should be considered acute and transferred to an acute care setting. Patients with a neurologic event that occurred more than 2 to 3 days prior to presentation and who have a nondisabling deficit can be evaluated in the urgent care setting. If the patient is stable, consultation with the primary care physician or a neurologist is appropriate to determine the course of treatment. If the patient is to be discharged, aspirin therapy should be initiated, along with CT scanning and carotid ultrasound evaluation if indicated. If there has been any worsening of the symptoms or deficit since the onset of symptoms, triage to the acute care setting is appropriate.

TRAUMA IN THE URGENT CARE SETTING

Tanise I. Edwards

In the urgent care setting, the trauma seen may present anywhere from an isolated sprain to a major, life-threatening injury. Ideally, major trauma is self-selected out of the urgent care setting, but in reality, major traumas or multiple trauma victims do occasionally present for treatment. Depending on the location of the urgent care facility, more severe injuries may be seen on a routine basis. The duty of urgent care physicians, therefore, is to:

1. Be able to recognize and appropriately assess for potentially serious injuries
2. Know how to properly stabilize a patient for transport
3. Be able to treat presenting injuries as indicated

Any patient presenting with a history consistent with significant trauma or evidence of it requires immediate notification of emergency medical services (EMS) for transport while simultaneous assessment and stabilization are in progress. There is a fine balance between evaluation and stabilization and the need to transport without a full workup. *A trauma patient can decompensate very rapidly. It is always better to transport a stable patient than to attempt to stabilize and arrange transport for a deteriorating one.* All transport should occur in concert with EMS and the receiving hospital or, if indicated, a designated trauma center. Early consultation with the appropriate specialist should also be initiated.

All patients with multiple trauma or with a history of significant trauma should be evaluated as per Advanced Trauma Life Support (ATLS) protocols.[1] Most if not all of these patients will require direct emergency department transfer for further evaluation and observation. Under certain circumstances, depending on the skills of the urgent care physician and the capabilities of the urgent care center, more advanced trauma care may be provided in the urgent care facility. It is important, however, never to delay definitive care or attempt to provide care above the practitioner's individual skill level and expertise.

THE TRAUMA HISTORY AND PHYSICAL EXAMINATION

History taking is key in the assessment of trauma patients, since the history will often give more insight into possible injury than the physical examination itself. Key points to be elicited on history include:

- Timing of injury
- Mechanism of injury
- What occurred leading up to the injury
- Initial symptoms experienced
- What has occurred since the injury (i.e., self-treatment or change in symptoms)
- Any extenuating circumstances (i.e., antecedent chest pain, seizure activity, etc.)
- Any alcohol or drug use that may confuse the history or alter pain response on evaluation

The AMPLE mnemonic gives an easy means to remember key information that should be obtained in all trauma victims. This information is especially important should rapid deterioration occur and no further history be obtainable:

A: allergies
M: medications
P: past medical history (including last tetanus immunization)
L: last meal
E: events of injury[1]

Physical examination of the trauma patient is best achieved using an organized and systematic method. This approach obviates the potential for missed injuries, inappropriate stabilization, and improper treatment. Per ATLS protocol, the first-look evaluation and resuscitation of a trauma patient follows the ABCDEF approach to assessment and concomitant stabilization:

A: airway with stabilization of the cervical spine (C-spine)
B: breathing
C: circulation, with hemorrhage control
D: disability
E: exposure
F: finger in every orifice[1]

The purpose of this primary survey[1] is to identify any immediately life-threatening conditions related to the respiratory or circulatory systems and provide immediate treatment as needed for stabilization. The following are included in this primary survey.

Airway with Cervical-Spine Stabilization

- Assessment of patency and the ability to maintain an airway
- Treatment, when indicated:
  Chin lift/jaw thrust, suction, oral airway, nasal airway, or intubation
  Immobilization with hard collar, sandbags, and taping of the head to a backboard or the bed for C-spine stabilization

Errors to Avoid

- Failure to control C-spine during airway management
- Attempting to use an oral airway in an awake individual, as an oral airway will stimulate the gag reflex
- Attempting intubation without proper training (a patient can be ventilated with a bag-valve-mask device while awaiting properly trained personnel; improper technique can cause spinal cord injury.)

Breathing

- Assess breath sounds, adequacy of air exchange, and adequacy of chest wall mobility
- Identify tension pneumothorax, open pneumothorax/sucking chest wounds, flail chest
- Treat as indicated:
    Needle decompression for tension pneumothorax
    Occlusive dressing for sucking chest wounds

Circulation

- Assess adequacy of peripheral perfusion and evidence of exsanguinating bleeding (see Table 19-1: "Assessment of Palpable Pulses")
- Treatment:
    Pressure dressings to sites of bleeding or direct pressure to control rapid blood loss

Disability

- Assess the patient's level of consciousness and the capacity for spontaneous limb movement

Any patient with a possible spinal injury must be moved *only* with appropriate spinal stabilization. In addition to C-spine stabilization, this includes log rolling of patient to avoid any undue movement of the lower spine.

Exposure

- Assess for hidden injury

In theory, the resuscitation phase immediately follows the initial evaluation; in practice, however, it occurs in a more concomitant fashion, with any immediately life-

TABLE 19-1

ASSESSMENT OF PALPABLE PULSES

- Palpable radial pulse denotes systolic BP of at least 80 mmHg
- Palpable femoral pulse denotes systolic BP of at least 70 mmHg
- Palpable carotid pulse denotes systolic BP of at least 60 mmHg

threatening condition treated upon identification. Immediate resuscitative measures include the following:

- Application of supplemental oxygen
- Insertion of two large-bore intravenous lines for crystalloid fluids (blood is drawn concomitantly and *labeled* immediately)
- Electrocardiographic (ECG) monitoring
- Placement of urinary catheter and nasogastric tube as indicated

 Errors to Avoid

- Attempting to place a urinary catheter without evaluating for urethral transection (That is, if blood is seen at the meatus or in the scrotum, or a high-riding prostate is noted on rectal examination, *a catheter must not be placed.*)
- Attempting to place an nasogastric tube in a patient with a possible fracture of the cribriform plate (this can lead to intracranial insertion)

Patients who require this advanced level of care necessitate *immediate* emergency medical services (EMS) transfer to a trauma center.

THE KEY TO PROPER TRAUMA EVALUATION IS CONTINUAL REASSESSMENT OF THE PATIENT'S CONDITION.

The Secondary Survey

The next sequential step in trauma evaluation is the secondary survey, which immediately follows the primary and resuscitation phases. In the secondary survey, a detailed evaluation is performed, assessing the entire body for injury. The secondary evaluation can begin while awaiting EMS transport for unstable patients and stable patients with potentially life-threatening injuries. The secondary survey should also be followed when patients deemed stable for further urgent care evaluation are being assessed [for example, patients who have been in a motor vehicle accident (MVA) some 24 h earlier, patients presenting with limited trauma, or those with isolated injuries].

Special Considerations

Motor Vehicle Accidents
In MVAs, key information must be elicited on history to help gain insight into the potential for serious yet sometimes inapparent injuries. The following questions should be asked regarding the circumstances of all MVAs:

- Was the patient restrained? What type of restraint was used? (Three-point restraint? Lap belt? Deployed air bag?)
- Where was the patient seated in the vehicle?

- Was the windshield broken?
- Was the steering wheel bent or damaged?
- Why did the accident occur?
- Where was the impact?
- What types of vehicles were involved?
- What was the extent of damage?
- Was the patient ejected?
- Did the vehicle roll over?

These questions help to assess the potential for significant injury by providing information on the mechanism of injury and the force with which the injury was sustained. For example, a patient presenting after head injury that occurred with force significant enough to break the windshield is at higher risk for associated C-spine injury.

IF: Broken windshield   **THINK:** Potential for major head trauma or cervical spine injury

IF: Damage to steering wheel   **THINK:** Potential for sternal fractures, myocardial contusion, major intraabdominal injury, great vessel injury

IF: Isolated lap belt restraint   **THINK:** Potential for intraabdominal or lumbar spine injury

IF: Deployed airbag   **THINK:** Potential for tympanic membrane rupture

IF: Unclear cause for accident   **THINK:** Possible underlying conditions
- Myocardial infarction
- Syncope/blackout
- Sleep deprivation
- Drug use

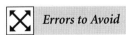 *Errors to Avoid*

- Not being prepared
- Placement of trauma patient in a small, poorly functional treatment area
- Failure to obtain a full, detailed history when patient's condition allows
- Failure to assess the patient fully
- Ignoring mechanisms of injury
- Underestimating how quickly changes can occur
- Delay in transport of a patient while attempting definitive diagnosis
- Failure to continually reassess a patient

CHEST TRAUMA

Injuries That May Be Seen in Chest Trauma

Life-Threatening Injury

- Pneumothorax (simple, open, tension)
- Hemothorax
- Flail chest
- Cardiac tamponade
- Aortic injury

Potentially Lethal Injury

- Myocardial contusion
- Pulmonary contusion
- Aortic injury
- Tracheobronchial injury
- Esophageal injury
- Diaphragmatic injury

Potentially Serious Injury

- Rib fractures

Chest injuries play a major role in the deaths that occur secondary to trauma. Patients sustaining life-threatening injuries, patients who have penetrating chest wounds, or those who, by history, have had trauma that could produce potentially lethal injuries should immediately be transferred to an acute care facility. It is important, therefore, to recognize these injuries and be knowledgeable about their stabilization.

During the clinical assessment of chest trauma, the presence or absence of the following should be evaluated and documented.

 ## History and Physical Examination

1. Respiratory distress
2. Cyanosis
3. Tachypnea
4. Tachycardia
5. Decreased breath sounds   **THINK:** pneumothorax
6. Tracheal deviation   **THINK:** tension pneumothorax
7. Hyperresonance on percussion   **THINK:** pneumothorax
8. Dullness on percussion   **THINK:** hemothorax
9. Abnormal chest wall mobility   **THINK:** flail chest
10. Beck's triad
    - Hypotension
    - Distended neck veins
    - Muffled heart sounds   **THINK:** cardiac tamponade
11. Subcutaneous emphysema   **THINK:** tracheobronchial or pulmonary parenchymal injury

Diagnostic Assessment

1. Oxygen saturation
2. X-ray evaluation:
   - Absent lung markings   **THINK:** pneumothorax
   - Tracheal deviation   **THINK:** tension pneumothorax
   - Effusion   **THINK:** hemothorax
   - Widened mediastinum   **THINK:** aortic injury
   - Mediastinal shift   **THINK:** tension pneumothorax, aortic injury
   - Obliteration of aortic knob   **THINK:** aortic injury
   - Subcutaneous emphysema   **THINK:** tracheobronchial or esophageal injury
   - Pneumomediastinum   **THINK:** esophageal injury
   - First- or second-rib fracture   **THINK:** major trauma
   - Rib fractures (single or multiple)
3. ECG abnormalities   **THINK:** cardiac contusion

Pneumothorax

A pneumothorax occurs when air is trapped in the pleural space. It may occur spontaneously or following blunt or penetrating chest trauma.

- Patients presenting with displaced rib fractures are at increased risk of developing a pneumothorax.

The presentation of a pneumothorax may range anywhere from symptoms of mild pleuritic chest pain to marked dyspnea and respiratory distress. Other presenting complaints may include shoulder pain or poorly localized back pain. Vital signs may be normal or the patient may be tachypneic and tachycardic. Breath sounds are typically decreased or absent over the area of the pneumothorax, and there is hyperresonance to percussion. There may also be evidence of subcutaneous air on palpation of the chest wall. A chest x-ray will typically show absence of lung markings, generally seen in the superior portion of the lungs on upright films. Small pneumothoraces may be difficult to see on x-ray studies (Table 19-2). Posteroanterior (PA) expiratory films often make a small pneumothorax more apparent.

Disposition
Advanced Life Support (ALS) transfer to emergency department for chest tube placement or, at a minimum, close observation and serial x-ray studies.

TABLE 19-2

ESTIMATING THE SIZE OF A PNEUMOTHORAX

- About 1 cm of intrapleural air is consistent with about a 10% pneumothorax
- About 2 cm of intrapleural air is consistent with about a 20% pneumothorax
- About 3 cm of intrapleural air is consistent with about a 30% pneumothorax

Management

1. Intravenous line placement
2. Monitoring of oxygen saturation
3. Supplemental oxygen via nasal cannula or simple face mask as indicated (i.e., hypoxia, older patients, patients with cardiac disease)
4. ECG monitoring as indicated by age, underlying conditions, and patient status
5. EMS transport
6. Continual assessment for conversion from a simple pneumothorax to a tension pneumothorax

 Errors to Avoid

- Failure to recognize progression to a tension pneumothorax
- Failure to obtain an expiratory film, thereby missing the diagnosis of a pneumothorax

Tension Pneumothorax

A tension pneumothorax occurs when the air trapped in the pleural cavity is unable to escape and pressure builds within the intrapleural space. *Tension pneumothorax is an acute life-threatening condition.* Clinically, patients will present in acute respiratory distress with hypotension, tachycardia, absent breath sounds on the affected side (secondary to complete collapse of the affected lung), tracheal deviation, and distended neck veins.

 Immediate Management

Immediate insertion of a large caliber needle into the second intercostal space at the midclavicular line on the involved side. This procedure will convert the tension pneumothorax into a simple pneumothorax. Treatment should occur immediately upon identification and should not be delayed while awaiting x-ray confirmation.

- If symptoms are not relieved after proper needle decompression, other causes for symptoms should be sought, including cardiac tamponade.

Disposition

ALS transfer to emergency department for chest tube placement *after* needle decompression.

 Management

1. Intravenous line placement
2. Monitoring of oxygen saturation

3. Supplemental oxygen via nasal cannula or simple face mask
4. ECG monitoring as indicated by age, underlying conditions, and patient status
5. ALS transport

 Errors to Avoid

- Failure to treat immediately
- Delay in treatment while awaiting confirmatory chest x-ray

Open Pneumothorax or Sucking Chest Wound

An open pneumothorax or sucking chest wound is an injury that occurs secondary to external penetration of the chest cavity. There will be air entering and exiting the chest cavity from a defect in the chest wall.

Disposition
ALS transfer to emergency department for repair.

 Management

1. Placement of sterile occlusive dressing secured on three sides
2. Intravenous line placement
3. Monitoring of oxygen saturation
4. Supplemental oxygen via nasal cannula or simple face mask
5. ECG monitoring as indicated by age, underlying conditions, and patient status
6. ALS transport

 Errors to Avoid

- Taping occlusive dressing on all four sides, which can convert an open chest wound into a tension pneumothorax

Flail Chest

A flail chest occurs when two or more ribs are fractured in two or more places, causing disruption of normal chest wall movement. On examination, there will be evidence of multiple rib fractures, and the patient may exhibit paradoxical movement of the flail section.

Disposition
ALS transfer to emergency department. This injury requires reexpansion of the lung and can require intubation for ventilatory failure or hypoxia.

Management

1. Intravenous line placement
2. Monitoring of oxygen saturation
3. Supplemental oxygen via nasal cannula or face mask (can potentially require ventilatory support—i.e., intubation)
4. ECG monitoring as indicated by age, underlying conditions, and patient status
5. Obtain a chest x-ray to evaluate for a pneumothorax if feasible
6. ALS transport

Cardiac Tamponade

Traumatic cardiac tamponade occurs when, as a result of blunt or penetrating trauma, blood accumulates in the pericardial sac and restricts mechanical cardiac function. On physical examination, the patient may present with *Beck's triad:*

1. Distended neck veins (may not occur in hypovolemic patients)
2. Hypotension
3. Muffled heart sounds

Although these presenting symptoms may be difficult to distinguish from a tension pneumothorax, breath sounds in cardiac tamponade are present bilaterally and the trachea remains midline. Treatment consists of the removal of blood from the pericardial sac.

Disposition
ALS transfer to emergency department.

 Management

1. Intravenous line placement with an initial fluid bolus for hypotension
2. Monitoring of oxygen saturation
3. Supplemental oxygen via nasal cannula or simple face mask
4. Continuous ECG monitoring
5. ALS transport

Hemothorax

The development of a hemothorax is the result of bleeding into the chest cavity. It may occur secondary to a laceration of the lung parenchyma, as a result of hilar or myocardial injury or injury to one of the small (intercostal or internal mammary) or major (aortic) blood vessels. Patients may present with dyspnea and shoulder, back, or pleuritic chest pain. They may be tachypneic or hypotensive if significant bleeding has occurred. Breath sounds of the involved area will be absent and dullness to percussion may also be present. An upright chest x-ray will show blunting of the costophrenic angle on the injured side if more than 200 to 300 mL of blood has collected in the chest cavity.

Disposition

ALS transfer to emergency department for chest tube placement or, at a minimum, close observation and serial x-ray studies.

 Management

1. Intravenous line placement (if significant findings, placement of two large-bore lines)
2. Monitoring of oxygen saturation
3. Supplemental oxygen via nasal cannula or face mask
4. ECG monitoring as indicated by age, underlying conditions, and patient status
5. ALS transport

Pulmonary Contusion

Pulmonary contusions occur following blunt chest wall trauma with injury to the pulmonary parenchyma. The severity of this injury increases over the first 48 to 72 h following trauma; these patients may therefore present several days after the initial injury. Patients often present with increasing dyspnea and tachypnea. Oxygen saturation will be decreased and chest films may show a dense infiltrate.

Disposition

ALS transfer for inpatient management.

 Management

1. Intravenous line placement
2. Monitoring of oxygen saturation
3. Supplemental oxygen via nasal cannula or face mask (can potentially require ventilatory support—i.e., intubation)
4. Continuous ECG monitoring
5. ALS transport

Myocardial Contusion

Myocardial contusion occurs following direct trauma to the anterior chest wall. This injury may be seen after an MVA when an unrestrained driver strikes the steering column or when an individual has sustained a significant blow directly to the anterior chest. Patients may complain of a midsternal, anginal type of chest pain and pressure or localized chest pain. There may be associated tachypnea and tachycardia as well as bruising and swelling of the anterior chest wall. Patients presenting with sternal fractures are at increased risk of myocardial injury. Patients with a history consistent with a potential myocardial contusion require ECG monitoring and serial cardiac enzymes. These patients are at increased risk for the development of sudden dysrhythmias including

TABLE 19-3

ELECTROCARDIOGRAPHIC FINDINGS ASSOCIATED WITH MYOCARDIAL CONTUSIONS

- Sinus tachycardia (the most frequent finding)
- ST-T abnormalities (T-wave flattening, ST-segment elevations)
- Dysrhythmias (particularly PVCs and atrial fibrillation)
- New RBBB or first-degree AV block

KEY: PVCs, premature ventricular contractions; RBBB, right bundle branch block; AV, atrioventricular.

premature ventricular contractions (PVCs), atrial fibrillation, or bundle branch blocks (see Table 19-3: "Electrocardiographic Findings Associated with Myocardial Contusions").

Disposition
ALS transfer to emergency department.

 Management

1. Intravenous line placement (obtaining blood for serial enzymes)
2. Monitoring of oxygen saturation
3. Supplemental oxygen via nasal cannula or face mask
4. Continuous ECG monitoring with appropriate treatment of dysrhythmias
5. ALS transport

Aortic Injury

Aortic injuries occur following a significant deceleration, as seen in falls or high-speed MVAs. Patients may present with symptoms of chest pain radiating to the back, dyspnea, stridor, hoarseness or dysphagia, and hypotension. Cardiac auscultation may reveal a harsh systolic murmur. Upper extremity hypertension may be present and pulse defects or pulse differences between the upper and lower extremities may be noted on palpation. On chest x-ray, there may be widening of the mediastinum, tracheal deviation (to the right), effusions, or obliteration of the aortic knob (Table 19-4). Any suspicion of possible aortic injury necessitates immediate emergency department transfer for further workup and treatment.

Disposition
ALS transfer to emergency department.

TABLE 19-4

CHEST X-RAY FINDINGS ASSOCIATED WITH AORTIC INJURY

- Mediastinal widening
- Tracheal deviation to the right
- Left apical cap
- Depression of the left mainstem bronchus
- Pulmonary effusion
- Loss of the aorticopulmonary window

Management

1. Intravenous line placement with two large-bore lines
2. Monitoring of oxygen saturation
3. Supplemental oxygen via nasal cannula or simple face mask
4. Continuous ECG monitoring
5. ALS transport

Tracheobronchial Injury

Tracheobronchial injuries may be the result of blunt trauma (from a major deceleration or a direct blow) or the result of a penetrating injury. On history, patients may complain of chest pain, and on examination, physical findings may show respiratory distress, dyspnea, hoarseness, hemoptysis, subcutaneous emphysema, or Hamman's crunch. Table 19-5 lists x-ray findings often seen in tracheobronchial injury.

Disposition
ALS transfer to emergency department.

 Management

1. Intravenous line placement
2. Monitoring of oxygen saturation
3. Supplemental oxygen via nasal cannula or simple face mask
4. Continuous ECG monitoring
5. ALS transport

Esophageal Injury

Esophageal injury is most commonly due to penetrating trauma; injury due to blunt trauma is rare. Of primary importance with esophageal injury is early diagnosis and treatment in order to decrease the incidence of subsequent mediastinitis. Maintaining a high index of suspicion for this injury is key, since clinical symptoms are often subtle and the initial presentation may occur several days after the trauma. Subcutaneous air, pain out of proportion to injury, and pneumomediastinum should prompt consideration of this injury. In upper esophageal injuries such as those seen with neck trauma, complaints of dysphagia and dyspnea may also be noted.

Possible chest x-ray findings include pneumomediastinum, pneumothorax, left pleural effusion, and pneumopericardium.

TABLE 19-5

POTENTIAL CHEST X-RAY FINDINGS IN TRACHEOBRONCHIAL INJURY

• Subcutaneous emphysema	• Pneumomediastinum	• Pneumothorax

Disposition
EMS transfer to emergency department.

 Management

1. Intravenous line placement
2. Broad-spectrum intravenous antibiotics
3. Monitoring of oxygen saturation
4. Supplemental oxygen via nasal cannula or simple face mask
5. Continuous ECG monitoring
6. EMS transport

Rib Fractures

Rib fractures may occur secondary to blunt trauma, as from a fall or a direct blow, but they may also occur without external trauma following forceful coughing or sneezing, particularly in patients with underlying bone disease such as osteopenia or osteoporosis. Clinical findings include chest pain that is aggravated by movement, deep breathing, or coughing. Patients may have guarded respiration and associated dyspnea. On physical examination, palpation will elicit localized bony tenderness and possibly crepitance. Evaluation must include a detailed lung and abdominal examination to assess for potentially serious associated injuries, including pneumothorax, hemothorax, splenic injury, and liver trauma.

- Some 10 percent of patients with right lower rib fractures have associated liver injuries, while 20 percent of patients with left lower rib fractures have associated splenic injury.[2]

Additionally, fractures involving the lower posterior ribs should prompt concern for potential renal injury, which may not be readily detectable on physical examination.

X-ray Evaluation
Chest films are the more important tool in evaluating patients with rib injuries in order to exclude an associated pneumo- or hemothorax. Rib films are not always sensitive in the evaluation of acute, nondisplaced fractures and may miss up to 50 percent of rib fractures.[2] Repeat films 7 to 10 days after injury will often show evidence of fractures that were not visible initially. Fractures of the anterior cartilage or at the costochondral junction will not be visible on x-ray. *Fractures of the first and second ribs* require special attention, as they indicate that a significant force was responsible for the injury.

- Fractures of the first and second ribs are frequently associated with concomitant head, neck, great vessel, or spinal injuries, and there exists a 36% mortality due to associated injuries.[2]

Laboratory Evaluation
If indicated by fracture location, a urinanalysis should be performed to check for hematuria and evidence of renal injury.

Disposition
- Emergency department transfer for fractures of the first, second, or third rib
- Emergency department transfer for associated injuries—i.e., pneumothorax, hemothorax, splenic injury, liver injury, or renal injury

 Management

- First, Second, or Third Rib Fractures
- Fractures with Associated Injuries

1. Intravenous line placement (if significant findings, placement of two large-bore lines)
2. Monitoring of oxygen saturation
3. Supplemental oxygen via nasal cannula or face mask
4. ECG monitoring as indicated by age, underlying conditions, and patient status
5. ALS transport

 Management of Simple Rib Fractures

1. Associated injuries ruled out
2. Adequate pain medication administered [nonsteroidal anti-inflammatory drugs (NSAIDs) if not contraindicated, narcotic pain medication as indicated]
3. Instructions on frequent deep breathing to prevent atelectasis
4. Home application of cold therapy for first 24 to 48 h, followed by heat therapy after first 48 h
5. Discharge instructions reviewing symptoms that mandate immediate reevaluation
   - Abdominal pain
   - Shortness of breath
   - Light-headedness
   - New or worsening symptoms
   - Hematuria
6. Follow-up with primary care physician (PCP) (Intercostals rib blocks may sometimes be used for pain control.)

 Management of General Chest Trauma

Minor chest wall injuries and intercostal muscle strains:

1. Associated injuries ruled out
2. Adequate pain medication administered (NSAIDs if not contraindicated, narcotic pain medication as indicated)
3. Instructions on frequent deep breathing to prevent atelectasis
4. Home application of cold therapy for first 24 to 48 h, followed by heat therapy after first 48 h

5. Discharge instructions reviewing symptoms that mandate immediate reevaluation
   - Abdominal pain
   - Shortness of breath
   - Light-headedness
   - New or worsening symptoms
   - Fever
   - Coughing up blood
6. Follow-up with PCP

SOFT TISSUE NECK TRAUMA

Injuries That May Be Seen in Soft Tissue Neck Trauma

- Associated C-spine injury
- Major vessel injury (including carotid artery)
- Laryngeal injury
- Tracheal injury
- Pharyngeal injury
- Esophageal injury
- Muscle injury (strains and sprains)

The neck contains several major structures at risk for severe or lethal injury. Evaluation of this area can be hindered if the patient has been stabilized with a hard collar or has been placed in a soft collar. Although direct examination of this area is mandatory, any removal of immobilization devices in a patient whose C-spine has not been cleared requires alternative immobilization techniques such as end-line traction, sandbags, and head taping. This should be undertaken only by personnel skilled in these techniques in order to avoid potential spinal cord injury. Any penetrating trauma, once again, mandates immediate emergency department transfer. Penetration of the platysma muscle generally requires surgical consultation and possible operating room exploration. Blunt soft tissue neck trauma may occur secondary to a direct blow to the neck, strangulation (including attempted hanging), sports injuries (especially with hyperextension of the neck) or clothesline injuries. Attention to airway maintenance and potential C-spine injury is of prime concern.

 History and Physical Examination

During the clinical assessment of all soft tissue neck trauma, the following should be evaluated for their presence or absence along with the appropriate documentation.

1. Vital signs, especially fever   **THINK:** occult esophageal injury
2. Abrasions and ecchymosis
3. Lacerations and/or puncture wounds
4. Soft tissue swelling
5. Soft tissue crepitance/emphysema   **THINK:** tracheal injury

6. Palpable pain
7. Pain on active range of motion
8. Dyspnea
9. Hoarseness   **THINK:** tracheal or laryngeal injury
10. Change in voice
11. Stridor
12. Dysphonia
13. Dysphagia
14. Hemoptysis   **THINK:** tracheal injury
15. Pulsatile mass   **THINK:** vascular injury
16. Expanding hematoma   **THINK:** vascular injury
17. Bruits   **THINK:** vascular injury
18. Neurologic deficits [particularly Horner's syndrome or symptoms of a transient ischemic attack (TIA)]

Diagnostic Assessment

As indicated by history and physical examination:

1. Indirect laryngoscopy
2. C-spine films
3. Soft tissue neck films

Laryngeal Injuries

Laryngeal injuries may present with complaints of dysphagia, dysphonia (with change in voice), hoarseness, hemoptysis, or symptoms consistent with airway injury. Physical examination may reveal tenderness to palpation, stridor, subcutaneous emphysema, ecchymosis, and soft tissue swelling. On soft tissue x-rays of the neck, subcutaneous air or a fracture of a calcified larynx may be noted. In this injury, it is crucial that the practitioner be fully prepared to protect and maintain an adequate airway.

Disposition
ALS transfer to emergency department.

 Management

1. Intravenous line placement
2. Monitoring of oxygen saturation
3. Supplemental oxygen via nasal cannula or simple face mask
4. Continuous ECG monitoring as indicated
5. ALS transport

Esophageal Injury

See "Chest Trauma," above.

Vascular Injury

Vascular injuries (carotid and vertebral) associated with blunt neck trauma may present with symptoms of an expanding hematoma, a pulsatile mass, bruits, or neurologic deficits, including Horner's syndrome. However, these injuries may also be present with little clinical evidence of trauma. Vascular injuries are difficult to diagnose, in part because they may present several hours after the trauma has occurred. Any suspicion of vascular injury mandates emergency department transfer for further evaluation, usually including angiography.

Disposition
ALS transfer to emergency department.

 Management

1. Intravenous line placement
2. Monitoring of oxygen saturation
3. Supplemental oxygen via nasal cannula or simple face mask
4. Continuous ECG monitoring
5. ALS transport

Muscle Injury

Muscle injury (sternocleidomastoid, paracervical, and trapezius muscles) is by far the most likely neck injury to present in an urgent care facility. There may be a history of a whiplash type of injury, a sporting injury, or simply having "slept funny." Clinically, patients will complain of pain on range of motion (active and passive) secondary to stretching the injured muscle. There may be tenderness along the muscle to palpation or palpable muscle spasm. Mild soft tissue swelling may also be noted.

Disposition
Discharge to home.

 Management

1. Associated injuries ruled out.
2. Home application of cold therapy for first 24 to 48 h, followed by heat therapy after first 48 h.
3. Adequate pain medication (NSAIDs if not contraindicated).
4. Consideration of muscle relaxants such as cyclobenzaprine (Flexeril), metaxalone (Skelaxin), or chlorzoxazone (Parafon Forte) for spasm. Diazepam can be considered in selective patients with severe spasm.
   • Patients must be cautioned on side effects associated with the use of muscle relaxants.

5. Instructions reviewing symptoms that mandate immediate reevaluation, including:
    - Trouble swallowing
    - Trouble breathing
    - Neck swelling
    - Numbness, tingling, or weakness
    - Change in voice
    - Any new symptoms
    - Any worsening
    - Not improving as expected
6. Gentle stretching exercises can be started after 48 to 72 h and early referral to physical therapy considered if return to function has not returned during this time.

Abdominal Trauma

Injuries That May Be Seen in Abdominal Trauma

Intrathoracic and True Abdomen

- Splenic injury
- Liver injury
- Small bowel injury
- Bladder injury
- Colon injury
- Diaphragm injury
- Stomach injury

Retroperitoneal Abdomen

- Kidney injury
- Pancreatic injury
- Retroperitoneal duodenal injury
- Vascular injury (abdominal aorta)

Injury to the abdominal cavity can occur secondary to either penetrating or blunt trauma. Any *penetrating abdominal trauma* beyond epidermal or superficial dermal involvement warrants emergency department transfer for further evaluation and definitive care.

Blunt abdominal trauma can present with symptoms ranging from hypovolemic shock to minor abdominal muscle strain. Mechanisms of injury frequently encountered in abdominal trauma include seat belt injuries with deceleration forces, injury from falls, and injury from direct blows. Injury (ruptures or lacerations) can occur to any of the solid organs in the intraabdominal cavity, the hollow viscera (less frequently), the genitourinary system, or retroperitoneal structures. (Genitourinary injuries are addressed under "Genitourinary Trauma," below.)

During the clinical assessment of abdominal trauma, evaluation of the following should be performed.

History and Physical Examination

1. Vital signs, especially noting any tachycardia, tachypnea, and orthostatic changes
2. Ecchymoses (especially seat belt ecchymosis) **THINK:** mesenteric, bowel, or lumbar spine injuries
3. Abrasions
4. Swelling
5. Abdominal distention **THINK:** stomach injury
6. Quality of bowel sounds
7. Peritoneal signs (guarding, rigidity, rebound, percussion tenderness)
8. Localized tenderness
9. Organomegaly
10. Kehr's sign (left shoulder pain secondary to hemoperitoneum) **THINK:** splenic injury
11. Rectal examination (particularly for position of prostate and for blood) **THINK:** urethral injury if high-riding, nonpalpable, or boggy prostate
12. Abnormal distal pulses **THINK:** vascular injury

Diagnostic Assessment

1. Initial hematocrit (HCT) (even if patient is to be transferred). If an intravenous line is placed, blood can be drawn simultaneously for baseline HCT
2. Urinalysis (with special attention to hematuria) **THINK:** renal injury
3. Test for fecal occult blood **THINK:** colon or rectal injury
4. Abdominal series (particularly the upright chest x-ray for free air)

Further emergency department evaluation may require amylase, blood chemistries, computed tomography (CT) scanning, and/or peritoneal lavage (less commonly).

In the assessment of abdominal trauma, evaluation of the clinical picture at one point in time is not nearly as important as what the clinical picture shows over a continuous period of time. Many injuries may not be readily apparent initially but become manifest over time. Special concerns in delayed diagnosis include retroperitoneal injuries, which may be particularly difficult to diagnose. The limited usefulness of the physical examination in assessing these injuries mandates a high index of suspicion for their diagnosis. Any patient who exhibits use of alcohol or mind altering drugs may have an unreliable examination. These patients require closer attention and a higher index of suspicion for injuries.

SERIAL EXAMINATIONS ARE OF KEY IMPORTANCE FOR ANY PATIENT WITH ABDOMINAL TRAUMA.

Disposition

Emergency department transfer. Transfer should be initiated for all penetrating trauma and all patients with unstable or abnormal vital signs, positive findings on examination or diagnostic testing, a history consistent with significant force, or the potential for significant injury. Transfer should be done in consultation with a general surgeon in order to expedite specialty evaluation.

 Management for Emergency Department Transfer

1. Intravenous line placement with administration of crystalloid fluid (two large-bore lines, as indicated)
2. Monitoring of oxygen saturation as indicated
3. Supplemental oxygen via nasal cannula or face mask as indicated
4. ECG monitoring as indicated by age, underlying conditions, and patient status
5. Consideration of nasogastric tube placement
6. Consider urinary catheter placement (this *always* requires antecedent rectal examination in cases of abdominal trauma)
7. EMS transport

Disposition

Discharge to home. Patients with minor abdominal trauma, stable vital signs, and an unremarkable examination may potentially be discharged home.

 Management for Discharge Home

Observation is key. Initially, observation in the urgent care setting is required to assess for any change in the examination over time. If the patient remains stable without change in examination (including repeat orthostatics and possibly repeat HCT), he or she may be discharged home for continued home observation. Patient must be given *detailed* discharge instructions with criteria for reevaluation and follow-up treatment (for sample instructions, see Table 19-6).

TABLE 19-6

DISCHARGE INSTRUCTIONS FOR PATIENTS WITH ABDOMINAL TRAUMA

1. Obtain immediate repeat evaluation in the emergency department for:
   - Any new symptoms
   - Any worsening or change in symptoms
   - Light-headedness
   - Persistent pain
   - Abdominal pain or distention
   - Vomiting or anorexia
   - Fever or shaking chills
   - Blood in urine or bowels
   - Back pain
   - Shoulder pain
   - Yellow color to skin or eyes
2. Avoid pain medication stronger than acetaminophen (Tylenol)
3. Avoid aspirin, as it will prolong bleeding time
4. Apply cold therapy for first 24 to 48 h, followed by heat therapy after first 48 h for strains or sprains
5. Follow up with primary care physician in 24 to 48 h for recheck

GENITOURINARY TRAUMA

Injuries That May Be Seen in Genitourinary Trauma

- Kidney injury (contusion, laceration, fractures)
- Urethral injuries [least common renal injury, typically seen with penetrating trauma, after surgery (iatrogenic), or associated with other intraabdominal injury]
- Bladder injury
- Prostate injury
- Penile injury
- Scrotal or testicular injury

Injury to the genitourinary system may occur in association with other trauma such as abdominal and/or back injuries or in isolation secondary to blunt or penetrating trauma. In general, in the urgent care setting, genitourinary trauma will present as isolated injuries—that is, usually as a result of a direct blow, as is frequently seen with sporting injuries. Renal injury may also be seen secondary to deceleration forces associated with MVAs. Any patient presenting with hematuria following trauma must be evaluated for possible renal injury. Hematuria may be noted grossly or only on microscopic evaluation. It is important to realize that the degree of microhematuria does not always correlate with the severity of injury. Hematuria may be indicative of injury anywhere in the renal system. Although opinions vary as to the necessity for immediate workup of microscopic hematuria, patients with gross hematuria should be referred for computed tomography (CT) of the abdomen and retroperitoneum.

All *penetrating trauma* warrants emergency department transfer for more extensive evaluation.

During the clinical assessment of genitourinary trauma, the following should be evaluated for their presence or absence, along with the appropriate documentation.

 History and Physical Examination

1. Abnormal vital signs
2. Orthostatic position changes
3. Flank tenderness
4. Flank ecchymosis or swelling
5. Abdominal tenderness (particularly suprapubic tenderness)
6. Inability to void
7. Scrotal/penile/perineal ecchymosis, swelling, or hematomas
8. Blood at meatus   **THINK:** ureteral injury *(do not catheterize!)*
9. Prostate examination for position   **THINK:** ureteral injury if high-riding or boggy *(do not catheterize!)*
10. Lower posterior chest wall injury
11. History of underlying kidney disease (polycystic, etc.)

Diagnostic Assessment

As indicated by history and physical examination:

1. Urinalysis for blood (gross and microscopic)
2. Chest x-ray for lower rib fractures   **THINK:** kidney injury
3. Lumbar spine for transverse   **THINK:** kidney injury
   process fractures

    Emergency department evaluation may require further assessment through cysto-grams, intravenous pyelography (IVP), retrograde urethrograms, CT scanning, and urologic consultation.

Disposition

Emergency department transfer. Transfer should be initiated for patients with gross hematura following trauma, microscopic hematuria with significant trauma history, abnormal vital signs, positive physical findings on examination as listed above, or presence of associated injury (rib or lumbar transverse process fractures).

 Management

1. Intravenous line placement with crystalloid fluid administration (two large-bore lines as indicated)
2. Monitoring of oxygen saturation as indicated
3. Supplemental oxygen via nasal cannula or face mask as indicated
4. ECG monitoring as indicated by age, underlying conditions, and patient status
5. ALS transport

Microscopic Hematuria

Microscopic hematuria following trauma requires investigation for possible renal tract injury. Patients who are stable with normal vital signs, no associated injuries or positive physical findings, unremarkable ancillary studies, and low-impact trauma by history do not necessarily require renal imaging. At times, these patients may be followed conservatively with repeat urinalysis in 24 h. This decision should always be made in consultation with the urologist to whom the patient will be referred for follow-up care.

Testicular Injury

Injury to the testicle or scrotum is usually the result of a direct blow. Generally patients will give a history of trauma and subsequent testicular pain. There may be a hematocele (which presents as a tender, blue scrotal mass) on examination or isolated testicular swelling. A testicular ultrasound or color Doppler, as indicated, may be needed in order to rule out testicular rupture; urologic consultation should be obtained.

- Testicular swelling noted after a minor injury may be a sign of severe rupture.

Penile Injury

Penile injury may be due to fracture, entrapment, contusion, zipper trauma, or amputation. Fractures of the penis are due to injury to the penile tunica albuginea. These injuries generally occur during sexual intercourse; the patient will give a history of having heard a snapping sound along with development of severe pain and swelling of the penile shaft. These patients require immediate urologic consultation.

Zipper injuries should, if possible, be treated by breaking the bridge (median bar) of the zipper, thereby disrupting the zipper mechanism and freeing the penile tissue. If this approach cannot be used, the skin will have to be anesthetized (*no use of epinephrine*) and a limited excision of the entrapped skin performed.

Entrapment injuries are generally related to rings placed around the penis. (In children, a fine hair may also work its way around the shaft of the penis.) Removal of ring objects may be attempted in the urgent care center depending on the offending object, but specialty consultation should be sought early as needed. Prolonged entrapment can lead to venous engorgement and occlusion of the arterial blood supply. Because the integrity of the urethra and blood supply should be checked, urologic consultation and emergency department transfer may be warranted.

HEAD TRAUMA

Injuries That May Be Seen in Head Trauma

- Scalp laceration (see Chap. 23)
- Soft tissue hematomas
- Skull fractures
    Linear
    Depressed
    Basilar
- Intracranial hematomas

Closed Head Trauma

Patients with mild degrees of head trauma commonly present to urgent care facilities, and even though most patients seen urgently have only mild trauma, there is always the concern that a serious injury could have occurred. The severity of head injury is dependent on a number of factors, including the mode and circumstances of the injury. All patients with a head injury should be suspected of also experiencing a C-spine injury until proven otherwise.

 History and Physical Examination

1. Mechanism of injury
2. History of unconsciousness or being dazed
3. Abnormal behavior

4. Ataxia
5. Seizure activity
6. Repeated vomiting
7. Severity of headache if present
8. Neck pain or injury
9. Focal neurologic findings
10. Lacerations, hematomas, or soft tissue swelling
11. Blood from ears or nose
12. Clear fluid from nose or ears
13. Battle's sign (bruising at mastoid area)
14. Raccoon eyes (periorbital ecchymosis)
15. Hemotympanum

Diagnostic Assessment

As indicated by history and physical examination:

1. C-spine x-rays
2. Skull x-rays
3. CT scan

The term *concussion* refers to a temporary alteration in mental functioning caused by a head injury. This may occur with or without clear loss of consciousness. *Mild head trauma* is used operationally to describe confusion or other symptoms seen in head injury with no loss of consciousness and a normal neurologic examination. With this degree of trauma, there are no focal abnormalities and the patient is awake, alert, and oriented, perhaps after a brief period of confusion (15 min or less = grade 1 concussion). Headache and dizziness are common in the initial evaluation.

- In general, patients with mild head injuries are frequently amnesic for the event and only eyewitnesses can clearly comment on whether loss of consciousness actually occurred.

Loss of consciousness suggests a moderate or severe head injury. *Moderate or severe head injury* is associated with confusion lasting longer than 15 min (grade 2 concussion), loss of consciousness (grade 3 concussion), focal neurologic signs, skull fracture, seizure, Glasgow Coma Scale (Table 19-7) score of 14 or less, vomiting, or the presence of drugs or alcohol. Therefore head injuries in the setting of alcohol or drugs should be considered moderate to severe until proven otherwise.

General Evaluation of Head Trauma

The general medical examination should immediately assess airway, breathing, and circulation, carefully documenting vital signs. The C-spine should be immobilized when indicated and cleared with x-rays. The skull should be palpated for fractures, and scalp wounds should be digitally examined with a sterile gloved hand to assess for bony ridges, step-offs, or any palpable deformities. Hematoma formation may complicate this assessment, since the associated swelling can make skull palpation difficult.

- If the mechanism of injury suggests the possibility of a depressed skull fracture (i.e., a direct blow from an object such as a hammer, bat, or golf ball), x-rays should be

TABLE 19-7

GLASGOW COMA SCALE

MEASURE	RESPONSE	SCORE
Eye opening	Opens:	
	Spontaneously	4
	To verbal command	3
	To pain	2
	No response	1
Verbal	Oriented and converses	5
	Disoriented and converses	4
	Inappropriate words	3
	Incomprehensible sounds	2
	No response	1
Motor	Obeys verbal command	6
	To painful stimulus:	
	Localizes pain	5
	Flexion-withdrawal	4
	Abnormal flexion (decorticate rigidity)	3
	Extension (decerebrate rigidity)	2
	No response	1

SOURCE: Tintinalli J et al: *Emergency Medicine: A Comprehensive Study Guide*, 5th ed. New York: McGraw-Hill; 2000, with permission.

obtained prior to digital examination. If films are positive for a fracture, digital examination should be avoided.

The remainder of the head, ear, nose, and throat (HEENT) examination should check for signs suggestive of a basilar skull fracture, including hemotypanum, cerebrospinal fluid (CSF) rhinorrhea, otorrhea, Battle's sign, and raccoon eyes.

On neurologic examination, mental status testing is important, documenting attention, orientation, and memory. The patient is asked for details regarding the event, the first things remembered after the trauma, and the last thing remembered before the event in order to assess the presence of amnesia. The pupils are examined for any inequality in size or responsiveness, and this is recorded. Pupillary dilators should not be used for examination of the fundi because of the subsequent inability to follow pupillary changes related to an intracranial lesion. Extraocular movement should be checked, since diplopia can occur secondary to sixth nerve trauma, and unilateral nystagmus may be secondary to a cerebellar lesion. The motor examination and reflexes are assessed for any asymmetry. The gait is observed to ensure that it is normal. The Coma Scale is a way to standardize the recording and evaluation of patients. Any changes in the examination after the initial evaluation or any focal signs or symptoms must be recognized and assessed with emergent CT scan. Worsening in mental state, in particular a progressive decline in consciousness, is a bad prognostic sign and suggests an expanding intracranial lesion.

Key Points of Documentation

- Ear examination for the presence or absence of hemotympanum or otorrhea
- Results of palpation of skull for depressed skull fractures (bony ridges, step-offs, deformity)
- Results of direct palpation of C-spine for tenderness
- X-ray clearance of C-spine as indicated
- The presence or absence of alcohol or mind altering drugs
- A detailed neurologic examination
- Evaluation for associated injuries

 Errors to Avoid

- *Depending on pupillary changes as a sign of worsening. The earliest sign of neuro-logic involvement is often a subtle change in mental status.* Pupillary changes herald ominous events.

Disposition

Moderate to Severe Head Injuries   Patients with moderate to severe head injury as described above require immediate transfer to an acute care setting for imaging and observation.

Head Injury with Associated Skull Fractures

The clinical implications of skull fractures are dependent on the type of fracture, the location, and whether the fracture is open or closed. Patients with uncomplicated linear fractures or simple closed stellate fractures require, at the minimum, observation; consultation with a neurosurgeon is prudent.

Increased risk of brain injury is associated with the following:

- Linear or stellate fractures that are open
- Depressed fractures
- Linear fractures that cross the middle meningeal artery or a major venous sinus
- Occipital fractures (which carry an increased risk of complications including subarachnoid hemorrhage)
- Basilar skull fractures

These patients require emergency department transfer for CT scanning, direct observation, and neurosurgical consultation.

 Management

1. Intravenous line placement with D_5W ¼ normal saline
2. Continuous observation with neurologic checks

3. EMS transport
4. Neurosurgical consultation

Minor Closed Head Trauma

In patients with mild head trauma as defined above, if their evaluation is unremarkable and no changes have occurred during a period of observation in the urgent care setting, these patients can be sent out for observation by family or others for 24 h (see Table 19-8 for criteria for discharge). Simple analgesics can be used for headache. Follow-up with a primary care physician should be arranged for the following week in order to address any late complications associated with the head injury, such as persistent headache, dizziness, or difficulties with concentration.

Patients who are discharged home should be instructed to return for evaluation if they encounter a decline in consciousness, worsening headache or vertigo, focal deficits, or intractable vomiting. Worsening in mental state or the development of focal signs or symptoms in the first week after the injury requires CT scanning to exclude an intra-cranial hemorrhage or contusion. It is important that these patients be discharged to the care of a family member or friend, as continued observation is key.

Discharge Instructions for Head Trauma

- Patient must be awakened every 2 h to check on status for the first 24 h following injury.
- All alcohol intake must be avoided.
- Any analgesic pain medications stronger than Tylenol must be avoided.
- Use of aspirin or aspirin-containing products must be avoided.

Patients should be counseled to be rechecked immediately in the emergency department setting for any of the following:

- Change in level of consciousness, including restlessness, confusion, or difficulty arousing (*often the first evidence of serious injury is mild abnormal behavior*).
- Worsening headache
- Vertigo
- Focal neurologic deficits (weakness, numbness, trouble walking, trouble with speech, etc.)
- Visual changes (double vision, blurred vision, etc.)
- Repeated vomiting
- Neck stiffness
- Discharge from ears or nose (may be clear or bloody)
- Any new symptoms

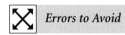 *Errors to Avoid*

- Discharging a patient with head injury to an environment without someone to observe for changes
- Underestimating the severity of head trauma in the elderly

TABLE 19-8

CRITERIA FOR DISCHARGE HOME

- *Minor* head injury with no history of loss of consciousness
- Normal neurologic examination
- No associated injuries
- No indication of drug or alcohol use
- Reliable patient
- Reliable family members or friend who can observe patient for any changes
- No underlying complicating conditions such as bleeding disorders, use of warfarin, previous head injury, etc.

FACIAL TRAUMA

Injuries That May Be Seen in Facial Trauma

- Facial lacerations (see Chap. 23)
- Mandibular fractures
- Midface fractures
- Orbital floor fractures
- Zygomatic arch fracture
- Dislocation of the temporomandibular joint (TMJ)
- Nasal fractures (see Chap. 8)
- Parotid duct injury
- Seventh nerve injury

Facial trauma can range in presentation from the isolated superficial laceration to multiple midface fractures secondary to blunt force from an MVA. In general, facial injuries are not acutely life-threatening unless they are associated with other major injuries such as spinal injury or airway compromise. Patients presenting with injury secondary to significant force should be assumed to have a potential C-spine injury until proven otherwise. Airway patency may be affected secondary to swelling, bleeding, or abnormal positioning of bone.

 Errors to Avoid

- Attempting to perform nasal intubation in the presence of a midface fracture
- Attempting to insert a nasogastric tube in the presence of a midface fracture

 History and Physical Examination

- Airway patency
- Intraoral lesions
- Dental trauma
- Malocclusion   **THINK:** Mandibular fracture
- Abnormal deviation on opening mouth   **THINK:** Mandibular fracture

- Range of motion of mandible
- Facial symmetry
- Localized bony tenderness
- Facial anesthesia

THINK: seventh nerve injury or mental nerve injury depending on location of anesthesia

- Localized soft tissue swelling
- Ecchymosis
- Depression of cheekbone
- Extraocular movement
- Diplopia
- Abnormal mobility of maxillary alveolar process
- CSF rhinorrhea

Diagnostic Assessment

As indicated by history and physical examination:

- C-spine x-rays
- Waters' view (for evaluation of Le Fort fractures, orbital floor fractures, zygomatic arch fractures)
- Zygomatic arch/submental/jug handle x-rays
- TMJ films
- Mandibular films (Panorex x-rays are more accurate when available)

Mandibular Injuries

Mandibular injuries include fractures as well as TMJ dislocations. Dislocation of the TMJ may occur without a history of trauma. Antecedent events seen with nontraumatic TMJ dislocations include yawning or opening of the mouth wide. Dislocations secondary to trauma usually occur with direct blows to the chin while the mouth is in an opened position. If the dislocation is bilateral, patients may present with a partially open mouth and an inability to close the anterior teeth. In contrast, unilateral dislocations tend to present with deviation of the jaw toward the dislocated side when the mouth is open. Swelling may be noted just anterior to the tragus secondary to the abnormal position of the condylar head. (For management of TMJ dislocations, see Chap. 8.)

Mandibular fractures present with pain (either localized or on biting down), swelling, and decreased range of motion of the jaw. There may be an inability to open the mouth fully or deviation noted on opening the mouth. Patients may also complain of a new malocclusion.

On physical examination, the mandible should be palpated for localized tenderness or palpable step-offs along the entire course of the bone. Sensation of the lower lip should be checked and documented to assess the integrity of the inferior alveolar and mental nerves. Next, range of motion of the jaw, including lateral excursion, should be evaluated. Any malocclusion, intraoral injuries, or dental injuries should be noted. If asked to bite down on a tongue depressor, patients with a fracture may be unable to do so or, if able, may have marked pain. On x-ray evaluation, mandibular films may reveal a fracture line; however, Panorex x-rays are better at detecting fractures that may not be evident on plain x-rays.

 Errors to Avoid

- *Failure to assess for multiple fractures.* Mandibular fractures are often multiple due to the ring-like shape of the mandible. The most common sites for fractures are the angle, the molar and mental regions of the body, and the condyle.

 Management

1. ENT or oral surgeon telephone consultation for directed care. Emergent specialty evaluation is generally not needed unless marked deformity or marked associated soft tissue injury is present.
2. May require antibiotic for associated soft tissue or intraoral wounds and should be discussed with the consultant who will provide aftercare for the patient.
3. Appropriate management of subluxed, avulsed, or fractured teeth.
4. Tetanus prophylaxis if indicated.

Midface/Maxillary Fractures

Midface fractures are categorized by the Le Fort classification, which defines midface fractures by the location of the fracture line.

Le Fort I: Transverse fracture across the inferior maxilla (Fig. 19-1)

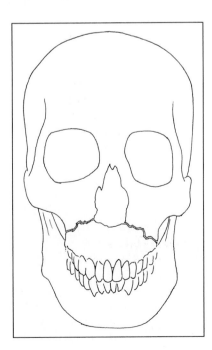

FIGURE 19-1 Le Fort I fracture. (From Scaletta TA: *Emergent Management of Trauma.* New York: McGraw-Hill; 1996, with permission.)

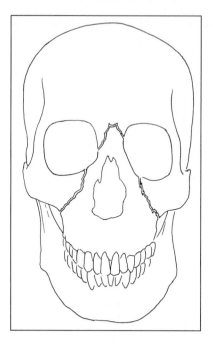

FIGURE 19-2 Le Fort II fracture. (From Scaletta TA: *Emergent Management of Trauma.* New York: McGraw-Hill; 1996, with permission.)

Le Fort II: Pyramidal fractures extending from the maxilla through the maxillary sinus and infraorbital rim and across the nasal bridge (Fig. 19-2)

Le Fort III: Craniofacial disjunction with fractures involving the maxilla, the nasal complex and zygoma, and extending through the orbits, nasal septum, and pterygoid plates (Fig. 19-3)

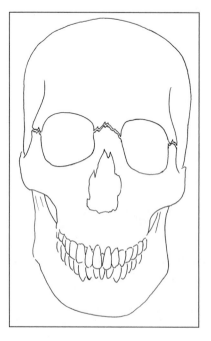

FIGURE 19-3 Le Fort III fracture. (From Scaletta TA: *Emergent Management of Trauma.* New York: McGraw-Hill; 1996, with permission.)

- On clinical examination, abnormal mobility of the maxilla will be noted in all Le Fort fractures.

Waters' views should be obtained to help confirm the diagnosis.

Management

1. All Le Fort fractures require direct surgical (ENT or maxillofacial) consultation.
2. If CSF rhinorrhea is present or suspected secondary to clear nasal discharge (i.e., in cribriform plate fractures), emergent neurosurgical consultation is required.

Zygomatic Arch Fractures

Isolated zygomatic arch fractures are usually secondary to a direct blow to the arch. Patients with these fractures will present with localized tenderness and cheekbone depression (which may be obscured if significant soft tissue swelling is present). On occasion, limitation of mouth excursion may also be present.

Tripod fractures or fractures of the zygomaticomaxillary complex involve the zygomatic arch, the lateral and inferior orbital rims, and the anterior and lateral walls of the maxillary sinus. These patients will present with facial flattening (which may also be obscured if significant soft tissue swelling is present), circumorbital ecchymosis, and infraorbital nerve anesthesia or hypesthesia of the upper lip, cheek, and gum. Diplopia, subconjunctival hemorrhages, as well as injuries to the globe may also occur. Waters' view x-rays should be obtained, which may reveal fracture lines as well as air-fluid levels in the maxillary sinus. Other x-ray studies that may be useful include Caldwell, Towne, and submental vertex views.

Management

- Consultation with an ENT or maxillofacial surgeon

Dental injuries

Tooth Injury

- Avulsion
- Intrusion
- Subluxation
- Fracture

Dental trauma is usually the result of a direct blow to the face and mouth area, as seen in falls, altercations, or sporting injuries. Trauma may also result from a seemingly minor insult such as biting a hard object while eating. All tooth trauma requires follow-up with either a dentist or oral surgeon, though some temporizing actions on initial examination can increase the probability of a good outcome.

Avulsions

A tooth that has been completely avulsed from its socket represents a true dental emergency. Timely reimplantation is critical for a good outcome. If the tooth has not been recovered, x-rays should be obtained to evaluate for intrusion into the gingiva or inadvertent ingestion or aspiration. Avulsed primary teeth do not require replacement into their sockets, as this increases the likelihood for the development of fusion with the bone. In contrast, permanent teeth should be replaced into the socket *as soon as possible*; the longer an avulsed tooth is out of its socket, the less the likelihood of viable reimplantation. It is critical that an avulsed tooth be handled *only* by its crown. The root of a tooth should never be handled. The tooth should be *gently* rinsed with saline and then reimplanted into its socket. Any clot present in the socket must be cleaned away prior to implantation. Teeth that have been avulsed require stabilization, which can be done initially by having the patient bite on gauze while awaiting dental consultation.

If reimplantation is not possible, avulsed teeth can be transported either in moist gauze, a glass of milk, saliva (including under the patient's tongue—but not if patient presents a risk for ingesting or aspirating the tooth), or ideally in a commercially available medium known as Hank's solution. This solution maintains the viability of the periodontal ligament cells, which is key to successful reimplantation; in fact, it has been found to restore cell viability in teeth that have been out of their sockets for longer than 30 min.[3]

If a tooth is not recovered, persistent bleeding can be treated with direct pressure, i.e., biting on saline-soaked gauze or gauze impregnated with 2% lidocaine with epinephrine (if not contraindicated) for 20 min.

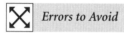 *Errors to Avoid*

- Delay in reimplantation of an avulsed tooth
- Handling of tooth by the root, which can damage periodontal ligament fibers
- Overzealous cleaning of an avulsed tooth

Intruded Teeth

Teeth that have been intruded have been displaced upward into the gingiva. This type of injury is usually seen following a fall. Primary teeth that have been intruded are given a period of time (about 6 weeks) to reerupt. Permanent teeth generally require surgical repositioning. Intruded teeth can be diagnosed by x-ray studies, which should be performed on any patient presenting with a history of tooth avulsion but without recovery of the tooth. Patients should be treated with warm saline rinses four times daily and arrangements should be made for timely dental follow-up.

Subluxation

Subluxed teeth are teeth that have become loose as a result of injury. The diagnosis is made by eliciting mobility during examination of the tooth or noting the presence of blood at the gingival crevice. Significant mobility requires urgent dental consultation for stabilization. Patients with minimally subluxed teeth can be discharged home on a soft diet with arrangements for prompt dental follow-up.

Fractures

Fractured teeth are teeth that have become chipped or broken due to mouth trauma. Tooth fractures can be classified using the Ellis fracture classification (Table 19-9).

Ellis Class I

Ellis class I fractures are of immediate significance only if a sharp edge is causing discomfort or soft tissue injury. Sharp edges can be treated urgently with filing to reduce the immediate sharpness. Dental consultation will be needed for any cosmetic repair.

Ellis Class II

Patients with Ellis class II fractures may present with complaints of sensitivity and pain on exposure to heat, cold, and air. Additionally, pain may also be elicited on percussion. This injury is of increased significance in children and in patients with more severe class II injuries. In both situations, there is less dentin overlying the pulp to protect it from infection.

Management of Ellis Class II Fractures   Treatment requires covering the exposed dentin with a glass ionomer cement compound or, if not available, a calcium hydroxide dressing. It is prudent to speak with a dentist at the time of evaluation, as these patients require evaluation within 24 h. They should be instructed to avoid ingesting food and liquids at the extremes in temperature. Pain medication should also be prescribed as needed for comfort. Improper treatment of these injuries increases the need for future root canal therapy.

Ellis Class III

Ellis class III fractures can present either with severe pain or no pain at all if the neurovascular supply has been disrupted.

Management of Ellis Class III Fractures   These fractures require *emergent* dental consultation. As with Ellis class II fractures, the tooth should be covered with a glass ionomer compound or a calcium hydroxide dressing as a temporizing measure while dental consultation is arranged. Delay in treatment is likely to result in abscess formation.

TABLE 19-9

ELLIS FRACTURE CLASSIFICATION	
Class I	Fractures involving enamel only (white surface seen at broken edge)
Class II	Fractures involving the enamel and dentin (white and yellow surface seen at broken edge)
Class III	Fractures involving enamel, dentin, and pulp (red or pink color noted in center of the dentin or frank blood may be noted at broken edge of tooth)

Burns

Burns can be classified as thermal (caused by heat), electrical, or chemical. Any patient presenting with a burn should be questioned regarding the mechanism of the burn. Burns requiring special consideration include those sustained in a fire in an enclosed space; these burns may be associated with smoke inhalation or exposure to toxic fumes. All patients sustaining burns should also be questioned regarding their tetanus status, which should be updated as indicated.

Classification of Burn by Depth

Burns can further be classified as first-, second-, or third-degree, depending on the depth of injury.

First degree: Partial thickness, involving only the epidermis. There is no blistering. The involved area is reddened and painful. Example: mild sunburn.

Second degree: Includes superficial partial thickness as well as deeper partial thickness.

Superficial partial-thickness burns involve the epidermis and upper dermal layer. These are exquisitely painful and hypersensitive wounds; the area blanches with pressure and blistering of the skin occurs. Examples: scalds and burns caused by hot metals or chemicals.

Deep partial-thickness burns involve the epidermis and lower dermis. These burns appear mottled white, with edema and sloughing. Blisters have generally ruptured. The area is minimally painful initially. Examples: burns caused by flames or hot oil.

Third Degree: Full-thickness injury involving epidermis and all dermal layers.

Hair follicles, sweat glands, and nerves are destroyed. Area may appear mottled or waxy or pearly white. The surface is painless due to nerve destruction. Examples: burns due to flames or hot oil.

- The development of infection in a burn can advance the depth of tissue involvement, thereby changing a first-degree burn into a second-degree burn or converting a second-degree burn into a third-degree burn.

The extent of surface involvement in burns can be determined using the "Rule of Nines" (for adults), however, a simpler approach is to use the size of the patient's palm (which represents 1 percent of the body surface) to estimate burn size (Fig. 19-4). It is important to assess the involved surface area accurately not only for the classification of burn depth, but also in order to treat the patient properly and arrange for his or her disposition. *Minor burns* can easily be managed in the urgent care setting, but any patient with a burn classified as *moderate or major* must be transferred for presumptive inpatient care.

Major Burns

Major burns should be transferred to the hospital setting for presumed inpatient management. Major burns are classified as follows:

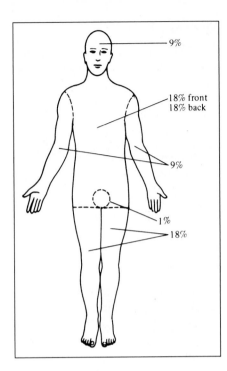

FIGURE 19-4 **Rule of nines for estimation of percentage of burn.** (From Tintinalli J et al: *Emergency Medicine: A Comprehensive Study Guide*, 5th ed. New York: McGraw-Hill; 2000, with permission.)

- Partial-thickness burns involving more than 25 percent of the total body surface area in patients 10 to 50 years of age
- Partial-thickness burns involving more than 20 percent of the total body surface area in patients under 10 or over 50 years of age
- Full-thickness burns of more than 10 percent of the total body surface.
- Burns involving the hands, face, feet, perineum
- Circumferential limb burns
- Electrical burns
- Burns involving inhalational injury (see Table 19-10)
- Burns crossing major joints
- Burns with associated trauma
- Burns in infants, the elderly, or high-risk patients (particularly those with underlying medical disease)

TABLE 19-10

PHYSICAL FINDINGS SUGGESTIVE OF INHALATIONAL INJURY

• Facial burns	• Carbonaceous sputum or soot
• Singed nasal hair	• Wheezing on lung examination
• Intraoral or pharyngeal burns	

Moderate Burns

Moderate burns also warrant transfer to an inpatient facility. Moderate burns can be classified as burns not involving the hands, face, feet, or perineum or the extremities circumferentially and that are:

- Partial-thickness burns involving 15 to 25 percent of the total body surface area in patients 10 to 50 years of age
- Partial-thickness burns involving 10 to 20 percent of the total body surface area in patients under 10 or over 50 years of age
- Full-thickness burns of less than 10 percent of the total body surface area

Disposition of Major and Moderate Burns

Hospital transfer for emergency department and inpatient care.

 Management

1. The ABCDE guidelines for trauma evaluation are followed.
2. A *sterile* saline dressing is applied to the burn area. (If the burn area is large, the burns are covered with clean dry sheets to avoid hypothermia.)
3. Supplemental oxygen at 100% is administered for any suspected inhalational injuries.
4. Intravenous line placement and normal saline is administered (hydration helps avoid complications of rhabdomyolysis).
5. All jewelry and clothing distal to the involved area is removed.
6. Tetanus prophylaxis is administered.
7. EMS transport to emergency department or burn unit as indicated.

Patients with major and moderate burns should typically be sent for inpatient treatment. In certain circumstances it may be acceptable to obtain specialty consultation with either a general surgeon or a plastic surgeon for directed care. In that case, the specialist may want to evaluate the patient in the office setting before deciding on the course of treatment. Common sense should also be exercised. For instance, a superficial partial-thickness burn to the hairline by a curling wand obviously does not warrant emergency department transfer, nor would a small, localized, superficial partial-thickness burn on the hand sustained from an oil splash or inadvertent contact with a hot pot while cooking. If there is any doubt, it is always more prudent to obtain consultation or to transfer the patient to a burn unit (see Table 19-11).

Minor Burns

Minor burns are classified as burns that are not associated with any other injuries and that:

- Involve less than 15 percent of the total body surface area in patients 10 to 50 years of age
- Involve less than 10 percent of the total body surface area in patients under 10 years or over 50 years of age
- Are full-thickness burns involving less than 2 percent of total body surface area

TABLE 19-11

BURN CENTER REFERRAL CRITERIA

1. Second- and third-degree burns > 10 percent TBSA in patients under 20 or over 50 years of age
2. Second- and third-degree burns > 20 percent TBSA in any age group
3. Second- and third-degree burns involving the face, hands, feet, genitalia, perineum, and major joints
4. Third-degree burns > 5 percent TBSA in any age group
5. Electrical burns, including lightning injury
6. Chemical burns
7. Inhalation injury
8. Burns of any size in patients with preexisting medical disorders that could complicate management, prolong recovery, or affect mortality
9. Burns with concomitant mechanical trauma (e.g., fractures) where the burn injury poses the greatest risk of morbidity or mortality (If the trauma poses the greater immediate risk, the patient should be treated initially and stabilized in a trauma center and then transferred to a burn center, in accord with established regional triage protocols.)
10. Burns in children if there are no qualified personnel or equipment for pediatric care at the initial hospital
11. Burns in patients requiring special social, emotional, and/or long-term rehabilitative support, including cases of suspected child abuse, substance abuse, etc.

SOURCE: Schwartz, S. et al: *Principles of Surgery Companion Handbook,* 7th ed. New York: McGraw-Hill, with permission.

 Management of Minor Burns

1. The involved area is elevated if feasible.
2. All jewelry and clothing distal to the involved area is removed.
3. Cool, sterile, saline-soaked dressings are applied for 10 to 30 min, depending on the patient's response.
4. Any broken blisters are debrided. Intact blisters are left intact.
5. Burn dressings: Bulky silver sulfadiazine (Silvadene cream) dressing with non-adherent material is used for the first layer. Neosporin or Bactroban is applied to burns involving the face.
6. Pain medication is given as indicated (the patient may need a prescription upon discharge).
7. Specific discharge instructions on burn care are given (Table 19-12).

 Errors to Avoid

- Use of Silvadene cream in a patient with a sulfa allergy, a pregnant patient, or an infant
- Use of Silvadene cream on the face, which can cause discoloration

TABLE 19-12

DISCHARGE INSTRUCTIONS FOR MINOR BURNS

1. Elevate area of burn
2. Perform dressing changes twice daily (wash area with water with each dressing change to remove burn ointment)
3. Do not attempt to pop intact blisters
4. Use narcotic pain medication as prescribed
5. Recheck in 24 h
6. Recheck immediately for:
   Increased pain
   Numbness
   Coldness
   New symptoms
   Signs of infection

Electrical Burns

Electrical burns are burns sustained secondary to injury from an electric current. These burns are different from typical thermal burns in that surface injury may not accurately represent the true extent of injury. Electrical injuries may occur from low-voltage (typical household injuries) or high-voltage exposure, as seen in occupational injury. The current can be classified as alternating current (which, at a certain amperage, can cause sustained muscle contractions that inhibit the patient from releasing the source) or direct current. Direct current exposures require high voltage in order to cause injury. Lightning is a unique example of direct current with exposure of up to 2 billion volts.

In electrical injuries, the current may be carried throughout the body. There may be an entrance wound and one or more exit wounds; the location of these wounds may give some indication of the path through which the current flowed. In patients with electrical burns, the lower extremities and heels should always be examined for evidence of exit wounds. Exit wounds tend to have larger surface areas than entrance wounds. High-acuity injuries are associated with currents that pass through the heart or the head. Nerve tissue is the best conductor of electricity, followed in descending order by blood, muscle, skin, tendon, fat, and bone.

Because electrical injuries can cause extensive internal injury, any patient with more than an insignificant exposure should be transferred for further evaluation and ongoing monitoring. Some of the complications for which these patients are at risk include dysrhythmia secondary to injury to the conductive system, rhabdomyolysis and myoglobinuria, electrolyte disturbances, and skin burns. Cardiac disturbances that may occur include immediate asystole (AC current), ventricular fibrillation (direct current), atrial fibrillation, ventricular tachycardia, bundle branch block, sinus tachycardia, and ST-segment elevations. Several of these rhythm disturbances may not occur until up to 12 h following exposure. Changes may also be noted secondary to hyperkalemia and acidosis. Neurologic symptoms that can occur as a result of electrical injuries include headache, amnesia, focal weakness, tinnitus, seizures, paresthesias, or loss of consciousness. Additionally, patients who sustain electrical burn injuries may also sustain injury related to blunt trauma from falls or being thrown at the time of injury.

Management

- ABCDE assessment
- Intravenous line placement with normal saline or lactated Ringer's solution, with adequate hydration in those patients at risk for rhabdomyolysis
- Continuous cardiac monitoring
- Blood drawn for baseline cardiac enzymes
- Urine check for hematuria
- Documented detailed neurologic examination
- Documented detailed vascular examination
- Burn wound care
- EMS transfer

Factors to Be Documented That May Affect Severity of Injury

- Type of current (AC versus DC)
- High- or low-voltage exposure
- Length of contact with electrical source
- Associated exposure to water/sweat (which decreases the resistance to current and leads to more severe injury)
- Amperes delivered

Another type of electrical injury that may be seen in young children is an oral burn sustained by chewing on a live wire. In this injury, the current is carried via the saliva and causes burns at the corners of the mouth. The commissure, alveolar ridge, and tongue may also be affected. These children must be evaluated and treated as dictated by the severity of the burn and any associated injuries, though generally no systemic involvement occurs. Delayed bleeding from the labial artery may occur 5 days to 2 weeks after the initial injury. These children therefore require close follow-up and consultation with a plastic surgeon or their primary care physician. Follow-up is important, given the possibility of delayed bleeding from the site of injury, poor healing, or the development of scarring that could limit range of motion of the mouth.

Chemical Burns

Chemical burns can be caused by a variety of agents. They are frequently seen with home exposure as well as with occupational exposures. The most frequently involved areas are the extremities (especially the upper extremities) and the face. Chemical burns can be due to acid or alkali compounds. *Acid compounds* typically cause coagulation necrosis with eschar formation, which limits tissue involvement. *Alkali compounds*, on the other hand, cause a liquefaction necrosis, which leads to deeper tissue penetration and injury.

- Information on the offending agent should be elicited as soon as possible and poison control assistance should be sought as needed to determine the nature of the compound and required treatment.

Immediate removal of the substance is the initial and key step in stopping further injury. Generally, copious irrigation of the area should be initiated. Water, however, should *not* be used on dry compounds. Dry compounds should be removed initially by brushing or shaking off the substance; once the particulate matter has been removed, the area can be irrigated. Water also should *not* be used on any agent containing sodium metal, as its mixing with water can cause a marked exothermic reaction. Instead, these compounds should initially be treated with mineral oil. *Hydrofluoric acid* is another substance that requires special attention. Hydrofluoric acid can rapidly penetrate the skin, causing progressive tissue damage and severe pain. There may be a delay in the onset of symptoms following exposure to hydrofluoric acid and the patient may not appreciate the injury until several hours after exposure. Specific treatment for severe exposure involves use of calcium gluconate, which can be administered topically, subcutaneously, or intra-dermally. Unless the facility is fully equipped and knowledge-able about calcium administration, the patient should be transferred for ongoing treatment after initial irrigation.

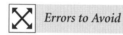 *Errors to Avoid*

- Using water for irrigating compounds that contain sodium metals
- Using water on dry compounds prior to removal of solid particles
- Discontinuing irrigation prior to complete neutralization of chemicals

Tar Burns

Tar burns are typically seen in patients with occupational injuries related to roofing tar or asphalt. At the time of evaluation, the tar will usually have cooled and the patient will have already suffered a partial thickness burn beneath the tar. For full evaluation, the tar must first be removed, which is best done using an emulsifying or dissolving agent such as that found in Neosporin. Other appropriate agents include Shur-Clens, mineral oil, or petroleum jelly. These ointments can be used initially in an effort to remove the tar or used as part of a dressing for later removal. Typically, the tar can easily be removed in about 2 to 3 days after treatment with a Neosporin dressing. Of note, removal of the tar will avulse the underlying tissue. Once exposed, tar burns should be treated like any other burn. Tar injuries that involve the face or large surface areas may require transfer and specialty consultation.

EXTREMITY TRAUMA

Trauma to specific extremities is covered in Chapter 15, "Orthopedics." General key points, however, that should be checked and documented with any extremity trauma, both before and after any manipulation, include the following:

- Presence/absence of deformity
- Presence/absence of abnormality of distal pulses

- Capillary refill time
- Pallor or cyanosis
- Mobility (either abnormal laxity or restricted motion)
- Range of motion (both active and passive as indicated)
- Sensation
- Skin integrity (presence or absence of associated wounds)
- Localized tenderness

SPECIAL CONSIDERATIONS

Care of an Amputated Part

Initial care of an amputated part in preparation for transport requires cleansing of any obvious dirt and debris. The amputated part should then be wrapped in a moistened sterile towel and placed into a sterile plastic bag. The plastic bag containing the amputated part should be immersed in a container of iced water or an insulated chest filled with crushed ice. It is vital that the part not be allowed to freeze, and it should never be placed directly on the ice. Specialty consultation should be arranged without delay, particularly if the patient must be transported to a designated facility with reimplantation capabilities.

REFERENCES

1. American College of Surgeons, Committee on Trauma: *Advanced Trauma Life Support Course (Student Manual)*, 6th ed. Chicago: ACS; 1997.
2. Scaletta TA, Schaider JJ: *Emergent Management of Trauma.* New York: McGraw-Hill; 1996: 131–132, 135.
3. Tintinalli J et al (eds): *Emergency Medicine: A Comprehensive Study Guide*, 5th ed. New York: McGraw-Hill; 2000:1547.

BIBLIOGRAPHY

American College of Surgeons, Committee on Trauma: *Advanced Trauma Life Support Course (Student Manual)*, 6th ed. Chicago: ACS; 1997.

Arient C, Caroli M, Balbi S: Management of head injured patients in the emergency department: a practical protocol. *Surg Neurol* 48:213, 1997.

Jelenko C: Chemicals that burn. *J Trauma* 14:65, 1974.

Johnson R: Descriptive classification of trauma: the injuries to the teeth and supporting structures. *J Am Dent Assoc* 102:195, 1981.

Manafo W: Initial management of burns. *N Engl J Med* 335:1581, 1996.

Roberts JR, Hedges JR, *Clinical Procedures in Emergency Medicine,* 2nd ed. Philadelphia: Saunders; 1991.

Schwartz D, Reisdorff E: *Emergency Radiology,* New York: McGraw-Hill; 2000.

Schwartz S, *Principles of Surgery Companion Handbook*, New York: McGraw-Hill; 1999.

Trope M: Clinical management of the avulsed tooth. *Dent Clin North Am* 39:93, 1995.

Zubair M Besner GE: Pediatric electrical burns: management strategies. *Burns* 23:413, 1997.

20

PSYCHIATRY

John Howell / Thom A. Mayer

Acute psychiatric illness is increasingly common in the outpatient setting. Approximately one-third of the patients in urban settings present to urgent care centers and emergency departments with psychiatric disorders. When the physician is confronted with such patients, his or her role is to control abnormal behavior and initiate therapy for life-threatening conditions. It is also important to determine whether a psychosis is due to a primary medical condition or mental disorder. This chapter discusses acute anxiety, depression, and suicidal ideation and distinguishing delirium (i.e., nonpsychiatric disorders) from acute psychiatric illness (e.g., psychosis).

Psychosis describes a dysfunction of thought processing and behavior that can be caused by schizophrenia, schizoaffective disorder, major affective disorders, delirium, dementia, and organic brain syndromes. Psychotic patients are extremely uncomfortable and have lost the demarcation between internal and external stimuli. The psychotic patient may act on any stimulus and become violent, combative, or manic. Psychosis may also be a symptom of a major medical problem, as discussed below.

In contrast to those who are psychotic, patients who are suicidal usually interpret external stimuli in an appropriate manner; however, they are generally very depressed and either are considering or have attempted harm to themselves. *Suicide* or *completed suicide* implies death, directly or indirectly consummated by an individual's willful activity. *Attempted suicide* requires the patient to perform some action that has caused injury or illness or has the potential to cause harm or death. *Suicidal ideation* refers to the patient's conscious thought process, which is occupied by suicidal imagery, ideas that life is not worth living, and possibly suicidal plans.

Acute anxiety is a relatively common disorder. Among patient visits to internists for apparently physical complaints, approximately 27 percent are attributable to psychiatric complaints, including depression and anxiety. Fifteen percent of patients seeing cardiologists have panic disorders. Acute anxiety may be viewed as either a functional disorder or a symptom attributable to multiple underlying causes. Nonpsychiatric causes of acute anxiety include endocrine and metabolic disorders, medications, and illicit drugs. In general, the management of psychiatric disorders mandates the ability to distinguish true psychiatric disorders from medical causes of abnormal behavior.

Distinguishing psychiatric illness from delirium

The examiner should remain nonaggressive and nonjudgmental when approaching a patient with possible delirium or acute psychiatric illness. This may pacify the patient with behavior-control problems. However, one should place oneself in a position to exit the examination area without coming into contact with the patient or crossing his or her path. Occasionally, a show of force or physical restraint is necessary to protect the patient, staff, and other individuals in the treatment area. If a psychiatric patient is combative and may harm members of the treatment team, emergency medical services (EMS) should be called and told to transport the patient to the closest appropriate emergency department. If, however, the patient is in control of his or her thoughts and actions and appears nonviolent, a full clinical assessment can proceed.

Clinical Assessment

Historical information must be obtained from all available sources including the patient, family, and medical records. Previous psychiatric illnesses, medications or illicit drug use, symptom onset and duration, and family history of psychiatric disorders must be documented, along with a description of the patient's social situation and any chronic medical problems. Treatable causes of acute psychosis are listed in Table 20-1, and medications that may mimic acute psychosis are listed in Table 20-2. Normal functioning before the onset of acute psychosis increases the likelihood of a medical cause. For example, infection may worsen the symptoms of a patient with chronic organic brain syndrome.

TABLE 20-1

TREATABLE CAUSES OF ACUTE PSYCHOSIS

Metabolic Causes
  Electrolyte imbalances
  Hypothyroidism
  Addison's disease
  Cushing's disease
  Hypocalcemia or
    hypercalcemia
  Vitamin deficiencies
  Pituitary dysfunctions
  Renal dysfunction or failure
  Hyperthyroidism
  Wilson's disease
  Diabetic ketoacidosis
  Hypoglycemia
  Hepatic dysfunctions
Neurologic Causes
  Chronic subdural hematoma
  Cerebral neoplasms

Intracranial aneurysms
Intracranial angiomas
Hypertensive encephalopathy
Cerebral abscess
Cerebral infections
Normal-pressure
  hydrocephalus
Seizure disorder (i.e.,
  temporal lobe and
  postictal states)
Cardiovascular Causes
Hypoxia
Anemias associated with
  chronic heart disease
Pulmonary insufficiency
Hypoperfusion
Infectious Causes
Pneumonia

Typhoid fever
Syphilis
Legionnaire's disease
Rocky Mountain spotted
  fever
Malaria
Sepsis
Diphtheria
Acute rheumatic fever
HIV-related infections
Other Causes
Substance abuse
Collagen vascular diseases
Depression
Substance withdrawal
Sensory deprivation

SOURCE: Howell JM et al (eds): *Emergency Medicine.* WB Saunders, Philadelphia, PA, 1998. With permission.

TABLE 20-2

MEDICATIONS THAT MAY CAUSE PSYCHOSIS

Cardiovascular agents	Antianxiety agents	Miscellaneous agents	Drugs of abuse
Digitalis	Diazepam	Corticosteroids	Alcohol
Disopyramide	Chlordiazepoxide	Disulfiram	Methamphetamine
Methyldopa	Ethchlorvynol	Antineoplastic drugs	Phencyclidine (PCP)
Captopril	Alprazolam	Cimetidine	Psilocybine
Procainamide	Clonazepam	Cycloserine	Locoweed (e.g.,
Reserpine	Antidepressants	Bromides	jimsonweed)
Propranolol	Amitriptyline	Heavy metals	Cocaine
Anticonvulsants	Doxepin	L-dopa	Amphetamines
Phenytoin	Protriptyline	Over-the-counter drugs	Lysergic acid
Ethosuximide	Imipramine	Antihistamines	diethylamide
Primidone	Trimipramine	Antitussives	(LSD)
Phenobarbital	Antibiotics	Decongestants	Mescaline
	Isoniazid	Diet or weight-loss	Marijuana
	Rifampin	drugs	

SOURCE: Howell JM et al (eds): *Emergency Medicine*. WB Saunders, Philadelphia, PA, 1998. With permission.

On physical examination, the vital signs are noted first. Tachycardia may reflect cocaine use, and an elevated temperature may mean that the patient is septic and has an infectious cause of psychotic behavior. A thorough physical examination is then performed looking for signs of trauma, *especially head trauma.* For example, the ears must be examined for hemotympanum and the patient screened for Battle's sign or raccoon eyes. These last two signs may reflect a basilar skull fracture. Pinpoint pupils suggest narcotic use and large pupils the use of anticholinergics (e.g., psychotropics or over-the-counter cold medications), which can produce signs similar to those of acute psychosis.

The chest and abdomen are next examined for signs of infection. A thorough neurologic examination is performed looking for focal deficits or evidence of structural brain disturbances. Myoclonus suggests a metabolic cause of acute psychosis. A normal neurologic examination and normal vital signs usually reflect a nonmedical cause of psychosis.

The mental status examination is critical. An initial screen may include the following questions:

- Where are you?
- What town are you in?
- What is the date?
- How old are you?
- When were you born and where?
- Who is the president of the United States?

Abnormal responses to these questions call for a more formal mental status examination and referral for a more formal psychiatric evaluation. The patient with a medical cause of psychosis is usually not oriented, has impaired recent memory, demonstrates nonauditory hallucinations, and has fluctuations in consciousness. The patient with an acute psychiatric psychotic episode is usually oriented and has fixed auditory hallucinations, good recent memory, and a lack of insight.

Diagnosis

The initial approach to patients with an acute psychotic presentation includes a basic metabolic panel and a search for infection and illicit drugs. Appropriate laboratory tests include a complete blood count, electrolytes, serum glucose, blood urea nitrogen (BUN), creatinine, urinalysis, a chest x-ray, and a urine drug screen. More advanced tests include computed tomography of the head and lumbar puncture. The latter tests are done at the physician's discretion, but usually, because of limitations in the urgent care setting, patients will require emergency department transfer in order to obtain laboratory results on an urgent basis.

Disposition

Patients with a medical cause of acute psychosis generally require referral to an emergency department or admission to a hospital. Alternatively, acute psychiatric psychosis may require admission to an inpatient psychiatric facility. When patients are referred directly to a psychiatric facility, any medical conditions must be identified and properly treated prior to transfer. Acute psychiatric psychoses may require admission when:

- Patients are experiencing a first psychotic episode
- Patients are a danger to themselves or others
- Patients are unable to care for themselves
- Patients have a poor social support team
- Patients are experiencing fluctuating psychoses that appear unstable

Transport of an acutely psychotic patient is often difficult; EMS, along with police backup, may be required. It is important never to place other patients or staff of the urgent care center in danger. At times, a court order may be necessary to initiate transport, particularly for persons who are not actively threatening harm to themselves or others.

Depression and Suicide

Most patients with suicidal ideation or those who have attempted suicide are acutely depressed. In these patients, the first step is to treat any medical or surgical emergencies, such as the suturing of lacerations. With drug overdoses, emergency department transfer will often be necessary for complete evaluation, treatment, and monitoring. Any psychiatric evaluation must be deferred until the patient is hemodynamically stable.

The next task is to identify the continued risk of suicide. Typically, patients with a high risk of suicide are male, above the age of 45 years, estranged or divorced, depressed, drinking alcohol, and have previously attempted suicide. The examining physician must at this point assess the patient's degree of hopelessness and the resources that he or she has for coping and obtaining social support.

During the history it is typically helpful to ask direct questions. For example, "Did you want to kill yourself?" "Do you want to kill yourself now?" "Do you have a present relationship with unresolved issues?" "Did you believe that your action would result in death?" In attempting to determine hopelessness on the part of the patient, suggested questions include "Do you have anything to live for?" "Do you have any hope?" "How do you see your future?"

It is important to obtain a past medical history because chronic illness is also a risk factor for depression and suicide. The patient's medications must be listed, as specific medications may predispose to depression and suicide (e.g., benzodiazepines, barbiturates). The patient's social history and family structure are explored, including supportive relationships outside the family (e.g., coworkers, employers, teachers, ministers). A full review of systems helps screen for occult medical problems and determines the stability of known health problems.

A thorough physical examination is vital. Specifically, a neurologic examination is necessary to exclude acute neurologic causes of the patient's illness.

Diagnosis

The history and physical examination guide any laboratory tests. Appropriate studies may include a complete blood count, electrolytes, pulse oximetry, urinalysis, and a urine toxicology screen, serum glucose, creatinine, and BUN. Chronic alcoholics may benefit from liver function studies and a serum ammonia level.

Disposition

Depressed patients generally require transfer for admission when:

- The patient has ongoing suicidal ideation.
- This was a serious suicide attempt in terms of lethality.
- The patient has ongoing feelings of hopelessness.
- The patient is irrational.
- The patient's judgment is impaired by disease, depression, psychosis, alcohol, or drugs.

If there is doubt, it is best to err on the side of caution by having the patient evaluated by a psychiatrist or transferred to an emergency department for psychiatric intervention. Patients who are suicidal or who require further evaluation in order to determine their potential for suicidal behavior must be transported via ambulance with continuous monitoring or under the care of a reliable family member. Depending on the circumstances, it is often prudent to be cautious and arrange ambulance transport.

ANXIETY

Clinical Presentation

Acute anxiety may mimic serious medical conditions (e.g., myocardial infarction or pulmonary embolus). Consequently, the history and physical examination should be thorough and cognizant of the potential for underlying medical problems. During the history, the patient should be asked about the time of symptom onset, aggravating and alleviating factors, prior psychiatric illness and medications, and medical history. Individuals experiencing a panic attack frequently feel overwhelmed by a variety of symptoms, including palpitations, sweating, shaking, shortness of breath, chest pain, nausea, dizziness, and a sense of impending doom. Panic attacks are different from generalized anxiety in that they are generally more intense and discrete, usually lasting only briefly.

TABLE 20-3

COMMON MEDICAL PROBLEMS THAT MASQUERADE AS PANIC OR ANXIETY

Cardiovascular Conditions
  Angina pectoris
  Congestive heart failure
  Dysrhythmia
  Hypovolemia
  Intra-aortic balloon pump
  Myocardial infarction
  Syncope
  Valvular disease, especially
    mitral valve prolapse
Endocrine Conditions
  Hyperadrenalism
  Hypocalcemia
  Hyperthyroidism
  Hypothyroidism
Immunologic Conditions
  Anaphylaxis
  Systemic lupus erythematosus
Metabolic Conditions
  Anemia
  Hypoglycemia
  Hyponatremia
  Hyperkalemia
  Hyperthermia
  Porphyria
Neurologic Conditions
  Akathisia

Encephalopathy
Essential tremor
Postconcussive syndrome
Restless leg syndrome
Seizure disorder, especially
  temporal focus
Vertigo
Respiratory Conditions
  Asthma
  Chronic obstructive
    pulmonry disease
  Pneumonia
  Pneumothorax
  Pulmonary edema
  Pulmonary embolus
  Respiratory dependence
Secreting Tumors
  Carcinoid
  Insulinoma
  Pheochromocytoma
Drugs
  Alcohol (withdrawal)
  Amphetamines
  Aminophylline
  Anticholinergics
  Antihypertensives: reserpine
    and hydralazine

Antituberculous agents:
  isoniazid and cycloserine
Barbiturates (withdrawal)
Benzodiazepines
  (withdrawal)
Caffeine
Cocaine
Digitalis (toxicity)
Dopamine
Epinephrine
Levodopa
Lidocaine
Methylphenidate
Monosodium glutamate
Neuroleptics
Nonsteroidal anti-
  inflammatory agents
Nicotinic acid
Phenylpropanolamine
Procarbazine
Pseudoephedrine
Salicylates
Steroids
Theophylline
Thyroid preparations

SOURCE: Adapted from Gehringer ES, Stern TA: Anxiety and depression in the medically ill. *Probl Crit Care Med* 1:39, 1988.

Patients experiencing an acute stress disorder have generally been exposed to a traumatic event in which there was a threat of serious injury or death to self or others. Symptoms include numbing and detachment, derealization, amnesia, flashbacks, marked anxiety, and impairment in social or occupational functioning.

Given the wide range of medical problems that may masquerade as anxiety (Table 20-3), a thorough physical examination is suggested. Specifically, an in-depth neurologic examination is extremely helpful.

Diagnosis

Diagnostic studies are suggested by the history and physical examination. Possible studies include a complete blood count, electrolytes, calcium, chest radiograph, electrocardiogram, pulse oximetry, a urine toxicology screen, and serum levels of specific medications.

TABLE 20-4

ANXIOLYTIC OPTIONS PROFILE

Drug	Usual Daily Dose	Onset of Action	Comments
Short-Acting Benzodiazepines (half-life 2–20 h)			
Midazolam (Versed)	5–10 mg	Fast	Very short half-life, may require more than one dose in ED; builds tolerance, abstinence syndromes can occur, can have paradoxical response or cause falls in elderly; use shorter forms for elderly patients
Alprazolam (Xanax)	1–5 mg	Intermediate	
Long-Acting Benzodiazepines (half-life 20–200 h)			
Lorazepam (Ativan)	1–5 mg	Intermediate	Long-acting (e.g., Valium, Klonopin, Librium) builds tolerance, abstinence syndromes can occur, can have paradoxical response or cause falls in elderly; use shorter-acting drugs in elderly; IM and IV forms available for Valium, Ativan
Clonazepam (Klonopin)	0.5–4.0 mg	Slow	
Diazepam (Valium)	1.0–20 mg	Fast	
Nonbenzodiazepines			
Buspirone (BuSpar)	15–40 mg	Slow	Little efficacy in acute state; more useful in long-term treatment of anxiety
Hydroxyzine (Atarax)	50–100 mg	Intermediate (oral within 1 h)	Anticholinergic effects and sedation; growing reports of anticholinergic abuse
Diphenhydramine (Benadryl)	50-100 mg		Anticholinergic effects and sedation; used in low dose in children; available in IM and IV form; contraindicated in patients with narrow-angle glaucoma, urinary retention, hyperthermia, congestive heart failure
Monoamine Oxidase Inhibitors			
Phenelzine (Nardil)	15–60 mg	Slow	Hypertensive emergency when combined with many foods and drugs; more useful in longer-term treatment of anxiety; little use in emergency setting
Tranylcypromine (Parnate)	30-60 mg	Slow	
Isocarboxazid (Marplan)	10–30 mg	Slow	
Selective Serotonin Reuptake Inhibitors			
Fluoxetine (Prozac)	20 mg		Antidepressants may worsen anxiety in some; expensive; 3–6 weeks for results
Sertraline (Zoloft)	10–40 mg	Slow	
Barbiturates			
Phenobarbital	100–200 mg	Fast	Because of their propensity to produce addiction, withdrawal, and danger in overdose, should not be prescribed for anxiety.
Beta Blockers			
Propanolol (Inderal)	40–120 mg		Worsens asthma, slows heart rate, may cause depression; used for stage fright; one 10–20 mg dose before speaking can help
Tricyclic Antidepressants			
Imipramine (Tofranil)	70–150 mg	Intermediate	Dangerous in overdose; useful in longer-term treatment of panic
Other			
Trazodone (Desyrel)	50–300 mg	Intermediate	Antidepressant useful in low dose for insomnia
Zolpide (Ambien)	5–10 mg	Fast	Should be used in time-limited (i.e., 10-day) fashion

SOURCE: Howell JM et al (eds): *Emergency Medicine*, WB Saunders, Philadelphia, PA, 1998. With permission.

Treatment

Table 20-4 lists a number of drugs that are useful as anxiolytics; these are usually prescribed in consultation with the patient's primary care physician. If a patient is discharged from a treatment area, a small prescription of either lorazepam (Ativan) or alprazolam (Xanax) may be helpful until the patient can see his or her primary care provider or following clinician.

Disposition

Most acute anxiety disorders are self-limiting and do not require admission. Referral to a primary care physician is frequently appropriate, with a short-term prescription for an anxiolytic, as described above. Admission should be considered for patients who exhibit substantial anxiety and active suicidal ideation.

BIBLIOGRAPHY

American Psychiatric Association: *Diagnostic and Statistical Manual of Mental Disorders*, 4th ed. Washington, DC: American Psychiatric Association; 1994.

Dubovsky SJ, Weissberg MP (eds): *Anxiety in Clinical Psychiatry in Primary Care*, 3d ed. Baltimore: Williams & Wilkins; 1986:83–86.

Jones PK, Jones SL, Yoder L: How urgent is the psychiatric patient in the emergency room? *J Psychiatr Treat Eval* 4:243, 1982.

Rund DA, Hutzler JC: N SAD CAGES: a mnemonic for depression. *Am J Psychiatry* 140:641, 1983.

GENITOURINARY DISORDERS

John Howell

Urgent care physicians evaluate and treat patients with acute genitourinary disorders on a daily basis. However, a complete list of the disorders that might fall into this chapter is myriad; consequently, this chapter focuses on common infectious and noninfectious disorders of the genitourinary tract. The common infectious disorders that are covered include urethritis, epididymitis, prostatitis, cystitis, and pyelonephritis. Mechanical disorders that are covered include urinary retention and testicular torsion.

URINARY TRACT INFECTIONS

Clinical Assessment

The clinical assessment of patients presenting with urinary tract complaints requires focused questions during the history to differentiate among the various types of genitourinary infections. Urgency, frequency, and dysuria are consistent with simple cystitis. The dysuria that is present with cystitis is usually complete (i.e., present throughout the stream). Constitutional symptoms of fever, chills, and nausea may point in the direction of an upper tract infection, or pyelonephritis. Urethritis is suggested by initial dysuria, penile discharge, and penile itching. Initial dysuria is also consistent with acute prostatitis. However, perineal pain, difficulty initiating the stream, and frequent urination are more specific for acute prostatitis. It is important to obtain a thorough past medical history. For example, diabetes and human immunodeficiency virus infection (HIV) increase the chance that patients with genitourinary infections will become more seriously ill (e.g., acute sepsis).

On physical examination, the patient's hydration status (e.g., mucous membranes, skin turgor), and degree of pain (e.g., tachycardia and diaphoresis) are noted. In a male, a distended bladder may reflect cystitis from acute prostatitis due to a urethral obstruction. Also, inspection of the external genitalia is required, because acute epididymitis also may cause cystitis. There is some controversy as to whether a digital rectal examination to evaluate the prostate is warranted. If the prostate is palpated, it should be done very gently to identify a potential prostatic abscess. Massaging of an infected prostate may increase the risk of bacteremia and sepsis.

Diagnosis

The diagnosis of acute cystitis is usually made with a urine dipstick, either alone or in combination with microscopic analysis. If the urine dipstick method is utilized, both leukocyte esterase and nitrite should be tested. Leukocyte esterase alone has a sensitivity of 72 to 89 percent and a specificity of 68 to 92 percent. Nitrite alone has a lower sensitivity at 40 to 75 percent but a higher specificity of 93 to 98 percent. The chance of a false-positive result if both leukocyte esterase and nitrate are positive is only 4 percent. Also, if both leukocyte esterase and nitrate are negative, the sensitivity is reasonably high (i.e., the false-negative rate is low). On microscopic urinalysis, more than 10 white blood cells per high-power field has a sensitivity of 82 percent and a specificity of 80 percent for a positive urine culture with more than 50,000 colony-forming units per milliliter.

Urinalysis and urine dipstick examination may be performed in patients with possible urethritis, prostatitis, and epididymitis, but they are less helpful in this regard since these three diagnoses generally are made clinically. In patients with suspected urethritis, a gram stain may be performed in an attempt to identify gonococci; however, this test is infrequently performed in the acute outpatient setting. Urethral swabs, therefore, should be obtained and sent to the laboratory to be tested for gonorrhea and chlamydia. Various methods are available; however, DNA probes are particularly helpful. All patients who engage in high-risk behavior or who are positive for sexually transmitted urethritis should be counseled regarding HIV testing. Many practitioners will either initiate or schedule such testing. Likewise, patients who exhibit high-risk behavior or who have urethral swabs sent to the laboratory with a high clinical suspicion for sexually transmitted disease (STD) should also have blood drawn and sent to be tested for syphilis.

Treatment

Simple Cystitis

Patients with simple cystitis may be treated with either a single dose or a 3-day course of an antimicrobial. These patients have generally been ill for a relatively brief period of time, are not pregnant, are not immune-compromised, do not exhibit signs and symptoms of upper tract disease, and have no evidence of urinary obstruction or urethral calculus.

In patients who are not allergic to either sulfa or trimethoprim, trimethoprim/sulfamethoxazole may be given either as a one-time dose or for a longer period of time. Typically, the double-strength tablets are prescribed. An effective alternative drug is nitrofurantoin in the form of Macrobid. Nitrofurantoin may be given in the dose of 100 mg twice a day. Up to 7 to 10 days of antimicrobial may be necessary. Fluoroquinolones are very effective alternatives to nitrofurantoin and trimethoprim/sulfamethoxazole. Some centers prescribe fluoroquinolones as first-line drugs due to increasing resistance of *Escherichia coli* to trimethoprim/sulfamethoxazole. Do not give fluoroquinolones to children.

Bacterial Prostatitis

A more prolonged treatment period is necessary for acute bacterial prostatitis. The organisms primarily responsible for bacterial prostatitis are gram-negative bacilli. *E. coli*

TABLE 21-1

TREATMENT OF ACUTE URETHRITIS—ALTERNATE DRUG REGIMENS

Gonorrheal infection	Ceftriaxone, 250 mg IM
Ciprofloxacin, 500 mg PO	Spectinomycin, 2 g IM
Ofloxacin, 400 mg PO	**Chlamydial infection**
Norfloxacin, 800 mg PO	Azithromycin, 1 g PO
Cefixime, 400 mg PO	Doxycycline, 100 mg PO bid for 7 days
Cefuroxime axetil, 1 g + probenecid	Tetracycline, 500 mg PO qid for 7 days
1 g PO	Erythromycin, 500 mg PO qid for 7 days

causes more than 80 percent of these cases. Sexually transmitted organisms such as *Neisseria gonorrhoeae* and *Chlamydia* are less frequent causes of acute prostatitis. Sexually transmitted causes of prostatitis are more common in younger males; it may be treated either with double-strength trimethoprim/sulfamethoxazole tablets twice a day or a fluoroquinolone. Such antimicrobial therapy must continue for approximately 30 days.

Bacterial Epididymitis

For acute bacterial epididymitis, males younger than 35 years may be treated as if they had a STD because of the frequency of *N. gonorrhoeae* and *Chlamydia* in the younger age group. Single-dose therapy is not warranted. In older patients, either trimethoprim/sulfamethoxazole double-strength tablets or a fluoroquinolone may be used for at least 10 days.

Treatment regimens for acute urethritis are listed in Table 21-1.

Disposition

Patients who appear toxic, are unable to take oral medication due to nausea and vomiting, have intractable pain, or have a home situation that does not allow them to be managed as outpatients should be admitted. Hospital admission should also be considered for patients who are immune-compromised (e.g., diabetes, HIV).

Those patients who can be treated on an outpatient basis should have a referral made to a primary care physician or urologist for follow-up. Discharge instructions should include specific criteria for urgent reevaluation.

URINARY RETENTION

Clinical Assessment

Acute urinary retention in males is most frequently caused by infection (e.g., acute bacterial prostatitis), benign prostatic hypertrophy (BPH), or medication side effects. Difficulty starting one's urine stream, hesitancy, decreased force of stream, and dribbling suggest urinary outlet obstruction from BPH. These patients should be asked about symptoms of infection—including dysuria, fever, nausea, and chills—as well as any new medications or changes in their existing medications. Pharmacologic agents that precipitate acute urinary retention are listed in Table 21-2. A history of any associated neurologic symptoms should also be sought and documented, since a spinal cord lesion

TABLE 21-2

PHARMACOLOGIC AGENTS THAT PRECIPITATE URINARY RETENTION

Sympathomimetics (alpha-adrenergic agents)
Ephedrine sulfate (Marax, Tedral)
Phenylephrine HCl (Neo-Synephrine)
Phenylpropanolamine HCl (Contac, Ornade)
Pseudoephedrine HCl (Sudafed, Actifed)

Sympathomimetics (beta-adrenergic agents)
Isoproterenol
Metaproterenol
Terbutaline

Antidepressants
Imipramine (Tofranil)
Nortriptyline (Aventyl)
Amitryptyline (Elavil)
Doxepin (Adapin)
Amoxapine (Asendin)
Maprotiline (Ludiomil)

Antiarrhythmics
Quinidine
Procainamide
Disopyramide

Anticholinergics (selected)
Atropine
Scopolamine hydrobromide
Belladonna
Homatropine methylbromide
Anisotropine methylbromide (Valpin)
Clidinium bromide (Quarzan)
Glycopyrrolate (Robinul)
Mepenzolate bromide (Cantil)
Methantheline bromide (Banthīne)
Oxyphenonium bromide (Antrenyl)
Propantheline bromide (Pro-Banthīne)
Dicyclomine HCl (Bentyl)
Oxybutynin (Ditropan)
Flavoxate HCl (Urispas)
Hyoscyamine sulfate (Anaspaz)

Antiparkinsonian Agents
Trihexyphenidyl HCl (Artane)
Benztropine mesylate (Cogentin)
Antihistamines (e.g., Benadryl)
Amantadine HCl (Symmetrel)
Levodopa (Dopar, Sinemet)
Bromocriptine mesylate (Parlodel)

Hormonal Agents
Progesterone
Estrogen
Testosterone

Antipsychotics
Haloperidol (Haldol)
Thiothixene (Navane)
Thioridazine (Mellaril)
Chlorpromazine (Thorazine)
Fluphenazine (Prolixin)
Prochlorperazine (Compazine)

Antihistamines (selected)
Diphenhydramine HCl (Benadryl)
Chlorpheniramine (Chlor-Trimeton)
Brompheniramine (Dimetane)
Promethazine (Phenergan)
Cyproheptadine (Periactin)
Hydroxyzine (Atarax, Vistaril)

Antihypertensives
Hydralazine (Apresoline)
Trimethaphan (Arfonad)

Muscle Relaxants
Diazepam (Valium)
Baclofen (Lioresal)
Cyclobenzaprine (Flexeril)

Miscellaneous
Nifedipine (Procardia)
Indomethacin (Indocin)
Carbamazepine (Tegretol)
Amphetamines
Mercurial diuretics
Dopamine
Vincristine
Morphine sulfate

SOURCE: Fontanarosa PB, Roush WR: Acute urinary retention. *Emerg Med Clin North Am* 6:428, 1988, with permission.

may precipitate urinary retention due to a change in innervation, not mechanical obstruction. A full differential diagnosis of urinary retention is listed in Table 21-3.

On physical examination, distention of the abdomen should be sought and the abdomen percussed and palpated for a distended bladder. Also, the patient's general habitus is assessed for signs of acute toxicity and hydration. The prostate is carefully palpated to ascertain whether it is enlarged, but this is done at the risk of seeding the blood with gram-negative bacilli.

Diagnosis

Diagnostic studies are ordered at the discretion of the care provider. Certainly, no diagnostic studies may be required in some cases. For example, bladder catheterization may be all that is needed in patients with mechanical obstruction due to BPH and no evidence of infection. However, a urinalysis is generally necessary to exclude infection. If urinary obstruction has been prolonged, electrolytes, blood urea nitrogen, creatinine, glucose, and radiologic studies may be warranted. A helical computed tomography scan of the abdomen and kidneys may be required to exclude ureteral calculus (see Chap. 17,

TABLE 21-3

DIFFERENTIAL DIAGNOSIS

	URINARY RETENTION	**URINARY INCONTINENCE**
Mechanical causes	Benign prostatic hypertrophy	Overflow incontinence
	Prostatic cancer and infections	Detrusor instability
	Urethral strictures	External spincter incontinence
	Bladder neck contractures	
	Phimosis or paraphimosis	
	Foreign bodies	
Neurologic dysfunction	Cerebral lesions or infections	Cerebral lesions or infections
	Spinal cord trauma	Suprasacral spinal cord lesions
	Disk herniation	Dementia
	Nerve root compression	Delirium
	Systemic neurologic disorders (such as MS, ALS)	
Infections	Cystitis and/or urethritis	Same as for retention
	Prostatitis	
Miscellaneous	Urinary tract malignancy or metastic involvement	Bladder or prostate carcinoma
	Urinary tract calculi	Urinary fistulas
	Blood clots	
	Sickle cell syndrome	
	Psychologic disorders	
	Functional disorders	

KEY: MS, multiple sclerosis; ALS, amyotrophic lateral sclerosis.
SOURCE: Fontanarosa PB, Roush WR: Acute urinary retention. *Emerg Med Clin North Am* 6:428, 1988, with permission.

"Evaluation and Treatment of Nontraumatic Abdominal Pain"). Ultrasonography is an acceptable alternative.

 Management

In general, patients with acute urinary obstruction are managed very effectively with bladder catheterization. Foley catheters, generally between 13 and 18 F, are used. Alternatives for more difficult catheterizations are Coudé and suprapubic catheters. Urinary tract infections are treated as noted above and medications that may have precipitated urinary obstruction are discontinued.

Disposition

The great majority of patients with urethral obstructions are discharged with a catheter in place and a leg bag. Timely follow-up is necessary. Consequently, most dispositions should be made following a phone call to either the urologist or primary care physician. Of note, patients become more dependent upon a bladder catheter the longer it is in place. Therefore it is important for patients discharged with bladder catheters to be reevaluated within 2 to 3 days.

TESTICULAR TORSION

Clinical Assessment

All patients with acute testicular pain represent a potential surgical emergency with the attendant risk of loss of anatomy and fertility. Acute testicular torsion may occur even though the patient has had a prior orchiopexy or is experiencing intermittent pain. A brief history targeting evidence of urinary infection—such as dysuria, urgency, frequency, and fever—should be performed and any history of trauma or previous episodes of testicular pain obtained. Young males with testicular torsion can present at times with symptoms of abdominal pain and gastroenteritis; therefore a testicular examination should be a part of the evaluation of all males presenting with complaints of abdominal pain.

On physical examination, the torsed testicle is generally tender, may be high-riding, and may have a transverse orientation. A hydrocele also may be present. There may also be a loss of the cremasteric reflex.

Isolated torsions of either the appendix epididymis or appendix testis may occur. In these cases, there is focal tenderness either in the area of the epididymis or more anteriorly on the testicle.

Diagnosis

In-depth diagnostic studies are not indicated. Patients with suspected testicular torsion must be referred immediately to an emergency department or a urologist for diagnostic studies and rapid management. These diagnostic studies may include either a Doppler ultrasound or nuclear scintigraphy. It is inappropriate to wait for the results of a urinalysis and electrolyte panel to refer a patient with possible testicular torsion.

Treatment

As noted above, patients with suspected testicular torsion are referred immediately to either an emergency department or a urologist. Manual detorsion may be attempted if this referral will be delayed. To perform this technique, the testicle is carefully grasped and then turned laterally as if one were opening a book. If there is no immediate improvement in symptoms, turning the testicles in the opposite direction may be attempted.

 Timely Diagnosis and Management

Any delay in this referral may result in loss of function and anatomy.

BIBLIOGRAPHY

Bowie WR: Effective treatment of urethritis. *Drugs* 44:207–215, 1992.
Hooton TM, Stamm WE: Management of acute uncomplicated urinary tract infection in adults. *Med Clin North Am* 75:339–357, 1991.
Prater JM, Overdorf BS: Testicular torsion: a surgical emergency. *Am Fam Physician* 44:834–840, 1991.
Stewart C: Prostatitis. *Emerg Med Clin North Am* 6:391–402, 1988.

22

ANAPHYLAXIS AND ACUTE ALLERGIC REACTIONS

Thom A. Mayer

Anaphylaxis is an acute, dramatic, and life-threatening systemic reaction manifest most commonly by angioedema, urticaria, bronchospasm, hypotension, upper airway obstruction, and gastrointestinal disturbances. These features may be present to varying degrees, and anaphylaxis may initially present as symptoms such as lip swelling or postural hypotension. Anaphylaxis is caused by chemical and IgE mediators released from mast cells in reponse to a foreign antigen to which previous sensitization has occurred but of which the patient is usually unaware (except in cases of bee-sting or medication allergy). Antigen-specific IgE binds to the cell membranes of mast cells and basophils, resulting in the release of a "witches' brew" of chemicals, including histamine, leukotrienes, platelet-activating factor, kallikreins, prostaglandins, and chemotactic factors. These substances cause vasodilatation and increased vascular permeability, with resultant tissue swelling and edema. The most serious and life-threatening symptoms from anaphylaxis are airway obstruction, bronchospasm, and hypotension due to widespread vasodilatation and third spacing of extracellular fluid. The most common causes of anaphylaxis are penicillin allergies, Hymenoptera stings, and reactions to radiopaque contrast material, although food allergies (including peanut allergies) and reactions to a wide variety of medications can also be responsible (Table 22-1).

In the past, the term *anaphylactoid reaction* was used to describe responses that are clinically identical to anaphylaxis, but that were found to be mediated by non-IgE factors and did not require presensitization exposure to the antigen. However, recent studies have shown that the final pathway is identical in anaphylactic and anaphylactoid reactions. Therefore they are treated clinically in the same fashion. *Hypersensitivity or classic allergic reactions* are at the opposite end of the spectrum of anaphylaxis and result from an immune system response to specific antigens. It is important to recognize that even mild acute allergic reactions should be evaluated carefully to make sure that such reactions do not progress to severe anaphylaxis.

TABLE 22-1

COMMON CAUSES OF ANAPHYLAXIS AND HYPERSENSITIVITY REACTIONS

DRUGS

Haptens	Prostaglandin inhibitors
Penicillin	Aspirin
Cephalosporins	Nonsteroidal anti-inflammatory drugs
Trimethoprim sulfamethoxazole	Complement activators
Vancomycin	Local anesthetics
	Radiopaque contrast media

FOODS AND ADDITIVES

Shellfish	Milk	Nitrates and nitrites
Nuts	Monosodium glutamate	Tartrazine dyes
Wheat	(MSG)	

VENOMS AND OTHER AGENTS

Hymenoptera (bee stings)	Exercise-induced anaphylaxis
Other insect and snake venoms	Cold-induced urticaria and anaphylaxis

CLINICAL PRESENTATION

In its classic and full-blown form, anaphylaxis is an easy diagnosis to make in that the patient presents with respiratory or cardiovascular collapse and is often resistant to initial treatment. Patients classically present with symptoms within 15 to 30 min of antigen exposure, with a clear predilection toward a more severe reaction when symptoms present immediately following antigen exposure. Although delays of up to 2 to 3 h may occur with some antigens (usually those taken by the oral route), most anaphylactic reactions occur within minutes of the exposure. Symptoms include airway obstruction, laryngeal edema, bronchospasm, urticaria, angioedema, rhinitis, conjunctivitis, and symptoms of acute, often dramatic, gastroenteritis. As mentioned previously, anaphylactoid reactions are clinically indistinguishable from anaphylaxis and should be treated similarly. Hypersensitivity or acute allergic reactions present with milder symptoms, most commonly related to urticaria, pruritus, or isolated angioedema. Nonetheless, these patients must be observed closely to make sure that their symptoms do not progress.

The principal cause of death in patients with anaphylaxis is laryngeal edema and subsequent respiratory failure. Profound hypotension and cardiovascular collapse are the second most common causes of death. Although skin involvement presenting as urticaria or angioedema is the most common symptom, this is clearly the least life-threatening one. "Cardiac anaphylaxis" involves a syndrome of findings including ventricular arrhythmias, ST-T–wave changes on the electrocardiogram, chest pain, and prolonged ventricular irritability. However, all of those findings are almost undoubtedly secondary to the hypoxia, hypotension, and cardiovascular response seen in anaphylaxis and do not represent a distinct clinical entity.

TABLE 22-2

DIFFERENTIAL DIAGNOSIS OF ANAPHYLAXIS

Status asthmaticus	Hereditary angioedema	Drug reactions
Epiglottitis	Foreign-body airway obstruction	Vasovagal reactions
Seizures	Mastocytosis	Myocardial ischemia

Diagnosis

The diagnosis of classic anaphylaxis is straightforward and direct; it should take only moments to make. Patients presenting in profound respiratory distress and cardiovascular collapse, with or without cutaneous symptoms, should be assumed to be in anaphylaxis until proven otherwise. During the initial phase of therapy, it is not necessary to identify the antigen itself, since in a vast majority of cases the exposure has already occurred and the focus should be on treating the patient aggressively. While a wide variety of diseases may produce symptoms similar to anaphylactic reactions, aggressive treatment is indicated, with a lesser emphasis on differential diagnosis until the patient can be stabilized. Table 22-2 lists additional diseases that may present similarly to anaphylaxis.

There is effectively no role for laboratory studies in the diagnosis and management of patients with anaphylactic reactions except to confirm acid-base and electrolyte status following initial stabilization. These are not diagnostic tests, however; they simply confirm the extent of disease and the response to therapy. Similarly, radiology has a limited role except to rule out other problems such as airway obstruction or epiglottitis.

Treatment

Patients presenting with anaphylactic reactions require immediate stabilization and treatment, as symptoms that are allowed to progress may become irreversible. Although it is uncommon for patients with anaphylactic reactions to present to urgent care centers, each facility must be prepared to manage such patients in an aggressive fashion, particularly since there is little time to arrange for transport via emergency medical services to the nearest emergency department. Thus all urgent care centers should have not only the equipment but also the training to help assure that such patients can be cared for. Further, urgent care centers should stage "mock codes" on a regular and routine basis to assure that the staff is well prepared to deal with the eventuality of an anaphylactic reaction, which is among the most common life-threatening emergencies presenting to urgent care centers.

The most important priority is securing the airway, particularly if there are signs of laryngeal edema, angioedema, bronchospasm, or other signs of respiratory compromise. The patient should be given 100% oxygen by bag-valve-mask at the same time that preparations for endotracheal intubation are made. A pulse oximeter should be placed on the patient to assure adequate oxygenation ($\geq$92% saturation). If the patient undergoes further respiratory compromise or respiratory failure, or if angioedema or laryngeal edema is noted on airway examination, an endotracheal tube of appropriate size should be placed. If there is time to give sedating agents or to perform rapid sequence induction (RSI), these methods should be undertaken. However, in the majority of patients with true anaphylactic reactions, there may not be time to perform even a "crash" RSI, and the tube must simply be placed as rapidly as possible, since laryngeal edema and airway swelling can proceed quite dramatically. Once the endotracheal tube is placed, 100% oxygen should be maintained, with the goal of obtaining a pulse oximetry value greater than 92%.

One of the main cornerstones of therapy for anaphylactic reactions is epinephrine, specifically for patients with moderate to severe symptoms. Severe symptoms include upper airway obstruction, significant bronchospasm, laryngeal edema, respiratory arrest, hypotension, or signs of impending shock. The beta-agonist effect on mast cells stimulates release of intracellular cAMP, which inhibits further release of vasoactive mediators. In addition, it increases bronchodilation and positive chronotropic and inotropic cardiac effects. The alpha-adrenergic effects of epinephrine primarily result in an increase in systolic and diastolic blood pressure through vasoconstriction and a decrease in vascular permeability, reducing angioedema. In severe cases of anaphylaxis, epinephrine should be given intravenously, although caution must always be taken because of the potential for creating malignant ventricular arrhythmias. However, epinephrine should never be withheld in patients with severe symptoms; the physician should simply be prepared to deal with any resultant ventricular arrhythmias. The initial dose should be 1.0 mL of 1:10,000 epinephrine, which should be further diluted in 10 mL of normal saline and given by slow intravenous push over 3 to 5 min. If shock or airway obstruction does not improve during this time, the intravenous dose may have to be repeated up to three or four times, with cautious monitoring throughout for the development of chest pain or ventricular arrhythmias. Some patients require ongoing intravenous epinephrine, which can be given by drip. This is prepared by adding 1.0 mg of epinephrine to 250 mL of normal saline, which is infused at a rate of 1 to 4 μg/min. Once a clinical response has been demonstrated and the patient's airway and cardiovascular status has improved, the drip can be discontinued and further epinephrine given by the subcutaneous route.

In patients with moderate symptoms of non–life-threatening bronchospasm and limited angioedema or borderline hypotension, epinephrine can be given subcutaneously in a dose of 0.3 to 0.5 mL of 1:1000 epinephrine, repeated every 5 to 10 min according to response. For pediatric patients with severe symptoms, the dose is 0.1 mL/kg per 5 mL 1:10,000, given over 3 to 5 min. The pediatric dose for mild to moderate symptoms is 0.01 mL/kg of 1:1000 epinephrine given subcutaneously. These treatment guidelines are summarized in Table 22-3.

Once the airway has been secured through appropriate means and treatment with epinephrine has begun, an intravenous line should be placed during the acute stage of anaphylaxis and an isotonic solution such as normal saline or lactated Ringer's solution started at a sufficient rate to maintain the blood pressure. In children, this should constitute a bolus of 20 mL/kg for mild hypotension, and 40 mL/kg for profound shock. In adult patients, a minimum of 1 L of isotonic solution should be given aggressively, to be followed by appropriate fluids as indicated by clinical progress.

In addition to aggressive isotonic fluid therapy, antihistamines, corticosteroids, albuterol, and glucagon may have to be given. All patients who present with signs and symptoms of anaphylaxis should receive corticosteroids. Adults should be given 125 mg of methylprednisolone intravenously and children should be given 1 to 2 mg/kg of

TABLE 22-3

STABILIZING MEASURES FOR ANAPHYLAXIS AND ALLERGIC REACTIONS

Airway control and support with 100% oxygen and breathing	Circulatory support for hypotension: Adults, 1–2 L of normal saline or Ringer's solution
If clinically indicated:	Children, 20 mL/kg of normal saline or Ringer's solution
Bag-valve-mask assisted ventilation	
Endotracheal intubation	Cardiac monitoring

methylprednisolone intravenously. Most patients should also receive an H_1 histamine blocker such as diphenhydramine intravenously in a dose of 50 mg for adults and 1 mg/kg for children. In patients with less severe hypersensitivity reactions, diphenhydramine may be given by mouth. If an intravenous line has not been established, diphenhydramine may be given intramuscularly, although there may not be adequate perfusion in such cases to allow absorption of the drug. H_2 histamine blockers should also be given to patients in anaphylaxis, since research has shown that such blockers may be effective in patients who are in shock and are refractory to the above measures. The safest H_2 blocker is ranitidine, which is given as a 50-mg intravenous bolus over 5 min. Children should be given 0.5 mg/kg intravenously over 5 min. In the past, cimetidine was used to treat anaphylactic reactions, but there is strong evidence to indicate that this agent prolongs the metabolism of beta blockers and may interfere with the metabolism of other drugs. If cimetidine is given, the dose is 300 mg by mouth or intravenously for adults and 10 mg/kg by mouth or intravenously for children.

Where wheezing and shortness of breath are a part of the initial presentation, a bronchodilator such as albuterol should be given via nebulizer. In patients weighing more than 20 kg, 2.5 mg of nebulized albuterol (0.5 mL of 5% solution) can be given in a continuous nebulization, while patients weighing less than 20 kg should receive a dose of 1.25 mg of nebulized albuterol (0.25 mL of 5% solution).

In patients with anaphylactic reactions due to beta blockers, glucagon should be given in a dose of 1 mg intravenously every 5 min until hypotension resolves, followed by an infusion of 5 to 15 µg/min until the patient fully stabilizes. Glucagon may cause hyperglycemia, dizziness, nausea, vomiting, and hypochloremia, but it is an effective agent in patients with anaphylaxis due to the ingestion of a beta blocker. The pediatric dose is 50 µg/kg IV every 5 min.

In patients with hypersensitivity reactions that do not progress to anaphylaxis and do not involve hypotension or significant respiratory symptoms, a less dramatic treatment regimen is indicated. Epinephrine and intravenous fluids should be reserved for patients who show significant respiratory compromise, bronchospasm, and hypotension. In patients without these symptoms, symptomatic treatment is indicated. If bronchospasm occurs, nebulized albuterol may reverse the symptoms without the need for intravenous or subcutaneous epinephrine. Whenever possible, the causative agent should be identified and discontinued. For example, in a patient with bee-sting allergy, it is important to remove the stinger (without using forceps—it should be "brushed" off), irrigate the wound site, and apply cold compresses. Diphenhydramine should be given to these patients, usually by the oral route, although intramuscular or intravenous diphenhydramine can also be utilized in the doses listed in Table 22-4. The patient

TABLE 22-4

TREATMENT MEASURES

TREATMENT	ADULTS	CHILDREN
Epinephrine		
Moderate/severe	1.0 mL of 1:10,000 in 10 mL NS IV over 3–5 min	0.01 mL/kg 1:10,000 in 5 mL NS IV over 3–5 min
Mild/moderate	0.3–0.5 mL of 1:1,000 SC every 15 min	0.01 mL/kg 1:1,000 SC every 15 min
Allergic reaction	0.3 mL of 1:1,000 SC as needed every 15 min	0.01 mL/kg 1:1,000 SC as needed
H_1 Antagonists		
Diphenhydramine		
Moderate/severe	50–100 mg IV	1–2 mg/kg IV
Mild/allergic reaction	25–50 mg PO	1 mg/kg PO
H_2 Antagonists		
Ranitidine (preferred)		
Severe/moderate	50 mg IV	0.5 mg/kg IV
Mild	150 mg PO	2 mg/kg PO
Steroids		
Methylprednisolone (severe/moderate)	125 mg IV	2 mg/kg IV
Prednisone (mild)	60 mg PO	1–2 mg/kg PO
Albuterol	>20 kg: 2.5 mg (0.5 mL of 5% solution)	<20 kg: 1.25 mg (0.25 mL of 5% solution)
Glucagon	1 mg IV push every 3–5 min	50 μg/kg IV every 5 min

KEY: NS, normal saline; IV, intravenously; SC, subcutaneously; PO, by mouth.

should be observed for a minimum of ½ h following allergic symptoms, and there should be a clear demonstration both clinically and in the chart that the patient has improved with appropriate symptomatic therapy. A careful search for potential sources of the hypersensitivity reaction should be undertaken, including identifying patients with latex allergies, reactions to angiotensin-converting enzyme (ACE) inhibitors, food allergies, and drug reactions.

DISPOSITION

In patients with anaphylactic reactions, admission to the emergency department and into the hospital in most cases will be necessary. While the initial priorities are clearly resuscitation and stabilization, a staff member should be instructed to contact emergency medical services and the nearest emergency department at the earliest possible time for transfer of the patient as soon as possible. In addition, the "extra hands" of the EMS crew may be helpful during initial stabilization, particularly since these crews deal with such emergencies on a fairly routine basis.

Many patients with milder symptoms of anaphylaxis (bronchospasm and postural hypertension) may respond quickly to appropriate therapy. Nonetheless, they should all be transferred to an emergency department for observation over a period of several hours, since some of these patients can dramatically reverse course, particularly if there is ongoing exposure to the antigen.

For patients with hypersensitivity reactions that are mild and are largely limited to cutaneous symptoms, immediate treatment and advice to avoid the allergen are appropriate. In most cases, an adult or pediatric Epi-pen prescription should be given with clear instructions for its use if serious allergic reactions occur. When known allergies have been identified, a Medic Alert bracelet should be suggested. If a patient has reacted to an ACE inhibitor or beta blocker, the primary care physician should be informed of the allergy and arrangements made to make sure that the patient is switched to a different, more appropriate antihypertensive drug.

It should be noted that the pathophysiology of angioedema due to ACE inhibitors differs from the classic hypersensitivity reaction. For that reason, such patients' cutaneous symptoms are often refractory to antihistamines, steroids, and—in many cases—even epinephrine. If symptoms are mild and limited to local angioedema, the patient can simply be removed from treatment with the ACE inhibitor and referred for careful follow-up. However, if severe swelling, respiratory distress, bronchospasm, or difficulty in swallowing occurs, these patients should be referred to the emergency department for close observation.

Common Errors and Pitfalls

Because airway compromise can progress rapidly, even isolated airway symptoms should be observed carefully. Uvular, lip, and palatal edema may be an early warning sign of laryngeal edema and respiratory failure.

- Any signs of hoarseness, difficulty in swallowing, or airway compromise should be treated rapidly and aggressively.
- Hypersensitivity reactions that could progress to anaphylaxis must always be treated aggressively.
- In the differential diagnosis of patients who present with sudden, otherwise unexplained hypotension, respiratory compromise, or respiratory arrest, anaphylaxis must always be considered.
- Patients experiencing hypersensitivity reactions must be questioned carefully for all events in the hours leading up to the reaction to help identify possible causative agents.
- Cephalosporin antibiotics must never be prescribed in patients with a documented severe systemic reaction to penicillin despite the fact that the risk may be low.

 Key Points of Documentation

Regardless of the severity of symptoms and a hypersensitivity reaction, the chart should clearly document the patient's improvement prior to discharge, clear discharge instructions, and instructions for follow-up in the event of recurrence or worsening of symptoms.

- The chart should reflect an appropriate search for the potential allergen, with instructions to avoid such allergens in the future.
- The chart should clearly reflect all procedures and treatments given to the patient as well as the patient's response at the urgent care center.

BIBLIOGRAPHY

Anderson JA: Allergic reactions to drugs and biological agents. *JAMA* 268:2845–2857, 1992

Atkinson TP, Kaliner MA: Anaphylaxis. *Med Clin North Am* 76:841–855, 1992.

Bochner BS, Lichtenstein LM: Anaphylaxis. *N Engl J Med* 324:1785–1790, 1991.

Friday GA, Fireman P: Anaphylaxis. *Ear Nose Throat J* 75:21–26, 1996.

Roberts JR, Wuerz RC: Clinical characteristics of angiotensin-converting enzyme inhibitor–induced angioedema. *Ann Emerg Med* 20:555–558, 1991.

WOUND REPAIR PROCEDURES IN THE URGENT CARE CENTER

Thom A. Mayer/Michael Mortiere

INTRODUCTION

A number of wound repair procedures are routinely performed in the setting of the urgent care center (UCC); all providers should be familiar with them, knowledgeable about them, and able to handle them confidently. These include routine laceration repairs, local anesthesia, and basic nerve blocks. Each of these items is addressed in this chapter, which includes a discussion of general principles through more advanced techniques that may be performed by some providers in the UCC setting, depending upon familiarity, experience, and exposure to certain procedures during the course of training. Procedures that are specific to certain body areas are not discussed here but are covered in the appropriate chapters (e.g., ophthalmology; ear, nose, and throat procedures; obstetrics and gynecology, etc.).

WOUND REPAIR

Clinical Assessment

In the UCC setting, wound assessment should always be conducted in a systematic fashion, eliciting the mechanism of injury and examining the whole of the patient instead of concentrating on obvious wounds or injuries in isolation. A thorough and complete history and physical examination should be performed, including an elucidation of the mechanism of injury, amount of time elapsed from the initial injury, predisposing underlying illnesses or injuries (diabetes, hypertension, steroid therapy, etc.), immunization status, and initial care performed prior to evaluation in the UCC. Further information that must be elicited includes a detailed account of the mechanism of the injury, whether the injury was work-related, the type of activity normal to the patient (for referral and work reasons), and any prior history of wounds and their pattern of healing, infection, scarring, keloid formation, etc.

A wound should be typified by shape, length, mechanism of injury, depth, location, wound borders, and neurovascular status. In most cases the wound should be examined while the patient is supine and in a comfortable position. In some cases the patient may be more comfortable on a stretcher in a seated position, particularly if an extremity has been injured.

Key Points of Documentation

- Length—the wound should be measured in centimeters and recorded on the chart.
- Location—described as precisely as possible, with drawings whenever possible.
- Wound edges—clean, sharp, crushed, abraded, macerated, etc.
- Depth—partial skin thickness, full skin thickness, subcutaneous tissue, muscle fascia, muscle belly, bone, etc.
- Foreign bodies—a detailed examination should be performed and any foreign bodies noted.
- Associated injuries—fractures, tendon injuries, dislocations, crush injuries to soft tissue, etc.
- Neurovascular and motor function—in addition to a description of the wound site, function proximal and distal to the wound site should be examined and documented on the chart, which should be done prior to the administration of anesthesia or nerve blocks. Capillary refill proximal and distal to wound should be documented.

All of this information should be carefully documented on the chart; in most cases, a wound/laceration form should be utilized to make sure that this is captured efficiently (see "Documentation," below, and Fig. 23-1).

STERILE TECHNIQUE AND INFECTION CONTROL

All health care providers in the UCC setting should be familiar with and utilize the Universal Precautions Guidelines established by the Centers for Disease Control. The institution should have a specific policy indicating adherence to the CDC guidelines and new staff should be oriented to these policies. The following recommendations are intended to help to reduce the risk of contamination during wound closure:

- Careful hand washing should be performed between patients and before all procedures.
- A surgical mask should be worn to prevent aerosol/droplet contamination of wounds.
- Sterile or nonsterile gloves should be worn while examining the wound prior to repair. Sterile gloves should always be worn when sterile instruments or sterile trays are being used and should be changed between wound preparation and suturing.
- If there is any possibility of contamination by the provider's hair, it should be contained by a surgical cap or tieback.
- Eye protection should be worn in all cases to prevent droplet contamination.

HISTORY

MECHANISM OF INJURY: _____

Time Lapse From Injury to Repair: _____ Work Related? ❏ No ❏ Yes Patient is: ❏ Right handed ❏ Left handed

PHYSICAL EXAMINATION

Location of wound(s) _____

_____

TOTAL Wound length: _____ cm

Wound Margins: ❏ Tidy ❏ Untidy

Wound Depth: ❏ Superficial (dermal) ❏ Full-thickness

❏ Muscle/facia involvement ❏ to Bone

Fracture Present? ❏ No ❏ Yes

Foreign Body Present? ❏ No ❏ Yes

Burn Description: _____ % TBSA ❏ 1° ❏ 2° ❏ 3°

Distal Sensory Function: ❏ Normal ❏ Abnormal _____

2 point discrimination _____ mm (radial)

_____ mm (ulnar)

Motor Function	❏ Normal	❏ Abnormal _____	
Tendon Laceration	❏ No	❏ Yes	❏ N/A
Joint Stable?	❏ No	❏ Yes	❏ N/A
Active Bleeding?	❏ No	❏ Yes	
Capillary Refill	❏ Good	❏ Poor	
Pulse Deficit?	❏ No	❏ Yes	

NARRATIVE / ADDITIONAL COMMENTS: _____

_____

PROCEDURE NOTE

TIME PROCEDURE BEGAN / ENDED	TOURNIQUET TIME BEGAN / ENDED	ANESTHETIC AGENT	AMOUNT	ADMINISTRATION ROUTE	PREPARATION ❏ STANDARD Betadine scrub Normal saline irrigation 50-100 cc/cm	❏ OTHER

REPAIR PROCEDURES

❏ DEBRIDEMENT ❏ DRAINAGE ❏ FB EXTRACTION ❏ OTHER: _____

❏ EXCISION ❏ UNDERMINING ❏ NAIL PLATE REMOVAL _____

❏ EXTENSION ❏ DRAIN/PACKING INSERTED ❏ NAIL BED REPAIR _____

❏ INCISION ❏ FB SIMPLE REMOVAL ❏ TREPHINATION OF SUBUNGUAL HEMATOMA

CLOSURE METHOD

❏ SUTURES ⟶

❏ TAPE

❏ STAPLES

(NUMBER USED _____)

❏ DERMABOND

❏ NONE

SIZE	TYPE	NUMBER	TISSUE LAYER

REPAIR TYPE:
❏ SIMPLE
❏ INTERMEDIATE
❏ COMPLEX

TETANUS PROPHYLAXIS
❏ Td
❏ TIG
❏ None

DRESSING APPLIED: ❏ NONE ❏ BACITRACIN ❏ ADAPTIC ❏ XEROFORM ❏ GELFOAM ❏ SURGICEL ❏ KLING ❏ KERLEX ❏ TUBE GAUZE ❏ SILVADENE CREAM ❏ BANDAID ❏ OTHER: _____

SPLINT APPLIED: ❏ NONE ❏ METAL/ALUMINUM FINGER ❏ STACK FINGER ❏ VELCRO VOLAR ❏ VOLAR (fiberglass) ❏ RADIAL GUTTER ❏ ULNAR GUTTER ❏ DORSAL HAND ❏ POSTERIOR ANKLE ❏ POSTERIOR ARM ❏ SUGAR TONG ARM ❏ SUGAR TONG ANKLE ❏ KNEE IMMOBILIZER ❏ AIRCAST ❏ SLING/SWATHE ❏ SLING ❏ CAST SHOE ❏ CRUTCHES WITH INSTRUCTION ❏ OTHER: _____

FOLLOW-UP WITH: ❏ E.D. ❏ PMD ❏ PLASTICS ❏ ORTHO ❏ OTHER _____ in _____ DAYS

Procedure performed by: ❏ PA ❏ Resident ❏ Student ❏ Attending Physician **Splint Checked by:** ❏ PA ❏ Physician

_____ _____
E.D. PA / RESIDENT SIGNATURE E.D. ATTENDING PHYSICIAN SIGNATURE

PATIENT IDENTIFICATION

INOVA FAIRFAX HOSPITAL

EMERGENCY DEPARTMENT
WOUND RECORD

CAT #82553 / R11-99 • PKGS OF 100

FIGURE 23-1 Wound care record. Preprinted wound care records can assist in documentation of wound extent, repair procedures, closure methods, and appropriate additional treatment, which assures that detailed information is kept on each patient. Reproduced with permission.

- A laboratory coat or jacket should be removed prior to wound preparation and repair to prevent dragging sleeves across the sterile operating field as well as cross-contamination between patients. Ties and/or jewelry should be restrained from potential contamination of the wound.
- One should never attempt to place a cover back onto contaminated sharps (needles, scalpels, sutures, etc.).
- Once a wound has been prepared, the sterility of the wound field should be protected; if it is violated, the wound will have to be reprepped and a separate suture tray utilized.
- All contaminated wound items should be discarded in a nearby trash receptacle and treated as contaminated material during disposal.

Wound Classification

Soft tissue injuries should be classified by their appearance, causative mechanism, and degree of trauma to the tissues. Each wound should be addressed individually and examined carefully, since the amount of underlying trauma may not be reflected by a skin examination alone. Many wounds may appear small, clean, and incision-like on the surface when in fact the wound may extend deep into the subcutaneous tissues and have caused major contamination of those tissues. For example, puncture wounds to the foot that have traversed a sock and the sole of a tennis shoe often introduce pieces of both the shoe and the sock deep into the tissue. In such cases, the superficial appearance of the wound may indicate that a minimal wound has occurred when in fact aggressive irrigation and treatment are necessary to prevent infection and the foreign body must be removed from the tissue to prevent complications. Similarly, stab wounds (even with mechanisms as simple as kitchen knives) must be treated and assessed aggressively to assure that there has been no underlying trauma or disruption to subcutaneous tissues, tendons, and neurovascular structures. The following offers a simple classification system for wounds.

Lacerations

A laceration is a wound resulting from the tearing or shredding of tissue by blunt, penetrating, or sharp forces. In some cases, the term *incision* is used to refer to wounds made by sharp instruments, although most such wounds are generically referred to as lacerations. Lacerations may be described as clearly defined, linear, stellate, L-shaped, T-shaped, or any combination thereof. The wound margins should be carefully described as sharp, jagged, abraded, contused, grossly contaminated, or other appropriate descriptions.

Abrasions

Wounds in which the dermis and/or epidermis has been removed by friction are referred to as abrasions. The most common example of this injury is the child's scraped knee, usually resulting from a fall while running, bicycling, scootering, or skateboarding. More serious abrasions can occur from contact with the pavement after motorcycling or bicycling (also known as "road rash") and involve larger areas of skin. Road rash may even involve full-thickness injuries through the subcutaneous tissue. There is a tendency for inexperienced providers to assume that abrasions will heal easily when in fact deep abrasions and those with significant debris can result in permanent scarring and "tattooing" of the skin. In addition, such wounds are at high risk for infection and should be treated in the same aggressive fashion as a burn injury. Abrasions are akin to second-degree or partial-thickness burns at a minimum.

Avulsions

An avulsion is a loss of soft tissue, which may involve various structures from the epidermis to subcutaneous tissue or even muscle. However, most avulsions are confined to the epidermis or dermis and most commonly result from falls, motor vehicle accidents, or food preparation injuries. Most avulsions are oblique in nature, resulting from an impact and a shearing force transmitted to the epidermis, dermis, subcutaneous tissue, or muscle layer, depending upon the force and direction of injury. Incomplete avulsions are also known as *flap lacerations* and may present difficult management problems, particularly with regard to those wounds that have compromised the vascular supply to the avulsion (see below).

Puncture Wounds

Puncture wounds can be caused by a wide variety of objects and most commonly involve the hands and the soles of the feet. The wounding objects typically penetrate the skin into the deeper tissues; they may introduce foreign bodies or the inoculum for infection into those deep tissues and for that reason require a careful evaluation. The most common side effect of puncture wounds is infection, the incidence of which depends upon the puncturing instrument, location, and introduction of inoculum. Infection occurs in 6 to 12 percent of patients with puncture wounds and is usually due to gram-positive organisms, typically *Staphylococcus aureus*, although many other microorganisms have been isolated from puncture wound infections. In puncture wounds to the foot where the wounding object has traversed sneakers or in penetration to bone, *Pseudomonas aeruginosa* is the most frequently isolated pathogen. Puncture wounds that are more likely to become infected include those in patients with poor resistance to infection, punctures of the forefoot, those that occur outdoors, those involving penetration through footwear, large lesions with deep penetration and large inoculum, and presentations more than 6 h after injury (Table 23-1).

TABLE 23-1

POSTPUNCTURE WOUND INFECTION: INCREASED INCIDENCE

Immunosuppression	Poor wound repair
Diabetes	Elderly
Chemotherapeutic agents	Malnourished
Steroids	Connective tissue disorder
Chronic renal failure	Wound factors
Hematologic malignancies	Crush injury
Congenital immunodeficiencies	Tissue loss
Tissue ischemia	Contamination
Peripheral vascular disease	Foreign bodies
Anemia	Location
Vasculitis	

SOURCE: From Martin J, Herfel R: Methods for wound closure, in Tintinalli JE, Kelen GD, Stapczynski JS (eds): *Emergency Medicine: A Comprehensive Study Guide,* 5th ed. New York: McGraw-Hill; 2000, with permission.

The presence of a foreign body must be excluded to the best extent possible in puncture wounds, given the nature of the wound itself. In patients with typical sneaker injuries, following adequate anesthesia, the wound should be examined and irrigated aggressively. It is not uncommon that pieces of the tennis shoe or sock float out of the wound when this more aggressive technique is utilized. For any wound where radiopaque material is suspected (metal, gravel, glass), plain-film radiographs (including three views) should be utilized. Radiopaque foreign bodies greater than 0.5 to 1.0 mm are usually identifiable and are seen in 80 to 90 percent of plain films. Other common foreign-body substances include cactus spines, thorns, vegetable matter, and wood splinters, which have a radiodensity so close to that of soft tissue that plain-film radiographs may not identify them. In these cases, ultrasound, computed tomography (CT), magnetic resonance imaging (MRI), and xeroradiograpic studies may be helpful.

Treatment of puncture wounds remains one of the most controversial areas of wound therapy. While cleansing the wound is helpful, soaking has no proven benefit whatsoever. Low-pressure irrigation of wounds is always recommended to assist in cleansing and for better visualization for possible foreign bodies. However, high-pressure irrigation (greater than 7 psi) has been shown to lead to deeper displacement of foreign-body material and dissemination of bacteria deeper into the wound and surrounding tissue. For this reason, high-pressure irrigation should not be undertaken.

Wound exploration, debridement, or "coring" of the wound track has sometimes been recommended but should be limited to those cases in which large objects or particularly contaminated ones have been introduced into the wound. While there is no proven benefit to routine prophylactic antimicrobial therapy in the management of clean, uncontaminated, nonplantar puncture wounds, there is in fact some evidence to suggest that this may contribute to the rise of secondary infections with gram-negative organisms in the wound. Plantar puncture wounds, especially those in high-risk patients with forefoot punctures or those that have gone through soft-soled shoes, should be treated with antibiotics. Since the ability of antibiotics to decrease infection is related to the achievement of appropriate antimicrobial blood levels, intravenous or intramuscular administration of a cephalosporin, an aminoglycoside, or both is widely utilized. However the development of the fluoroquinolone class of antibiotics has resulted in the ability to administer broad-spectrum antibiotics by mouth, thus achieving appropriately high blood levels in a short time. Ciprofloxacin and levofloxacin are the most commonly used antibiotics in these settings, although they are not approved by the U.S. Food and Drug Administration (FDA) for use in children because of their potential effect on cartilage. In children, an alternate possibility is the use of amoxicillin/clavulanate.

Mammalian Bites

Human bites carry with them a high rate of infection and commonly occur on the hands and upper extremities, followed by the head and neck, trunk, and lower extremities. They usually result from intentional bites, fights, or sports injuries. Human bites to the hands have particularly serious consequences, including infection and loss of function. These bites typically produce a crushing or tearing force with tissue destruction and some degree of devitalization. The most common serious complication from human bites is infection from both aerobic and anaerobic oral flora. Patients who present more than 24 h after injury often already exhibit signs of infection, including swelling, warmth, redness, and a purulent discharge. In these patients, cultures should be obtained and the wound irrigated copiously; radiographs should be taken to determine whether there is extension further into soft tissues. All such wounds should be examined under anesthesia to assure that the extent and delineation of injury are clearly documented. If wounds extend into the joint space or bone, referral to the emergency department (ED) for evaluation by a plastic or hand surgeon should be undertaken. If the wound is limited to the soft tissues and signs of infection are already present, antibiotics should be started regardless of the site of the wound. Prophylactic antibiotics should be started with all human bites of the hands and with bites to other locations in high-risk patients. Antibiotics that can be helpful include amoxicillin/clavulanate, a cephalosporin plus penicillin, dicloxacillin plus penicillin, or a fluoroquinolone.

Patients who are allergic to penicillin can be treated with clindamycin plus trimethoprim/sulfamethoxazole. For prophylactic treatment, 5 days of therapy is appropriate, whereas 10 to 14 days of therapy will be necessary for patients who have already developed signs of infection.

Dog bites occur frequently and are responsible for up to 90 percent of reported animal bites in the United States. Dog bite injuries occur most commonly in the upper extremities and more commonly in males. When infection occurs in dog bites, it is usually due to organisms inoculated into the wound by the animal's teeth, as opposed to bacterial flora on the skin driven into the wound. Such infections are usually caused by multiple organisms, including aerobic and anaerobic bacteria. While there is some controversy regarding primary closure of dog bite wounds, the majority of such wounds can be closed provided they are:

- Less than 8 h old
- Not involved with deep structures such as muscle, joint, or bone
- Not infected at the time of presentation
- Not in patients prone to infection (diabetic, immunocompromised, and geriatric patients, etc.)

Some authorities recommend not closing dog bite lacerations of the distal extremities, but others have done so and have data to support the practice of closure following copious irrigation of the wound. Regardless of whether the wound is closed by primary or secondary intention, patients with dog bites should be given careful instructions regarding the potential for infection and the signs and symptoms thereof. In patients with infections in the first 24 h after injury, *Pasteurella multocida* is the most likely organism, and treatment with penicillin, fluoroquinolones, or trimethoprim/sulfamethoxazole is recommended. In patients seen after 24 h, *Staphylococcus* and *Streptococcus* are the more common organisms and a penicillinase-resistant penicillin or a cephalosporin should be utilized. Despite the relatively low rate of infection with well-irrigated and rapidly diagnosed and treated dog bite wounds, most authorities recommend prophylactic treatment with antibiotics for 3 to 5 days, simply because of the potential for infection with organisms that can cause dramatic infections, including *Pasteurella multocida,* *Staphylococcus aureus,* and *Capnocytophaga canimorsus.*

Cat bites are also often seen in UCCs and account for 10 to 18 percent of reported animal bites in the United States. The majority of these injuries occur on the distal extremities, including the hands, forearms, and arms. Because of the cat's teeth, most cat bites result in smaller but deeper puncture wounds, and up to 80 percent of cat bites become infected. *Pasteurella multocida* is the major pathogen and is found in up to 80 percent of patients with infections following cat bites. Infections with this pathogen are usually typified by a fairly rapidly developing and intense inflammatory response, with pain, swelling, and minimal discharge. Bites over joints are particularly prone to develop septic arthritis. All cat bites should be aggressively cleansed, dressed, and splinted.

The majority of cat bite wounds are either puncture wounds or small lacerations and most commonly do not require wound closure. Lacerations over 2 cm in length can be closed after aggressive irrigation without increased risk of infection. Prophylactic antibiotics should be administered to patients with puncture wounds of the hand or over joints and in immunocompromised or elderly patients. In fact, the majority of emergency physicians treat all cat bites with prophylactic antibiotics for 5 days, including either penicillin, amoxicillin/clavulanate, cefuroxime, or doxycycline, all of which are effective against *Pasteurella multocida*.

WOUND PREPARATION

Wound preparation and cleansing are extremely important but underrated steps in abetting the process of wound healing. In the past, many institutions soaked injured wounds in a basin of povidone-iodine, hydrogen peroxide, or some other antiseptic solution. However, numerous clinical studies have proven that soaking in any solution other than normal saline or lactated Ringer's solution inhibits normal healing processes and may increase the risk of infection. It also produces an inflammatory response, particularly when agents such as povidone-iodine are utilized.

Almost without exception, anesthesia and pain control should be obtained prior to extensive wound preparation and irrigation. This not only is more sensitive to the patient's needs but also ensures better preparation and treatment as well as evaluation of the patient for potential foreign bodies. As mentioned previously, prior to the administration of local or nerve block anesthesia, the sensory, motor, and vascular examination should be performed and documented.

Similarly, hemostasis should be obtained for proper evaluation of the wound. Most blood loss usually occurs from superficial veins in the subdermal plexus, bleeding from which can be controlled with direct pressure in most cases. Bleeding from deeper or larger vessels may require clamping of the vessel and suture ligation with absorbable synthetic suture. Most vessels are small enough that 5-0 suture material can be utilized. In deeper wounds, superficial venous or arterial vessels may retract into the wound margin, making it impossible to visualize the tip of the vessel for clamping. In most cases, tension on the wound and appropriate retraction will allow visualization of the vessel, followed by careful clamping and suture ligation. Figure-of-eight or mattress sutures blindly placed are to be avoided whenever possible, both because of the potential for nerve damage and because such sutures obstruct blood flow more than a carefully placed suture ligature.

For abrasions or avulsions, chemical hemostasis with topical epinephrine, Gelfoam, Actifoam, Surgicel, or Oxycel may be utilized. While topical epinephrine does not work well on wounds to the subcutaneous tissue, it can be quite effective in superficial abrasions that continue to bleed. Epinephrine should never be used in end organs such as fingers, toes, ears, the penis, the vulva, or the tip of the nose. In some cases, electrocautery may be necessary to achieve hemostasis from blood vessels, but this should not be too widely or extensively applied, since tissue necrosis may occur. Small battery-powered, hand-held cautery units are available and may be utilized to produce coagulation in small vessels.

Facial, scalp, and body hair can act as a foreign body, which can increase the possibility of wound infection. Shaving of hair should be limited to those instances when the wound is obscured or extensive. Numerous studies show that shaving the hair allows considerable bacterial invasion and is associated with up to a 10-fold increase in infection rates when compared with clipping hair close to the skin. In addition, scalp hair can often be pulled back away from the wound edges by using antibiotic ointment or water-soluble lubricant. Obviously, hair should never be shaved from the eyebrows for any reason, since in a small but identifiable percentage of patients the eyebrow hair will not regrow.

Wound Preparation Agents

Over the years there has been considerable controversy concerning which wound cleansing solution is the most beneficial and least cytotoxic. A classic adage has been "Any solution that would not be placed in the eye should not be placed in an open wound." While the veracity of that adage is questionable, research has more clearly delineated several facts. First, agents such as isopropyl alcohol, hydrogen peroxide, chlorhexidine, and hexachlorophene cause injury to healthy tissues and retard wound healing. Similarly, deeply pigmented or concentrated solutions such as undiluted povidone-iodine stain tissues and thus make the identification of viable tissue difficult; they may also retard wound healing. Further, it is increasingly clear that no wound prep solution will sterilize a wound completely, nor should it be expected to. Instead, it is now accepted that proper solutions such as polaxamer 188, pluronic F-68, or dilute povidone-iodine solution can be used to clean the skin but should always be followed by normal saline irrigation under low pressure to remove it from the skin and from any contact with the wound itself.

Wound irrigation decreases the bacterial count and helps to remove macroscopic and microscopic foreign bodies, which helps decrease the risk of wound infection. Wound soaking is not effective and should not be utilized. Studies have shown that irrigation pressures of 5 to 8 psi are recommended for appropriate wound irrigation, which can be accomplished with forceful thumb pressure utilizing either a 30- or 60-mL syringe and a 19-gauge needle/catheter. Commercially available irrigation sets and splash shields are also effective at these pressure levels. However, sufficient pressures cannot be generated using either a bulb syringe or fluid directly from intravenous fluid bags. The following minimum wound irrigation guidelines are recommended.

- If the wound is relatively clean and the margins are sharp and intact, 50 mL/cm length and depth
- If the wound is contaminated or the wound margins are ragged or macerated, 100 mL/cm length and depth

Following appropriate skin prep and wound irrigation, the wound is covered with sterile 4 × 4's. Then, prior to wound repair, the provider's gloves should be changed.

Wound Debridement and Excision

Debridement is the removal of dead or contaminated tissue to provide better approximation and a better cosmetic result and to lessen the likelihood of infection. This should always been done without damaging underlying structures, and with the consideration that some areas, such as the face, lend themselves to debridement more readily than do areas where there is little redundant tissue, such as the hand or the fingers. In the vast majority of cases, debridement should be limited to no more than 1 to 2 mm from the wound edge and should be done in a cosmetic and anatomically appropriate fashion. Prior to sharp excision of the wound margins, the provider should always be aware of the skin tension patterns in the area and the underlying anatomy. Devitalized tissue should be removed from both the superficial and deep structures, which ensures that there is a discrete, viable margin for better wound approximation. In most cases in the UCC, the use of sharp iris scissors is sufficient for debridement and is effective at removing irregular skin margins or devitalized subcutaneous tissue.

Excision is a surgical method used to revise large, irregular wounds or to remove skin lesions. Excision uses sharp tissue dissection, most commonly with a no. 15 scalpel blade and/or iris scissors and Adson forceps (either with or without teeth, depending upon the preference of the provider). Figure 23-2 illustrates wound excision techniques in patients with irregularly shaped wounds. In general, the length of the elliptoid incision should be three times the width of the wound. In most cases, incisions with less than three times the width will result in a dog-ear deformity.

Appropriate methods of wound excision should be rigorously followed. With firm tension applied by the provider's fingers along the wound axis, a light "marking" incision is made into the dermis, taking into account the shape of the wound and skin tension lines. The skin should bleed only slightly after this "marking" incision is made. The purpose of the marking incision is to give the provider a path to follow in removing the tissue and to maintain appropriate tissue-plane relationships. Once this marking incision is made, the devitalized tissue inside the marking incision can be grasped with forceps and either iris scissors or a scalpel can be used to trim away devitalized tissue down to the subcutaneous fat. The resulting wound margins should be perpendicular to the skin's surface to allow for easier wound margin apposition and ensure the symmetry of the

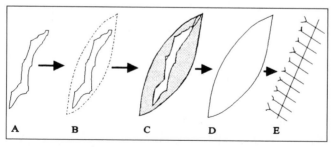

FIGURE 23-2 Wound excision technique. *A.* Untidy wound. *B.* Wound with light "marking" incision around margins. *C.* Shaded area represents tissue to be removed. *D.* "New" wound with fresh margins. *E.* Sutured wound. (From Mortiere MD: *Principles of Primary Wound Management—A Guide to the Fundamentals.* Clifton, VA: Clifton Publishing; 1996, with permission.)

wound. Following excision and debridement of the wound, it can be closed in a linear fashion for a better cosmetic and anatomic result.

Suture Material

The simplest classification of suture material is nonabsorbable versus absorbable, to which the category of cyanoacrylate polymers must be added. All suture materials, regardless of their composition, are foreign bodies that are being introduced into the wound, which means that suture bulk and mass should be kept to a minimum. The body reacts to varying degrees to these foreign bodies and attempts to degrade the suture by enzymatic, hydrolytic, and phagocytic activity.

Within the categories of absorbable and nonabsorbable suture, each suture varies by relative tissue reactivity, handling features, and composition. The absorbable sutures are further characterized by their absorption and tensile strength retention over time. All sutures in these two groups are either braided or monofilament materials (Table 23-2).

Any suture that is enzymatically degraded or hydrolyzed by tissue fluids is considered absorbable or temporary. The most commonly used absorbable suture materials are plain, catgut, fast-absorbing plain gut, chromic gut, polyglactin 910 (or polyglycolic acid), and polydioxanone. The first three materials are natural collagen substances while the others are synthetic absorbable materials.

Absorption times for absorbable suture materials vary from tissue to tissue and even from patient to patient. For example, a suture can lose its tensile strength quickly but be absorbed slowly, or vice versa. Table 23-3 summarizes the average total absorption and tensile strength times for commonly used absorbable sutures.

While no suture is totally unabsorbable, many sutures are so resistant to tissue enzymes that they become, in effect, permanent or semipermanent foreign bodies if they are not removed. When placed internally during surgery, these sutures are encapsulated by fibrous tissue instead of being digested and may remain present for many years following surgery. When used as percutaneous sutures, they must be removed to prevent unnecessary and unsightly scarring or foreign-body reaction. Nonabsorbable suture materials include nylon, polypropylene, polyester, and silk. Suture material is graded by government regulation on the basis of the size of the suture strand. Thus,

TABLE 23-2

SUTURE REACTIVITY (LEAST TO MOST REACTIVE)

Absorbable sutures	Nonabsorbable sutures
Polydioxanone (PDS)	Polypropylene (Prolene)
Polyglactin 910 (Vicryl)	Nylon
Polyglycolic acid (PGA)	Polyester
Poliglecaprone 25 (Monocryl)	Silk
Chromic gut	
Plain gut	
Fast-absorbing plain gut	

SOURCE: From Mortiere MD: *Principles of Primary Wound Management—A Guide to the Fundamentals.* Clifton, VA: Clifton Publishing; 1996, with permission.

TABLE 23-3

ABSORPTION AND RETENTION PROFILES FOR ABSORBABLE SUTURES

ABSORBABLE SUTURE TYPE	TOTAL ABSORPTION TIME (DAYS)[a]	RETENTION TIME OF 50% TENSILE STRENGTH (DAYS)
Plain gut:		
Fast-absorbing	21–42 days[b]	3–4 days[b]
Regular	70 days[b]	7–10 days[b]
Chromic gut	60–90 days[b]	21–30 days[b]
Polyglactin 910		
Coated Vicryl	90–120 days	21 days
Vicryl *RAPIDE*	42 days	5 days
Polydioxanone (PDS)	180 days	30 days

[a]Times are for implanted suture material.
[b]Absorption and tensile strength times are shortened in the presence of infection.
SOURCE: From Mortiere MD: *Principles of Primary Wound Management—A Guide to the Fundamentals.* Clifton, VA: Clifton Publishing; 1996, with permission.

zero (0) suture is much larger than 6-0 suture (which is shorthand for 000000). Table 23-4 summarizes the handling characteristics of suture materials and their appropriate uses. While a variety of types of surgical needles are available, conventional cutting or reverse cutting needles (which terms simply refer to the direction of the upward point of the needle's triangular tip) are utilized in the ED and UCC setting, whether the suture is absorbable or nonabsorbable and whether it is being placed in deep tissue or percutaneously.

BASIC SUTURING PRINCIPLES

Suturing is designed to accomplish four basic purposes:

- To achieve hemostasis
- To speed wound healing
- To decrease the risk of wound infection
- To afford the best possible cosmetic result

In most cases, all of these results can be accomplished by selecting the proper suture material and technique and conscientiously and skillfully employing certain basic principles. The fundamental tenets of wound care and suturing are:

1. The provider should work slowly and precisely, not accepting any result that would not be acceptable on a family member.
2. It is vital to prepare carefully and assure that there is good light into the wound.
3. The provider must make sure that all proper materials have been assembled ahead of time and that the suture tray is appropriate for the type of procedure to be done, including debridement and excision of the wound where appropriate.

TABLE 23-4

HANDLING CHARACTERISTICS AND USES FOR SUTURE MATERIALS

TYPE OF SUTURE MATERIAL	INDICATIONS FOR SUTURE USE	COMMENTS
Absorbables		Ideal for repair where infection potential is high.
Plain gut: Regular	Vascular ligation Intraoral laceration repair	Monofilament; bristle-like knot.
Fast-absorbing (FAPG)	Only for skin repair—*never* for internal tissues! Ideal for repair of facial wounds on children.	Rinse FAPG suture strand gently with saline before using; removes some preservative residue.
Chromic gut	Vascular ligation Muscle repair, dermal approximation	Same as above
Polyglactin 910/PGA		Used in tissues with low infection potential and wounds closed without tension.
Coated Vicryl	Muscle repair, dermal approximation	Braided, soft knots.
Vicryl *RAPIDE*	Skin and mucosal repair	Same as above but can be used for *nonfacial* skin closure.
Polydioxanone (PDS)	Muscle repair, dermal approximation	Same as above except monofilament. Bristle-like knot.
Nonabsorbables		Braided, very soft knot. Elicits moderate to high tissue reaction due to natural protein composition. Braid "wicks."
Silk	Intraoral lacerations, repair of eyelid laceration at gray line	
Polyester	Same as above	Same as above for handling. Less tissue reaction because synthetic material.
Nylon	Primarily for percutaneous (skin) closure	Black monofilament. Bristle-like knot. Relatively inert.
Polypropylene (Prolene)	Primarily for percutaneous (skin) closure—also for tendon repair	Blue or clear monofilament. Bristle-like knot. Ideal for dark-haired or skin areas. Inert.

SOURCE: From Mortiere MD: *Principles of Primary Wound Management—A Guide to the Fundamentals.* Clifton, VA: Clifton Publishing; 1996, with permission.

4. All layers that have been lacerated are repaired individually, such as the galea, the muscle fascia, the dermis, and the skin.

5. In closing the skin, it is important to evert the wound edges (Fig. 23-3) and to avoid wound edge inversion at all costs, as wound retraction will produce a larger, depressed scar.

6. The rule is "Approximate—do not strangulate." The tissue margins should touch each other gently. Avoid tying sutures too tightly.

7. Suturing can either be carried from one end to the other or the "halving" technique, by placing a suture in the middle of the wound to decrease wound tension during closure, can be used.

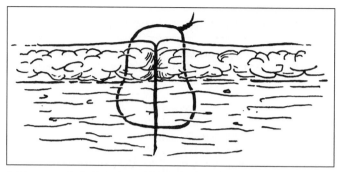

FIGURE 23-3   A single interrupted percutaneous suture with everted edges. [From Martin J, Herfel R: Methods for wound closure, in Tintinalli JE, Kelen GD, Stapczynski JS (eds): *Emergency Medicine: A Comprehensive Study Guide,* 5th ed. New York: McGraw-Hill; 2000, with permission.]

8. The most gentle tissue handling technique possible should always be used, depending upon the location and friability of the tissue.
9. The number of suture needle punctures through the skin with each bite should be kept to a minimum; the suture should be placed correctly the first time.
10. Suture types and sizes appropriate to the tissue must be used (see Table 23-5).
11. Each suture should be placed with the needle point perpendicular to the skin's surface.
12. The arc of the needle should be followed and, with gentle pressure on the needle holder, the needle is allowed to drive itself through the tissue.
13. In most cases, the suture should be advanced halfway through the wound, removed with smooth Adson forceps, and guided through the second half of the wound in a separate bite, observing appropriate tissue planes and suture angles.
14. Whether tied by hand or using an instrument tie, secure flat, square knots should be tied. Knot security and tension should be checked with each suture.
15. The knots must be pulled to the side of the wound margin to adjust for wound eversion.
16. The number of sutures must be kept to a minimum while at the same time assuring that there are no gaps or dog ears in the wound.
17. *The provider must know his or her limitations and should not hesitate to refer patients, even if the the wound closure has been completed. If it looks bad now, it will look worse later.*

As indicated above, tissue should be closed in layers in most instances. While some lacerations involve only the skin itself and minimal soft tissue, if soft tissue has been involved to a substantial degree, it should be closed appropriately and anatomically, usually with "buried" absorbable sutures tied at the bottom of the wound (Fig. 23-4). The placement of intradermal and subcutaneous sutures allows for more rapid wound healing and places less tension on the skin's surface and the collagen-rich dermis.

There are several ways to achieve appropriate wound edge eversion. First, the needle should be placed near one wound margin, entering the skin's surface at a perpendicular angle through the skin and taking more tissue "bite" at the bottom of the suture path than

TABLE 23-5

RECOMMENDED CLOSURE GUIDELINES BY ANATOMIC LOCATION AND TISSUE LAYER

ANATOMIC WOUND LOCATION	TISSUE LAYER TO BE SUTURED	SUTURE MATERIAL RECOMMENDATION	SUTURE TECHNIQUE
Face and neck	Skin	6-0 FAPG,[a] nylon, polypropylene	Simple
	Dermis	6-0, 5-0 Vicryl, PDS	Inverted
	Muscle	4-0, 5-0 Vicryl, PDS	Simple
	Perichondrium	6-0 Vicryl	Simple
Mouth	Tongue	4-0, 5-0 Vicryl, chromic gut	Simple, inverted
	Mucosa	Same as above	Simple, inverted
Scalp	Skin	4-0 Nylon, polypropylene	Simple
	Dermis	4-0 Vicryl, PDS	Inverted
	Muscle, galea	3-0, 4-0 Vicryl, PDS	Simple
Arms and legs except hands and feet	Skin	4-0, 5-0 Nylon, polypropylene	Simple, mattress
	Dermis	4-0, 5-0 Vicryl, PDS	Inverted
	Fascia	3-0, 4-0 Vicryl, PDS	Simple
Hand	Skin	5-0 Nylon, polypropylene	Simple
	Nail bed	6-0 Vicryl	Simple
	Dermis	5-0 Vicryl; nothing in fingers	Inverted
Foot	Skin, dorsum	4-0, 5-0 Nylon, polypropylene	Simple, mattress
	Sole	4-0, 5-0 Nylon, polypropylene	Simple
	Nailbed	6-0 Vicryl	Simple
	Dermis	5-0 Vicryl; nothing in toes	Inverted

[a]FAPG = fast-absorbing plain gut.
KEY: Simple = simple interrupted loop suture; inverted = inverted loop (intradermal) suture; mattress = horizontal or vertical mattress suture.
SOURCE: From Mortiere MD: *Principles of Primary Wound Management—A Guide to the Fundamentals.* Clifton, VA: Clifton Publishing; 1996, with permission.

at the top. The suture needle should then be reloaded and placed in the opposite wound margin at the same tissue level and with the same depth of bite as on the previous side. When the suture is gently tied, the wound margins should gently evert, which produces less scarring (see Fig. 23-3). The natural process of wound healing is for the wound to retract slightly, which is the reason the wound edges should be minimally everted.

In areas of the body where there is excess redundant tissue—as the elbow, the dorsum of the hand, the foot, or web spaces—either vertical or horizontal mattress sutures can be placed. The technique of those sutures is discussed below. The "tails" of percutaneous sutures should be left long enough to allow ease of grasping when suture

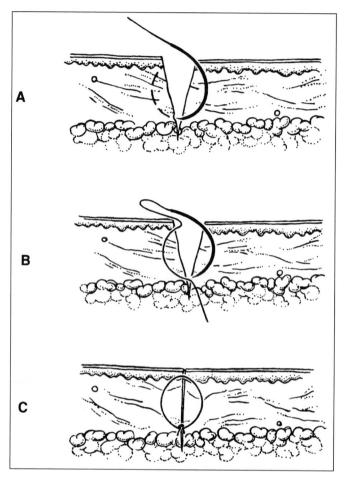

FIGURE 23-4   Dermal suture. *A.* Entry is at base of wound on one side and exit at the dermal-epidermal junction. *B.* Entry on the opposite side is at the dermal-epidermal junction with exit at the base. *C.* The tied loop has the knot buried in the wound away from the skin surface. [From Martin J, Herfel R: Methods for wound closure, in Tintinalli JE, Kelen GD, Stapczynski JS (eds): *Emergency Medicine: A Comprehensive Study Guide,* 5th ed. New York: McGraw-Hill; 2000, with permission.]

removal occurs but no longer than about 1 to 2 cm. With absorbable subcutaneous sutures, minimal tails should be left so there is less foreign body in the wound.

SPECIFIC SUTURING TECHNIQUES

Simple Interrupted Dermal Sutures

For most simple lacerations including facial lacerations, the wound can be adequately closed with interrupted dermal sutures. The distance between sutures varies by location on the body and may be as short as 1 to 2 mm for facial lacerations, and up to 5 to 10 mm in areas such as the scalp, where a "looser" closure allows for appropriate wound drainage. In general, lacerations on an extremity fall between and require sutures every 3 to 7 mm for appropriate cosmetic, hemostatic, and tension reasons. So-called running or continuous sutures can be utilized in cases where adequate closure can be obtained and there is a small enough wound tension to make breakage of the continuous suture unlikely. In addition, continuous sutures should be utilized only with those who are comfortable with the cosmetic results obtainable with this procedure, which requires somewhat more experience to execute proficiently. It should be reiterated that this technique should be used only for extremely clean wounds in which the chances of infection are minimal. In placing continuous sutures, care should be taken that tension is distributed evenly and that the final knot is not placed too tightly so that the tissue is not strangulated instead of approximated. In areas of the body where hemostasis is important, a locking running suture technique can be utilized (Fig. 23-5).

Subcuticular Sutures

Subcuticular or continuous dermal sutures are often used in areas where wounds are subjected to strong skin tensions, in patients prone to keloid formation, or in those children to whom suture removal is extremely frightening. It is a particularly effective technique for facial lacerations but should be utilized only by those who are extremely proficient and comfortable in its use. Subcuticular sutures begin as an interrupted dermal stitch with the knot buried in the subcutaneous tissue, after which the free end of the knot is cut and the suture is used as a continuous closure passed horizontally through the superficial dermis. This suture is usually placed as an absorbable suture and may be augmented with several reinforcing interrupted dermal absorbable sutures. Again, this technique requires some experience and should be utilized only by those who are proficient and comfortable in its use.

Mattress Sutures

There are two types of mattress sutures, vertical and horizontal, each of which provides anatomical eversion of the tissue when correctly executed. Mattress sutures are ideal for surfaces in which there is excess or redundant tissue or areas where there is particular stress on the laceration, as over the kneecap. Mattress sutures should *never* be used on

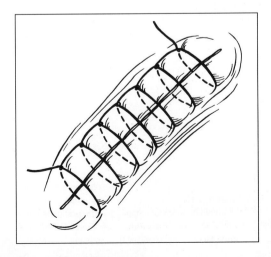

FIGURE 23-5 Running lock suture. **The suture helps reduce wound tension and may be valuable where hemostasis is important. It differs from a simple running suture in that a needle is passed back through each horizontal stitch, thereby "locking" the suture in place. Care should be taken in placing the suture to avoid undue tension.** [From Martin J, Herfel R: Methods for wound closure, in Tintinalli JE, Kelen GD, Stapczynski JS (eds): *Emergency Medicine: A Comprehensive Study Guide*, 5th ed. New York: McGraw-Hill; 2000, with permission.]

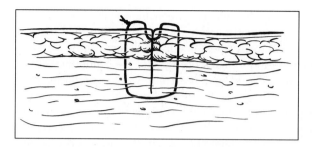

FIGURE 23-6 Vertical mattress suture. [From Martin J, Herfel R: Methods for wound closure, in Tintinalli JE, Kelen GD, Stapczynski JS (eds): *Emergency Medicine: A Comprehensive Study Guide,* 5th ed. New York: McGraw-Hill; 2000, with permission.]

the face for any reason. Vertical mattress sutures are placed in a single location on the skin and incorporate an initial pass through the skin, dermis, and subcutaneous layers, which is repeated on the opposite side. A second pass of the suture catches the superficial layer of the skin on each side, resulting in anatomic closure and good wound eversion (Fig. 23-6). Care must be taken not to tie vertical mattress sutures too tightly, as this may strangulate the tissue and overevert the wound margins. Rather, anatomic eversion should be easily attainable with this technique if properly utilized. The first bite is usually a large one, starting approximately 1 to 1.5 cm away from the wound edge and crossing through the wound at an equal distance on the opposite side. A shallow (2- to 3-mm) bite is taken at the epidermal/dermal edge on each side of the wound.

Horizontal mattress sutures can be more rapidly placed and in general achieve better wound eversion than vertical mattress sutures. The technique is faster because it covers more linear distance in a shorter period of time and can be helpful in areas where there is dramatically increased skin tension, including areas over joints or in web spaces. With horizontal mattress sutures, the individual sutures must also be tied loosely to avoid strangulation of the tissue. The first stitch is similar to a simple interrupted suture, but instead of tying the suture, a second bite is taken approximately 5 mm adjacent to the first exit on the same side and directed back toward the initial side, maintaining an anatomic position of similarity with regard to the opposite side (Fig. 23-7).

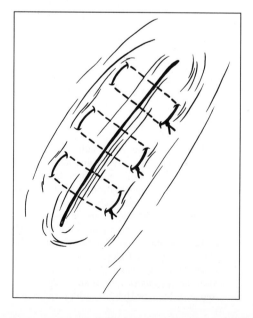

FIGURE 23-7 Horizontal mattress suture. [From Martin J, Herfel R: Methods for wound closure, in Tintinalli JE, Kelen GD, Stapczynski JS (eds): *Emergency Medicine: A Comprehensive Study Guide,* 5th ed. New York: McGraw-Hill; 2000, with permission.]

Purse-String Sutures

Purse-string sutures can be helpful to approximate multiple flap tips created in stellate wounds. They may be placed either as absorbable sutures buried in the subcutaneous tissue or as partially buried absorbable sutures that can later be removed. The purse-string suture is helpful in maintaining blood supply and gaining initial approximation of wound margins, which can be augmented with interrupted dermal stitches to provide cosmetic closure (Fig. 23-8).

Cyanoacrylate Tissue Adhesive Closure

Cyanoacrylate tissue adhesives have been widely utilized in Europe and in Canada for a number of years and have more recently been approved for use in the United States. The most commonly used adhesive, Dermabond (2-octylcyanoacrylate), is produced by Ethicon Inc. This tissue adhesive, like superglue, polymerizes rapidly when applied to the skin and allowed to bond. However, all cyanoacrylate products create an intense inflammatory reaction when exposed to any tissue below the skin's surface; they should therefore never be applied within wounds. They also cannot be used on mucous membranes or mucosal surfaces, on infected areas, on wounds that are wet or exposed to body fluids, in areas with dense hair, or at any location near the eye. However, when they are used on appropriately selected surfaces, cosmetic results have been similar to those obtained when experienced providers have used interrupted dermal or subcuticular skin closures.

In general, results are best when the wound edges are clean and sharp and when the closure occurs on nonmobile areas with little skin tension. In general, if a wound is wider than 5 to 10 mm prior to closure, use of tissue adhesives may be less successful.

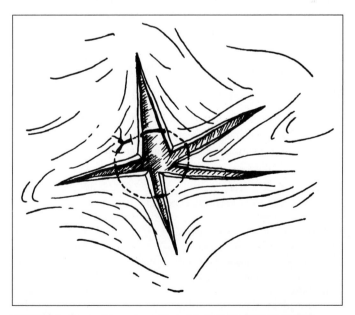

FIGURE 23-8 Purse-string suture. [From Martin J, Herfel R: Methods for wound closure, in Tintinalli JE, Kelen GD, Stapczynski JS (eds): *Emergency Medicine: A Comprehensive Study Guide,* 5th ed. New York: McGraw-Hill; 2000, with permission.]

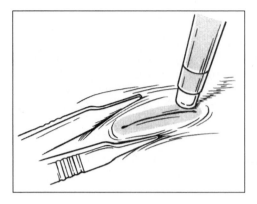

FIGURE 23-9 Tissue adhesives are applied in several light coats over the wound, carefully avoiding entry of the adhesive into the wound. [From Martin J, Herfel R: Methods for wound closure, in Tintinalli JE, Kelen GD, Stapczynski JS (eds): *Emergency Medicine: A Comprehensive Study Guide,* 5th ed. New York: McGraw-Hill; 2000, with permission.]

Dermabond is available as a single-use vial with an applicator tip, which is violet in color to make it visible during the process of application. The included instructions are very clear, but the wound should be cleaned and hemostasis obtained before the tissue adhesive is placed, although complete absolute dryness is not required. The wound should be held together and its edges slightly everted with tissue forceps, recognizing the principles of wound closure mentioned previously (Fig. 23-9). The adhesive is applied approximately 5 mm beyond the wound margins, taking care to be sure that it is not applied to the subcutaneous tissue itself; three to four layers should be applied on each side. The wound edges are held together for about 1 to 2 min after the last adhesive application. Once the adhesive has dried, it should not be covered with ointment, bandages, or dressing and the patient should be instructed not to use such items. The adhesive spontaneously exfoliates in 5 to 10 days, but the patient should be instructed to return immediately if the wound reopens.

SPECIAL CONSIDERATIONS IN WOUND CLOSURE

Wounds That Require Consultation

Table 23-6 lists wounds that should be considered for referral for consultation, since specialty care is usually indicated. This includes wounds involving an open fracture or joint space; lacerations of the tarsal plate of the eyelid or lacrimal duct; amputations;

TABLE 23-6

WOUNDS THAT REQUIRE CONSULTATION

Wounds involving an open fracture	Wounds that involve blood vessels
Wounds involving a joint space	Wounds in which a significant loss of
Lacerations of the tarsal plate of the eyelid	epidermis has occurred
Lacerations of the lacrimal duct	Wounds that require substantial wound
Amputations	revision for anatomic closure
Wounds with associated loss of function	Any facial laceration with which the provider
Wounds that involve tendons	is uncomfortable
Wounds that involve nerves	

wounds with associated loss of function; wounds that involve tendons, nerves, or blood vessels; wounds in which a significant loss of epidermis has occurred; wounds that require substantial wound revision for anatomic closure; and any facial laceration with which the provider is uncomfortable. In all of these cases, referral to the appropriate on-call physician or to the nearest ED should be arranged and physician-to-physician contact established regarding the reasons for the consultation.

Facial Wounds

Closure of facial wounds depends upon the experience and proficiency of the provider. However, most simple, superficial facial lacerations can easily be closed using appropriate suture material (6-0), absorbable or nonabsorbable suture, or cyanoacrylate adhesive when appropriate. Wounds that require debridement and excision of wound margins up to approximately 5 mm of excision and not crossing major anatomic landmarks can usually be closed in the UCC setting if the provider is comfortable with such procedures. Wounds involving periorbital tissues, particularly the lacrimal duct, and penetrating wounds to the face are usually referred for appropriate subspecialty closure and follow-up.

Lip Lacerations

Lacerations extending across the vermilion cutaneous border of the lip should be carefully and accurately repaired but can usually be handled in the UCC setting as long as the provider is experienced and proficient in such closure. Meticulous technique must be utilized to make sure that precise alignment of the vermilion border occurs, because of the ease of recognition of a nonanatomic closure when scarring occurs. For those who are experienced at performing infraorbital or mental nerve blocks, these techniques can be utilized to avoid distortion of the tissue. However, small wounds to the lip can still be locally infiltrated assuming that they are handled in a symmetrical fashion. Excision of the wound at the vermilion border should be avoided whenever possible. If the wound edge is ragged or avulsed along this border, the patient should be referred for plastic surgical closure.

The first step of repair for vermilion border lacerations is to place a single nonabsorbable suture exactly across the margins of the vermilion border itself to obtain precise anatomic alignment of this critical area. If the initial suture placement does not result in precise alignment, the suture should be removed and replaced with an accurate suture. The dermis and skin should then be sutured in the usual cosmetic fashion with interrupted sutures (Fig. 23-10). Lacerations to the mucosal (red) tissue of the lip should be closed with a fast-absorbing 6-0 suture, which is much more comfortable for the patient. The "tails" of these knots should be cut as short as possible, as long "tails" in or near the mouth can be very annoying to the patient.

Tongue Lacerations

Small tongue lacerations and puncture wounds to the tongue bleed profusely but do not usually require sutures. They heal rapidly and extremely well without surgical intervention; patients should be instructed to rinse or swab the tongue wound several times a day

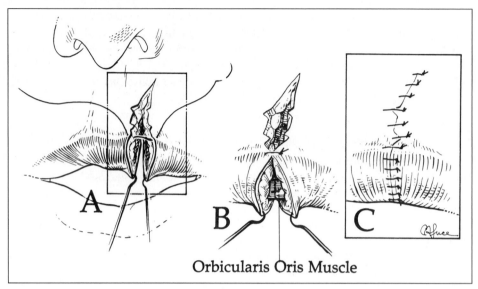

FIGURE 23-10   Closure of torn upper lip.   [From Martin J, Herfel R: Methods for wound closure, in Tintinalli JE, Kelen GD, Stapczynski JS (eds): *Emergency Medicine: A Comprehensive Study Guide,* 5th ed. New York: McGraw-Hill; 2000, with permission.]

with a half-strength hydrogen peroxide solution. Patients should also be instructed to avoid highly acidic or salty foods, as they will irritate the wound and produce an inflammatory reaction.

Larger tongue lacerations often need to be sutured primarily to control hemostasis and for the comfort of the patient. In such cases, absorbable material of either 4-0 or 5-0 size should be utilized and, whenever possible, the knots should be buried as opposed to being exposed. All tongue lacerations should be closed in a fairly loose fashion to allow for drainage.

Scalp Lacerations

In addition to requiring an adequate examination for a closed head injury and foreign bodies, scalp lacerations pose unique issues. Until the clinician proves otherwise through physical examination and appropriate radiographic studies, where indicated, it must be assumed that a foreign body is present and that a closed head injury has occurred with any scalp laceration. Once it is clear that there is no foreign body in the wound and there have been no penetrating injuries, the extent of injury should be documented after careful anesthesia, including making sure that there is no galeal laceration. If a galeal laceration is found, the galea and any superficial muscles should be sutured with absorbable sutures, followed by closure of the subcutaneous tissue and the skin itself.

In patients with dark hair, it is almost always preferable to close the scalp with blue polypropylene sutures, so that they can be easily identified when suture removal occurs. In some UCCs, staples are utilized for closure of scalp lacerations, as these are capable of providing both hemostasis and adequate anatomic closure. When the scalp is sutured, this is the one area of the body where closing the wound somewhat more tightly to achieve hemostasis is acceptable, particularly if the scalp is lacerated in areas that are normally covered by skin. This does not mean that anatomic closure and wound eversion are not necessary but simply that somewhat more tight knots may be acceptable in this area for hemostasis.

Atrophic Skin Wounds—Elderly Patients

In many patients with atrophic skin, including elderly patients and those on chronic steroid therapy, the skin does not have sufficient tensile strength to allow for adequate repair of the laceration with sutures or tissue adhesives. An alternate method of treatment for these skin lacerations involves application of tincture of benzoin in parallel strips along the axis of the laceration. Once the benzoin has become "tacky," Steri-Strips can be applied across the wound to help provide skin closure. If necessary, after the Steri-Strips have been applied, the wound may be sutured, with each suture passing through the Steri-Strips themselves, which reinforces the edges and often prevents tearing of thin skin. Alternate methods of closing wounds in atrophic skin include placing pledgets or skin bolsters through the sutures to help reinforce the skin. However, closure with Steri-Strips with or without sutures is usually obtainable in most cases.

Care after Wound Closure

Regardless of the method of wound closure chosen, the wound should be kept sterile; in cases where laceration repair has occurred, a dressing will usually be applied. Wound dressing should not be occlusive and should never compromise circulation or the wound's ability to drain. Studies from the plastic surgical literature have shown that a slightly moist wound heals better than a completely dry one. However, heavy application of ointment followed by multiple layers of nonadhering gauze may actually produce wound maceration. Maceration, or the retention of excessive moisture on and in the skin, can lead to the tracking of bacteria into the wound, wound dehiscence, and wound infection. The following general principles apply to nonfacial wound dressings, which should consist of three layers:

- The contact layer—a single thickness of xeroform, adaptic, etc.
- The absorbent layer—4 × 4's, 2 × 2's, or other appropriate material
- The outer layer or protective layer—consisting of roll gauze, tube gauze, Ace wrap, splint, etc.

Facial wounds closed with sutures generally do not require bulky dressings but can be covered with an antibacterial ointment and a sterile bandage. If there is significant likelihood of hematoma formation, a light pressure dressing can be used for 24 h but should be checked after that time.

General guidelines for follow-up care include keeping the sutured area elevated as much as possible, placing cold compresses on the area to help reduce swelling and bleeding, and maintaining appropriate wound cleanliness. Suture removal depends upon the type and location of the injury but varies from 3 to 5 days for cosmetic facial lacerations to 12 to 14 days for sutures placed over lower extremities in areas of high tension, as over the knee joint or the foot.

LOCAL ANESTHETICS AND NERVE BLOCKS

Local anesthetics are divided into two classes: the esters and the amides. Local anesthetics of the amide linkage group are used almost exclusively; however, in some cases, institutions may continue to use the ester-linked local anesthetic agents. Amides include lidocaine hydrochloride, bupivacaine hydrochloride, and mepivacaine hydrochloride. Ester-type local anesthetics include procaine hydrochloride and chloroprocaine hydrochloride, but these agents are rarely used in UCC settings. All local anesthetics prevent the conduction and generation of nerve impulses by preventing a large transient increase in the permeability of nerve cell membranes of sodium ions. Pain sensation is usually the first to disappear, followed by temperature perception, deep pressure sensation, and rarely motor activity. Regression or "wearing off" of the anesthetic agent occurs in the reverse order.

Prior to administration of any anesthetic agent, the patient should be carefully questioned regarding allergies to these agents. Allergic reactions to the amide anesthetics are usually linked to a preservative, methylparaben, which is utilized in multiple-dose vials. Methylparaben-free single-dose vials are available for patients with such allergies and should be kept at all UCCs. However, allergic reactions to amide anethetics are extremely rare and usually result from inadvertent intravascular injection of the drug or overdosage. Local reactions to the agent may include urticaria or pruritus.

The most commonly used agent for local or field blocks is lidocaine hydrochloride, which is available in 0.5, 1, and 2% solutions with or without epinephrine. In most cases, 1% lidocaine is adequate for wound preparation, irrigation, debridement, and closure. In cases where more prolonged anesthesia may be necessary, other agents such as mepivacaine or bupivacaine can be utilized. The use of epinephrine with lidocaine decreases the rate at which the anesthetic is absorbed and may improve hemostasis through vasoconstriction. This hemostatic action takes about 10 min to occur. No anesthetic agent with epinephrine should be administered to the digits, the tip of the nose, the penis, or any area with end arteries or poor collateral circulation. Some recent clinical studies have looked at utilizing buffering agents such as sodium bicarbonate (1 meq/mL) to reduce the pain of injection of local anesthetic agents. The addition of 1 mL of sodium bicarbonate to 10 mL of lidocaine or mepivacaine has been shown to be effective in reducing the patient's pain perception; this is attributable to the buffering of the acidic anesthetic solution (from a pH of 6.5 to a more neutral pH of 7.35). However, buffering does decrease the stability of the anesthetic agent and reduces its shelf life to about 72 h.

There are some alternative local anesthetic agents, including diphenhydramine hydrochloride, which may be injected into the wound after dilution of 1 mL of diphenhydramine with 4 mL of normal saline.

Topical anesthetic agents such as TAC (an acronym for tetracaine, adrenaline, and cocaine) have been shown to be as effective as infiltration anesthesia for facial lacerations. The solution or gel is applied firmly to the wound and the surrounding skin for approximately 20 min, with achievement of anesthesia evidenced by blanching of the surrounding skin. If anesthesia is incomplete or there is not adequate blanching, TAC can be augmented by the use of a local anesthetic.

In many UCCs, the difficulty of storing a cocaine-containing derivative has prevented its widespread use. In such settings, alternative topical anesthetic agents include

LET [which stands for lidocaine (4%), epinephrine (0.1%, 1:1000), and tetracaine (0.5%)]. In addition, EMLA cream can also be utilized for painful procedures, but this agent requires up to 1 h to take effect and should not be used in open wounds, which renders it far less practical in the UCC setting.

NERVE BLOCK ANESTHESIA

Peripheral nerve blocks can be of advantageous use in the UCC environment but are usually utilized primarily for extremity lacerations. By far the most common nerve block used in the UCC is the digital nerve block. Digital nerve blocks provide excellent anesthesia for fingers and toes and have an extremely rapid onset of action. They are most commonly used for laceration repair of the hands or toes as well as for incision and drainage of paronychia or nail removal. The technique for the digital nerve block involves using a 27- or 30-gauge needle inserted through the skin in the web spaces of the affected finger and injecting approximately 1 mL of 1% lidocaine or 0.5% bupivacaine superficially in the subcutaneous tissue. The injection should include both the dorsal and volar surfaces of the extensor tendon to make sure that both branches of the nerve are blocked. In general, 1 mL of the anesthetic solution should be injected in each of the dorsal and volar aspects. The technique is then repeated on the opposite web space to ensure complete anesthesia of the digit.

Since the thumb is innervated by branches of both the radial and the median nerves, each of those nerves must be blocked separately in order to accomplish a complete thumb block. The superficial branch of the radial nerve is blocked by drawing 3 mL of 2% lidocaine or mepivacaine without epinephrine into a syringe. A 27-gauge 1¼-in. needle should be used to subcutaneously inject over the distal radius at the level of the distal wrist crease, with a subcutaneous wheal of anesthetic extended over the dorsum of the wrist toward the extensor carpi radialis longus and brevis tendons. Extreme care should be taken to be sure that no bolus of anesthetic is injected intravascularly into the artery. The volar aspects of the thumb and distal phalanx are innervated by the recurrent branch of the median nerve, which is blocked by using 3 mL of 2% lidocaine and a 27-gauge, ½-in. needle, with the anesthetic placed on either side of the thumb at the level of the metacarpophalangeal crease. It is important to remember that the digital nerves of the thumb lie more volarly and closer together than those in the fingers. Additional anesthetic blocks that are sometimes used include blocks of the median nerve, the radial nerve, and various facial nerves. However, these are less commonly used in the UCC setting; interested readers are referred to texts in emergency medicine to familiarize themselves with these agents and procedures.

DIFFERENTIAL DIAGNOSIS OF COMMON PRESENTING COMPLAINTS

Tanise I. Edwards

The complaints listed in the following section represent a group of frequently encountered symptoms seen in the urgent care setting. These are complaints with extensive differentials, from immediate life-threatening conditions to benign disease entities. The charts are designed to help formulate a differential for patients presenting with the selected complaint. The diagnoses are listed by organ system. In evaluating patients who present with one of the listed complaints, the history, physical examination, and ancillary studies ordered should be directed toward determining a definitive diagnosis. If a definitive diagnosis cannot be made, then the evaluation must rule out potentially life-threatening conditions and those conditions requiring acute intervention. When any of the acute diagnoses cannot be reasonably eliminated by history or physical examination, further evaluation of the patient is needed. This additional evaluation may require further urgent care assessment and testing, specialty consultation (including emergency department transfer for more extensive evaluation), or possible hospital admission. In other words, if the patient is to be discharged home, any of the life-threatening conditions listed in the differential should have been either appropriately treated and triaged or ruled out as a possible cause for the patient's complaint. Evaluating patients using this type of approach, along with appropriate supporting chart documentation, can markedly decrease the liability associated with providing episodic care.

ABDOMINAL PAIN

Gastrointestinal

- Appendicitis
- Pancreatitis
- Peritonitis
- Biliary disease
    - Cholangitis
    - Biliary colic
    - Acute cholecystitis
- Splenic disease (rupture, infarct, enlargement)
- Diverticulitis
- Crohn's disease
- Bowel obstruction
- Peptic ulcer disease
- Bowel infarction
- Perforated viscus (ulcer, intestinal, etc.)
- Mesenteric adenitis
- Gastritis
- Gastroenteritis
- Liver disease (hepatitis, abscess, enlargement)
- Ulcerative colitis
- Irritable bowel
- Volvulus
- Hernia
- Psoas abscess
- Intussusception
- Constipation

Gynecologic

- Ectopic pregnancy
- Pelvic inflammatory disease
- Ovarian cyst
- Mittelschmerz
- Ovarian torsion
- Endometriosis
- Spontaneous abortion

Cardiovascular

- Cardiac ischemia
- Acute myocardial infarction
- Aortic aneurysm
- Mesenteric ischemia/thrombosis

Genitourinary

- Renal colic
- Urinary tract infection
- Testicular torsion
- Seminal vesiculitis
- Prostatitis

Other

- Abdominal wall musculature
- Metabolic (diabetic ketoacidosis, etc.)
- Sickle cell disease
- Poisoning (lead)
- Henoch-Schönlein purpura
- Strep throat
- Scorpion envenomation

Pulmonary

- Pneumonia
- Pleural effusion

BACK PAIN

Musculoskeletal

- Fractures
- Muscle strain
- Arthritis (spinal, hip)
- Bone disease (ankylosing spondylitis, sarcoma, etc.)
- Osteomyelitis
- Tumor (bony)
- Osteoporosis

Gynecologic

- Ectopic pregnancy
- Dysmenorrhea
- Mittelschmertz
- Endometriosis
- Pelvic inflammatory disease

Cardiovascular

- Abdominal aortic aneurysm
- Dissecting thoracic aneurysm
- Acute myocardial infarction
- Arteriovenous malformation

Renal

- Renal calculi
- Pyelonephritis
- Prostatitis
- Tumor

Neurologic

- Herniated disk
- Spinal cord disease
- Spinal stenosis
- Tumor (neural)

Gastrointestinal

- Peptic ulcer disease
- Pancreatitis
- Cholecystitis

Pulmonary

- Pneumonia
- Pneumothorax

Other

- Herpes zoster
- Paget's disease
- Infectious (abscess, tuberculosis, disk-space infection, meningitis)
- Lymphoma
- Sickle cell disease
- Hyperparathyroidism

CHEST PAIN

Cardiac

- Acute myocardial infarction
- Angina (stable, unstable, variant)
- Aortic dissection
- Pericarditis
- Valvular disease
  - Aortic stenosis
  - Hypertrophic cardiomyopathy
  - Mitral valve prolapse
- Pulmonary hypertension
- Myocarditis

Gastrointestinal

- Pancreatitis
- Biliary disease
- Peptic ulcer disease
- Gastroesophageal reflux disease/dyspepsia
- Esophageal spasm
- Esophageal tears/perforation

Other

- Herpes zoster
- Tumor
- Nonspecific
- Pyschogenic (anxiety/stress)

Pulmonary

- Bronchitis
- Pneumonia
- Pneumothorax
- Tracheobronchitis
- Pneumomediastinum
- Pleurisy
- Tumor
- Pulmonary embolism

Musculoskeletal

- Costochondritis
- Arthritis (spine, shoulder)
- Muscular strain
- Fractures
- Thoracic outlet syndrome
- Degenerative disk disease

DIZZINESS AND VERTIGO

Otologic

- Otitis media (acute, serous, chronic)
- Labyrinthitis
- Ménière's disease
- Acoustic neuroma
- Foreign body
- Benign positional vertigo
- Vestibular neuronitis
- Cholesteatoma
- Perilymphatic
- Trauma

Neurologic

- Head injury
- Encephalitis
- Malignancy
- Abscess

Vascular

- Brainstem infarct
- Cerebellar infarct/hemorrhage
- Vertebrobasilar insufficiency

Miscellaneous

- Orthostatic hypotension
- Medication induced
- Motion sickness
- Temporomandibular joint dysfunction
- Diabetes
- Hypertension
- Toxins
- Psychogenic

DYSPNEA

Pulmonary

- Asthma
- Chronic obstructive pulmonary disease (COPD)
- Pneumonia
- Bronchitis
- Pneumothorax
- Aspiration
- Toxic exposure
- Pulmonary effusion
- Tumor
- Bronchiolitis (in children)
- Foreign body
- Croup

Ear/Nose/Throat

- Angioedema
- Epiglottitis
- Foreign body

Metabolic

- Acidosis (including diabetic keto-acidosis)
- Salicylates
- Toxins

Cardiac

- Congestive heart failure
- Pulmonary edema
- Cardiac ischemia
- Arrhythmias
- Emboli
- Tamponade

Other

- Anaphylaxis
- Sepsis
- Hyperthyroidism
- Anemia
- Obesity
- Myasthenia gravis
- Hyperventilation
- Guillain-Barré syndrome
- Sickle cell disease
- Sarcoidosis
- Tick paralysis

HEADACHE

Vascular

- Migraine
- Cluster headache
- Subarachnoid hemorrhage
- Hematoma (subdural, epidural, cerebellar)
- Temporal arteritis
- Hypertensive crisis

Other

- Fever
- Muscle tension
- Arthritis
- Glaucoma
- Optic neuritis
- Temporomandibular joint dysfunction
- Hypoglycemia
- Post–lumbar puncture
- Postconcussion
- Drug-induced
- Hypoxia
- Carbon monoxide exposure
- Monosodium glutamate
- Preeclampsia

Infectious

- Meningitis (viral, bacterial)
- Abscess
- Encephalitis
- Sinusitis
- Dental abscess

Neurologic

- Trigeminal neuralgia
- Tumor
- Pseudotumor cerebri

HYPOTENSION

Cardiac

- Acute myocardial infarction
- Dysrhythmia (tachy- or bradyarrhythmia)
- Cardiac tamponade

Gastrointestinal

- Dehydration
- GI bleed
- Pancreatitis (hemorrhagic)
- Liver failure

Trauma

- Splenic injury
- Fractures (femur, pelvis)
- Lacerations (major)
- Intraabdominal injury
- Hemothorax
- Retroperitoneal injury
- Myocardial contusion

Vascular

- Aneurysm (ruptured, leaking, dissecting)
- Arteriovenous malformation
- Epistaxis

Pulmonary

- Pneumothorax (tension)
- Pulmonary embolism

Genitourinary

- Vaginal bleeding
- Ruptured ectopic pregnancy
- Ruptured ovarian cyst
- Abruptio placentae

Other

- Adrenal insufficiency
- Anaphylaxis
- Heat stroke
- Sepsis
- Poor oral intake
- Anemia
- Hypothermia
- Toxins
- Medications

SYNCOPE

Cardiac

- Arrhythmia (brady- or tachyarrhythmia)
- Aortic stenosis
- Mitral regurgitation
- Hypertrophic cardiomyopathy
- Subclavian steal syndrome
- Left atrial myxoma

Neurologic

- Epilepsy

Other

- Vasovagal
- Micturition
- Postprandial
- Postdefecation
- Orthostatic
- Hypovolemia (dehydration, blood loss, ectopic pregnancy, etc.)
- Pulmonary embolism
- Medication (vasodilators, antiarrhythmic agents)
- Hypoglycemia
- Hyperventilation

VAGINAL BLEEDING

Non-Pregnancy-Related

- Menstruation
- Abnormal menstrual bleeding
- Infection (vaginitis, cervicitis, endometritis)
- Vaginal trauma
- Ulcerative lesions
- Polyps
- Malignancy
- Dysfunctional uterine bleeding
- Breakthrough bleeding secondary to contraceptive use
- Retained foreign body
- Intrauterine device
- Postprocedural
- Coagulopathy

Pregnancy-Related

- Implantation
- Spontaneous abortion (threatened, incomplete, inevitable)
- Ectopic pregnancy
- Placenta previa
- Abruptio placentae
- Retained products of conception

Apparent Vaginal Bleeding of Nonvaginal Origin

- Hematuria
- Hemorrhoids
- Anal fissures
- GI bleed

VOMITING

Gastrointestinal

- Gastroenteritis
- Food poisoning
- Gastritis
- Obstruction
- Intraabdominal processes
  - Appendicitis
  - Pancreatitis
  - Hepatitis
- Peptic ulcer disease
- Dysmotility disorders

Neurologic

- Hemorrhage (cerebellar, cerebral)
- Intracranial process (tumor, abscess)
- Meningitis
- Head trauma
- Migraine
- Labyrinthitis
- Ménière's disease

Cardiac

- Myocardial infarction or ischemia

Genitourinary

- Renal calculi
- Pregnancy
- Hyperemesis gravidarum
- Ovarian torsion
- Testicular torsion
- Dysmenorrhea

Other

- Medication (side effect, toxic levels)
- Bulimia
- Stress
- Motion sickness
- Glaucoma
- Vertigo/labyrinthitis
- Uremia
- Metabolic (diabetic ketoacidosis, alcoholic ketoacidosis, etc.)
- Postnasal drip
- Pain
- Reye's syndrome
- Toxic exposure
- Hyper- or hypocalcemia
- Thyrotoxicosis
- Hyperparathyroidism
- Hypoadrenalism

RADIOGRAPHIC SIGNS AND FINDINGS

Tanise I. Edwards

This appendix provides an overview of commonly ordered x-rays in the urgent care setting and specific radiographic findings that may be seen. It is not meant to provide a comprehensive text on radiology but rather is meant to be an overview. Not all x-ray studies are included or all radiographic findings. The reader is referred to a radiology text for more comprehensive teaching.

The information provided under the sections headed "Evaluation of" will help outline a method that can be used to analyze radiographs for the specific area identified. Reading of all x-rays should be approached in a systematic manner in order to minimize missed findings.

As noted, under each section entitled "Radiographic Findings by Disease Entities," any, all, or none of the findings listed may be present for a particular disease process or injury. X-ray findings and pertinent pearls helpful in diagnosing an entity are listed, but additional findings that are not listed may be seen in clinical practice, depending on the circumstances.

STANDARD AND ADDITIONAL RADIOGRAPHIC VIEWS

Chest Films

Standard Views	• AP
	• Lateral
Additional Views	
Oblique	Use to better delineate parenchymal findings such as nodules
Apical lordotic	Use to evaluate lung apices, particularly with suspected tuberculosis

Lateral decubitus	Use to evaluate effusions or bronchial obstruction with air trapping (as seen with bronchial foreign bodies) in patients unable to cooperate with expiratory films
Expiratory	Use to evaluate for small pneumothorax or bronchial obstruction with air trapping (as seen with bronchial foreign bodies)

Abdominal Films

Standard Views
- Flat plate of the abdomen
- Upright abdomen
- Upright chest

Additional Views

Left lateral decubitus	Used to evaluate for free air in patients who are unable to stand for an upright chest film
Cross-table lateral	Use to evaluate abdominal aortic aneurysm

Facial Films

- Nasal • Facial • Orbits • Mandible

Nasal Films

Standard Views
- Left lateral
- Right lateral
- Waters'

Facial Films

Standard Views
- Waters'
- Caldwell
- Lateral
- Submental vertex (jug-handle)

Orbit Films

Standard Views
- Waters'
- Caldwell
- Obliques

Mandibular Films

Standard Views
- PA
- Bilateral obliques
- Towne

Additional View

Panorex	Use to evaluate fractures, particularly nondisplaced fractures or fractures that are difficult to assess on plain films

Soft Tissue Lateral of the Neck

Standard Views	• AP
	• Lateral

Cervical Spine

Standard Views	• Odontoid
	• Cross-table lateral or upright lateral
	• AP
	• Bilateral obliques
Additional Views	
Swimmer's view	Use to better visualize the lower cervical spine, particularly C7-T1
Flexion/extension	Use in specific circumstances to help diagnosis cervical instability

Thoracic Spine

Standard Views	• AP
	• Lateral
Additional Views	
Thoracolumbar junction	Use to better assess the T-12 and L-1 region

Lumbar Spine

Standard Views	• AP
	• Lateral
Additional Views	
Obliques	
Cone-down lumbosacral	

Fingers

Standard Views	• PA
	• Lateral
	• Pronation oblique

Thumb

Standard Views	• PA
	• Lateral
	• Obliques
Additional Views	
AP Thumb (Robert view)	

Hand

Standard Views	• PA
	• Lateral
	• Pronation oblique
Additional Views	
Supination oblique	Use for evaluation of the metacarpal bases of the fourth and fifth fingers
Brewerton view	Use for evaluation of the metacarpal base

Wrist

Standard Views	• PA
	• Lateral
	• Pronation oblique
Additional Views	
Scaphoid/navicular view	Use for evaluation of the scaphoid
Supination oblique	Use for evaluation of the pisiform
Carpal tunnel view	Use for evaluation of fractures at the hook of the hamate, trapezium fractures (volar surface), and pisiform fractures

Forearm

Standard Views	• PA
	• Lateral

Elbow

Standard Views	• AP
	• Lateral
Additional Views	
Obliques	Use for evaluation of the medial or lateral condyles and the radial head (lateral oblique)
Olecranon view	Use to evaluate the olecranon
Capitellum view	Use to evaluate the capitellum and radial head

Shoulder

Standard Views	• AP (internal rotation)
	• AP (external rotation)
	• Lateral
Additional Views (May Be Standard in Some Facilities)	
Axillary view	Use to evaluate possible dislocations; use to evaluate the head of the humerus, the glenoid, and the acromion
Y view	Use to evaluate possible dislocations
Posterior oblique	Use to evaluate the glenohumeral joint

Humerus

Standard Views	• AP
	• Lateral

Clavicle and Acromioclavicular Joint

Standard Views	• AP
	• Angled AP
Additional Views	
AC joint with weights	Use to evaluate second- and third-degree AC separation

Pelvis

Standard Views	• AP
Additional Views	
Anterior and posterior Judet views	
Inlet and outlet views	
Lateral sacrum	

Hip

Standard Views	• AP pelvis
	• Lateral hip
Additional Views	
Frog-leg view	Use to evaluate intertrochanteric fractures, femoral fractures; use to evaluate slipped capital femoral epiphysis in children
Oblique (anterior)	Use to evaluate the acetabulum
Oblique (posterior)	Use to evaluate the acetabulum and proximal femur

Knee

Standard Views	• AP
	• Lateral
	• Obliques
Additional Views	
Sunrise view	Use to evaluate patella for nondisplaced fractures
Tunnel view	Use to diagnose tibial spine fractures

Ankle

Standard Views	• AP
	• Lateral
	• Ankle mortise
Additional Views	
Obliques (internal and external)	Use for posterior tibial fractures and to evaluate the distal fibula

Foot

Standard Views
- AP
- Lateral
- Oblique (internal)

Additional Views
Talus   Use to evaluate the dome of the talus
Calcaneus   Use to evaluate the calcaneus for fractures

Toes

Standard Views
- AP
- Lateral
- Oblique (internal)

 General Radiographic Errors to Avoid

- *Failure to adhere to the ABC's of radiographic evaluation:*
    Alignment
    Bone
    Cartilage
    Soft Tissue
- *Failure to examine the entire film.* Often significant incidental findings may be diagnosed, as well as unsuspected additional injury or pathology.
- *Failure to obtain additional views as needed for a complete radiographic evaluation.*
- *Failure to repeat a film if quality is not adequate.* Poor quality may be due to under- or overpenetration, poor positioning, or patient movement.
- *Failure to treat the patient and not the film.* Always evaluate the clinical picture. Radiographs may be confirmatory, but if not, treat the patient, not the film!

CHEST

Evaluation of the Chest

Lung fields   Evaluate for the presence of infiltrates, consolidations, abnormal interstitial markings, vascular markings, cavitations, masses or nodules, pneumothorax. Check apices, periphery, and retrocardiac space.

Cardiac silhouette   Evaluate size and shape.

Mediastinum   Evaluate size and shape of aorta and hilum, including any evidence of hilar adenopathy or increased vascularity.

Diaphragm   Evaluate shape and position; check for effusions and free air.

Bony structures   Evaluate ribs, clavicles, thoracic spine, and shoulder joint for bony disease, fracture, or abnormal contours.

Pearls

- The cardiac silhouette on PA projection should measure less than half of the lung diameter at its greatest point.
- The dome of the right hemidiaphragm is usually 1.5 to 2.5 cm higher than that of the left hemidiaphragm.
- The width of the normal mediastinum should typically be less than 7.5 cm on a PA film.
- On the lateral projection, the vertebral bodies should become more radiolucent (i.e., darker) in the lower positions, since there will be less overlying soft tissue structures to penetrate.
- On lateral films, increased radiodensity of the lower vertebral bodies may signify the presence of an infiltrate.
- For adequate inspiratory effort, typically there should be *at least* 9 to 10 posterior ribs noted above the diaphragm.
- In a nonrotated film, there should be equidistance between the spinous processes and each of the medial ends of the clavicles.
- Expiratory and lateral decubitus films can be used to help indicate the presence of a nonradiopaque foreign body. Air trapping occurs through a ball-valve effect, which can be noted on forced expiratory films or on lateral decubitus films (affected side down) in patients such as children, who are unable to cooperate with end-expiratory films.

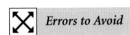 *Errors to Avoid*

- Underpenetrated films, which can cause falsely prominent lung markings
- Overpenetrated films, which can darken pulmonary infiltrates and may lead to a failure in diagnosis
- A poor inspiratory effort, which may falsely distort the cardiac silhouette and mediastinum, making them appear enlarged
- Rotation, which will make the cardiac silhouette and mediastinum appear enlarged

TABLE A2-1

FOREIGN BODIES THAT CAN AND CANNOT BE VISUALIZED ON X-RAY

VISUALIZED		NOT VISUALIZED
Glass if greater than 1 mm	Painted wood	Wood (unpainted)
Coins	Painted plastic	Organic matter
Batteries	Sand	peanuts
Metal	Teeth	fishbone
Gravel greater than 1 mm	Pencil graphite	Unpainted plastics

Common Differentials on Chest X-ray

See Tables A2-2 to A2-6.

TABLE A2-2

COMMON DIFFERENTIAL DIAGNOSIS OF INFILTRATES OR CONSOLIDATIONS

Pneumonia	Tuberculosis
Atelectasis	Pulmonary infarct (pulmonary embolism)
Pulmonary edema	Pulmonary hemorrhage
Tumor	

TABLE A2-3

COMMON DIFFERENTIAL DIAGNOSIS OF INCREASED INTERSTITIAL MARKINGS

Congestive heart failure	Collagen vascular disease
Viral pneumonia	Pneumoconiosis
Pulmonary fibrosis	Milary tuberculosis
Sarcoidosis	Hypersensitivity pneumonosis

TABLE A2-4

COMMON DIFFERENTIAL DIAGNOSIS OF MULTINODULAR DISEASE

HIV disease	Lymphoma
Fungal infections	Septic emboli
Parasitic infections	Inflammatory disorders (rheumatoid disease,
Tumors (particularly metastatic)	tuberculosis, Wegener's granulomatosis)

TABLE A2-5

COMMON DIFFERENTIAL DIAGNOSIS OF ATELECTASIS

Hypoventilation	Tumor
Foreign body	Mucous plugging

TABLE A2-6

COMMON DIFFERENTIAL DIAGNOSIS OF HILAR ADENOPATHY

Lymphoma	Tumor
Sarcoidosis	Infection (fungal, viral, tubercular)

CHEST FILMS

Radiographic Findings by Disease Entities

All, some, or none of the listed findings may be present for each disease entity.

Asthma

- Normal chest x-ray
- Hyperinflation
- Flattened diaphragms
- Increased lung volume
- Hyperlucency
- Narrowed cardiac silhouette

Chronic Obstructive Pulmonary Disease

- Cardiomegaly (may be obscured secondary to hyperinflation)
- Increased bronchovascular markings
- Increase in retrocardiac space
- Hyperlucency

Emphysema

- Hyperinflation
- Increased anterior-to-posterior chest wall diameter
- Flattened diaphragms
- Thin, elongated cardiac silhouette
- Bullae

Congestive Heart Failure with Progression to Pulmonary Edema

- Cardiac enlargement
- Cephalization (redistribution of blood flow to the upper lung regions and to the vasculature of the upper hilum)
- Presence of Kerley A, B, or C lines
- Peribronchial cuffing
- Pleural effusions
- Thickening of the fissures
- Bat-wing opacification of the perihilar region

Pneumonia

- Consolidation or infiltrates that may be as follows:
  - Lobar
  - Lobular (bronchopneumonia)
  - Interstitial
  - Patchy
- Air bronchograms
- Silhouette sign
- Hilar adenopathy (more likely with viral or atypical pneumonias)

- With retrocardiac involvement:
  - Opacification in the retrocardiac space on lateral films
  - Increased radiodensity (i.e., more opacified) in the lower vertebral bodies
- Pleural effusions
- Cavitations (particularly associated with *Staphylococcus aureus*)
- Lobar involvement with bulging fissures (particularly associated with *Klebsiella pneumoniae*)
- Bilateral interstitial infiltrates (bat-wing pattern associated with PCP pneumonia)

  - *The right lower lobe is the most common area for aspiration pneumonia when aspiration occurs in the upright position.*
  - *Findings of pneumonia on x-ray often lag behind the clinical picture.*
  - *X-ray findings in patients with Mycoplasma pneumoniae infection will often appear much worse than the clinical appearance.*
  - *X-ray findings of pneumonia may be less prominent in a patient who is dehydrated.*

Pneumomediastinum

- Air dissecting into the soft tissues of the neck
- Outlining of the mediastinal parietal pleura as it runs parallel to the mediastinum

Pneumothorax

- Absent lung markings at the periphery
- Separation of the parietal pleura from the visceral pleura noted as a radiolucent line
  - *End-expiratory films allow better visualization of small pneumothoraces.*

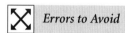 *Errors to Avoid*

- *Mistaking the scapular border or a skin fold for the pleural line of a pneumothorax.* Check for lung markings. Lung markings should not be present beyond the pleural line when a pneumothorax is present.

Tension Pneumothorax

- Mediastinal shift away from the side of the collapsed lung
- Tracheal shift away from the side of the collapsed lung
- Hyperlucency of the involved side
- Depression of the hemidiaphragm

Pulmonary Abscess

- Cavity with air-fluid levels seen in the lung parenchyma

Pulmonary Contusion

- Dense pulmonary infiltrate in the area of injury

Pulmonary Effusions

- Seen on upright films or lateral decubitus films
- Effusions can be visualized when 200 to 300 mL of fluid is present in the chest cavity

Pulmonary Embolus

- Normal chest x-ray
- Nonspecific findings:
  - Discoid atelectasis or infiltrate
  - Elevated hemidiaphragm
  - Pleural effusion
- *Westermark sign:* a relative lack of vascular markings associated with a dilated pulmonary artery and distal oligemia
- *Hampton's hump:* A wedge-shaped opacification secondary to intraparenchymal hemorrhage (occurs with pulmonary infarction)

Thoracic Aortic Aneurysm

- Mediastinal widening
- Calcium sign (separation of intimal calcium from the aortic wall)
- Tracheal deviation to the right
- Downward depression of the left mainstem bronchus
- Left pleural effusion
- Change in shape and size of aorta from previous films

When associated with a rupture due to trauma, one may also see the following:

- A left apical cap
- Indistinct or obliteration of the aortic knob
- Loss of the aorticopulmonary window
- Obliteration of the paravertebral stripe

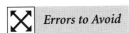 *Errors to Avoid*

- *Failure to diagnose a thoracic aneurysm because of a tortuous aorta.* In older patients, the aorta may become elongated and dilated. If possible, compare findings with previous films.

ABDOMEN

Evaluation of the Abdomen

Stomach	Evaluate location, size, presence of air-fluid level.
Diaphragm	Check for evidence of free air under the diaphragm. Evaluate the shape and position of the diaphragm
Intestines	Evaluate location, mucosal markings, distribution of gas and gas pattern, luminal size, distention, presence of air-fluid levels, presence of gas in the bowel wall
Solid Organs	Evaluate size, presence of abnormal air (i.e., air in the gallbladder wall or in the biliary tree), loss of properitoneal fat line or psoas margin, presence of stones (gallbladder, renal)
Vasculature	Check for abnormal calcifications, evidence of widening, or abnormal positioning

Pearls

- Abdominal series are good for evaluation of possible obstruction, perforation, or radioopaque foreign bodies.
- The upright chest x-ray is the best film for detecting free air. Look for free air visualized under the diaphragm.
- The presence of a sentinel loop (a localized dilated loop of small bowel) may be indicative of pancreatitis, cholecystitis, or appendicitis, depending on its location.

ABDOMINAL FILMS

Radiographic Findings by Disease Entities

All, some, or none of the listed findings may be present for each disease entity.

Abdominal Aortic Aneurysm

- Eccentric aortic calcifications in an enlarged aortic wall

Appendicitis

- Calcified appendicolith (occurs in approximately 10 percent of adults)
- Nonspecific gas pattern
- Localized ileus
- Loss of the psoas margin
- Air-filled appendix with a dilated lumen

Cholecystitis

- Gallstones
- Sentinel loop in the right upper quadrant
- Scoliosis with concavity to the right
- Gas in the gallbladder wall (emphysematous gallbladder)
- Air in the biliary tree (seen in biliary-enteric fistulas; a stone in the small bowel may also be visualized)
- Only 15 percent of gallstones are radiopaque.

Coin Foreign Bodies

- In the esophagus, coins will be "en face" on AP films and on edge on lateral views
  - *Coins that are lodged in the trachea will be visualized "en face" on the lateral view and visualized on edge on AP films.*
  - *Always obtain both AP and lateral films to evaluate the presence of foreign bodies. A lateral view will sometimes show the presence of more than one coin that may not be seen on the AP view.*

Ileus (Adynamic)

- Dilated loops of bowel
- Upright films with air-fluid levels of equal heights

Ileus (Gallstone)

- Small bowel obstruction
- Gallstone visualized in the intestine
- Air within the biliary tree

Obstruction (Small Bowel)

- Centrally located dilated loops of small bowel (>3 cm)
- Differential air-fluid levels on upright films
- Paucity of bowel gas distally (there may be a total absence of gas distally if obstruction is complete)
- "Stack of coins" appearance of the valvulae conniventes

Obstruction (Large Bowel)

- Peripherally located dilated loops of large bowel
- Haustral indentations
- Fluid-filled bowel
- Thickened colonic wall

Perforation

- Air under the diaphragm on upright chest film (may be more easily identified under the right hemidiaphragm)
  - *To increase visibility of small amounts of free air, the patient should be upright for longer than 5 min prior to taking the x-ray.*
- Free air may also be visualized on left lateral decubitus films between the right hepatic margin and the right hemidiaphragm.
- Free air may not be visible with an appendiceal perforation.

Pancreatitis

- Sentinel loop
- Elevated left hemidiaphragm
- Left lower lung atelectasis
- Calcifications (if chronic)

Renal Calculi

- Stones (sites of impaction: pelvic brim, ureteropelvic junction, ureteovisceral junction)
  - *90 percent of kidney stones are radioopaque.*
  - *Stones typically present with an irregular shape, which helps differentiate them from phleboliths (which are rounded and have a lucent center).*

Toxic Megacolon

- Massively dilated colon
- Loss of haustration
- Nodular indentation of the mucosa

Volvulus

- Massively dilated loop of bowel
- Absent haustration
- Closed loop dilatation, which may lead to a "coffee bean" appearance of the dilated loop
  - *Volvulus involving the cecum usually occurs in the elderly; in the younger population, volvulus of the sigmoid colon is more common*

THE SOFT TISSUE NECK
EVALUATION OF THE SOFT TISSUE LATERAL OF THE NECK

Radiographic Findings by Disease Entities

All, some, or none of the listed findings may be present for each disease entity.

Croup

- "Steeple sign" of the trachea on AP
- Narrowed subglottic trachea
- Normal epiglottis on lateral films

Epiglottitis

- Swelling of the epiglottis, which may appear in the shape of a thumb print on lateral films
  - *The normal epiglottis appears as a thin, soft tissue structure. X-rays taken during inspiration or without full hyperextension of the neck will falsely enlarge the epiglottis on the lateral film.*

Pneumomediastinum

- Air streaks noted in the soft tissues of the neck that extend up from the mediastinum
- May also be diagnosed on chest x-ray

Retropharyngeal Abscess

- Swelling of the retropharyngeal soft tissue just anterior to the second and third cervical vertebrae

CERVICAL SPINE

- *Up to 20 percent of cervical spinal fractures may be missed in the traditional three-view series (AP, lateral, odontoid)*[1]

Evaluation of the Cervical Spine
ANY ABNORMALITY OR UNCERTAINTY IN EVALUATION REQUIRES CONTINUED IMMOBILIZATION AND TRANSFER FOR FURTHER EVALUATION

- On the lateral view, check that all seven cervical vertebrae are visible, including the C7-T1 interspace and complete superior margin of T1

Errors to Avoid

- *Failure to visualize all seven cervical vertebrae and the full C7-T1 junction.* The cervical spine cannot be cleared unless the entire cervical spine, including the full cervicothoracic junction, has been evaluated. If this cannot be achieved, the patient must be kept properly immobilized and transferred for further evaluation

- On the lateral view, check alignment. There should be four curvilinear lines that are smooth and continuous, without step-offs or angulation (Fig. A2-1)
    1. The anterior vertebral body line
    2. The posterior vertebral body line
    3. The spinolaminar line
    4. The tips of the spinous processes

- Check the odontoid view for fractures of the dens (base, body, and tip); check that the dens is centered between the lateral masses of C1. Check for fractures of the articular masses of C1 and fractures of the body of C2.

- Check that the lateral masses of C1 are vertically aligned with the lateral borders of C2.
    - *The alignment of C1 on C2 will be affected by rotation of the head or lateral tilting.*

- Check for fractures of the posterior arch of C1 and neural arch of C2 (lateral view).

- Evaluate each vertebral body and its endplate. (C3 through C7 should be rectangular and of uniform height.) Check for fractures, displacement, subluxation, angulation, and compression. Evaluate the laminae and articular masses. Check for subluxation and interfacetal dislocations.

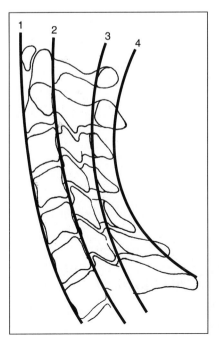

FIGURE A2-1 Vertebral alignment in the lateral cervical spine radiograph. The four curves of alignment are shown: (1) anterior vertebral body line; (2) posterior vertebral body line; (3) spinolaminar line, and (4) tips of spinous processes. (From Schwartz DT, Reisdorff E: *Emergency Radiology.* New York: McGraw-Hill; 2000, with permission.)

- Check for fractures of the spinous processes. Check that the spinous processes are midline (AP view.) Check for evidence of widening between the tips of the spinous processes.
- Check disk spaces, which should be uniform and parallel to the adjacent endplates; evaluate the interfacetal joint and the interlaminar space.
- On obliques: Check the inferior and superior facets. Check for facet overriding or vertebral body rotation.
- Check the soft tissue, particularly the predental and prevertebral soft tissue, for bulging and widening.

> **Indirect Evidence of Fractures:** Prevertebral soft tissue swelling

- *While prevertebral soft tissue swelling may be indicative of a cervical spinal injury, the lack of soft tissue swelling does not exclude a fracture.*

The characteristics of the normal cervical spine are described in Table A2-7.

Radiographic Findings by Disease Entities

All, some, or none of the listed findings may be present for each disease entity.

Anterior Subluxation

- Normal film
- Posterior disk space widening
- Increased distance/widening between the spinous processes
- Anterior disk space narrowing
- Interspace angulation > 11 degrees[2]

Clay Shoveler's Fracture

- Avulsion of the spinous process (usually of the lower cervical spine)
- Occurs most frequently at C7

TABLE A2-7

NORMAL CERVICAL SPINE

Basion–dental interval <12 mm
Predental space < 3 mm in adults (greater than 3.5 mm suggests instability)
        < 5 mm in children
Prevertebral soft tissue: C1 < 10 mm
           C2 < 5 mm
           C3 < 5 to 7 mm or less than one-half the width of the vertebral body
           C7 < 22 mm
  Additionally, there should be no prevertebral soft tissue bulging
Lateral masses of C1 should be vertically aligned with the lateral borders of C2
Dens of C2 should be centered between the lateral masses of C1
Angle of the superior surface of adjacent vertebral borders <11 degrees
Mild lordotic curvature of C3 to C7

SOURCE: Tintinalli et al.,[2] with permission.

Wedge Fractures

- Wedged compression of anterior aspect of vertebral body
- Widening of spinous process

Unilateral Interfacetal Dislocation

- Malalignment of the spinous process with deviation toward the dislocation (AP view)
- Anterosuperior displacement of the articular facet in relation to subjacent facet (lateral view)

Extension Teardrop Fracture

- Triangular avulsion of the anterior vertebrae at the inferior edge
- Occurs most commonly at C2

THORACOLUMBAR SPINE

- *Most fractures of the thoracic and lumbar spine occur between T-12 and L-2.*

Evaluation of the Thoracic and Lumbar Spine

- Check for a smooth, continuous alignment on the lateral film along the following:
    Anterior vertebral line
    Posterior vertebral line
    Apophyseal joints
    Tips of the spinous processes
- Check alignment on the AP film for scoliosis.
- Check alignment on the lateral film for kyphosis (T spine) and lumbar lordosis (L spine).
- Check the vertebral bodies and their endplates. Check for fractures, displacement, compressions, subluxation, and dislocations. Check for loss or disruption of the pedicles.
- Check for fractures of the spinous processes, the transverse processes, and the laminae.
- Check disk spaces, which should be uniform and parallel to the adjacent endplates.
- Check the interpedicular distance for evidence of widening.
- On obliques: Evaluate the "Scotty dog." Check the inferior and superior facets. Check for facet overriding or vertebral body rotation. Check for spondylolysis of the pars interarticularis and spondylolisthesis.
- On the AP view, check for the paraspinous line (usually at the level of T10 to the left of the spine) and psoas margin.

LUMBAR SPINE

Radiographic Findings by Disease Entities

All, some, or none of the listed findings may be present for each disease entity.

Compression Fractures[1]

- Wedge compression of the anterior vertebral body with < 50 percent compression
- Loss of height of the anterior aspect of the vertebral body only

- < 20 percent compression angle
- Posterior body vertebral angle < 100 percent

Burst Fractures[1]

Loss of anterior and posterior vertebral body height with compression > 50 percent (lateral view)

- Increased interpedicular space
- > 20 percent compression angle
- Posterior body vertebral angle > 100 percent

Distraction Injuries

- Widening of interspinous distance
- Horizontal fracture through the spinous process, vertebral body, or posterior arch
- Loss of height of the anterior aspect of the vertebral body

> **Indirect Evidence of Fractures of the Transverse Process:** Loss of the psoas margin or new scoliosis may be indicative of a transverse fracture.

Spinal Disk Space Infections

- Narrowed disk space
- Erosion of vertebral endplates
- Loss of vertebral height (advanced)

Spondylolysis

- Defect of the pars interarticularis (neck of the "Scotty dog")

Spondylolisthesis

- Anterior slippage of a vertebra secondary to bilateral spondylolysis

MUSCULOSKELETAL SYSTEM
NONTRAUMATIC INJURY

Radiographic Findings by Disease Entities

All, some, or none of the listed findings may be present for each disease entity.

Gout

- Punched out bony lesions
- Joint space narrowing
- Tophus calcification
  - *Gout most commonly occurs at the first metatarsal-phalangeal joint, the knee, and the ankle.*
  - *X-ray findings of gout occur later in the disease process.*

High-Pressure Injury

- Radiolucent streaks visualized in the soft tissue extending away from the site of injection

Osteoarthritis

- Asymmetrical joint space narrowing
- Osteophytes/bone spurs
- Increased bone density with subchondral sclerosis

Osteomyelitis

- Normal films (early)
- Periosteal elevation
- Evidence of new bone formation
- Erosion and destruction of cortical bone (lytic lesions)
    - *There must be at least 50 percent bone destruction before x-ray changes of osteomyelitis can be noted on plain films.*[1]

Chronic Osteomyelitis

- Sclerotic bone
- Irregular bony margins
- Thickened periosteum
- Areas of radiolucency

Osteoporosis

- Cortical thinning
- Loss of interconnective trabeculae
- Accentuation of structural trabeculae

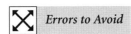 *Errors to Avoid*

- *Failure to diagnose a fracture in a patient with osteopenia.* Nondisplaced fractures may be difficult to visualize.

Sesamoid Bone

- Small, smooth, rounded bones embedded in the flexor tendons
- Usually bilateral
- Fractures can occur in sesamoid bone
- Common sites:
    - metacarpophalangeal joint of the volar thumb
    - interphalangeal joint of the volar thumb
    - metacarpophalangeal joints of the volar index and little fingers

Vascular Grooves

- Oblique radiolucent lines with smooth sclerotic margins that are typically found at the midshaft metaphysis of the phalanges
- No associated cortical disruption

Errors to Avoid in Fracture Diagnosis

- Failure to examine the entire film for multiple fractures
- Failure to x-ray the joint above and the joint below the site of injury. *This may lead to a failure to diagnosis fractures or dislocations associated with the primary area of injury such as those seen with Galeazzi fractures, Monteggia fractures, and fibular head fractures associated with ankle injuries.*
- Failure to obtain additional or special views when clinical suspicion for a fracture is high but no fracture is visualized on routine films. *Obtain at least three views: AP, lateral, and oblique.*
- Failure to obtain a postreduction film
- Failure to appropriately treat and immobilize an injury based on a "normal" x-ray. *If a normal x-ray is not consistent with the clinical examination, the injury should be properly immobilized and the area re-x-rayed in 10 days to 2 weeks.*
- Failure to diagnose a fracture at the epiphysis of a growth plate (i.e., a Salter I fracture)
- Failure to diagnose a fracture by mistaking it for an accessory ossicle
- Failure to diagnose a fracture by mistaking it for a sesamoid
- Failure to diagnose an oblique fracture by mistaking it for a vascular groove
- Failure to diagnose a torus fracture. *The only evidence of a fracture may be a small abnormal angulation of the cortex without evidence of a fracture line.*
- Failure to consider the etiology of fracture to be due to a bone lesion or a pathologic process (i.e., failure to diagnose a pathology fracture)
- Failure to diagnose a small avulsion fracture. *Knowledge of common sites of avulsions will help in identifying fractures at those sites.*

Tables A2-8, A2-9, and A2-10 list common sites of avulsion fractures, radiographic findings that mimic fractures, and accessory ossicles and their locations, respectively.

TABLE A2-8

COMMON SITES FOR AVULSION FRACTURES

Proximal interphalangeal joints
Volar surface of the middle phalanx
Site of insertion of the ulnar collateral ligament of the thumb (gamekeeper's thumb)
Base of the distal phalanx (mallet finger)
Olecranon at the site of the triceps insertion
Anterior superior iliac crest of the pelvis (site of insertion of the sartorius)
Anterior inferior iliac crest of the pelvis (site of insertion of the rectus femoris)
Ischial tuberosity apophysis of the pelvis (site of insertion of the hamstrings)
Apophysis of the lesser trochanter of the femur (site of insertion of the iliopsoas)

TABLE A2-9

RADIOGRAPHIC FINDINGS THAT MIMIC FRACTURES

Growth plates	Vascular grooves/nutrient arteries
Accessory ossicles	Mach bands

ACCESSORY OSSICLES AND THEIR LOCATIONS

ACCESSORY OSSICLE	LOCATION
Os peroneum	Adjacent to cuboid
Os supranaviculare	Superior surface of navicular
Os supratalare	Superior surface of the talus
Os trigonum	Posterior tubercle of talus
Os vesalianum	Adjacent to the base of the fifth metatarsal

TRAUMATIC INJURY

Radiographic Findings by Disease Entities

All, some, or none of the listed findings may be present for each disease entity.

Torus Fractures (occur in children)

- This is the most common fracture in children.
- A buckle or bulge usually occurs at the metaphysis without an identifiable cortical fracture line.
- It may be noted on one or both sides of the metaphysis on x-ray.

Greenstick Fractures (occur in children)

- Usually occurs at the diaphysis of the bone
- Incomplete fractures with a break and angulation of one side of the bone

Stress Fractures

- Fractures that occur secondary to repeated stresses.
- X-rays are generally negative early on.
- May show evidence of new callus formation or fracture line if evaluated later in the course of the injury.
- May be seen in the metatarsals (march fractures), navicular, femoral neck, calcaneus.

Fingers and Hand

Evaluation of the Fingers and Hand

Bones Outline and evaluate cortex of each phalanx and metacarpal on all views; evaluate base of metacarpals carefully for fractures obscured by overlapping bone; check for subluxation, dislocation, and joint widening or narrowing; check for avulsion fractures at sites of tendon insertions (mallet finger, volar plate injuries); check the fourth and fifth metacarpal heads for impacted boxer's fractures.

Bennet Fracture

- Intraarticular fracture
- Fracture-dislocation at the base of the thumb
- Dorsal and radial displacement of the base of the metacarpal

Boxer's Fracture

- Fracture at the neck of a metacarpal (generally the fourth or fifth metacarpals)

 Errors to Avoid

- *Failure to diagnose a subtle impacted boxer's fracture.* Cortical disruption may not be easily visible if the fracture is impacted.

Gamekeeper's Thumb

- Normal x-ray (ulnar collateral ligament injury)
- Avulsion fracture at the site on insertion of the ulnar collateral ligament at the metacarpophalangeal joint of the thumb
- May need stress views performed

Mallet Finger

- Normal x-ray (partial or complete rupture of the extensor tendon)
- Dorsal avulsion fracture of the base of the distal phalanx (intraarticular)

Phalanx Fractures

- Can be transverse, oblique, or comminuted.
- May be angulated or nondisplaced (which may be visible on one view only).
- Distal phalanx fractures are the most common fractures of the hand.

Volar Plate Fractures

- Most commonly occur at the proximal interphalangeal joint
- May visualize an avulsion fracture off the volar surface at the base of the middle phalanx

Wrist

Evaluation of the Wrist

- Evaluate both rows of carpal bones, the distal radius, and the distal ulna.
- Check for a smooth contour of the arches of the radiocarpal joint, the carpocarpal joint, and the carpometacarpal joint.
    Proximal carpals row: proximal articular margin
    Proximal carpals row: distal articular margin
    Distal carpals row: proximal articular margin
- Check intercarpal joint spaces, which should uniformly be 2 mm.
- Outline bony cortex, evaluating for fracture lines, buckles, and deformities.
- Check for chip fractures of the triquetrum (dorsally).
- Check for the normal trapezoidal shape of the lunate.
- Check for scaphoid fractures (use scaphoid view if snuff-box tenderness is elicited).
- Check for the presence of the pronator quadratus fat stripe (should be present and not displaced or bulging).

- Check the alignment of the capitate in the lunate cup and the lunate in the radial cup.
- *There should be 1 to 2 mm of joint space between all the intercarpal joints.*

Scapholunate Dissociation

- Greater than 4 mm widening of the scapholunate joint
- Scapholunate angle greater than 60 degrees on lateral view
- "Signet ring" shape of the scaphoid bone on the PA view
- Transverse rotation of the scaphoid

Colles Fracture

- Fracture of the distal radius with dorsal displacement
- Must check for carpal bone fractures (especially the scaphoid) and for associated elbow injury
- Usually best seen on lateral views

Distal Radioulnar Joint Disruption

- Radial shortening (>5 mm)
- Widening of the distal radioulnar joint space
- Fracture of the ulnar styloid
- Disruption of the normal alignment of the ulnar in relation to the carpal bones

Perilunate Dislocation

- Dorsal dislocation of capitate in relation to the lunate
- Normal positioning of the lunate in relation to the distal radius
- "Crowding" of the two rows of carpal bones
- Triangular shape of the lunate

Lunate Dislocation

- Anterior dislocation of the lunate in relation to the distal radius
- Lunate rotates, forming a "spilled teacup" appearance
- "Crowding" of the two rows of carpal bones

Scaphoid (Navicular) Fracture

- May only be visible on scaphoid view of the wrist

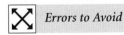 *Errors to Avoid*

- Failure to identify a nondisplaced tuft fracture associated with soft tissue injury (i.e., an open fracture)
- In the face of a suspicious clinical examination, failure to properly immobilize a potential scaphoid fracture based on a normal x-ray
- Failure to diagnose a dorsal chip fracture of the triquetrum. *These fractures may be visible only on the lateral film.*

- Failure to diagnose associated injuries with distal radial fractures, including ulnar styloid fractures, scaphoid fractures, elbow injuries, or scapholunate dissociation.
- Failure to diagnose a nondisplaced fracture of the distal radius. *Nonvisualization or bulging of the pronator quadratus fat stripe may be the only radiographic indication of a fracture.*

Forearm and Elbow

Evaluation of the Forearm and Elbow

Bones	Evaluate the proximal shaft of the radius and ulna; evaluate the distal humeral shaft; evaluate the radial head and neck as well as the olecranon and coronoid process and the humeral condyles, epicondyles, and the supracondylar area; evaluate the positioning of the bones, including measuring the anterior humeral line and the radiocapitellar line.
Soft Tissue	Examine the joint space of the articulation of the radius, ulna, and humerus; check for the presence of an anterior fat pad, posterior fat pad, and the supinator fat stripe.

Anterior Humeral Line

- Is measured on the lateral view.
- A line from the anterior shaft of the distal humerus that extends through the capitellum (Fig. A2-2).
- The line should intersect the middle third of the capitellum.

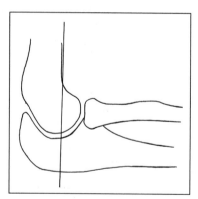

FIGURE A2-2 Normal anterior humeral line. (From Scaletta TA, Schaider JJ: *Emergent Management of Trauma.* New York: McGraw-Hill; 1996, with permission.)

Radiocapitellar Line

- A line drawn down the middle of the radius should normally intersect the middle of the capitellum (Fig. A2-3)

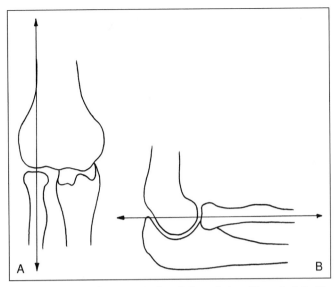

FIGURE A2-3   The elbow. *A*. AP view. *B*. Lateral view. (From Scaletta TA, Schaider JJ: *Emergent Management of Trauma*. New York: McGraw-Hill; 1996, with permission.)

- Anterior fat pads should normally be seen on a true lateral view of the elbow. When a joint effusion is present, a sail sign can be noted, in which there is elevation and bulging of the anterior fat pad.
- Posterior fat pads are visualized only when a joint effusion is present.
- Overread films with a "bright" light (i.e., hot-light the films), particularly when evaluating for a fat pad or fracture.
- Supracondylar fractures are the most common elbow fractures in children.
- Radial head fractures are the most common elbow fractures in adults.
- Epicondylar fractures may sometimes be visible only on oblique views.

Indirect Evidence of Fractures of the Radial Head

- Positive posterior fat pad
- Distended anterior fat pad on lateral views
- Nonvisualization or bulging of the pronator quadratus fat stripe

---

- The pronator quadratus fat stripe is normally parallel to the volar surface of the distal radius.

Indirect Evidence of Supracondylar Fractures

- Positive posterior fat pad.
- Distended anterior fat pad on lateral views.
- Posterior displacement of the capitellum is noted on the anterior humeral line.

Galeazzi Fracture

- Fracture of the distal radius with an associated dislocation of the distal radioulnar joint

Monteggia Fracture

- Ulnar shaft fracture with an associated dislocation of the radial head

 Errors to Avoid

- Failure to diagnose a radial head fracture or supracondylar fracture because no fracture line can be identified
- Failure to diagnose a radial head dislocation secondary to not assessing the radiocapitellar line
- Failure to identify a supracondylar fracture secondary to not assessing the anterior humeral line
- Failure to identify a fat-pad sign secondary to overpenetration of the x-ray

SHOULDER, HUMERUS, CLAVICLE, AND ACROMIOCLAVICULAR (AC) JOINT

Evaluation of the Shoulder, Humerus, Clavicle, and AC Joint

Bones Evaluate the head of the humerus, including the greater and lesser tuberosities, humeral neck, and glenoid fossa; check for abnormal relation between the head of the humerus and its position in the glenoid fossa, which could suggest dislocation; evaluate the clavicle, acromion and coracoid process; check for any abnormal trabecular patterns.
Evaluate entire length of the clavicle.

- *Most clavicular fractures occur in the middle third of the clavicle.*

Soft Tissue Check for calcifications; check for widening or narrowing of the glenohumeral joint.
Evaluate the AC joint for widening; evaluate the coracoclavicular space for widening; evaluate the sternoclavicular joint space.

- *There should be appropriate overlap of the humeral head in the glenoid fossa[1]*
- *The average AC joint space should be < 3 to 5 mm; it should not exceed 8 mm[1]*
- *The space between the coracoid process and the clavicle should be < 11 mm*

 Errors to Avoid

- Failure to diagnose a shoulder dislocation. If there is clinical suspicion of a dislocation, a Y view and/or an axillary view should be ordered.

Anterior Dislocations

- Displacement of the humeral head in relation to the glenoid fossa
- Fixed external rotation of the humeral head
- There may be an associated Hill-Sachs deformity (fracture of the posterolateral surface of the humeral head) or a Bankart lesion (fracture of the glenoid rim).
  - *Anterior dislocations account for 95% of shoulder dislocations.*

HIP

Evaluation of the Hip

Evaluate the cortical margin and trabeculae of the femur; evaluate the femur along its entire course—head/neck/shaft; evaluate the position of the femur in the acetabulum and the joint space; evaluate the greater and lesser trochanters for avulsions and the intertrochanteric area; check for acetabular fractures; evaluate the structure of the pelvis.

- *The medial half of the femoral head should overlap the acetabulum*
- *Femoral neck fractures can occur in the elderly with only a history of minor trauma*

Subcapital Fractures

- Abnormality of cortical structure
- Abnormal trabecular pattern
- Shortening of the femoral neck with an abnormal angle
- Increased density at the femoral neck at fracture line

Avascular Necrosis

- Normal films (early)
- Abnormality of the femoral head with areas of increased density and lucencies
- "Crescent sign" of the shape of the femoral head
- Collapse of femoral head (late)

KNEE

Evaluation of the Knee

Bones

Evaluate the patella, proximal fibula, proximal tibia, distal femur, and femoral condyles; evaluate cortical margins and trabecular pattern; evaluate the tibial plateaus and intercondylar spines.

Soft Tissue

Check for effusions; evaluate the patellofemoral joint space; check the positioning of the patella.

- *A patellar tendon rupture may show a high-riding patella.*
- *A quadriceps tendon rupture may show a low-riding patella.*

Patellar Fractures

- May be transverse, vertical, or comminuted
- Nondisplaced fractures of the patella may be missed on standard views and only be visible on the sunrise view. This is particularly true for vertical fractures.

ANKLE

Evaluation of the Ankle

Bones	Evaluate tibia, fibula, ankle mortise, and base of fifth metatarsal; check for fractures of the medial/lateral/posterior malleoli; evaluate for bimalleolar and tri-malleolar fractures; check for fractures of the talus, navicular, and calcaneus; order films to evaluate the head of the fibula as indicated by physical examination.
Soft Tissue	Evaluate the joint space of the ankle mortise; check for the presence of an effusion.

- *Fractures of the lateral malleolus are the most common type of ankle fracture.*
- *The joint space surrounding the ankle mortise should be uniform.*

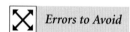 **Errors to Avoid**

- Failure to diagnose a chip fracture of the talus or navicular. *This area often requires bright-light evaluation for fractures to be visible.*

FOOT

Evaluation of the Foot

Bones	Assess each metatarsal (head, neck, shaft, and base); check base of fifth metatarsal; check each tarsal bone (talus, navicular, cuboid, and the cuneiforms); evaluate the calcaneous; check Bohler's angle.
Soft Tissue	Assess each metatarsal phalangeal joint; evaluate the talonavicular and calcaneocuboid joint.

- *Bohler's angle should be between 20 and 40 degrees (Fig. A2-4).*

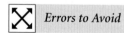 **Errors to Avoid**

- Failure to diagnose a fracture at the base of the fifth metatarsal associated with a lateral ankle injury.

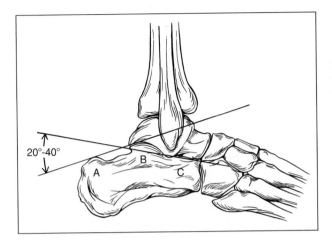

FIGURE A2-4   Bohler's angle. This is formed by two lines, one between the posterior tuberosity (*A*) and the apex of the posterior facet (*B*) and the other between the apex of the posterior facet (*B*) and the apex of the anterior process (*C*). An angle less than 20 degrees suggests a calcaneal compression fracture. (From Tintinalli J et al: *Emergency Medicine: A Comprehensive Study Guide,* 5th ed. New York: McGraw-Hill; 2000, with permission.)

- Failure to diagnose a calcaneal fracture. These fractures may be difficult to assess. *Any patient with a possible calcaneal fracture should have Bohler's angle measured and documented.*
- Failure to diagnose associated injuries. *Patients who present with calcaneal fractures secondary to falls from a height may also have injuries to the wrist and lumbar spine.*

Navicular Fractures

- Dorsal chip
- Tubercle fracture
- Fracture of the body

Jones Fracture

- Transverse fracture of the base of the fifth metatarsal

Avulsion Fracture

- Must be distinguished from an unfused apophysis

FACIAL BONES

Evaluation of the Facial Bones

Bones	Evaluate orbital rims, orbital floor, orbital walls, zygomatic arch, nasal bones, mandible, and lateral walls of the maxillary sinus.
Sinuses	Check for air-fluid levels, opacification, prolapse of infraorbital tissue, fractures of the sinus walls.
Soft Tissue	Check for soft tissue swelling and emphysema.

> **Indirect Evidence of Orbital Fractures:** Air-fluid level in the maxillary sinus and orbital emphysema

Orbital Rim Fractures

- Seen on Waters' and Caldwell views

Orbital Blowout Fracture

- "Teardrop" sign (herniation of soft tissue into the maxillary sinus)
- Disruption of the orbital floor with a downward displacement
- Air-fluid level in the maxillary sinus
- Orbital emphysema
- Widening of > 2 mm between the orbital rim and the orbital floor

Tripod Fracture

- Air-fluid level in the maxillary sinus
- Orbital emphysema
- Diastasis of the frontozygomatic suture
- Interruption of the zygomaticotemporal junction at the arch
- Fracture of the orbital floor and infraorbital rim
    - *The zygomatic arch is a rigid ring; therefore, if one fracture is identified, there should be at least one other fracture of either the zygoma or another midface bone. With an isolated zygomatic injury, the zygoma is usually broken in three places.*

Nasal Fractures

- Usually transverse fractures of the nasal bones

 Errors to Avoid

- Misdiagnosing a nasomaxillary suture as a fracture

Mandibular Fractures

- The body of the mandible is the most common area for fractures, followed by the angle.
    - *Because the mandible is a ring-like structure, the mandible usually fractures in more than one place.*

 Errors to Avoid

- Failure to diagnose a nondisplaced fracture secondary to a negative plain film. *If clinical suspicion for a fracture is high, a negative plain film should be followed up with a Panorex.*

REFERENCES

1. Schwartz DT, Reisdorff E: *Emergency Radiology*. New York: McGraw-Hill; 2000: 22, 123, 271, 283–285.
2. Tintinalli J et al: *Emergency Medicine: A Comprehensive Study Guide*, 5th ed. New York: McGraw-Hill; 2000: 1795.

BIBLIOGRAPHY

Scaletta TA: *Emergent Management of Trauma*. New York: McGraw-Hill; 1996.

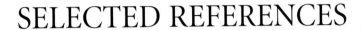

SELECTED REFERENCES

Cardiology

Cardiology in Primary Care
Branch WT et al: *Cardiology in Primary Care.* New York: McGraw-Hill; 2000.
Advances in Cardiology 2001
Braunwald E: *Advances in Cardiology 2001.* New York: McGraw-Hill; 2001.

Dermatology

Color Atlas and Synopsis of Clinical Dermatology
Fitzpatrick TB et al: *Color Atlas and Synopsis of Clinical Dermatology.* New York: McGraw-Hill; 1997.
Fitzpatrick's Dermatology in General Medicine
Freedberg IM, Eisen AZ, Wolff K, et al (eds): *Fitzpatrick's Dermatology in General Medicine,* 5th ed. New York: McGraw-Hill; 1999.
Color Atlas and Synopsis of Pediatric Dermatology
Kane K et al: *Color Atlas and Synopsis of Pediatric Dermatology.* New York: McGraw-Hill; 2001.

Emergency Medicine

Infectious Disease in Emergency Medicine
Brillman JC, Quenzer RW (eds): *Infectious Disease in Emergency Medicine,* 3d ed. Philadelphia: Lippincott Williams & Wilkins; 1998.
EMRA 2000 Guide to Antibiotic Use in the Emergency Department
Bryan J, Jui J, Dirk K: *EMRA 2000 Guide to Antibiotic Use in the Emergency Department.* New York: McGraw-Hill; 2000.

Clinical Practice of Emergency Medicine
Harwood-Nuss A, Wolfson AB, Linden CH, et al (eds): *Clinical Practice of Emergency Medicine*, 3d ed. Philadelphia: Lippincott Williams & Wilkins; 2001.
Atlas of Emergency Medicine
Knoop K, Stack LB, Storrow AB: *Atlas of Emergency Medicine*. New York: McGraw-Hill; 1997.
Clinical Procedures in Emergency Medicine
Roberts JR, Hedges JR (eds): *Clinical Procedures in Emergency Medicine*, 3d ed. Philadelphia: Saunders; 1998.
Emergency Care of the Woman
Perlman MD, Tintinalli JE (eds): *Emergency Care of the Woman*. New York: McGraw-Hill; 1998.
Emergency Medicine: A Study Guide
Tintinalli J, Kelen GD, Stapczynski JS (eds): *Emergency Medicine: A Study Guide*, 5th ed. New York: McGraw-Hill; 2000.

Geriatric Medicine

Essentials of Clinical Geriatrics
Kane RL, Ouslander JG, Abrass IB: *Essentials of Clinical Geriatrics*, 4th ed. New York: McGraw-Hill; 1999.

Neurology

Basic Neurology
Gilroy J: *Basic Neurology*, 3d ed. New York: McGraw-Hill; 2000.

Ophthalmology

General Ophthalmology
Vaughn D, Asbury T, Riordan-Eva P: *General Ophthalmology*, 15th ed. Stamford, CT: Appleton & Lange; 1999.

Orthopedics

Clinical Sports Medicine
Brukner P, Khan K: *Clinical Sports Medicine*, 2d ed. New York: McGraw-Hill; 2000.
Handbook of Fractures
Perry CR: *Handbook of Fractures*, 2d ed. New York: McGraw-Hill; 2000.
Emergency Orthopedics
Simon R, Koenigsknecht S: *Emergency Orthopedics*, 4th ed. New York: McGraw-Hill; 2000.

Otorhinolaryngology

Ear, Nose and Throat Disorders in Primary Care
Woodson GE: *Ear, Nose and Throat Disorders in Primary Care*. Philadelphia: Saunders; 2001.

Pediatrics

Current Pediatric Diagnosis & Treatment
Hay WW, Hayward AR, Levin MJ, et al (eds): *Current Pediatric Diagnosis & Treatment,* 15th ed. Stamford, CT: Appleton & Lange; 2001.
Harriet Lane Handbook
Siberry GK, Iannone R. (eds): *Harriet Lane Handbook,* 15th ed. St. Louis: Mosby; 2000.
Pediatric Emergency Medicine
Strange G. et al (eds): *Pediatric Emegency Medicine.* New York: McGraw-Hill; 2001.

Radiology

Emergency Radiology
Schwartz DT, Reisdorff E (eds): *Emergency Radiology.* New York: McGraw-Hill; 2001.

Surgery

Advanced Trauma Life Support Course (Student Manual)
American College of Surgeons, Committee on Trauma: *Advanced Trauma Life Support Course (Student Manual),* 6th ed. Chicago: ACS; 1997.
Principles of Surgery Companion Handbook
Schwartz SI (ed): *Principles of Surgery Companion Handbook,* 7th ed. New York: McGraw-Hill; 1999.
Emergent Management of Trauma
Scaletta TA: *Emergent Management of Trauma,* 2d ed. New York: McGraw-Hill; 2001.
Smith's General Urology
Tanagho EA, McAninch JW (eds): *Smith's General Urology.* New York: McGraw-Hill; 2000.

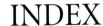

INDEX

Note: Page numbers followed by the letter "t" indicate tables; those followed by the letter "f" indicate figures.